Clinical Allergy

Clinical Allergy

Second Edition

Editor

Rajendra Prasad

MD DTCD FAMS FCCP (USA) FRCP (Glasgow) FRCP (London)
FNCCP FICS FCAI FIAB FIMSA FCCS DSc (Honoris Causa)

Director (Medical Education) and Professor
Department of Respiratory Medicine
Era's Lucknow Medical College and Hospital
Era University, Lucknow, Uttar Pradesh, India

Emeritus Professor
National Academy of Medical Sciences (India)

Former Director
Vallabhbhai Patel Chest Institute
University of Delhi, New Delhi, India

Director
UP Rural Institute of Medical Sciences and Research
Saifai, Etawah, Uttar Pradesh, India

Professor and Head
Department of Pulmonary Medicine
King George's Medical University
Lucknow, Uttar Pradesh, India

Associate Editors

VK Jain

MD DTCD FCCP (USA) FNCCP FCAI FIAB
Emeritus Professor
Department of Respiratory Medicine
Mahatma Gandhi Medical College and Hospital
Jaipur, Rajasthan, India

Nikhil Gupta

MBBS MD (Medicine) MAMS FIMSA DAA DFID (CMC Vellore)
Associate Professor
Department of General Medicine
Dr Ram Manohar Lohia Institute of Medical Sciences
Lucknow, Uttar Pradesh, India

Foreword

Vijay Kumar Arora

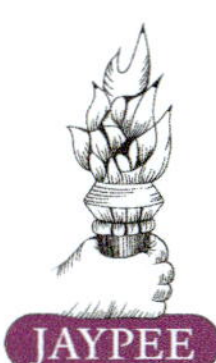

JAYPEE BROTHERS MEDICAL PUBLISHERS

The Health Sciences Publisher

New Delhi | London

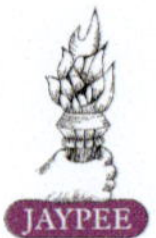

Jaypee Brothers Medical Publishers (P) Ltd

Headquarters
Jaypee Brothers Medical Publishers (P) Ltd
EMCA House, 23/23-B
Ansari Road, Daryaganj
New Delhi 110 002, India
Landline: +91-11-23272143, +91-11-23272703
+91-11-23282021, +91-11-23245672
Email: jaypee@jaypeebrothers.com

Corporate Office
Jaypee Brothers Medical Publishers (P) Ltd
4838/24, Ansari Road, Daryaganj
New Delhi 110 002, India
Phone: +91-11-43574357
Fax: +91-11-43574314
Email: jaypee@jaypeebrothers.com

Overseas Office
JP Medical Ltd
83 Victoria Street, London
SW1H 0HW (UK)
Phone: +44 20 3170 8910
Fax: +44 (0)20 3008 6180
Email: info@jpmedpub.com

Website: www.jaypeebrothers.com
Website: www.jaypeedigital.com

Inquiries for bulk sales may be solicited at: jaypee@jaypeebrothers.com

Clinical Allergy

First Edition: 2020

Second Edition: **2024**

ISBN: 978-93-5696-658-1

Printed in India

Dedicated to

My teachers for their guidance, wisdom and inspiration
My parents, wife and children for their love and patience

Contributors

AB Singh PhD
Former Scientist Emeritus
CSIR-Institute of Genomics and Integrative Biology
New Delhi, India

Abhimanyu Garg MD
Department of Respiratory Medicine
Mahatma Gandhi Medical College
Jaipur, Rajasthan, India

Aditya Goyal MBBS
Sawai Man Singh Medical College
Jaipur, Rajasthan, India

Alladi Mohan
MD FAMS FRCP (Edin) FCCP (USA) FICP
Professor and Head
Department of Medicine
Sri Venkateswara Institute of Medical Sciences
Tirupati, Andhra Pradesh, India

Amrutha D Holla MD
Consultant
Allergy, Asthma and Chest Center
Mysuru, Karnataka, India

Ankita MS
Department of Ophthalmology
King George's Medical University
Lucknow, Uttar Pradesh, India

Ankita Mishra PhD
Research Associate
Allergy and Immunology Laboratory
CSIR-Institute of Genomics and Integrative Biology
New Delhi, India

Anura Weerasinghe MD (Col) DCH (Col) DTM&H (Lond) MRCP (UK) FRCP (Edin) PdD (Niigata-Japan)
Fellow of the Ceylon College of Physicians
Professor of Medicine and Immunology
Sri Lanka

Anurag Agrawal MD PhD
Director
Translational Research in Lung Disease
CSIR-Institute of Genomics and Integrative Biology
New Delhi, India

Arun Raja V MD
Assistant Professor
Department of Medicine
Sri Venkateswara Institute of Medical Sciences
Tirupati, Andhra Pradesh, India

Asha Khandelwal PhD
Birbal Sahni Institute of Paleobotany
Lucknow, Uttar Pradesh, India

Ashok Shah MD
Former Director Professor
Department of Pulmonary Medicine
Vallabhbhai Patel Chest Institute
University of Delhi
New Delhi, India

B Vidyasagar
MD DTCD DNB FNCCP FIAA FCCP (USA)
Professor and Head
Department of Pulmonary Medicine
JJM Medical College
Davangere, Karnataka, India

Bharti Arora PhD
Research Associate
Allergy and Immunology Section
CSIR-Institute of Genomics and Integrative Biology
New Delhi, India

BJ Arun DNB DTCD FCCP (USA)
Assistant Professor
Department of Pulmonary Medicine
JJM Medical College
Davangere, Karnataka, India

BV Balachandra
MD (Pediatrics) Fellowship in Pediatric Intensive Care Diploma in Allergy Asthma and Immunology
Pediatrician, Allergist/Immunologist
Consultant Pediatrician and Allergist
Manipal Hospital
Bengaluru, Karnataka, India

Chandni Mathur PhD
Former Research Associate
Allergy and Immunology Section
CSIR-Institute of Genomics and Integrative Biology
New Delhi, India

Girish Jain MD
Department of Respiratory Medicine
Mahatma Gandhi Medical College
Jaipur, Rajasthan, India

Harshveer Singh Malhi MD
Medical Advisor
Allergopharma
Merck Specialities Private Limited
Mumbai, Maharashtra, India

Jacob N Abraham MD
Otolaryngologist
Tucsan, Arizona, USA

Kiran Vishnu Narayan
MD DNB DM
Assistant Professor
Pulmonary Medicine
Government Medical College
Kottayam, Kerala, India

Komarla Nagendra Prasad MD
Allergy Physician
Bengaluru Allergy Center
Bengaluru, Karnataka, India

Mahesh Goyal
MBBS MD
Jaipur Allergy and Asthma Center
Manipal Hospital
Jaipur, Rajasthan, India

Major K Nagaraju MD DCH
Pediatric Allergist
Saveetha Medical College
and Hospital
Apollo Children's Hospital
Chennai, Tamil Nadu, India

Manila Khatri MBBS
Department of Ophthalmology
King George's Medical University
Lucknow, Uttar Pradesh, India

MK Agarwal PhD
Professor and Head
Respiratory Allergy and Immunology
Metro Center for Respiratory Diseases
Metro Group of Hospitals
Noida, Uttar Pradesh, India
Former Professor and Head
Department of Respiratory Allergy
and Applied Immunology
Vallabhbhai Patel Chest Institute
University of Delhi
New Delhi, India

Mona PhD Medical Biochemistry
Associate Professor
Department of Biochemistry
Saraswati Medical College
Unnao, Uttar Pradesh, India

N Karthik MD (Pulmonary Medicine)
Consultant Pulmonologist
VN Hospital
Chennai, Tamil Nadu, India

Narmada Ashok DNB (Ped) MRCPCH
Director and Consultant Pediatrician
Nalam Medical Center and Hospital
Vellore, Tamil Nadu, India

Naveen Arora PhD
Senior Scientist
Allergy and Immunology Section
CSIR-Institute of Genomics and
Integrative Biology
New Delhi, India

Naveen K Bhatraju PhD
Research Associate
CSIR-Institute of Genomics
and Integrative Biology
New Delhi, India

Nikhil Gupta
MBBS MD (Medicine) MAMS FIMSA DAA
DFID (CMC Vellore)
Associate Professor
Department of General Medicine
Dr Ram Manohar Lohia Institute
of Medical Sciences
Lucknow, Uttar Pradesh, India

PA Mahesh
DTCD DNB Respiratory Diseases
Professor
Department of Chest and Tuberculosis
JSS Medical College
Mysuru, Karnataka, India

PC Kathuria MD DTCD
Senior Consultant
National Allergy Center
BLK Superspecialty Hospital
New Delhi, India

PK Vedanthan MD
Clinical Professor of Medicine
University of Colorado
Denver, Colorado, USA

PS Shankar MD FAMS
Emeritus Professor of Medicine
Rajiv Gandhi University of
Health Sciences
Director, MR Medical College
Kalaburagi, Karnataka, India

Raj Kumar
MD (Pul Med), MNASc FAMS FICAAI FICS
FNCCP (I) MAAAAI MACAAI
Professor and Head
Pulmonary Medicine
National Center of Respiratory Allergy,
Asthma and Immunology (NCRAAI)
Director
Vallabhbhai Patel Chest Institute
University of Delhi
New Delhi, India

Rajendra Prasad
MD DTCD FAMS FCCP (USA) FRCP (Glasgow)
FRCP (London) FNCCP FICS FCAI FIAB FIMSA
FCCS DSc (Honoris Causa)
Director (Medical Education) and
Professor
Department of Respiratory Medicine
Era's Lucknow Medical College and
Hospital, Era University
Lucknow, Uttar Pradesh, India
Emeritus Professor
National Academy of Medical
Sciences (India)
Former Director
Vallabhbhai Patel Chest Institute
University of Delhi, New Delhi, India
Director
UP Rural Institute of Medical Sciences
and Research
Saifai, Etawah, Uttar Pradesh, India
Professor and Head
Department of Pulmonary Medicine
King George's Medical University
Lucknow, Uttar Pradesh, India

Ramji Gupta
MBBS MD (Dermatology, Venereology
and Leprosy)
Consultant Dermatologist
Indraprashtha Apollo Hospital
New Delhi, India

RC Saxena
MD Dip Clin Pharmacol (UK) MNAMS MNASc FIAMS FIMSA
Former Professor and Head
Department of Pharmacology and Clinical Pharmacologist
King George's Medical University
Lucknow, Uttar Pradesh, India

Richa Gupta MD FCCP
Professor
Department of Pulmonary Medicine
Christian Medical College
Vellore, Tamil Nadu, India

Roopam Sehajpal MBBS MD
Department of Respiratory Diseases and Tuberculosis
SMS Medical College
Jaipur, Rajasthan, India

Sagar L Kale PhD
Allergy and Immunology Section
CSIR-Institute of Genomics and Integrative Biology
New Delhi, India

Sandeep Saxena MS FRCSEd FRCS FRCOphth FAcadTM FAICO FAMS
Professor and Chief of Retina Services
Department of Ophthalmology
King George's Medical University
Lucknow, Uttar Pradesh, India

Shally Awasthi MD (Ped) DNB (Ped) MMSc (Clinical Epidemiology) FAMS FIAP FASc FNASc FRCPCH (Hony)
Professor
Department of Pediatrics
King George's Medical University
Lucknow, Uttar Pradesh, India

Shambhavi Mishra MD (Ped)
Senior Resident
Department of Pediatrics
King George's Medical University
Lucknow, Uttar Pradesh, India

Shashi Chawla MSC PhD
Associate Professor
Department of Microbiology
Gargi College
University of Delhi
New Delhi, India

Shripad N Agashe PhD
Professor
Emeritus in Botany
Bangalore University
Bengaluru, Karnataka, India

Shubhra Jain MD
Assistant Professor
Department of Respiratory Medicine
Sawai Man Singh Medical College
Jaipur, Rajasthan, India

Sitesh Roy
MD (USA) FAAP FAAAAI FACAAI
Consultant
Dr Roy Health Solution Clinic
Mumbai, Maharashtra, India

SN Gaur MD
Former Director-Professor and Head
Department of Pulmonary Medicine
Vallabhbhai Patel Chest Institute
University of Delhi
New Delhi, India

Srishti Sareen MBBS
Ravindra Nath Tagore Medical College
Udaipur, Rajasthan, India

Suneetha P MD
Assistant Professor
Department of Medicine
Sri Venkateswara Institute of Medical Sciences
Tirupati, Andhra Pradesh, India

Suresh Koolwal MD DNB
Professor
Respiratory Medicine
Sawai Man Singh Medical College
Jaipur, Rajasthan, India

Surya Kant MD DTCD
Professor and Head
Department of Respiratory Medicine
King George's Medical University
Lucknow, Uttar Pradesh, India

Swati Priyadarshini MBBS
Department of Ophthalmology
King George's Medical University
Lucknow, Uttar Pradesh, India

Swati Sharma PhD
Senior Research Fellow
CSIR- Institute of Genomics and Integrative Biology
New Delhi, India

VK Jain
MD DTCD FCCP (USA) FNCCP FCAI FIAB
Emeritus Professor
Department of Respiratory Medicine
Mahatma Gandhi Medical College and Hospital
Jaipur, Rajasthan, India

Foreword

Allergic diseases are most common worldwide and there have been growing number of reports that the prevalence and severity of various allergic diseases have increased in the last two decades. It is estimated that 20–30% of the world's population is affected by one or more forms of allergic disease. The major portion of allergy practice is currently in the hands of General Practitioner and of Specialist whose practice is not limited to allergy and who does not devote much of their time to this important field of medicine. Therefore, there is a need for a comparatively simple textbook which doctor can use and refer to while dealing with different allergic diseases.

Against this backdrop, the publication of this textbook on *Clinical Allergy* by Professor Rajendra Prasad is a timely and useful addition to the existing literature. The book summarizes the current status of knowledge on every aspect of allergy. There are 54 chapters in this textbook. Chapters practically cover all the aspects of allergy ranging from epidemiology, varying presentation of allergy, diagnosis, and practical approach to the treatment of various allergic diseases. It also covers practical approach to prevention of allergy and pediatric issues in management of allergic diseases. Chapters also include allergic rhinitis, ocular allergy, urticaria, angioedema, atopic dermatitis, drug allergy and food allergy. Special chapters on latex allergy, human seminal plasma allergy, aspirin allergy, anticonvulsant hypersensitivity syndrome, hymenoptera allergy, radiocontrast allergy, local and general anesthetic allergy, cow milk allergy. Chapters on sublingual immunotherapy, cluster immunotherapy and future of immunotherapy are also included. This book also contains chapters on the pollen calendar with the use of photographs of allergenic plants mainly found in India. The chapters have been written on the basis of vast and rich clinical experience gained by authors from day-to-day patient management.

Rajendra Prasad MD DTCD FAMS FCCP (USA) FRCP (Glasgow) FRCP (London) FNCCP FICS FCAI FIAB FIMSA FCCS DSc (Honoris Causa), currently Director (Medical Education) and Professor, Department of Respiratory Medicine, Era's Lucknow Medical College and Hospital, Era University, Lucknow; Emeritus Professor, National Academy of Medical Sciences (India); Former Director, Vallabhbhai Patel Chest Institute, University of Delhi, New Delhi; Director, UP Rural Institute of Medical Sciences and Research, Saifai, Etawah; Professor and Head, Department of Pulmonary Medicine, King George's Medical University, Lucknow, Uttar Pradesh, India, did his MBBS in 1974 and MD in 1979 from King George's Medical College, Lucknow, India. Currently, he is Vice Chairman, National Task Force for involvement of medical colleges in Revised National Tuberculosis Control Program in India and Vice President of South Asia Association of Allergy, Asthma, and Applied Immunology. He has been International Governor of American College of Chest Physicians, USA. He has unique distinction of being President of all major scientific bodies in the field of pulmonary medicine in India including Indian College of Allergy, Asthma and Applied Immunology. Besides several prestigious fellowships of reputed National and International Organization, he was awarded fellowship of the National Academy of Medical Sciences, India; American College of Chest Physicians, USA; and Royal College of Physicians and Surgeons, Glasgow. He has supervised about 180 researches, and published 340 original articles, reviews, and book chapters. He also authored 8 books including 4 books on Tuberculosis and an Atlas on Fiber Optic Bronchoscopy based exclusively on Indian patients. He has presented over 1,600 guest lectures and scientific papers at various national and international meetings. Apart from being a clinician par excellence, he is also a very popular Medical Teacher in pulmonary medicine and allergy. His dynamic leadership in academic, research, and administrative areas has earned him 50 awards from various National Scientific Societies. He is recipient of Dr BC Roy National Award.

This comprehensive, well-referenced textbook contains a plethora of knowledge and would be a valuable source for general practitioners, specialists, undergraduate and postgraduate medical students will find this book as a practical guide.

I am quite hopeful that his textbook will help in better understanding towards alleviating the suffering of millions from various allergic diseases. This textbook deserves a place in the library of every medical college and healthcare providing institutions.

I wish Professor Rajendra Prasad all the success.

Vijay Kumar Arora
Former Vice-Chancellor, Santosh University
Former Additional DGHS Government of India, New Delhi
Former Director, NITRO Institute of TB and Respiratory Diseases, New Delhi (LRS)
Former Director and Professor, TB and CD, JIPMER, Puducherry
Former Director and Principal, Santosh Medical College and Hospital, Ghaziabad
Emeritus, Director, New Delhi TB Center
Former President, Indian Chest Society, National College of Chest
Physician and President, Indian Geriatric Society
President, JIPMER Scientific Society
President, NATCON
Former Chairman, Delhi Medical Council Disciplinary Committee
Presently Vice-Chairman (P&R)
Honorary Treasurer and Trustee, TB Association of India
Senior Consultant
TB and Respiratory Diseases, Noida (NCR Delhi)

Preface

Throughout the 47 years of my clinical practice in pulmonary medicine and allergy, I look upon allergy as a very special entity and learnt that there are lots of issues in the diagnosis and treatment of various allergic disorders. Allergic diseases are most common worldwide and there have been growing number of reports that the prevalence and severity of various allergic diseases have increased in the last two decades. It is estimated that 20–30% of the world's population is affected by one or more forms of allergic diseases.

The major portion of allergy practice is currently in the hands of general practitioners and of specialists whose practice is not limited to allergy and who does not devote much of his/her time to this important field of medicine. Therefore, there is a need for a comparatively simple textbook, which doctor can use and refer to while dealing with different allergic diseases. This textbook on clinical allergy is designed to serve the healthcare professionals in the understanding of diagnosis and treatment of allergic diseases. The contributors of this book were chosen for their specific expertise and interest in their respective areas. I wish to thank all my associate editors and contributors for giving their considerable amount of time and effort to write their respective chapters and complete this book.

This textbook consists of 54 chapters, which practically cover all the aspects of allergy ranging from epidemiology, varying presentation of allergy, diagnosis, and practical approach to the treatment of various allergic diseases. This also includes chapter on aerobiology and pollen calendar with the use of photographs of allergenic plants mainly found in India. The information in this book has been completed using the latest research, current medical updates and a wealth of experience the authors have gained while treating allergic diseases.

This comprehensive, well-referenced textbook contains a plethora of knowledge and would be a valuable source for general practitioners; specialists; undergraduate and postgraduate medical students will find this book as a practical guide.

Rajendra Prasad

Acknowledgments

As an editor of this textbook, I wish to acknowledge my indebtedness to a number of people who significantly contributed to the publication of this book. The individuals to whom I would like to acknowledge first are my teachers, Late Professor BK Khanna, Late Dr MS Agnihotri, Professor PK Mukherjee, Late Dr Jafar Jameel and Late Dr J Nath from Department of Tuberculosis at King George's Medical College, Lucknow, Uttar Pradesh, India while I was a postgraduate student in that department, markedly stimulated my interest in field of allergy. I am also indebted to Professor PN Tandon, then the Chairman governing body, Vallabhbhai Patel Chest Institute, New Delhi for his inspiration under whom I have honor to work as the Director, Vallabhbhai Patel Chest Institute, New Delhi whose tremendous knowledge and wisdom set an example of thoughtfulness and meticulousness, which I have always tried to emulate. I am greatly indebted to the many postgraduate students who have been trained with me in the department at King George's Medical College, Lucknow, Vallabhbhai Patel Chest Institute, New Delhi and Era's Lucknow Medical College Hospital Lucknow, especially Dr Sanjay Verma, Dr Kiran Vishnu Narayan, Dr Suneesh C Anand, Dr Giridhar BH, Dr Abhijeet, Dr Abhishek Agrawal, Dr Saurabh Karmakar, Dr Shailendra Singh, Dr Mandeep Singh and Dr Pawan Gupta, Dr Visweswaran Balasubramanian, Dr Faizan Ahmad, Dr Ahbab, Dr Amitabh Banka, Dr Sakshi Batra, Dr Kashif Raza, Dr Haris Gulraize, Dr Ronal Naorem, Dr Saurav Pandey, Dr Asna Khan, Dr Rishabh Kacker, Dr Jaskirat Singh, Dr Harsh Saxena, Dr Huda Shamim, and Dr Syed Ahmad. The efforts of these postgraduate students in part responsible for generating much of the data that can be incorporated in making the chapters in book more evidence based.

I also wish to express my appreciation to Professor VK Jain, Dr Nikhil Gupta (Associate Editors) and all other contributors for giving their considerable amount of time and efforts to write their respective chapters and their help in completing this book. I also wish to express my thanks to Mr PP Sharma, Mr Ashish Yadav, Mr Gyan Prakash, Mr Mithun, and Miss Seema Shukla for their invaluable help in the preparation, typing of manuscript and other help in bringing out this book. I am also thankful to all my patients, who gave me experience in the field of allergy.

I am especially thankful to Shri Jitendar P Vij (Group Chairman), Mr Ankit Vij (Managing Director), Mr MS Mani (Group President), Ms Chetna Malhotra (Senior Director—Professional Publishing, Marketing, and Business Development), Ms Pooja Bhandari [Director—Production (Books and Journals)], and Mr Priyansh Saxena (Development Editor) of M/s Jaypee Brothers Medical Publishers (P) Ltd, New Delhi, India, for giving a go-ahead at the very beginning and helping us in every way possible to bring out this book.

Contents

CHAPTER 1

Immune Response in Health and Allergic Diseases: An Overview

MK Agarwal, Shashi Chawla

INTRODUCTION

Human body is continuously under attack from an array of pathogenic microorganisms and other foreign substances and cancer cells generated within. Protection against these antagonists (called antigens) is provided by a large number of cells and molecules generated by the immune system of the body. The coordinated reaction of these cells and molecules against a particular antigen constitutes an immune response. This response provides immunity against various antigens and is essential for our ability to survive in an environment that is full of various pathogens. However, malfunction of immune response may result in various immunoinflammatory disorders such as hypersensitivity, autoimmunity, and/or immunodeficiency.

There are two components of immunity against an antigen—innate and adaptive.

INNATE IMMUNITY

The innate immune response is present in the body since birth, is nonspecific, and provides protection against the environmental microbes. Therefore, innate immunity forms the first line of defense. It consists of those defenses that are ready for immediate action against an attack by a pathogen. Various components of innate immunity include (1) anatomical or physical barriers (skin, cilia on mucous membranes), (2) physiologic barriers (acid in the stomach, digestive enzymes in the stomach and small intestine, chemicals such as lysozymes in tears and saliva), (3) cellular barriers [phagocytic cells such as macrophages and neutrophils, and natural killer (NK) cells], and (4) soluble inflammatory barriers [antimicrobial peptides such as defensins, cathelicidins, and interferons (IFNs); acute-phase proteins such as C-reactive protein, complement proteins, mannose-binding lectin (MBL), and some cytokines].[1-3]

Both physical and physiologic barriers are able to prevent the entry of pathogens in the body, thereby controlling many infections. However, if a pathogen is able to cross these primary barriers, then the cellular and inflammatory barriers generate a quick counter-response within minutes of invasion by the pathogen. The tissue damage by a pathogen induces a complex sequence of events called the inflammatory response. This response results in the accumulation of fluid (edema) and the movement of circulating white blood cells (leukocytes) through the blood capillaries (extravasation) in the affected tissue. Soluble effectors such as antimicrobial peptides,[4] complement components,[5] and acute-phase proteins[6] also get accumulated. The leukocytes phagocytose the pathogen as well as release mediators. The mediators not only attract more cells to the site of infection but also bring about conformational changes in the molecules present on the surface of various leukocytes collected at the site of infection.

Among leukocytes, the major phagocytes are neutrophils[7] and monocytes. These cells ingest and destroy microbes, other injurious agents, and one's own dead and damaged cells. A neutrophil is a type of granulocyte and has a multilobed nucleus and a granulated cytoplasm. It is also called polymorphonuclear leukocyte. Neutrophils are the first cells to reach the site of inflammation. They respond rapidly to foreign stimuli and to injury; their activation leads to acute inflammation.

When blood monocytes enter tissues, they mature and are called macrophages. Macrophages[8] are professional phagocytes and are present under epithelia, in connective tissues, and in all organs. Some of the macrophages stay in particular tissues where microbial invasion or exposure to foreign particles is likely and are called fixed macrophages. They are named according to their location, e.g., intestinal macrophages in the gut, alveolar macrophages in the lung, Kupffer cells in the liver, and microglial cells in the brain. Together they form the mononuclear phagocyte system in the body. However, other macrophages remain motile and are called free or wandering macrophages. In general, macrophages respond more slowly than neutrophils but for longer duration; this reaction is typical of chronic inflammation. Macrophages also help in repairing damaged tissue.

The response generated by all the components of innate immunity is not specific for a particular pathogen but for structures shared by a group of related pathogens. Also it is able to discriminate between the self and nonself molecules. For this purpose, some soluble mediators and cell membrane-bound molecules of the host possess pattern recognition receptors (PRRs).[9] These receptors recognize pathogens by their molecular patterns called pathogen-associated molecular patterns (PAMPs). PAMPs are structures that are highly conserved within a species of microbes, are not present on mammalian cells, and are often essential for survival of microbes, thus limiting the capacity of microbes to evade detection. Biochemically, PAMPs are combinations of sugars, certain proteins, some nucleic acid motifs, and a few lipid-bearing molecules. The engagement of PRRs with PAMPs activates soluble molecules and cells. When PRRs of soluble mediators identify PAMPs on pathogens, complement system (discussed later) gets activated. This system removes pathogen either through opsonization or lysis.

Cells like macrophages and dendritic cells have a variety of PRRs on their surface, such as Toll-like receptors (TLRs),[10] nucleotide-binding oligomerization domain (NOD) family receptors, and scavenger receptors (SRs). These receptors detect a broad spectrum of pathogens via the PAMPs present on their surfaces, thereby inducing the activation of the macrophages and dendritic cells (Table 1.1). Activated macrophages destroy the antigen by phagocytosis. They also secrete cytokines such as interleukin (IL)-1 (IL-1), IL-6, and tumor necrosis factor (TNF)-α, which produce inflammatory responses. However, dendritic cells internalize and process the antigen and then present it to T cells in lymphoid tissues. This activity of antigen processing and presentation helps in the initiation of the adaptive immune response and hence is considered as a bridge between the innate and adaptive immunity.

Table 1.1: Receptors of innate immunity and their location and targets.

Pattern recognition receptors (PRRs) in host	*Location of PRRs*	*Target (pathogen-associated molecular patterns)*
Toll-like receptors	Mostly cell surface	Microbial components not found in host
Nucleotide-binding oligomerization domain receptors	Intracellular	Bacterial cell wall components
Scavenger receptors	Cell membrane	Gram-positive and gram-negative bacteria

ADAPTIVE IMMUNITY

When a pathogen evades all the innate defenses, it is countered by a second system called adaptive or acquired immunity. *Adaptive/acquired immune response* recognizes and selectively eliminates specific microbes and molecules. It displays characteristic features such as self vs. nonself recognition, surveillance, specificity, diversity, tolerance, and immunologic memory. Generation of this response takes time—as much as a week or more before it is fully effective. Re-exposure of an individual, who has already developed primary immune response to a particular pathogen, results in generation of *secondary immune response*. Due to the presence of memory cells, it is rapid and higher in magnitude and avidity. Differences between innate and adaptive immunity[11] are listed in Table 1.2.

On the basis of the components generated by the immune system to provide immunity against different antigens, adaptive immune response can be divided into two types:

1. Humoral immune response (HIR)
2. Cell-mediated immune response (CMIR)

The initiation of these responses (described later in the chapter) occurs in peripheral lymphoid organs and requires interaction of a variety of cells through the molecules/receptors present on their surface. These cells develop and mature in central lymphoid organs. A brief description of the organs, cells, and their receptors involved in immune response is discussed in the following sections.

Table 1.2: Features of innate and adaptive immunity.

Feature	*Innate immunity*	*Adaptive immunity*
Response time	Minutes to hours	Days
Specificity	For structures shared by groups of related microbes	For all kinds of antigens
Diversity	Limited	Very large
Memory	None	Yes, faster and high-intensity response on subsequent encounters with antigen
Self vs. nonself discrimination	Perfect	Very good with occasional failure
Major cell types	Phagocytes, natural killer cells, dendritic cells	T and B lymphocytes
Soluble components	Acute-phase proteins and antimicrobial peptides	Antibodies

COMPONENTS OF THE IMMUNE SYSTEM

The immune system is made up of organs, tissues, and cells spread throughout the body.

Organs of the Immune System

The organs of the immune system are repositories for immune cells.[11] Central/primary lymphoid organs—bone marrow and thymus in human beings—are the sites for antigen-independent proliferation and maturation of immune cells. Peripheral/secondary lymphoid organs are the organs where antigen-dependent maturation of immune cells takes place. These include the lymph nodes and spleen. Besides these, lymphoid tissues associated with mucosa (mucosa-associated lymphoid tissue), bronchi (bronchus-associated lymphoid tissue), and gut (gut-associated lymphoid tissue) containing a large population of antibody-producing plasma cells are also part of secondary lymphoid organs.

Cells of the Immune System

All the cells of the immune system develop from pluripotent stem cells present in the bone marrow. These stem cells are called *hematopoietic stem cells*.[12] They differentiate along two separate pathways, giving rise to either a lymphoid or a myeloid progenitor cell. The lymphoid progenitor cells differentiate into different lymphocytes, i.e., T lymphocytes, B lymphocytes, or non-B non-T cells/NK cells. The myeloid progenitor cells give rise to dendritic cells, mast cells, granulocytes (basophils, neutrophils, eosinophils), monocytes, macrophages, megakaryocytes, and erythrocytes. After maturation, these cells enter the circulation to perform their respective functions. Dendritic cells and macrophages also participate as accessory cells in initiating lymphocyte responses to antigens.

All these cells have biologically active surface membrane proteins on their surface, which are very useful for identification, characterization, and immunophenotyping of the cells and their subpopulations. These molecules are recognized with the help of monoclonal antibodies and are called *cluster of differentiation (CD)* markers.[13] More than 370 CD clusters are described in humans till date. Each CD marker when identified is assigned a sequential number, e.g., CD4 and CD8 are expressed by two different phenotypes of T cells, T_H and T_C cells, respectively. CD3 is present on all the T cells and is known as a pan T-cell marker. B cells have CD19, CD20, CD21, and CD22 surface markers. Similarly, NK cells have CD16 and CD56, monocytes and macrophages have CD14 and CD33, and dendritic cells display CD11c. Now let us briefly discuss some of the cells important in immune response.

Lymphocytes

The most important cells of adaptive immunity are lymphocytes. There are two main classes of lymphocytes. B lymphocytes (so called because they mature in the bone marrow) secrete proteins called antibodies, which bind to and eliminate extracellular microbes. T lymphocytes (which mature in the thymus) function mainly to combat microbes that have learned to live inside cells (where they are inaccessible to antibodies).[14]

B cells: B cells are lymphocytes that are derived from those lymphoid progenitor cells, which mature in the bone marrow itself.[15] Mature B cells display approximately

1.5×10^5 molecules of membrane-bound immunoglobulins (mIgs). All these mIgs have an identical antigen-binding site, which serve as receptors for an antigen. They are part of the antigenic receptor present on the surface of B cells called the B-cell receptor (BCR). The binding of an antigen to the mIgs makes B cells divide rapidly and differentiate into memory B cells and plasma B cells (effector cells). Memory B cells continue to express the same BCR and are responsible for the immune memory required to combat the same antigen during subsequent encounters. Plasma cells, which are the major effector cells of humoral immunity, have a short lifespan and are highly specialized for secreting a large number of antigen-specific immunoglobulins.

T cells: These lymphoid progenitor cells that leave the bone marrow through the bloodstream and enter the thymus mature into T cells. During maturation, T cells express on their surface a unique antigen-binding receptor called T-cell receptor (TCR). TCR recognizes the antigen only when it is bound to cell membrane proteins called *major histocompatibility complex (MHC)* molecules. Two well-defined subpopulations of T cells are helper T cells (T_H) and T cytotoxic cells (T_C). They generally display CD4 and CD8 markers, respectively. Like B cells, T cells also differentiate into effector and memory cells after activation. T_H cells "help" B lymphocytes to make the antigen-specific antibodies (T_H2) and also "help" macrophages to kill ingested microbes (T_H1). T_H cells have been further classified into several functional subsets, which are as follows:[16,17]

- *T_H1 cells*: These cells promote cell-mediated immunity against intracellular invaders.
- *T_H2 cells*: These cells promote HIR and host defense against extracellular parasites.
- *T_H9 cells*: This subset of T_H cells is identified by the production of IL-9. These cells are thought to be involved in pathogen immunity and immune-mediated diseases.
- *T_H17 cells*: T_H cells producing IL-17 constitute a previously unknown subset of effector $CD4^+$ T cells. These cells provide protective immunity against extracellular bacteria and fungi. However, these cells promote autoimmune and inflammatory diseases. They may also be involved in neutrophil infiltration that occurs during acute phase of allergic reactions.
- *T_H22 cells*: These cells secrete IL-22, IL-13, and TNF-α, and have been implicated in the pathogenesis of inflammatory skin disorders such as psoriasis and atopic dermatitis.
- *T_{FH} cells*: These are a new subtype of T_H cells and are called T follicular helper cells. They play an important role in humoral immunity and in the regulation of B-cell development in the germinal center.

Participation of these subtypes of T_H cells in an immune response depends on the nature and type of the pathogen.

T_{reg} cells: Recently, much focus has been on an important subset of T cells called regulatory T cells (T_{reg}). They are identified by the presence of both CD4 and CD25 on their surface. Regulatory T-cell-mediated suppression serves as an important mechanism of regulation of immune-mediated inflammation. In other words, they are negative regulators of immune response and feature prominently in autoimmune diseases, allergy, acute and chronic infections, and cancer.

The effector T_C cells, called cytotoxic/cytolytic T lymphocytes (CTLs), kill infected host cells or target cells, and thus serve to eliminate virus-infected cells, tumor cells, and cells of transplanted tissue, which is incompatible to the host. These $CD8^+$ T cells play a very important role in CMIR.

NK cells: A small population of large granular lymphocytes and non-B non-T lymphocytes, called NK cells, possesses cytotoxic activity against tumor cells and some virus-infected cells. These cells mediate antibody-dependent cell-mediated cytotoxicity (ADCC) and even participate in T-cell-mediated responses.[18] NK cells possess two types of receptors: killer activator receptor and killer inhibitor receptors.

Accessory Cells

Antigen-presenting cells: For initiation of the adaptive (acquired) immune response, foreign substances have to be captured, processed, and presented to lymphocytes. The cells that perform these tasks are called antigen-presenting cells (APCs). The best-defined APCs are specialized types of cells called dendritic cells,[19] followed by macrophages,[20] and then by naïve B cells. All these cells display the processed antigen on their surface along with Class II MHC molecules (discussed later).

Besides lymphocytes and APCs, other cells such as *mast cells, basophils,* and *eosinophils* also help in the generation of immune response. Even though the functions of macrophages as phagocytes in the innate immunity and as APCs in the acquired immune response have already been discussed, they also play a very important role in the effector phase of adaptive immune response. In cell-mediated immunity, T cells activate macrophages to destroy phagocytosed antigen. In humoral immunity, antibodies coat the antigen and promote its phagocytosis by macrophage surface receptors for antibodies. This mechanism is called opsonization and is performed by neutrophils too.

Molecules of the Immune system

The three molecules involved in the recognition of antigens by B cells and T cells are immunoglobulin molecules, MHC molecules, and TCRs.

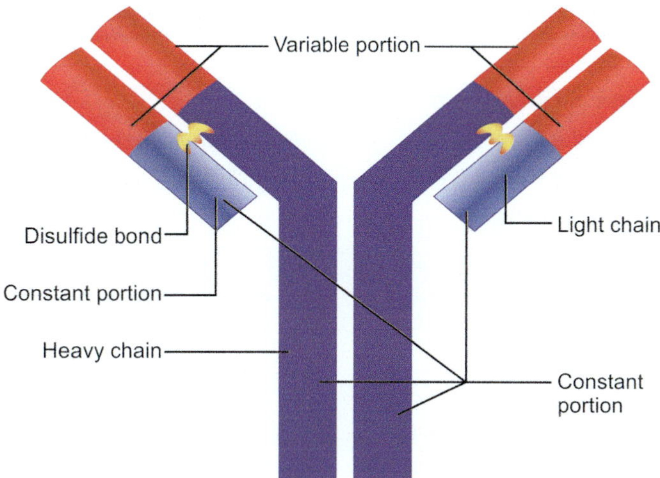

Fig. 1.1: Diagrammatic structure of an antibody molecule.
Source: https://commons.wikimedia.org/wiki/File:Antibody_svg.svg.

Immunoglobulins

Immunoglobulins or antibodies are glycoproteins produced by B lymphocytes that recognize a specific foreign antigenic determinant and facilitate clearance of that antigen. A normal human being synthesizes 10–100 millions of different immunoglobulin molecules, each with distinct specific antigen-binding capability. The antibody–antigen complex initiates a series of biologically important effector functions, such as opsonization to promote phagocytosis; complement activation; ADCC; transcytosis; and activation of mast cells, eosinophils, and basophils (exclusive to IgE).

Structure of immunoglobulins: Immunoglobulins include a heterogeneous group of proteins but have a similar structural organization. They may be classified into various groups and subgroups depending upon their antigenic activities and amino acid sequences. The core or monomeric unit of an immunoglobulin molecule has a total number of four polypeptide chains—two identical light chains (L) and two identical heavy chains (H). The light and heavy chains are held together by disulfide bonds and by noncovalent hydrophobic interaction (Fig. 1.1).

The basic structure of an immunoglobulin molecule was revealed by its enzymatic digestion carried out by different scientists.[11,21-23] A brief digestion with the proteolytic enzyme papain cleaved it into two identical Fab fragments (antigen-binding fragment) and one Fc (crystallizable) fragment. However, pepsin digestion generated one $F(ab)_2$ (two joined Fab-like fragments) only. The Fc fragment was not recovered from pepsin digestion as it got digested into multiple fragments. The molecule was also subjected to mercaptoethanol reduction and alkylation followed by filtration chromatography. The multichain structure could finally be deduced by raising antisera against all the products of various digestions and reacting them with each other.

Amino acid sequence and antigen-binding function of immunoglobulins: Amino acid sequencing has revealed that heavy and light polypeptide chains of immunoglobulins are composed of smaller units called homology units/domains.[24] Each homology unit contains about 110 amino acids. Two homology units are present in each light chain and, depending on the immunoglobulin class, four or five in the heavy chains (Fig. 1.1). The amino terminal regions of both heavy and light chains contain variable sequences of amino acids. These are called variable segments of light and heavy chains (V_L and V_H). Most of the variations are restricted to hypervariable/complementarity-determining regions on both light and heavy chains, which form the antigen-binding site of immunoglobulin. The carboxy terminal half of each light and heavy chain demonstrates a relatively constant class-specific amino acid sequence (C_L and C_H).

Depending on the γ, α, μ, δ, and ε classes of heavy chain constant regions, immunoglobulins have been divided into five major groups, namely, IgG, IgA, IgM, IgD, and IgE, respectively.[11,21] A comparison of the

Table 1.3: Properties of different classes of immunoglobulins.

Properties	*IgM*	*IgD*	*IgG*	*IgA*	*IgE*
Class of heavy chain	μ	δ	γ	α	ε
Molecular form	Pentamer, hexamer	Monomer	Monomer	Monomer, dimer	Monomer
Molecular weight (kDa)	950, 1,150	175	150	160, 400	190
C-region domains	4	3	3	3	4
Tailpiece	+	–	–	+	–
Accessory chains	J chain, secretory chain	–	–	J chain, secretory chain	–
Subclasses	–	–	G1, G2, G3, G4	A1, A2	–
Carbohydrate content (%)	10	9	3	7	13
Age of total serum immunoglobulins (%)	5–10	0.3	75–85	7–15	0.02
Average adult serum level (mg/mL)	0.7–1.7	0.04	9.5–12.5	1.5–2.6	0.0003
Serum half-life (days)	5	3	23	6	2.5
Placental transfer	–	–	+	–	–
Mast cell/basophil binding	–	–	–	–	+
Macrophage binding	–	–	+	+	–
Classical complement activation	+	–	+	–	–
Alternate complement activation	–	+	+	A1+, A2–	–

+ indicates present; – indicates absent.

properties of five classes of immunoglobulins is given in Table 1.3.

Major Histocompatibility Complex

The biologic basis for antigen recognition in the context of MHC allows distinction between self and nonself. The MHC gene complex is located on chromosome number 6 in human beings and comprises genes that code for Class I and Class II MHC molecules as well as other proteins.[25-28] The biologic role of MHC molecules is to display antigenic peptides that enable appropriate TCR to bind them. Class I MHC molecules are present on all nucleated cells. Their function is to present endogenously derived antigenic peptides like viral epitopes after antigen processing to CD8^{+} T_c cells. Interaction of the peptide–MHC complex with TCR of Tc cells leads to their activation and transformation into CTLs. These CTLs inactivate/eliminate the foreign antigens. However, Class II MHC molecules are expressed only by APCs, i.e., dendritic cells, macrophages, and B cells. They present exogenously derived antigenic peptides like soluble bacterial protein-derived peptides to CD4^{+} T_H cells (Fig. 1.2). The activated T_H cells are then called helper T cells.

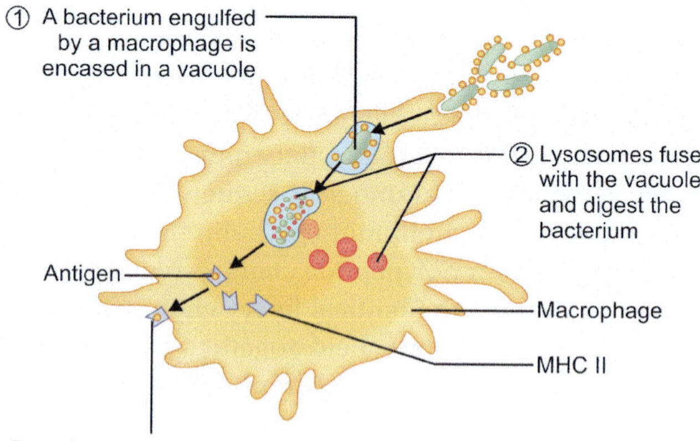

Fig. 1.2: Antigen-presenting cells (APCs), such as a macrophage, presenting peptides derived from phagocytosed and processed bacteria on its surface along with a Class II major histocompatibility complex (MHC) molecule.

Source: https://opentextbc.ca/biology/chapter/23-2-adaptive-immune-response.

T-cell Receptor

T-cell receptor (TCR) is a membrane-bound receptor of T cells. Unlike immunoglobulins, it does not exist in a secreted form. TCR is not just specific for the antigen but for the antigen–MHC complex.[29] In other words, it interacts with the processed antigen bound to the MHC molecule.

The TCR consists of two dissimilar polypeptides held together by noncovalent bonds and interchain disulfide bonds. The heterodimers have either α and β or γ and δ chains. Most of the T cells express $\alpha\beta$ TCR, whereas $\gamma\delta$ TCR is expressed by only a small subset. Each polypeptide chain has a constant and a variable domain. The variable domain of each chain contains three hypervariable regions that help in the recognition of the processed antigen–MHC complex.[11,21] Associated with TCR is a complex of polypeptide chains involved in signal transduction called CD3. CD3 is important for expression of the TCR, and together they are called the TCR–CD3 complex.

Cytokines

The interactions between various cells are mediated by a group of proteins called cytokines (*cyto* means "cell" and *kinen* means "to move"). Cytokines are low-molecular-weight regulatory proteins or glycoproteins secreted by leukocytes and other cells in response to various stimuli. These cytokines include lymphokines (secreted by lymphocytes), monokines (secreted by monocytes and macrophages), ILs (secreted by leukocytes), chemokines, etc.

Cytokines have some specific properties:[11,21]

- Cytokines mediate their activities in either an autocrine or a paracrine manner. Certain cytokines may exert an endocrine activity.
- Cytokines act by binding to high-affinity receptors present on the membranes of target cells.
- Cytokines that mediate innate immunity are produced by macrophages, e.g., IL-1, TNF, IL-12, and IFNγ.
- The cytokines that mediate adaptive immunity are produced mainly by T cells such as IL-2, IL-4, IL-5, and IFNγ.
- Cytokines regulate the magnitude and duration of the immune response by stimulating or inhibiting the activation, proliferation, and differentiation of various cells.

Even though all these components coordinate with each other to generate an immune response, the type of response generated against an antigen depends on its nature too.

ANTIGENS

Antigens are nonself substances (cells, proteins, polysaccharides), which were initially described as substances capable of producing and binding to antibodies produced against them by B cells. However, antigens are now defined as substances that can be specifically recognized by the receptors of T and B cells, thereby eliciting the immune response. It is estimated that an adult human being has the capability of recognizing at least 10^6–10^7 different antigens. While some antigens are small and simple, others are large and complex, containing many different sites that can be individually identified by receptor molecules present on the cell surfaces. These are known as *antigenic determinants* or *epitopes* (Fig. 1.3).[30]

Based on the way they stimulate and interact with the immune system, antigens may be categorized as immunogens and haptens. A substance that can initiate immune response and can specifically react with the antibodies or sensitized cells so produced is called an immunogen, and this property of a substance is called immunogenicity.[31] A hapten, however, is a low-molecular-weight substance incapable of initiating an immune response but can react with it. This property is called antigenicity. However, when a hapten is attached to a larger immunogenic molecule (a "carrier" molecule) forming a carrier–hapten conjugate, immune response is generated against both. Immunogenicity of a substance depends on its foreignness, molecular weight, chemical composition and complexity, and ability to be processed and presented

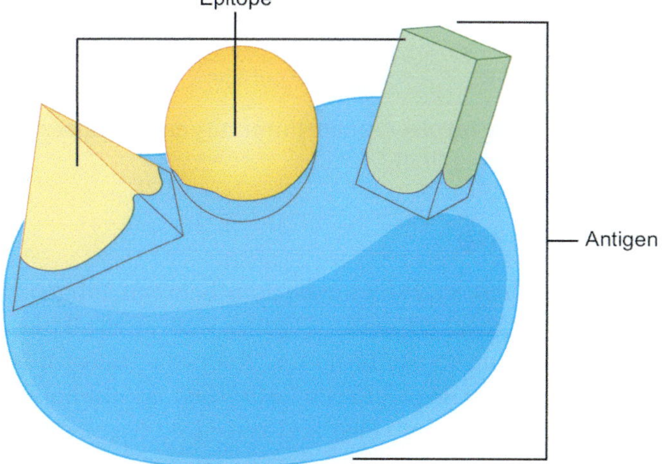

Fig. 1.3: An antigen displaying several epitopes.
Source: https://opentextbc.ca/biology/chapter/23-2-adaptive-immune-response.

with an MHC molecule on the surface of an APC or altered cell.[11,21,31] The ability of a substance to induce an immune response also depends on the genetic makeup of the host, dose of antigen, route of administration of the antigen, and the use of agents that enhance immunogenicity.

Some substances enhance the immune response when administered with an immunogen and are known as adjuvants. For example, colloidal suspension of mycobacterial proteins and oil (called complete Freund's adjuvant) aids in the initiation/enhancement of immune response by an antigen. It induces localized inflammation at the site of immunogen administration by the accumulation of phagocytic cells.

CELLULAR INTERACTIONS: DEVELOPMENT OF IMMUNE RESPONSE

The main function of the immune response is to protect the host against disease. The introduction of antigens such as bacteria, viruses, and fungi into an immunologically naïve host starts several events that lead to generation of an immune response. These mechanisms are classified as either cell-mediated or humoral immunity. Cell-mediated immunity mediates protection through sensitized T cells, and humoral immunity mediates protection strictly through antibodies. As already discussed (under the "Antigens" section), the type of the response that will be generated depends on the nature of the antigen as well as on the host.

Whether cell-mediated or humoral, an immune response develops sequentially. It can be divided into three sequential phases—initial, central, and effector.[21]

Initial Phase

The initial phase involves innate immunity and has already been discussed in detail.

Central Phase

The central phase includes interactions between antigens, B and T lymphocytes, and APCs, as well as cytokines generated during innate response. The net result of this phase is generation of effector cells such as antibody-secreting cells (plasma cells) and sensitized T cells and memory cells.

Usually if an extracellular antigen is protein, it is internalized and processed in the APCs to generate peptides. The peptides are then displayed on the surface of the APCs along with Class II MHC molecules. The TCR–CD3 complex of $CD4^+$ helper T lymphocytes interacts with this peptide–MHC complex and sends a stimulatory signal for initiation of T-cell activation. Activation also requires interaction of certain accessory molecules such as CD4 and CD28 on T cells and B7 on APCs, thereby generating a costimulatory signal. In the case of microbes, the innate immune response also activates APCs to express accessory molecules and secrete cytokines. During these interactions, the cytokines secreted by APCs stimulate the proliferation and differentiation of T lymphocytes. $CD4^+$ T cells, activated by this mechanism, function as T_H cells.[32] These cells are required for antibody production and will be discussed later. However, $CD8^+$ T lymphocytes recognize peptides derived from intracellular antigens and displayed bound to Class I MHC molecules. Their activation may also require help from $CD4^+$ cells.[33,34] The activated $CD8^+$ T cells function as CTLs.

Activation of both $CD4^+$ and $CD8^+$ T cells leads to the generation of effector and memory T cells. Effector T cells are short-lived and perform helper, cytotoxic, or other functions. Memory T cells are responsible for secondary responses.

The development of HIR requires cellular cooperation. B cells get activated by different routes depending on the biochemical nature of the antigen. In the case of most of the antigens, activation of B cells is thymus dependent, i.e., it requires T-cell help, and such antigens are called thymus-dependent antigens, e.g., soluble proteins. For these antigens, B-cell activation requires direct contact with T_H cell[35] involving engagement of BCR and costimulatory receptors (CD40, B7) of B cells with various receptors (TCR, CD40L, CD28) on T cells (Fig. 1.4). Like T cells, activated B lymphocytes generate antibody-producing plasma cells (effector cells) and memory cells (Fig. 1.5). Other antigens such as polysaccharides and other nonproteins are directly recognized by B lymphocytes and do not require T-cell help. These are called thymus-independent (TI) antigens and are divided into Type 1 [e.g., lipopolysaccharide (LPS)] and Type 2 (e.g., capsular polysaccharides). B lymphocytes that recognize TI antigens get activated by the cleavage products of complement produced during innate response and undergo proliferation and differentiation into plasma cells and memory cells.[11]

Both memory B and memory T cells are long-lived dormant cells that are capable of rapid recall responses to subsequent encounters with the antigen. Effector T cells

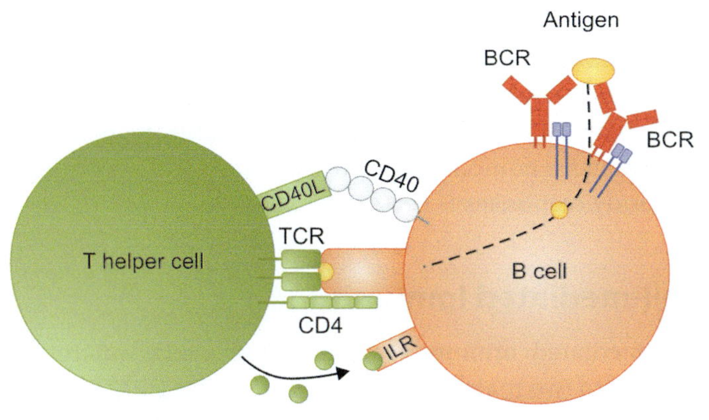

Fig. 1.4: Interactions between various receptors of a B lymphocyte and a helper T cell during their contact.

Source: https://commons.wikimedia.org/wiki/File:T-dependent_B_cell_activation.png.

exit the peripheral lymphoid organs, enter the circulation, and eliminate the antigen wherever present. Effector B lymphocytes (plasma cells) remain in the lymphoid organs or migrate to the bone marrow. The antibodies secreted by these cells enter the circulation and extravascular spaces and bind to the antigen. The response generated by the products of effector cells forms the effector function of T and B cells.

Effector Phase

The responses developed by effector B and effector T cells to remove the antigen constitute the effector phase of cell-mediated and humoral immunity. The response generated during first antigen encounter is called primary response. All subsequent encounters result in markedly enhanced secondary response that is characterized by the accelerated appearance of immunocompetent cells

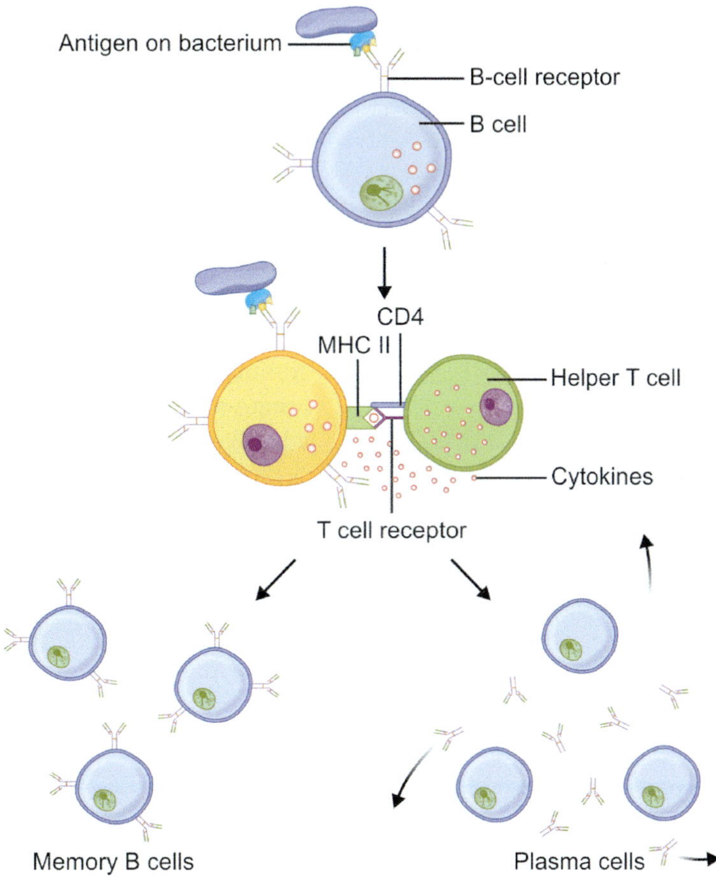

Fig. 1.5: Generation of plasma cells and memory B cells. After binding of an antigen to the B-cell receptor (BCR), B cell internalizes the antigen and presents it on major histocompatibility complex (MHC) II. A helper T cell recognizes the MHC II–antigen complex and activates the B cell, which then proliferates and differentiates into memory B cells and plasma cells.

Source: https://opentextbc.ca/biology/chapter/23-2-adaptive-immune-response.

and antibodies. The differences between the two can be easily studied in HIR as the kinetics of the response can be measured by serum antibody levels (Fig. 1.6). The primary response to an antigen is characterized by a lag phase. During this phase, naïve B cells undergo clonal selection, proliferation, and differentiation into memory cells and plasma cells. The lag phase is followed by a log increase in the serum antibody level, which reaches a peak or a plateau, and then declines. The length of lag and log phases varies with the nature, dose, and route of administration of antigen as well as the genotype of the individual. Activation of memory cells during second and subsequent exposures to antigen results in a secondary response. This response has a shorter lag phase, reaches a greater magnitude, and lasts longer. Even the antibodies secreted in the two phases are different in isotype, antigen affinity, etc.[11,21,31] An extensive comparison of the primary and secondary antibody responses is drawn in Table 1.4.

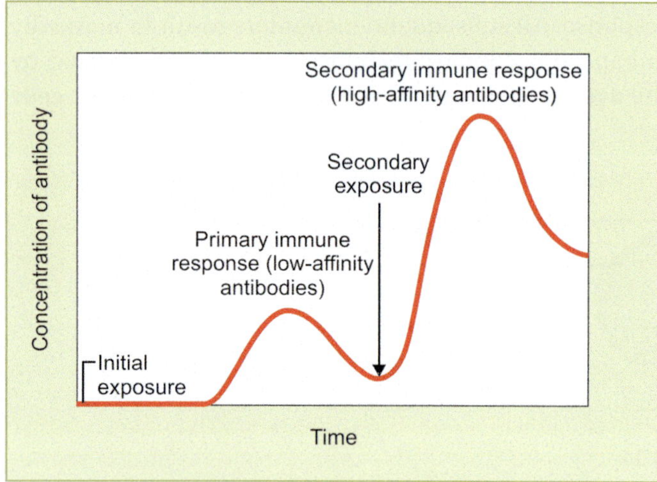

Fig. 1.6: Graph showing comparison between a primary and a secondary immune response.

Source: https://opentextbc.ca/biology/chapter/23-2-adaptive-immune-response.

Cell-mediated Immunity

Cell-mediated immunity against intracellular microbes consists of two main types of reactions:

1. The adaptive immune response to microbes residing within the phagocytes (mainly macrophages) is mediated by helper T cells of the T_H1 subset. In such cases, the specificity of the response is due to T cells, and the effector function is performed by macrophages. The infected macrophages produce IL-12, which helps in proliferation and differentiation of T_H cells. T cells recognize microbial antigens displayed by macrophages through their TCR and CD40L interactions with the antigen–MHC complex and CD40 of macrophages, respectively, and also produce cytokines (e.g., IFNγ) that activate phagocytes and stimulate inflammation. T-cell-dependent macrophage activation and inflammation may cause tissue injury. This reaction is called delayed-type hypersensitivity. The cooperation of T lymphocytes and phagocytes in this reaction is an important link between adaptive and innate immunity. Here, T cells stimulate the activity of nonspecific effector cells of innate immunity, thereby making these cells part of adaptive immunity.

Table 1.4: Differences between primary and secondary antibody responses.

Features	*Primary response*	*Secondary response*
Latent/lag period	Long (4–7 days)	Short (1–3 days)
Responding B cells	Naïve B cells	Memory B cells
Time of peak response (days)	7–10	3–5
Rate of antibody synthesis	Low	High
Peak antibody titer	Low	High
Persistence of antibody titer	Short	Long
Affinity and avidity of antibodies	Low	High
Presence of memory cells	Nil	High
Predominating isotype produced	IgM	IgG predominates
Antigens	Thymus dependent and thymus independent	Thymus dependent
Dose of immunogens to elicit	High	Low

2. CD8+ CTLs are effector T cells that recognize and kill target cells expressing peptides derived from intercellular nonself antigens in association with MHC I molecules. They kill target cells by the following three mechanisms:
    i. CTLs release perforin through granule exocytosis. Perforin is a membrane pore-forming protein that causes osmotic lysis of the target cell by polymerizing in its membrane.[36]
    ii. They also release serine proteases (called granzymes), which enter into the target cell through the perforin channel.[37] This triggers apoptosis in the target cell (Fig. 1.7).
    iii. CTLs start expressing FasL, which cross-links with Fas (CD95) on the target cell membrane, thereby delivering a death signal to the target cell and triggering its apoptosis.[38] Both FasL and Fas are cell surface proteins of the TNF receptor family present on many cells. Interaction of Fas with FasL initiates a signaling cascade leading to apoptosis of the cell.

Humoral Immunity

Humoral immunity helps in eliminating extracellular antigens and is mediated by antibodies secreted by antibodies. The effector functions of antibodies include neutralization of antigens, opsonization, and activation of a complement system.[11,21,31]

Neutralization: Antibodies block, or neutralize, the infectivity of microbes by binding to the microbes and sterically hindering interactions of the microbes with cellular receptors. Antibodies similarly block the pathologic actions of toxins by preventing binding of the toxins to host cells.

Opsonization: Phagocytes have receptors for Fc portion of the antibody molecules. Antibodies coat the antigens, and their Fc portions get attached to the Fc receptors on phagocytes. These attachments deliver signals that stimulate the phagocytic activity of phagocytes. When antibodies facilitate phagocytosis of the antigen by phagocytes, they are said to act like an opsonin, and the process of facilitated phagocytosis is called opsonization.

Activation of a complement system: The complement is a complex group of serum proteins that participate in an enzymatic cascade, ultimately resulting in a cytolytic membrane attack complex (MAC). Most of the complement factors are produced in the liver, with small contributions made by monocytes and fibroblasts. Complement components are designated by numerals (C1–C9) or by general names or letter symbols.

There are three pathways of complement activation resulting in C5b formation: *classical pathway, alternative pathway*, and *lectin activation pathway*. The classical pathway requires pre-existing immunoglobulins of the classes IgM and IgG. The alternative pathway is responsible for the complement system functioning in the absence of existing antibodies and provides early protection from pathogen. The lectin activation pathway depends on a protein called MBL to initiate the complement system. The final steps leading to the formation of final MAC are the same for all pathways.[39,40]

There are numerous effector functions of complement products. MAC mediates lysis of a wide array of microorganisms including bacteria and viruses.

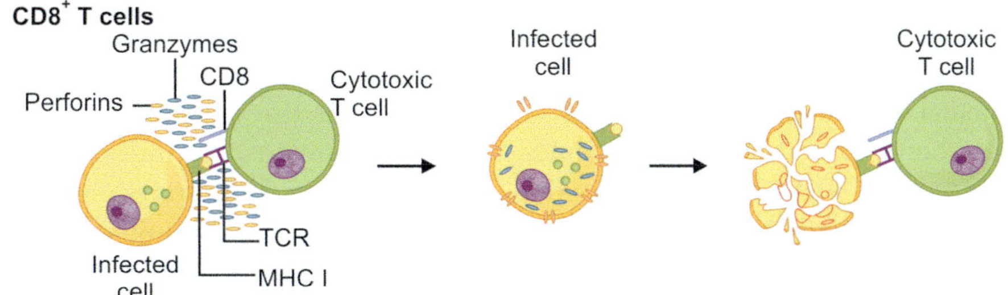

Fig. 1.7: Killing mechanism of cytotoxic T cells using perforins and granzymes.

Source: https://opentextbc.ca/biology/chapter/23-2-adaptive-immune-response.

Opsonization, i.e., coating the foreign cell with complement proteins, facilitates its ingestion by specific cellular components (phagocytosis). Complement protein-derived anaphylatoxins (C3a, C5a) bind to specific complement receptors on cells of immune system and act as potent inflammatory mediators.[41] Chemotactic factors formed during complement activation result in attracting neutrophils and monocytes to the sites of complement activation and form a part of the biological amplification system. The complement system also plays a crucial role in neutralizing viral infectivity. Various complement components are also important for immune clearance, which remove immune complexes from circulation and deposit them in the spleen and liver.

IMMUNOLOGICAL DISORDERS

The immune system is not infallible. Its malfunctioning may result in various immunologic disorders.

1. *Autoimmune diseases*: The immune response must recognize nonself from self-antigens (substances that are a normal part of the body). In normal conditions, the immune response is programmed to tolerate self-antigens. Whenever this delicate system fails, the immune system may attack the self-antigens, which results in autoimmune diseases such as systemic lupus erythematosus, psoriasis, rheumatoid arthritis, and some forms of diabetes.
2. *Immunodeficiency diseases*: Deficiency in any component of the immune system (stem cells, B lymphocytes, T lymphocytes, complement proteins, etc.) due to genetic, developmental, or acquired factors results in immunodeficiency diseases such as acquired immunodeficiency syndrome and tuberculosis.
3. *Hypersensitivity diseases*: The excessive and/or inappropriate immune response to a nonself-antigen results in hypersensitivity diseases. The typical examples are bronchial asthma and allergic rhinitis.

On the basis of mechanisms and effector molecules involved, Gell and Coombs (1963)[42] classified the hypersensitivity reactions into four types:

- Type I (immediate, IgE mediated)
- Type II (cytolytic or cytotoxic, IgG/IgM mediated)
- Type III (immune complex, IgG/IgM mediated)
- Type IV (delayed, T-cell mediated)

The two most commonly used terms with reference to hypersensitivity are allergy and atopy. The term "allergy" (*allos* means "altered" and *ergos* means "action") was coined by von Pirquet in 1906. Presently, it is defined as a hypersensitivity reaction initiated by specific immunologic mechanisms. Hypersensitivity describes objectively reproducible symptoms or signs initiated by exposure to a defined stimulus (allergen), which is well tolerated by a healthy person.[11] The localized (limited to a specific tissue or organ) hypersensitivity reactions are usually inherited. In 1923, Coca and Cooke coined the term "atopy" to describe this genetic predisposition of an individual to respond to environmental allergens with production of allergen-specific IgE antibodies.[43] In developed countries such as the United States, more than 54.3% of the population suffers from atopic allergies including a wide range of IgE-mediated disorders such as allergic rhinitis, asthma, atopic dermatitis, and food allergies.

TYPE I HYPERSENSITIVITY

In a sensitized individual, Type I or immediate reactions can affect almost any organ system of the body. The respiratory tract, gastrointestinal (GI) tract, and skin are most frequently affected organ systems. Clinically, Type I allergic symptoms are present as allergic rhinitis and/or bronchial asthma in the respiratory system; abdominal discomfort, vomiting, and/or diarrhea in the GI tract; and urticaria and/or eczema in the skin. The present chapter focuses on the allergic disorders of the respiratory system only.

Allergic Rhinitis

Allergic rhinitis, commonly known as hay fever, is an IgE-mediated reaction affecting the upper respiratory tract. It results from the interaction between aeroallergens with IgE on the sensitized mast cells in conjunctiva and nasal mucosa to induce mediator release and is manifested by symptoms, such as nasal congestion, sinus headache, running nose, watery eyes, itching, and sneezing.[44] The role of allergens in the etiology of allergic rhinitis was first identified by Blackley in 1867. The overall prevalence of allergic rhinitis in adult population ranges from 25% to 35% worldwide. The prevalence of allergic rhinitis in India has been found to be 11.69% in adult population.

Bronchial Asthma

Bronchial asthma is a common manifestation of IgE-mediated localized anaphylaxis in the lower respiratory tract. The resulting constriction of bronchioles and airway obstruction causes difficulty in breathing, often associated with wheezing.

Global Initiative for Asthma guidelines define asthma as a chronic inflammatory disorder of the airways in which many cellular elements play a role.[45] The chronic inflammation is associated with airway hyper-responsiveness that leads to recurrent episodes of wheezing, breathlessness, chest tightness, coughing, etc. These episodes are associated with widespread, but variable, airflow obstruction within the lung that is often reversible, either spontaneous or with treatment.

It is estimated that 300 million individuals throughout the world are affected with bronchial asthma alone. Based on the application of standardized methods, the prevalence of asthma has been reported to range from 1% to 18% of the population in different countries. In Delhi, India, the prevalence of bronchial asthma alone has been reported to be about 8–10% in children and 11% in adults. Allergens are one of the commonly identified agents involved as risk and trigger factors in extrinsic/allergic asthma.[46]

Historical Background

Hypersensitivity reactions have been mentioned as early as in 460–370 BC in Hippocratic writings.[16,43] Galen, in AD 131–201, also described allergic reactions in his writings. Another significant discovery that led to further research in the field was discovery of anaphylaxis in animals by Richet (1902). It was suggested that this was related to hay fever or asthma in humans. Mechanism of allergic reaction was first described by Prausnitz and Kustner (1921) who showed that serum from allergic subjects could produce an allergic reaction in healthy persons. This serum component was referred to as "reagin"-active substance. In 1967, Ishizaka and coworkers described gamma E globulin as the carrier of skin sensitizing activity. Simultaneously, Johansson and Bennich (1967) identified a unique myeloma protein called IgND having properties similar to the reagin. Collaborative studies by these two groups revealed that IgND and gamma E globulin were identical. In 1968, this molecule was designated as IgE by the World Health Organization Committee on Nomenclature for Human Immunoglobulins.

Factors Influencing Allergic Diseases

The susceptibility of developing an allergic disease is defined by the interaction of complex and multiple genetic factors and environmental stimuli.[47,48]

Genetic Factors

The ability to respond to allergen exposure is genetically determined. Various studies showed that allergy runs in the family. Some other studies showed that heritability of serum IgE levels was in the range of 50–84%. In twins raised together and apart, genetic factors were found to bear more influence on IgE levels than the environmental factors. Genetic control also appears to be more important in the determination of overall risk of allergy, while environmental influences determine the specific allergens to which a person will develop allergy. Several candidate genes have been identified; however, their actual linkage with asthma and atopy is still not clear. Linkage for atopy was found to genes on chromosomes 5, 6, 11, and 13. Only the linkage to chromosome 11 has been replicated and has been found to be associated with genes present on the 11q segment. Linkage of total serum IgE to chromosomes 1, 2, 4, 5, 6, 7, 9, 11, 12, 13, 14, 15, and 16 has been reported in several studies. However, results have been replicated only for chromosomes 5, 11, and 12. Linkage for specific IgE has been found to chromosomes 1, 2, 4, 6, 7, 9, and 12. However, a lot of research is still required to identify important genetic risk factors in a population and the mechanism by which they affect the pathology of atopy and asthma.

Environmental Factors

Environmental factors make an important contribution to the ultimate expression of the genetic potential for high IgE responder phenotype, the most important etiologic factor being allergen exposure. The sensitization to allergen depends on intensity and duration of exposure and potency of allergen. The other nonspecific adjuvant factors, that may enhance the immunogenicity of allergens presumably by increasing epithelial permeability and inflammation, include bacterial and viral infections, industrial and indoor pollutants, and cigarette smoking.

Mechanism of Allergic Reactions

To understand the mechanism of generation of Type I hypersensitivity, it is important to know the molecular and cellular participants involved in it. The main participants are allergens, IgE, and mast cells and basophils. In addition, other inflammatory cells such as eosinophils, macrophages and monocytes, neutrophils, lymphocytes, and platelets also play an important role in allergic inflammation. Besides these, changes in (1) activities of various pumps and (2) number and class of cell adhesion molecules on the surface of these cells have also been found to be associated with Type I hypersensitivity.

Allergens

Allergic reactions are initiated by certain types of antigens referred to as allergens. Allergens are harmless to general population. The common allergens include pollen, fungal spores, house dust mite and house dust, animal danders, insect emanations and detritus, drugs, foods, etc.

According to the routes of exposure, allergens have been classified into the following four types:[43]

1. Inhalants (e.g., pollen and fungal spores)
2. Ingestants (e.g., food articles and additives)
3. Injectants (e.g., insect bites and stings, injected medicines)
4. Contactants (e.g., cosmetics).

Of these, inhalants are the most important causative agents of Type I respiratory allergic disorders.

Chemical analysis of allergens has revealed that these are usually proteins or glycoproteins in nature with multiple epitopes per molecule. Till now, not many structural commonalities have been found among allergens to predict allergenicity of a given substance. Recent studies have reported a few features shared by allergens, which have provided some insight into the biological basis of their activity.[16] These features are as follows:

1. The presence of enzymatic activity in many allergens affects the cells and molecules of the immune system. For example, allergen extracts from dust mites, cockroaches, fungi, and bacteria are relatively high in protease activity. Some of these proteases are capable of disrupting the epithelial cell junctions, thereby allowing allergens to interact with the underlying cells and molecules of the innate and adaptive immune systems. A protease, Der p1, produced by the dust mite, cleaves and activates complement components at the mucosal surface. Still others cleave and stimulate protease-activated receptors on the surfaces of immune cells, enhancing inflammation.
2. Allergens may contain PAMPs, which when interact with receptors of the innate immune system initiate a cascade of responses leading to an allergic response. However, it is still not clear why this cascade is stimulated in certain individuals only.
3. Many allergens enter the host via mucosal tissues at very low concentrations. This tends to predispose an individual to generate activated T_H2 cells which, in turn, activate B cells leading to secretion of IgE.

Immunoglobulin E

The IgE is a serum protein (300 ng/mL), comprising less than 0.001% of total serum immunoglobulins. This is because some portion of the circulating amount is continuously removed and destroyed in endosomes. IgE is biologically very active, as it binds to high-affinity receptors on the surface of mast cells and basophils, rendering these cells highly sensitive to allergens, even when circulating IgE is very low.

Structure: The structure of IgE antibodies was first described by Bennich and Johansson (1971).[49] IgE comprises two heavy and two light chains linked by disulfide bonds, where the heavy chain has five domains. IgE is a glycoprotein (12% carbohydrate) with a sedimentation coefficient of 8S.

Characteristic features: The cell-binding site of IgE resides in its Fc portion, which is heat labile and is destroyed upon heating at 56°C for 40 minutes. This thermal sensitivity of IgE resides in Cε3/Cε4 regions of Fc. The serum half-life of IgE is 2.5 days but IgE bound to the mast cell surface may remain sensitized for weeks or even months due to high-affinity binding and consequent protection from proteolysis by serum proteases. IgE binds with high affinity to mast cells and basophils and with a much lower affinity to lymphocytes, eosinophils, macrophages, complement, etc.[50,51]

Concentration: Serum IgE levels are related to age, genetic predisposition, race, immune status, and some disease processes. The widely used unit for reporting IgE content is the international unit (1 IU = 2.4 ng/mL). The upper limit for IgE in normal adults, reported in the different studies, has been highly variable ranging from 40.9 to 200 IU/mL. In Indian population, due to helminthic infestations, the levels have been reported to be comparatively higher, i.e., 700 and 1025 IU/mL.[52,53]

The IgE levels have been found to be elevated in allergic diseases, parasitic infestations, smokers, and patients with pulmonary carcinoma.

Functions: IgE antibodies have the following two primary biological functions:

1. Mediate Type I hypersensitivity reactions. The mast cell degranulation mediated by IgE leads to release of pharmacologically active mediators, which cause tissue damage and inflammation.
2. Provide defense against parasitic infestations. High IgE concentrations are regularly found in patients with helminthic infestations, such as *Ascaris* and *Schistosoma*. The IgE-mediated parasite killing involves various effector cells, including mast cells, macrophages, monocytes, eosinophils, and platelets.[54]

Receptor for IgE on cells: IgE can bind to various cells through different types of receptors present on these cells:

- *High-affinity receptors (FcεRI)*: These receptors are present on the surface of mast cells and basophils. The IgE receptors are univalent with quite high affinity for IgE ($K_d \approx 10^{-9}$–10^{-10} M). The number of FcεRI receptors varies between 10^3 and 10^6 per cell in different cell preparations. FcεRI is a multimeric complex consisting of one α, one β, and two disulfide-linked γ chains.[55] The α-chain (45–60 kDa) has two immunoglobulin-binding domains (D1 and D2). IgE molecule binds to them by C_H3/C_H3 and C_H4/C_H4 domains present on the dimeric Fc fragment. The β-chain (33 kDa) has four transmembrane domains between its amino and carboxy terminals. Each γ-chain (15 kDa) has only one transmembrane domain. The amino terminals of both β and γ chains protrude out of the membrane surface, whereas their carboxy terminals remain in the cytoplasm. These C terminals have immunoreceptor tyrosine-based activation motifs (ITAMs), which have phosphoacceptors. Through these phosphoacceptors, these receptor subunits interact with the signaling proteins, which eventually lead to the cell activation. The intensity of signals perceived by γ-chain of the complex is further amplified (five- to sevenfold) by the β-chain.[56]
- *Low-affinity receptors (FcεRII)*: These receptors are present on B lymphocytes, T lymphocytes, eosinophils, platelets, and macrophages. The number of FcεRII receptors on these cells ranges from $10^3 \times 10^4$ to 6×10^4 per cell. They are specific for the C_H3/C_H3 domain of IgE. The amino terminal of these receptors is located in the cytoplasm, whereas carboxy terminal is directed toward the extracellular space. Based on the differences in the amino terminal of their cytoplasmic domain, two types of FcεRII receptors have been recognized: FcεRIIa and FcεRIIb. FcεRIIa, constitutively and exclusively expressed on B cells, regulates their growth and differentiation, whereas FcεRIIb is expressed only on stimulation with IL-4 on peripheral B and T cells, monocytes, and eosinophils in atopic individuals. These receptors seem to play an important role in regulating the intensity of IgE response.[57] The IgE receptors also exist in soluble form in serum. These soluble receptors are generated by autoproteolysis of the membrane receptors and have been shown to enhance IgE production by B cells.

Regulation of IgE production and role of cytokines: The IgE response is under the control of various regulatory factors, the most important being T cells.[58-61] As the APCs bind to resting T cells, IL-1, IL-4, IL-6, and TNF-β transform resting T cells to activated ones, which secrete IL-2. This IL-2 auto-stimulates T cells to express additional IL-2 receptors on T-cell surfaces, thus activating them further. Under the influence of IL-2, T cells become actively replicating cells that secrete other cytokines such as Il-3, IL-4, and IL-5.

The levels of IgE have been found to be regulated by these cytokines released by T_H1 and T_H2 cells. The T_H2 cells induce IgE synthesis by a cognate/noncognate T–B cell interaction and production of IL-4, which activates B cells and causes isotype switching of B cells into IgE-producing cells. It has also been observed that IL-4 induces and enhances IgE production. This production is further enhanced by IL-5. IL-6 also acts as a stimulant to the polyclonal production of immunoglobulins by B cells. In human and murine B cells, IgE production is also upregulated by IL-13. The cytokines secreted by Th1 cells, namely, IL-2, IFNγ, and TNF-α, antagonize the IgE responses. In addition to IL-2 and IFNγ, TGF-β and PGE_2 inhibit IgE synthesis. Ishizaka (1989) proposed that the regulation of IgE response occurs by two IgE-binding factors: IgE-potentiating and IgE-suppressive factors. The formation of these factors is in turn controlled by two T-cell factors: glycosylation-enhancing factor and glycosylation-inhibiting factor.

Mast Cells and Basophils

Both mast cells and basophils share significant structural and functional similarity, and play an important role in the development of allergies. The precursors of mast cells are released from the bone marrow into the blood, but they mature only after they leave the blood. Mast cells are found in a wide variety of tissues such as the skin, the connective tissue in various organs, and the mucosal epithelial tissue of the respiratory, urinogenital, and gastrointestinal tracts. The cytoplasm of these cells is full of granules that contain histamine and other pharmacologically active substances.[62] An apparent increase in mast cells in bronchoalveolar lavage (BAL) of asthmatics[63] and in nasal lavage of patients with allergic rhinitis[64] has been reported. Elevated levels of tryptase, a mast cell marker, have been observed in atopic asthmatics after allergen challenge.[65]

Basophils are nonphagocytic granulocytes containing large cytoplasmic granules filled with basophilic proteins. Very few basophils are present in the circulation but can be very potent. In response to the binding of IgE antibodies, basophils release the contents of their granules which are responsible for allergic manifestations.[66] Basophils also play an important role in helminthic infestations. They may secrete cytokines that modulate the adaptive immune response.

Mechanism

Hypersensitivity develops only after an initial exposure to the allergen. Thus, the mechanism can be divided into two phases: (1) primary encounter and (2) secondary encounter.

Primary encounter: Environmental allergens enter via mucosal surfaces and are taken up by local APCs. These APCs process the allergens and present them to naïve T_H2 cells. This is followed by selection and clonal expansion of T_H2 cells. These cells then interact with B lymphocytes, leading to their proliferation and differentiation into allergen-specific IgE-producing plasma cells and memory cells. The allergen-specific IgEs are then released in the circulation and bind to the FcεRI receptors on the surface of mast cells and basophils, thereby sensitizing them.

Secondary encounter: On a second or a subsequent exposure, allergen causes bridging of IgE molecules (bound on mast cells).[62] This initiates a cell-triggering signal leading to activation and degranulation of basophils or mast cells and release of mediators and cytokines, which are responsible for both early- and late-phase responses. The complete activation of these cells requires bridging of only a few (100 or lesser) IgE molecules (Figs. 1.8 A to E).[67]

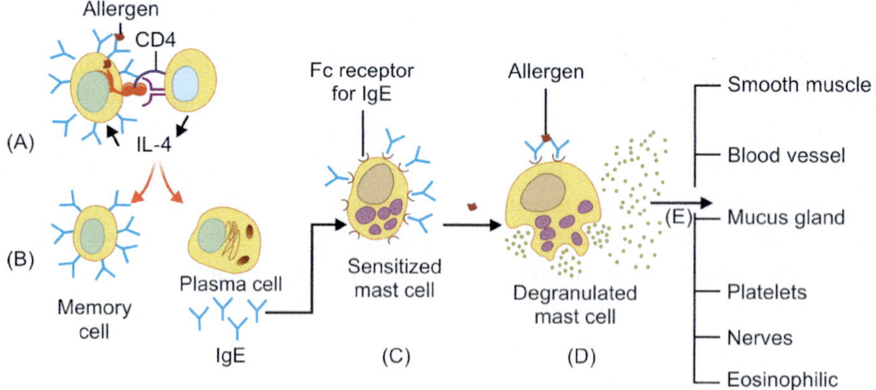

Figs. 1.8A to E: Mast cell degranulation. (A) Interaction of T and B cells [antigen-presenting cell (APC)] leading to activation of T cell and release of IL-4; (B) B cell differentiates into memory and IgE-producing plasma cell; (C) Binding of IgE to Fc receptors for IgE on mast cell; (D) Bridging of IgE receptors on mast cell followed by its degranulation upon subsequent exposures; (E) Effects of mediators.

The activation occurs due to cross-linking of IgE receptors in the plane of the plasma membrane of the sensitized cells. This brings about aggregation of their FcεRIα chains causing conformational changes in the α chain and activation of phosphotyrosine kinase (PTK). PTK phosphorylates the tyrosine residues of ITAM on β and γ chains, thereby activating the intracellular signaling cascades and complete activation of cells for cellular responses to occur. The cells undergo the following changes.

Intracellular changes: The major events that take place during the receptor–antigen aggregation and signaling are (1) activation of receptor-associated phospholipase C (PLC), (2) activation of serine protease to form serine esterase and of phosphomethyl transferases (PMT I and PMT II), and (3) increased influx of Ca^{2+} from extracellular milieu, which activates phospholipase A_2. Activated PLC hydrolyzes membrane phosphoinositides, namely, phosphatidyl inositol 4-5 bisphosphate (PIP_2), and generates two second messengers, inositol triphosphate (IP_3) and diacyl-glycerol (DAG).[67-69] IP_3 releases Ca^{2+} from intracellular stores (endoplasmic reticulum) and together with DAG activates protein kinase C, which phosphorylates proteins—a critical signal for cell secretion. DAG may also be acted upon by DAG lipase or monoglyceride lipase leading to the formation of arachidonic acid.[70]

The release of Ca^{2+} from intracellular stores (primarily from endoplasmic reticulum) depletes the stores, which are required to be refilled for sustained action of various Ca^{2+}-dependent events. This is replenished by influx of extracellular Ca^{2+}. As there are no voltage-dependent and/or ligand-gated calcium channels in mast cells, it is thought that a class of 'store-operated' calcium channels (SOCCs) mediates the influx.[71] In electrophysiological terms, depletion of calcium from intracellular stores is associated with a calcium release-activated current (I_{CRAC}), which is highly calcium cation selective.

The cell activation leads to the formation of serine esterase, which converts phosphatidyl serine into phosphatidyl ethanolamine (PE). PE undergoes methylation by stepwise action of PMT enzymes to form phosphatidyl choline (PC). PC accumulates on the exterior of plasma membrane causing an increase in membrane fluidity, leading to the formation of Ca^{2+} channels. The Ca^{2+} influx reaches a peak within 2 minutes of receptor cross-linkage.

Mediator release: Concomitant with phospholipid methylation and Ca^{2+} influx, there is a transient increase in membrane-bound adenyl cyclase activity leading to the generation of cyclic adenosine monophosphate (cAMP). It activates specific protein kinases, which cause phosphorylation of granule membrane proteins, changing their permeability to H_2O and Ca^{2+} ions leading to granule swelling.[72] In mast cells, the individual granular contents fuse by forming channels that open to the exterior by fusion with the plasma membrane, while in basophils the granular membranes fuse with the plasma membrane resulting in the extrusion of granular material to the outside. The fusion of granular membranes with plasma membrane is thought to be facilitated by lipids called Fusogens.[70] The movement of granules to plasma membrane is brought about by contraction of microfilaments, promoted by Ca^{2+} influx, changes in transmembrane potential, and rise in intracellular pH. Within 2–3 minutes of calcium influx and histamine release, the level of intracellular cAMP begins to drop. This drop in the levels of cAMP appears to be necessary for initiating degranulation leading to the release of both preformed and newly formed mediators.[67] The release reaction is temperature dependent with optimal release at 37°C. The optimal conditions for release of mediators depend on the concentration of allergen and allergen-specific IgE on cell membranes and affinity of IgE for allergen.

The increased levels of intracellular Ca^{2+}, achieved by SOCC-mediated influx or by increase in membrane fluidity, activate the enzyme phospholipase A_2, which promotes breakdown of PC into lysophosphatidyl choline and arachidonic acid. The arachidonic acid formed by various pathways is metabolized by either cyclo-oxygenase or lipoxygenase pathway to produce prostaglandins and leukotrienes, respectively.

Cyclo-oxygenase pathway: Specific membrane-bound cellular enzymes called cyclo-oxygenases catalyze the addition of two molecules of O_2 to arachidonic acid, leading to the production of prostaglandin PGG_2, a cyclic endoperoxide. PGG_2 is converted to PGH_2 by another peroxidase. PGH_2 is further converted to a variety of prostaglandins and thromboxanes (TXs) by selective enzymatic pathways.

Lipoxygenase pathway: The cytosolic enzymes called lipoxygenases introduce one molecule of O_2 at 5-, 12-, or 15- carbon atoms of arachidonic acid. As a result of oxygenation, 5-, 12-, and 15-hydroperoxy-eicosatetraenoic acids (HPETEs) are formed in different types of cells. These unstable compounds are rapidly converted to 5-, 12-, and 15-hydroxy-eicosatetraenoic acids. Besides, each HPETE serves as a precursor of complex mediators, i.e., leukotrienes (LTA_4, LTB_4, LTC_4, etc.) and lipoxins.

The mediators released by mast cells and basophils are pharmacologically active agents that act on local tissues as well as secondary effector cells including eosinophils, neutrophils, lymphocytes, monocytes, platelets, etc. They are classified as preformed (primary) mediators including histamine, proteases, etc. (Table 1.5) and newly formed (secondary) mediators including prostaglandins, TXs, and leukotrienes (Table 1.6).

Table 1.5: List of preformed mediators, their classes, and functions.

Mediator class	*Mediator*	*Function (s)*
Biogenic amines	Histamine	Effects on smooth muscle, endothelial cells, and nerve endings mediated by H_1 and H_2 receptors; causes vasodilation; stimulates mucus secretion; and increases vascular permeability
Neutral proteases	Chymase, carboxypeptidase, tryptase	Bronchial mucus secretion, degradation of blood vessel basement membrane, generation of complement split products
Acid hydrolases	Arylsulfatase	Hydrolyzes aromatic sulfate esters
	β-Glucuronidase	Removes β-linked glucuronic acid from complex carbohydrate chains
	β-D-Galactosidase	Hydrolyzes β-linked galactose from complex carbohydrates
	β-Hexosaminidase	Cleavage of β-linked hexosamines from carbohydrates and glycoproteins
Proteoglycans	Heparin	Increased vascular permeability, smooth muscle contraction
Oxidative enzymes	Superoxide dismutase	Converts O_2 to H_2O_2
	Peroxide	Converts H_2O_2 to H_2O, inactivates leukotrienes, generates lipid mediators
Chemotactic factors	Eosinophil chemotactic factor	Eosinophil chemotaxis and activation
	Neutrophil chemotactic factor	Neutrophil chemotaxis and activation

Table 1.6: List of newly formed mediators, their examples, and functions.

Mediator class	*Examples*	*Function (s)*
Prostaglandins	PGG2, PGH2	Vasodilation, contraction of pulmonary smooth muscles, platelet aggregation
Leukotrienes	LTC4, LTD4, LTE4	Increased vascular permeability, contraction of pulmonary smooth muscles
Bradykinin	–	Increased vascular permeability, smooth muscle contraction
Platelet-activating factor	PAF	Platelet aggregation and degranulation, contraction of pulmonary smooth muscles
Cytokines	IL-1 and TNF-	Systemic anaphylaxis, increased expression of adhesion molecules on venular endothelial cells
	IL-4 and IL-3	Increased IgE production
	IL-5, IL-6, IL-10, TGF-β, granulocyte-macrophage colony-stimulating factor	Various effects

Components of the Allergic Response

The chemotactic, inflammatory, and spasmogenic effects of the mast cell/basophil mediators are manifested in two phases.

Early-phase Reaction

The early-phase reaction (EPR) develops within minutes of allergen exposure and thus is also referred to as immediate reaction. The response is initiated by the release of preformed mediators from mast cells and basophils. These mediators result in various pathophysiologic changes by primarily increasing capillary permeability causing vasodilation and smooth muscle contraction.

Late-phase Reaction

In some subjects, after an immediate reaction to an allergen, a late response develops within 3–11 hours without any further exposure to the allergen. The magnitude of LPR is related to serum IgE concentration and amount of allergen administered or intensity of EPR. The chemotactic factors released during the EPR lead to infiltration of eosinophils, neutrophils, and mononuclear cells to the site of mast cell activation. These cells further release some newly formed mediators causing extensive and prolonged tissue damage.

Late-phase reactions (LPRs) are more prolonged than immediate responses and are associated with edema and erythema on skin[73,74] and increased resistance to air flow in nose and lungs.[75] The occurrence of LPR appears to be more relevant to clinical expression and severity of allergic reactions than EPRs.[76]

Role of Other Inflammatory Cells

Eosinophils

The association of eosinophilia with allergic diseases is well known.[77,78] Eosinophil infiltration is a characteristic feature of asthmatic and rhinitic airways. Increased numbers of eosinophils have been shown in lavage fluid and bronchial biopsies from asthmatics. Besides platelet-activating factor (PAF) and LTC_4, cytokines such as IL-5 and granulocyte-macrophage colony-stimulating factor (GM-CSF) and adhesion molecules such as integrins, intercellular adhesion molecules (ICAM)-1, and vascular cell adhesion molecules (VCAM)-1 also increase eosinophil recruitment into tissues. They contribute to pathogenesis by producing various cytotoxic and inflammatory mediators and superoxide anions. Eosinophils act as enhancers of tissue inflammation by generating cytokines including IL-1 and IL-3. Eosinophils also dampen the inflammatory response by releasing histaminase and aryl sulfatase, which inactivate histamine and slow-reacting substance of anaphylaxis. Eosinophils release eosinophil peroxidase, which inactivates LTC_4, LTD_4, and phospholipase D, which acts on PAF. The Charcot–Leyden crystal protein may be involved in the phagocytosis of mast cell granules and IgE–allergen complexes, further reducing inflammation.[79]

Lymphocytes

The role of B lymphocytes in the synthesis of IgE antibodies is well established. T cells play a vital role in generation of IgE response as they are required for cognate/noncognate interaction with B cells for IgE production. T cells are also involved in the regulation and coordination of IgE responses by production of various lymphokines. Although T cells are the major effector cells in an allergic response, $CD8^+$ T cells have also been found to have a role in IgE regulation.[80-82] The T-cell-derived lymphokines IL-4, IL-5, and IFNγ are involved in IgE regulation and cause eosinophil inflammation, expansion, and differentiation of mucosal mast cells. The presence of allergen-specific T_H2 type of T-cell clones in asthmatics has been demonstrated, indicating that T_H2 cells can play a central role in the pathogenesis of allergic inflammation.

Monocytes and Macrophages

Monocytes and macrophages have been suggested to participate in allergic inflammation by virtue of the presence of FcεRII receptors and their activation by allergen. These cells participate in allergic inflammation through release of mediators, which produce local effects and act as chemotaxins (LTB_4, PAF, TNF, PGD_2, and GM-CSF) and activators (IL-1, IL-6, and IL-8) for neutrophils, eosinophils, and fibroblasts. The mediators released by macrophages stimulate smooth muscle contraction and cause bronchoconstriction and mucus secretion, which leads to airway plugging.[82,83] Selective upregulation of cytokine production by monocytes and macrophages has been observed in asthma.

Neutrophils

Neutrophils have been found in airways and BAL fluid of asthmatics.[84] A marked increase in neutrophils has been noted in patients with severe asthma. However, there is no direct evidence to implicate neutrophils in causation of allergic inflammation.

Platelets

Bronchial biopsies of asthmatics show an evidence of platelet activation. After allergen challenge there is a significant decrease in the number of platelets in the circulation.[85] Chemokines associated with T_H2-mediated inflammation have been shown to activate and aggregate platelets. Only 10–20% of platelets from normal individuals can bind IgE, whereas more than 50% of platelets of allergic patients can bind IgE through FcεRII receptors on their surface. It has also been reported that platelet activation accompanies allergen-induced bronchoconstriction.

ROLE OF IMMUNOGLOBULIN G (IGG) IN ALLERGY

Even though Type 1 hypersensitivity is predominantly mediated by IgE antibodies, the role of other immunoglobulin classes such as IgG with its subclasses (mainly IgG4) has also been investigated in allergy research.[86] Some studies have reported an increase in the levels of allergen-specific IgG4 antibodies within the course of and after immunotherapy and named them "blocking antibodies". However, allergen-specific IgG4 may also play a role in the occurrence of anaphylactic events. Parish (1970), for the first time, demonstrated that some human sera contained IgG antibodies capable of sensitizing mast cells in the skin of monkeys and designated them as "short-term sensitizing IgG (IgG-S-TS)."[87] The evidence that IgE-deficient mice could still develop anaphylaxis added IgG in the group of allergy-promoting factors. At present, several reports on the effect of allergen-specific IgG4 in the pathogenesis of allergic diseases exist, but the overall results remain controversial and vary according to the antigen and exposure levels.[88] For example, the appearance and protective role of IgG antibodies in cat allergy was found to be related to the dose of exposure to the major allergen Fel d 1. Some studies reported parallel trends in the appearance of IgE, IgG, and IgG4 antibodies specific to various allergens, suggesting a complementary role. Jenmalm et al. (1999, 2001) reported a strong correlation between elevated IgG4 serum levels and atopic sensitization to birch, egg, and cat allergens in childhood.

TLR LIGANDS AND ALLERGY

The TLRs are a class of membrane-spanning noncatalytic receptors present on the surface of macrophages, monocytes, etc., that recognize structurally conserved molecules derived from microorganisms. They play a key role in innate immune responses to noninfectious immunostimulatory substances in the environment. About 13 TLRs have been identified (TLR 1-13) till date that recognize a variety of ligands.[16] TLR ligands have the potential of both protection from and precipitation of allergic manifestations.[89]

Various studies suggest that in addition to allergens, other substances that modulate immune response and influence the delicate homeostasis of immune system are also present in the environment. Endotoxin or LPS, a ligand for TLR4, is present in higher concentrations in homes with regular animal exposure.[90] Recently, a study proved that LPS (50 pg/mL) increased recombinant cat allergen-stimulated proliferation of human peripheral blood mononuclear cells (PBMCs) from subjects IgE-positive/IgE-negative to cat allergens. PBMCs from many of these subjects did not proliferate in response to stimulation with recombinant allergen alone but did so in the presence of LPS. In endotoxin-rich environments, levels of other components such as peptidoglycan (TLR2 ligand) and DNA sequences from bacteria and viruses (TLR9 ligand) also increase considerably. It has been observed that immunostimulatory activities of house dust extract were partially dependent on TLR2, TLR4, and TLR9.[91] They have been found to play an important role in mediating proinflammatory responses to particulates present in the air. However, more studies are required to develop a complete understanding of the effects of TLR ligands on immune response and allergic risk.

NEURAL PATHWAYS IN ALLERGIC REACTIONS

The neural control of airway function not only depends on a balance between cholinergic and adrenergic nervous systems but also on the non-cholinergic inhibitory and non-cholinergic excitatory nervous systems. Any imbalances in the autonomic nervous system in asthmatics lead to bronchospasm.[92]

Three groups of airway sensory receptors are involved in pathophysiology of allergic disorders: *C-fiber receptors, rapidly adapting receptors,* and *Aδ-nociceptive receptors,* which are sensitized by inflammatory and immunologic changes. C-fiber receptors may mediate axon reflex neurogenic inflammation. Activation of receptors also causes central nervous reflexes including bronchoconstriction, mucus secretion, etc.

C-fiber receptors also contain neuropeptides such as tachykinins, substance P, neurokinin A and B, and calcitonin gene-related peptide, which play an important role in the pathogenesis of asthma and airway inflammation. Substance P was found to increase in asthma and enhance vascular permeability, neutrophil adhesion and chemotaxis, mucus secretion, and smooth muscle contraction.[93] Mediators released by mast cells have been found to stimulate nerves present in the vicinity, leading to vascular edema and smooth muscle contraction.[94] However, most of these evidences are derived from studies on animal models, and the extent to which they apply to human beings needs to be investigated.

ROLE OF CELLULAR ADHESION MOLECULES IN ALLERGIC DISEASES

Adhesion molecules seem to play an important role in allergic diseases.[95,96] Increased expression of E-selectin, ICAM-1, lymphocyte function-associated antigen-1 (LFA-1), and VCAM-1 in airways and skin has been reported in extrinsic allergic asthma and atopic dermatitis.[97,98] However, some workers did not find statistical difference in the expression of adhesion molecules between patients with extrinsic asthma and normal control subjects. According to them, increased expression of these molecules may only be reflecting the degree of ongoing inflammation in the disease. Increased expression of ICAM-1/CD54 was also observed in conjunctival and nasal epithelium of all the allergic individuals investigated 30 minutes after allergen challenge. Conclusive evidence for the role of adhesion molecules in asthma requires the use of specific antagonists of adhesion molecules.[99] In a primate model of asthma, monoclonal antibodies to E-selection and ICAM-1 prevented antigen-induced airway hyper-responsiveness by inhibiting neutrophil and eosinophil infiltration, respectively.[100] However, further studies are needed to clarify the specificity of adhesion molecules for allergic diseases.

REFERENCES

1. Beutler B. Innate immunity: an overview. Mol Immunol. 2004;40:845-59.
2. Medzhitov R. Innate immune system. In: Paul WE, ed. Fundamental Immunology. 5th ed. Philadelphia, PA: Lippincott Williams & Wilkins; 2003:497-518.
3. Medzhitov R, Janeway C. Innate immunity. New Eng J Med. 2000;343:338-44.
4. Bulet P, Stoklin R, Menin L. Antimicrobial peptides: from invertebrates to vertebrates. Immunol Rev. 2004;198:169-84.
5. Carroll MC. The role of complement and complement receptors in induction and regulation of immunity. Ann Rev Immunol. 1998;16:545-68.
6. Ridiker PM, Cannon CP, Morrow D, et al. C-reactive protein and outcomes after statin therapy. New Eng J Med. 2005;352:20-8.
7. Nathan C. Neutrophils and immunity: challenges and opportunities. Nat Rev Immunol. 2006;6:173-82.
8. Taylor PR, Martinez-Pomares L, Stacey M, et al. Macrophage receptors and immune recognition. Annu Rev Immunol. 2005;23:901-44.
9. Kumagai Y, Takeuchi O, Akira S. Pathogen recognition by innate receptors. J Infect Chemother. 2008;14:86-92.
10. Uematsu S, Akira S. Toll-like receptors and innate immunity. J Mol Med. 2006;84:712-25.
11. Kindt TJ, Osborne BA, Goldsby RA, eds. Cells and organs of the immune system. In: Kuby Immunology. 6th ed. 2006;22-51.
12. Appelbaum FR. Hematopoietic stem cell transplantation. In: Dale D, Federman D, eds. Scientific American Medicine. New York, NY: Scientific American Publishers; 1996.
13. Engel P, Boumsell L, Balderas R, et al. CD nomenclature 2015: human leukocyte differentiation antigen workshops as a driving force in immunology. J Immunol. 2015;195: 4555-63.
14. Blom B, Spits H. Development of human lymphoid cells. Annu Rev Immunol. 2006;24:287-320.
15. Hardy RR. B-cell development and biology. In: Paul WE, ed. Fundamental Immunology. 5th ed. Philadelphia, PA: Lippincott Williams & Wilkins; 2003:159-94.
16. Judith AO, Jenni P, Sharon AS, Patricia PJ. Kuby Immunology. 7th ed. New York, NY: W. H. Freeman; 2012.
17. Golubovskaya V, Wu L. Different subsets of T cells, memory, effector functions, and CAR-T immunotherapy. Cancers (Basel). 2016;8:36-46.
18. Lanier LL. NK cell recognition. Annu Rev Immunol. 2005;23:225-74.
19. Banchereau J, Briere F, Caux C, et al. Immunobiology of dendritic cells. Annu Rev Immunol. 2000;18:767-811.

20. Gordon S. Macrophages and the immune response. In: Paul WE, ed. Fundamental Immunology. 5th ed. Philadelphia, PA: Lippincott Williams & Wilkins. 2003:481-96.
21. Elgert KD. Immunology: Understanding the Immune System. 2nd ed. Hoboken, NJ: John Wiley & Sons, Inc.; 2009.
22. Mazumdar PMH. Immunoglobulins: structure and function. In: Paul WE, ed. Fundamental Immunology. 5th ed. Philadelphia, PA: Lippincott Williams & Wilkins; 2003:47-68.
23. Abbas AK, Lichtman AH, Pober JS. Cellular and Molecular Immunology. 2nd ed. Philadelphia: W B Saunders Company; 2000.
24. Wu TT, Kabat EA. An analysis of the sequences of the variable regions of Bence-jones proteins and myeloma light chains and their implications for antibody complementarity. J Exp Med. 1970;132:211-50.
25. Benaceraff B. Role of major histocompatibility gene products in immune regulation. Science. 1981;212: 1229-38.
26. Snell GD. Studies in histocompatibility. Science. 1981;213:172-8.
27. Dausset J. The major histocompatibility complex in man. Science. 1981;213:1469-74.
28. Margulies DH, McCluskey J. The major histocompatibility complex and its encoded proteins. In: Paul WE, ed. Fundamental Immunology. 5th ed. Philadelphia, PA: Lippincott Williams & Wilkins; 2003:571-612.
29. Marrack P, Kappler J. The T cell and its receptor. Sci Am. 1986;254:36-45.
30. Laver WG, Air GM, Webster RG, Smith-Gill SJ. Epitopes on protein antigens: misconceptions and realities. Cell. 1990;61:553-6.
31. Berzofsky JA. Immunogenicity and antigen structure. In: Paul WE, ed. Fundamental Immunology. 5th ed. Philadelphia, PA: Lippincott Williams & Wilkins; 2003: 631-84.
32. Reiner SL. Development in motion: helper T cells at work. Cell. 2007;129:33-6.
33. Bevan MJ. Helping the $CD8^+$ T-cell response. Nat Rev Immunol. 2004;4:1-8.
34. Castellino F, Germain RN. Cooperation between $CD4^+$ and $CD8^+$ T cells. Ann Rev Immunol. 2006;24:519-40.
35. Lanzavecchia A. Antigen-specific interaction between T and B cells. Nature. 1985;314:537-9.
36. Voskoboinik I, Smyth MJ, Trapani JA. Perforin-mediated target-cell death and immune homeostasis. Nat Rev Immunol. 2006;6:940-52.
37. Kagi, D, Ledermann B, Burki K, et al. Cytotoxicity mediated by T cells and natural killer cells is greatly impaired in perforin-deficient mice. Nature. 1994;369:31-7.
38. Kischkel FC, Hellbardt S, Behrmann I, et al. Cytotoxicity-dependent APO-1 (Fas/CD95)-associated proteins form a death-inducing signaling complex (DISC) with the receptor. EMBO J. 1995;14:5579-88.
39. Arlaud GJ, Barlow C, Gaboriaud C, et al. Deciphering complement mechanisms: the contributions of structural biology. Mol Immunol. 2007;44:3809-22.
40. Muller-Eberhard HJ. Molecular organization and function of the complement system. Annu Rev Biochem. 1988;57: 321-47.
41. Guo RF, Ward PW. Role of C5a in inflammatory resposes. Annu Rev Immunol. 2005;23:821-52.
42. Coombs RRA, Gell PGH, eds. The classification of Allergic reaction underlying disease. In Clinical Aspect of Immunology. 1st ed. Philadelphia, PA: FA Davis Co.; 1963:317-37.
43. Jhamb S. Studies on the Allergen-specific Immune Response in Type-I Hypersensitivity of Respiratory System Including Observations on the Etiologic Role of Influenza Virus [PhD thesis]. New Delhi, India: University of Delhi; 1992.
44. Coleman RM, Lombard MF, Sicard RE. Hypersensitivity. In: Wheatley CH, ed. Fundamental Immunology. 2nd ed. Dubuque, IA: WMC Brown Publications; 1992:329-41.
45. National Heart, Lung and Blood Institute and World Health Organization (NHLBI/WHO). Global Strategy for Asthma Management & Prevention. NHLBI/WHO Workshop. NIH Publication No. 97;4051, Bethesda, MD; 1997.
46. Holt PG, Macaubas C, Stumbles PA, Sly PD. The role of allergy in the development of asthma. Nature. 1999; 402:B12.
47. Cookson W. The alliance of genes and environment in asthma and allergy. Nature. 1999;402:B5.
48. Feijen M, Gerritsen J, Postma DS. Genetics of allergic disease. Br Med Bull. 2000;56:894-907.
49. Bennich H, Johansson SGO. Structure and function of human immunoglobulin E. Adv Immunol. 1971;13:1-55.
50. Bennich H, Johansson SGO, Ishizaka K, et al. Biologic functions of the Fc fragments of E myeloma proteins. Immunochemistry. 1970;7:687-702.
51. Capron A. Functional study of monoclonal antibody to IgE Fc receptors (FεRII) of eosinophils, platelets and macrophages. J Exp Med. 1986;164:72-89.
52. Mittal OP, Katiyar SK, Prasad R. Serum IgE estimation in cases of respiratory allergy. ASP Allergy Appl Immunol. 1978;XI:92-100.
53. Saha K, Kulpati DDD, Padmini R. Serum immunoglobulins including IgE in patients of bronchial asthma with relation to the spectrum of the disease. ASP Allergy Appl Immunol. 1975;VIII:105-18.
54. Johanson SGO. The clinical significance of IgE. In: Franklin EC, ed. Clinical Immunology Update. New York, NY: Elsevier; 1981:123-45.
55. Kinet JP. The high affinity IgE receptor (FcεRI): from physiology to pathology. Ann Rev Immunol. 1999;17:931-72.
56. Turner H, Kinet JP. Signalling through the high affinity IgE receptor FcεRI. Nature. 1999;402:B24-30.
57. Corry DB, Kheradmand F. Induction and regulation of the IgE response. Nature. 1999;402:B18-23.

58. Vercelli D. Regulation of IgE synthesis in humans. J Biol Regul Homeost Agents. 1995;9:1-9.
59. Pene J, Rousset F, Briere F, et al. IgE production by normal human lymphocytes is induced by interleukin 4 and suppressed by interferon α, γ and prostaglandin E_2. Proc Natl Acad Sci USA. 1988;85:6880-4.
60. Mosmann TR, Coffman RL. T_H1 and T_H2 cells: different patterns of lymphokine secretion lead to different functional properties. Annu Rev Immunol. 1989;7:145-73.
61. Emson CL, Bell SE, Jones A, et al. Interleukin IL-4 independent induction of immunoglobulin E (IgE), and perturbation of T cell development in transgenic mice expressing IL-13. J Exp Med. 1998;108:399-404.
62. Ishizaka K. Mast-cells activation and mediator release. Prog Allergy. 1984;34:188-235.
63. Tomioko M, Ida S, Shibdoh Y, et al. Mast cells in bronchoalveolar lumen of patient with bronchial asthma. Am Rev Respir Dis. 1984;129:1000-5.
64. Pipkom U, Karisson G, Enerback L. The cellular response of the human allergic mucosa to natural allergen exposure. J Allergy Clin Immunol. 1988;86:1046-54.
65. Schwartz L, Huff T. Biology of mast cells and basophils. In: Middleton E Jr., Reed CE, Ellis EF, Adkinson NF Jr., Yunginger JW, Busse WW, eds. Allergy, Principles and Practices. 4th ed. St. Louis, MO: Mosby Year Book, Inc.; 1993:135-68.
66. Siracusa MC, Kim BS, Spergel JM, Artis D. Basophils and allergic inflammation. J Allergy Clin Immunol. 2013;132:789-801.
67. De Lisi C, Siraganian RP. Receptor cross-linking and histamine release. I. Quantitative dependence of basophil degranulation on the number of receptor doublets. J Immunol. 1979;122:2286-92.
68. Ishizaka T, Conrad DH, Schulman ES, et al. Biochemical analysis of initial triggering events of IgE-mediated histamine release from human lung mast cells. J Immunol. 1983;130:2357-62.
69. Siraganian RP. Mechanism of IgE-mediated hypersensitivity. In: Middleton E Jr., Reed CE, Ellis EF, et al., eds. Allergy, Principles and Practice. 4th ed. St Louis, MO: Mosby Year Book, Inc.; 1993:105.
70. Kennerly DA, Patricia AD. Activation mechanisms of mast cells and basophils. In: Holgate ST, Church MK, eds. Allergy. London: Gower Medical Publishing; 1993:4.1.
71. Putney JW Jr., McKay RR. Capacitative calcium entry channels. BioEssays. 1999;21:38-46.
72. Winslow CM, Austen KF. Role of cyclic nucleotides in the activation-secretion response. Prog Allergy. 1984;34: 236-70.
73. Solley GO, Gleich GJ, Jordan RE, Schroeter AL. The late phase of the immediate wheal and flare skin reaction: its dependence upon IgE antibodies. J Clin Invest. 1976;58: 408-20.
74. Lemanske RF, Kaliner MA. Late phase allergic reactions. In: Middleton E, Reed CE, Ellis EF, et al., eds. Allergy. Principles and Practice. St Louis, MO: Mosby-Year Book, Inc.; 1993:320.
75. Taylor G, Shivalkar PR. Changes in airway resistance on antigenic challenger in allergic rhinitis. Clin Allergy. 1971;1:63-73.
76. Durham SR. The significance of late response in asthma. Clin Exp Allergy. 1991;21:3-7.
77. Laitinen LA, Laitinen A, Heino M, et al. Eosinophil airway inflammation during exacerbation of asthma and its treatment with inhaled corticosteroid. Am Rev Respir Dis. 1991;143:423-7.
78. Reed CE. The importance of eosinophils in the immunology of asthma and allergic disease. Ann Allergy. 1994;72:376-80.
79. Kay AB. Eosinophils and neutrophils in the pathogenesis of asthma. In: Weiss EB, Segal MS, eds. Bronchial Asthma, Mechanism and Therapeutics. Boston, MA: Little, Brown & Co.; 1985:255.
80. Poulter LW, Power C, Burke C. The relationship between bronchial imunopathology and hyperresponsiveness in asthma. Eur J Respir Dis. 1990;3:792-9.
81. Walker C, Virchow JC Jr. T cells and endothelial cell in asthma. Allergy. 1993;48:24-31.
82. Damiani G. The role of macrophages and lymphocytes in bronchial asthma: perspectives for new research models. Eur Respir J. 1989;6:469s-472s.
83. Godard Ph, Damon M, Chanez P, Michel FB. Releasability of airway macrophages in bronchial asthma. Int Arch Allergy App Immunol. 1991;95:97-101.
84. Boschetto P, Mapp CE, Picotti G, Fabbri LM. Neutrophils and asthma. Eur Respir J. 1989;6:456-9.
85. Page C. The role of platelets in allergic disease. Clin Exp Allergy. 1990;20:339-40.
86. Hofmaier S, Comberiati P, Matricardi PM. Immunoglobulin G in IgE-mediated allergy and allergen-specific immunotherapy. Eur Ann Allergy Clin Immunol. 2014;46:6-11.
87. Agarwal MK, Chawla S, Singh P, Bansal SK. Immunity and allergy: an overview. In: Manual for course cum workshop on "Allergy and asthma", National conference on pulmonary diseases (NAPCON), Kanpur; 2000:15-41.
88. van de Veen W, Akdis M. Role of IgG4 in IgE-mediated allergic resposes. J Allergy Clin Immunol. 2016;138:1434-5.
89. Hammad H, Lambrecht BN. Dendritic cells and epithelial cells: linking innate and adaptive immunity in asthma. Nat Rev Immunol. 2008;8:193-204.
90. Hammad H, Chieppa M, Perros F, et al. House dust mite allergen induces asthma via TLR4 triggering of airway structural cells. Nat Med. 2009;15:410-6.
91. Boasen J, Chisholm D, Labet L, et al. House dust extracts elicit Toll-like receptor-dependent dendritic cell responses. J Allergy Clin Immunol. 2005;116:185-91.
92. Casale BT. Neurogenic control of inflammation and airway function. In: Middleton E, Reed CE, Ellis ET, et al., eds. Allergy: Principles and Practice. St Louis, Mo: Mosby Year Book Inc.; 1993:659.

93. Heaney LG, Cross LJM, Stanford CF, Ennis M. Substance P induces histamine release from human pulmonary mast cells. Clin Exp Allergy. 1995;25:179-86.
94. Barnes PJ. Neural control of human airways in health and diseases. Am Rev Respir Dis. 1986;134:1289-314
95. Bochner BS. Cellular adhesion and its antagonism. J Allergy Clin Immunol. 1997;100:581-5.
96. Baroody FM, Lee BJ, Lim MC, Bochner BS. Implicating adhesion molecules in nasal allergic inflammation. Eur Arch Oto-Rhino-Laryngol. 1995;252:550-8.
97. Bentley AM, Durham SR, Robinson DS, et al. Expression of endothelial and leukocyte adhesion molecules intercellular adhesion molecule-1, E-selectin, and vascular cell adhesion molecule-1 in the bronchial mucosa in steady-state and allergen-induced asthma. J Allergy Clin Immunol. 1993;92:857-68.
98. Ciprandi G, Buscaglia S, Pesce G, et al. Allergic subjects express intercellular adhesion molecule-1 (ICAMA or CD54) on epithelial cells of conjunctiva after allergen challenge. J Allergy Clin Immunol. 1993;91:783-92.
99. Ciprandi G, Pronzato C, Ricca V, et al. Evidence of intercellular adhesion molecule-1 expression on nasal epithelial cells in acute rhinoconjunctivitis caused by pollen exposure. J Allergy Clin Immunol. 1994;94:738-46.
100. Gundel RH, Wegner CD, Torcellini CA, et al. Endothelial-leukocyte adhesion molecule-I mediates antigen-induced acute airway inflammation and late-phase airway obstruction in monkeys. J Clin Invest. 1991;88:1407-11.

CHAPTER 2

Epidemiology of Allergy: Global

Nikhil Gupta, Rajendra Prasad

INTRODUCTION

The prevalence of allergic diseases worldwide is rising dramatically in both developed and developing countries. These diseases include asthma; rhinitis; anaphylaxis; drug, food, and insect allergy; eczema; urticaria (hives); angioedema; and occupational allergy.

This increase is especially problematic in children, who are bearing the greatest burden of the rising trend that has occurred over the last two decades. Secular trends in asthma and allergy have been studied most intensely in the Western countries. The rise in disease prevalence was particularly apparent between the 1960s and the 1990s, after which the rise evened out. The aim of this chapter is to review the global epidemiology of allergic diseases.

BURDEN OF ALLERGIC DISEASES

Allergic Rhinitis: It affects 10–30% of all adults and as many as 40% of children.[1] The World Health Organization has estimated that 400 million people in the world suffer from allergic rhinitis (AR). In the USA, the prevalence of AR ranges from 3% to 19%. Overall, it affects 30–60 million individuals annually. In childhood, affected males outnumber females, but the sex ratio is nearly equal in adults. AR develops before the age of 20 years in 80% of cases. Increased prevalence is observed in non-Whites, in some polluted urban areas, and in first-born children. In Europe, the European Community Respiratory Health Survey estimated the prevalence of AR to be from 4% to 32%. More than 40% of patients with AR have asthma, and more than 80% of asthmatic patients suffer from concomitant rhinitis. Also, patients with rhinitis have an increased risk of developing asthma. Other comorbidities that are observed with increased frequency in patients with AR include sinusitis, nasal polyposis, upper respiratory infections, otitis media with effusion, breathing through the mouth, sleep disorders, decreased quality of life, and impaired learning and attention in children.

Allergic Conjunctivitis: Allergic conjunctivitis is the most common cause of a red eye, affecting more than 1 billion people globally. The umbrella term "allergic conjunctivitis" includes distinct clinical entities, from mild but disturbing forms due to IgE sensitization to aeroallergens, to forms of keratoconjunctivitis, where the severe allergic inflammation, with corneal involvement, is more difficult to diagnose and treat and may lead to permanent ocular damage and even loss of vision. There are several clinical forms of allergic conjunctivitis: intermittent or seasonal allergic conjunctivitis (SAC), persistent or perennial Allergic conjunctivitis (PAC), vernal Kerato conjunctivitis (VKC), atopic Kerato conjunctivitis (AKC), and induced by contact lenses, contact lenses conjunctivitis (CLC).

Rhinosinusitis: It affects about 31 million subjects in the USA per year. It is about midway between rhinitis and asthma in frequency.

Asthma: Asthma is a serious public health problem throughout the world, affecting people of all ages. The World Health Organization estimates that 300 million individuals have asthma worldwide, and that with current rising trends this will reach 400 million by 2025. Approximately 250,000 people die prematurely each year from asthma; almost all these deaths are avoidable. There was a sharp increase in asthma prevalence, morbidity, and mortality in the early 1960s in the Western countries of the world. The best information on the prevalence of asthma throughout the world was obtained by the International Study of Asthma and Allergies in Childhood (ISAAC).[2] Questionnaires were completed by 463,801 children aged 13–14 years from 56 countries and by parents of 257,800 children aged 6–7 years from 38 countries in 1994 and 1995. Asthma was considered to be present if there was a positive response to the question "Have you had wheezing or whistling in the chest in the last 12 months?", translated into the appropriate local language. In the 13–14-year-old age group, the prevalence varied from 2.1% to 4.4% in Albania, China, Greece, Georgia, Indonesia, Romania, and Russia to 29.1–32.2% in Australia, New Zealand, Republic of Ireland, and the UK. Other countries with low prevalence were mostly in Asia, Northern Africa, Eastern Europe, and the Eastern Mediterranean regions, and others with high prevalence were in Southeast Asia, North America, and Latin America. Trends for the prevalence in the 6–7-year-olds were similar to those in the older children with the prevalence of wheezing varying from 4.1% to 32.1%.

The same survey was conducted 5–10 years later in 56 countries among children aged 13–14 years and in 37 countries among children aged 6–7 years. This study, termed ISAAC III, was primarily intended to assess changes in asthma prevalence over time. Overall, there was only a slight increase in asthma prevalence from 13.2% to 13.7% in the age group of 13–14 years and from 11.1% to 11.6% in the age group of 6–7 years. The most striking change was a decline in the prevalence of asthma in the English-speaking counties that formerly had the highest prevalence. Other areas such as Latin America, Eastern Europe, and North Africa that already had high to intermediate prevalence continued to show an increase, and, with the exception of India, all countries with low prevalence rates in ISAAC I reported increased prevalence in ISAAC III.[3] Thus, overall, the disparity in asthma prevalence found in ISAAC I was found to have diminished, perhaps due to the increasing urbanization in low- and middle-income countries. Annual worldwide deaths from asthma have been estimated at 250,000, and mortality does not appear to correlate well with asthma prevalence.

Atopic Eczema: With a lifetime prevalence of 15–30% in children and 2–10% in adults, the incidence of atopic eczema has increased by two- to threefold in industrialized countries during the last three decades. Atopic eczema is usually present during early infancy and childhood and can also persist or start in adulthood. The 12-month prevalence in 11-year-old children has been shown to vary from 1% to 20% with the highest prevalence typically found in Northern Europe (ISAAC).[1] In 45% of children, the onset of atopic eczema occurs during the first 6 months of life; during the first year 60% of these children are affected and 85% are affected before the age of 5. The prevalence of atopic eczema in rural areas is significantly lower, emphasizing the importance of lifestyle and environment in the mechanisms of atopic disease. Due to modern advances in genetics and immunology, much progress has been made in elucidating the pathophysiology of atopic eczema, yet the hygiene hypothesis is still one important and hotly debated feature.

FOOD ALLERGY

Worldwide, there is no study assessing the prevalence of food allergy and its time trends. The problem is complicated by the fact that only a small proportion of cases of perceived food allergy (i.e., the self-reported feeling that a particular food negatively influences health status) are true IgE-mediated food allergies or cell-mediated hypersensitivities. Thus, we can refer to two separate "food allergy epidemiologies":

- *Self-reported food allergy (12.4–25%)*: This does not represent the "true" epidemiology of food allergy, but gives an indication of the potential demand for allergy medicine.
- *Challenge-confirmed food allergy frequency (2.3–3.6%)*: This represents the real clinical dimension of the problem.

Food allergies are a cause of particular concern in young children, and the incidence of food allergy (often life-threatening) is estimated to be greater in young children (5–8%) than in adults (1–2%). The epidemiological knowledge of food allergy is crucial to the design of preventive strategies.[4]

In the USA, it has been estimated that food allergy is responsible for 30,000 anaphylaxis episodes/year, leading to 3,000 hospitalizations and 100 deaths. The following eight things cause about 90% of food allergy: *milk* (mostly in children); *eggs;* peanuts; tree nuts such as walnuts, cashews, almonds, pine nuts, *Brazil nuts*, and pecans; *soya, wheat,* and other grains with gluten, including *barley, rye,* and oats; fish; and *shellfish* (mostly in adults). Some common types of shellfish that cause food allergy are shrimp, lobster, crab, crayfish, and oysters. Among children, most allergic reactions to foods are caused by peanuts, milk, soybean, tree nuts, eggs, and wheat.

INSECT ALLERGY

Hymenoptera venom allergy is a common global medical problem and refers to subjects who have a sting-induced large local (LL) or systemic allergic reaction. LL reaction is defined as a reaction larger than 10 cm in diameter, which lasts over 24 hours in which the signs and symptoms are confined to tissues contiguous with the sting site. Systemic reactions include a spectrum of manifestations, ranging from mild to life-threatening. Mild systemic reactions may be limited only to the skin and consist of flushing, urticaria, and angioedema. More severe systemic reactions can involve bronchospasm, laryngeal edema, and hypotension. The prevalence of LL reactions ranges from 2.4% to 26.4% in the general population and up to 38% in beekeepers. The prevalence of allergic systemic reactions is between 0.3% and 7.5% in Europe; whereas in the USA, it is 0.5–3.3%. Allergic systemic reactions are less common in children, ranging from 0.15% to 0.8%. The latest population-based studies indicate that insect-induced allergic systemic reactions are responsible for 7.3–59% of all cases of systemic reactions in these subjects, being more frequent in adults than in children. The incidence of insect-sting mortality, secondary to anaphylaxis, ranges from 0.03 to 0.48 fatalities per million inhabitants per year.

OCCUPATIONAL ALLERGY

Occupational asthma (OA) is considered to account for approximately 25% of respiratory diseases due to the work environment.[5] It has been estimated that 15% of adult asthma is attributable to allergens encountered in the workplace.[6] Prospective cohort studies reported incidence rates of 0.2–3.5 per 100 person-years in workers exposed to laboratory animals, 4.1 per 100 person-years in bakers, and 1.8 per 100 person-years in dental care apprentices exposed to latex gloves.[5] Estimates of the incidence of OA in the general population ranged from 17 to 174 new cases per million active workers per year, suggesting that the disease is underestimated in most countries. Surveys of workforces exposed to sensitizing agents indicate that occupational rhinitis is 2–4 times more common than OA.[5]

Skin diseases account for 8–34% of all occupational diseases[7] Estimates of the annual incidence of occupational contact dermatitis in the general population range from 130 to 850 cases per million individuals.

Occupational allergic diseases are likely to be more prevalent and severe in some developing countries than in industrialized countries, since obsolete technologies are still extensively used and occupational diseases are even less recognized as a public health concern.[6]

The mortality due to respiratory diseases among workers with OA is higher than in generally healthy workers but similar to that observed in workers with asthma unrelated to work.[7] It has been estimated that 38,000 deaths and 1.6 million disability-adjusted life years result from work-related asthma each year worldwide.[8]

REFERENCES

1. Asher MI, Montefort S, Björksten B, et al. Worldwide time trends in the prevalence of symptoms of asthma, allergic rhinoconjunctivitis, and eczema in childhood: ISAAC phases one and three repeat multi-country cross-sectional surveys. Lancet. 2006;368:733-43.
2. Asher MI, Anderson HR, Stewart AW, Crane J. Worldwide variations in the prevalence of asthma symptoms: The International Study of Asthma and Allergies in Childhood (ISAAC). Eur Respir J. 1998;12:315-35.
3. Pearce N, Ait-Khaled N, Beasley R, et al. Worldwide trends in the prevalence of asthma symptoms: Phase III of the International Study of Asthma and Allergies in Childhood (ISAAC). Thorax. 2007:62:758-66.
4. Lack G. Epidemiologic risks for food allergy. J Allergy Clin Immunol. 2008;121:1331-6.
5. Gautrin D, Newman-Taylor AJ, Nordman H, Malo JL. Controversies in epidemiology of occupational asthma. Eur Respir J. 2003;22:551-9.
6. Balmes J, Becklake M, Blanc P, et al. American Thoracic Society statement: Occupational contribution to the burden of airway disease. Am J Respir Crit Care Med. 2003;167: 787-97.
7. Liss GM, Tarlo SM, Banks D, et al. Preliminary report of mortality among workers compensated for work-related asthma. Am J Ind Med. 1999;35:465-71.
8. Vandenplas O. Socio-economic impact of work-related asthma. Expert Rev Pharmacoeconomics Outcome Res. 2008;8:395-400.

CHAPTER 3

Epidemiology of Respiratory Allergy in India

Raj Kumar, Rajendra Prasad

Allergic disease is a spectrum of disorders identified by abnormal responses. The immune system reacts abnormally to normally harmless substances present in the environment. A substance that causes an allergic reaction is called an allergen. Allergy is formally called type I (or immediate) hypersensitivity and is one of the four or more forms of hypersensitivity. Allergy is one of the most common causes of rhinitis and asthma, which affects both children and adults.

The prevalence and burden of allergic diseases are increasing and vary globally, particularly in low- and middle-income countries. As per the World Health Organization, the number of asthma patients is expected to be increased by 300–400 million and to cause 250,000 deaths annually, by 2025. The effect of urbanization, industrialization, and also the workplace conditions with exposure to dust, gases, or fumes are responsible for about 11% of asthma worldwide. Approximately 15% asthma among adults is significantly contributed worldwide by occupational asthma. About 10–30% of the world population is affected by allergic rhinitis, which varies from country to country.[1]

The efforts are now targeted toward a common goal of reducing the burden of allergic diseases, but still the burden of allergic diseases has been on an uprising trend in terms of prevalence as well as severity. In India, about 20–30% of the total population suffers from allergic diseases such as asthma, rhinitis, anaphylaxis, drug, food and insect allergy, eczema and urticaria, and angioedema. Several studies have been conducted to find out the basic cause of respiratory allergy in India. A study in Delhi in 1964 reported around 10% allergic rhinitis and 1% asthma.[2] Further study in 1988 on school children in Delhi reported 20–30% of the population suffer from allergic rhinitis and that 15% of them develop asthma.[3] Recently, a multicentric population-based study conducted by Indian Study on Epidemiology of Asthma, Respiratory Symptoms and Chronic Bronchitis unveiled the prevalence of bronchial asthma at 2.05% (range, 0.4–4.8%). The study was done in 12 centers including rural and urban areas of the different parts of India. The study found the association of advancing age, smoking, indoor environmental tobacco smoke exposure, asthma in a first-degree relative, and use of unclean cooking fuels increased odds of asthma.[4] Prevalence of aeroallergens in asthma and allergic rhinitis patients with allergy in the north region (Delhi, Bihar, Haryana, Madhya Pradesh, and Uttar Pradesh) of India during the period of August 2008–July 2016 was studied and it was found that insects (mosquito, housefly and cockroach) are the most common sensitizing allergens in the younger age group (20–29 years).[5]

The etiology of respiratory allergic diseases is not clear so far. It is likely to be an alliance of genetic proneness and environmental factors, and also lifestyle changes with dietary habits play an important role. Recently, it has been found that diet has the potential to cause asthma and rhinitis. The link between diet and respiratory allergic diseases has been by and large driven from western literature. The change in sociodemographic factors has led to the increasing predilection toward fast foods; fried snacks are popular and consumed among the Indian population. The food pattern may be postulated as one of the unknown factors with a rise in the prevalence of asthma in India. Legumes such as peanuts, soybean, lentil, and chickpea have been identified as important triggers of food allergies in Europe and Asian countries.[6] Many food allergens from legumes family have been isolated and characterized in the past decades. IgE-mediated food allergy by black gram was established and eight major allergenic proteins of black gram were characterized by a double-blind placebo control food challenge test in asthma and rhinitis patients.[7] Further, a 28 kDa major allergen from black gram was also identified, which played a major role in the diagnosis of black gram allergy.[8]

A study was undertaken to investigate the relative prevalence of food allergens that causes IgE-mediated reactions in older children and adults with asthma, allergic rhinitis, or both. Of 1,860 patients screened, 1,097 (58.9%) gave a history of food allergy. Sensitization to food was significantly associated with asthma, whereas aeroallergens were strongly related to rhinitis. Food allergy is estimated to be 4.5% in adolescents and adults with asthma, rhinitis, or both. Rice, citrus fruits, black gram, and banana are identified as major allergens for inducing allergic symptoms. There is a great difference between perceived allergy and actual allergy to food.[9] In another study, the prevalence of food intolerance in asthma patients in India was examined and found that the asthma patients had highest food intolerance against vegetables and nuts. Food intolerance test among the asthma patients was found positive in descending order as cow milk (56%), casein (48%), tiger nut (48%), almond (46%), amaranth (46%), peanut (46%), soybean (44%), alga seaweed (44%), scallop (44%), and mulberry (42%) in asthmatic patients.[10] The inflammatory markers in asthma and rhinitis are very well known, and several studies have been conducted worldwide; subsequently a research on the inflammatory response to subcutaneous allergen-specific immunotherapy in patients with bronchial asthma and allergic rhinitis was elucidated.[11]

Whereas the prevalence rates of asthma in children in India have also been studied, and the mean prevalence has been found to be 7.2 ± 5.4%. The overall weighted mean prevalence from different studies has been observed to be 2.7%.[12] Childhood asthma among children of 13–14 years of age has been lower than that in younger children (6–7 years of age). In the sociodemographic analysis, urban children have higher general prevalence with male predominance. In another study done on schoolgirls (4–17 years), the prevalence of asthma was found to be 8.8%.[13] In a study pointing socioeconomic status of the family, the prevalence of asthma in children was 9.4% in the lower class, 7.3% in the middle class, 9.4% in the upper class in the urban areas of Delhi, and 3.9% in the village areas of Delhi.[14] A wide inter-regional variation in the prevalence of asthma has also been observed.

The Asthma Epidemiology Study Group of the Indian Council of Medical Research found the prevalence of allergic rhinitis is 3.5% of the population in India.[15] In the case of children, another multicentric study found that allergic rhino-conjunctivitis occurred in 3.3% of the children aged 6–7 years and 5.6% of the children aged 13–14 years in India. In a study, the prevalence of allergic rhinitis in schoolgirls (4–17 years) was found to be 21.27%. In another study,[16] the overall prevalence of allergic rhinitis was 26.1% in school children. When seen along with the socioeconomic status, the prevalence was 27.1% in the lower class, 33.3% in the middle class, 28.6% in the upper class in the urban area, and 11.1% in the rural areas of Delhi. Also, in a study it has been found that tobacco users had higher prevalence of rhinitis (55% of tobacco users compared to 12.8% non-tobacco users).[17] Studies have also found an association of indoor and outdoor air pollutant levels with respiratory problems among children. A study to identify the effect of indoor air pollution generated from fuel used for cooking on respiratory allergy in children was done in Delhi. The study concluded that biomass fuel increases the concentration of indoor air pollutants that may increase risk of asthma, rhinitis, and upper respiratory tract infection in children.[18,19]

The efficient diagnosis and treatment of the allergy can be done by knowing the prevalence, annual variations, and seasonal growth of aeroallergens of the particular area. The aeroallergens that are the bioparticles from different biological sources such as pollen grains, fungal spores, insect, and other materials are considered triggering factors for respiratory allergy. As India is a climatically diverse country with diversity in the flora and fauna, the pollens belonging to *Alnus nitida*, *Amaranthus spinosus*, *Argemone mexicana*, *Cocos nucifera*, *Betula utilis*, *Borassus flabellifer*, *Carica papaya*, *Cedrus deodara*, *Cassia fistula*, *Parthenium*, *Chenopodium album*, *Dodonaea viscosa*, *Mallotus philippensis*, *Plantago ovata*, *Prosopis juliflora*, *Ricinus communis*, and *Holoptelea integrifolia* are the allergenically important pollens of the country. Among the fungal aeroallergens, *Alternaria*, *Candida albicans*, *Aspergillus versicolor*, *Aspergillus terreus*, *Aspergillus japonicus*, *Cladosporium cladosporioides*, *Fusarium roseum*, *Ganoderma lucidum*, *Neurospora sitophila*, *Helminthosporium*, *Ustilago tritici*, and *Uromyces* are found in different parts of the country. Dust mites, cockroaches, beetles, mosquitoes, houseflies, and their dead or decayed parts also contribute toward the aeroallergens, which should be avoided. Other environmental risk factors like tobacco smoke and indoor air pollutions contribute to the rising trend.

Efforts targeting allergic diseases are still very shattered and vary from country to country. We need to come together to develop common strategies to find the solution at the level of policy healthcare delivery, health communication, and education under global association. To reduce the global burden of respiratory allergic diseases, some parameters should be set up such as increasing the trained personnel and clinical expertise to diagnose and treat allergic diseases, timely epidemiological studies for appropriate data, adopting environmental control measures to reduce triggers such as smoking and indoor-outdoor pollutants, and providing cost-effective pharmacotherapy or medication with public awareness program at both national and international levels. In this context, the VP Chest Institute is working tremendously for the past six decades. It is a premier government institute working toward diagnosis and management of respiratory diseases at national and international levels by a global coordination between international bodies.

REFERENCES

1. Bousquet J, Khaltaev NG, Cruz AA, World Health Organization. Global surveillance, prevention and control of chronic respiratory diseases: A comprehensive approach. Geneva: World Health Organization; 2007.
2. Viswanathan R. Definition, incidence, aetiology and natural history of asthma. Indian J Chest Dis. 1964;6:108-24.
3. Chhabra SK, Gupta CK, Chhabra P, Rajpal S. Prevalence of bronchial asthma in schoolchildren in Delhi. J Asthma. 1998;35:291-6.
4. Jindal SK, Aggarwal AN, Gupta D, et al. Indian study on epidemiology of asthma, respiratory symptoms and chronic bronchitis in adults (INSEARCH). Int J Tuberc Lung Dis. 2012;16:1270-7.
5. Kumar R, Kumar M, Bisht I, Singh K. Prevalence of aeroallergens in patients of bronchial asthma and/or allergic rhinitis in India based on skin prick test reactivity. Indian J Allergy Asthma Immunol. 2017;31:45-55.
6. Ibanez Sandin D, Martinez San Ireneo M, Alonso Lebrero E, et al. Specific IgE determinations to crude and boiled lentil (Lens culinaris) extracts in lentil-sensitive children and controls. Allergy. 1999;54:1209-14.
7. Kumari D, Kumar R, Sridhara S, et al. Sensitization to black gram in patients with bronchial asthma and rhinitis: clinical evaluation and characterization of allergens. Allergy. 2006;61:104-10.
8. Kumari D, Arora N, Kasera R, et al. Isolation and characterization of a 28 kDa major allergen from black gram (Phaseolus mungo). Immunobiology. 2012;895-904.
9. Kumar R1, Kumari D, Srivastava P, et al. Identification of IgE-mediated food allergy and allergens in older children and adults with asthma and allergic rhinitis. Indian J Chest Dis Allied Sci. 2010;52:217-24.
10. Kumar R, Singh M, Gupta N, et al. Prevalence of food intolerance in bronchial asthma in India. Indian J Allergy Asthma Immunol. 2013;27:121-8.
11. Kumar R, Gupta N, Bisht I. Inflammatory response to subcutaneous allergen-specific immunotherapy in patients with bronchial asthma and allergic rhinitis. Indian J Allergy Asthma Immunol. 2015;29:7-13.
12. Pal R, Dahal S, Pal S. Prevalence of bronchial asthma in Indian children. Indian J Commun Med. 2009;34:310-6.
13. Kumar R, Singhal P, Jain A, Raj N. Prevalence of bronchial asthma and allergic rhinitis in school girls in Delhi. Indian J Allergy Asthma Immunol. 2008;22:99-104.
14. Kumar R, Nagar JK, Raj N, et al. Impact of domestic air pollution from cooking fuel our respiratory allergies in children in India. Asia Pac J Allergy Immunol. 2008;20: 213-22.
15. Aggarwal AN, Chaudhry K, Chhabra SK, et al. Prevalence and risk factors for bronchial asthma in Indian adults: a multicentre study. Indian J Chest Dis Allied Sci. 2006;48:13-22.
16. Kumar R, Nagar JK, Raj N, et al. Impact of domestic air pollution from cooking fuel on respiratory allergies in children in India. Asian Pac J Allergy Immunol. 2008;26:213-22.
17. Kumar R, Mahakud GC, Nagar JK, Tabassum NG. Rhinitis and tobacco consumption: a brief study. Indian J Allergy Asthma Immunol. 2011;25:15-20.
18. Kumar R, Nagar JK, Kumar H, et al. Association of indoor and outdoor air pollutant level with respiratory problems among children in an industrial area of Delhi, India. Arch Environ Occup Health. 2007;62:75-80.
19. Kumar R, Nagar JK, Kushwah AS, et al. Indoor air pollution and respiratory function of children in Ashok Vihar in Delhi: an exposure-response study. Asia Pac J Public Health. 2008;20:36-48.

CHAPTER 4

Aeroallergens in India: Current Status

AB Singh

INTRODUCTION

Man is dependent on air. He breaths about 35 lb of air per day when compared to consumption of 3 lb of water and 1.5 lb of food. He cannot survive for a few minutes without air. Air carries an array of particles varying in size, shape, density, and other features, which poses burden on the respiratory tract of humans. These include a number of inorganic and organic contaminants. Airborne bioparticles (biopollutants) such as microorganisms, pollen grains, fungal spores, hyphae of fungi, spores of mosses and ferns, insect debris, animal dander, and mites are known to be the chief causative agents of allergic disorders such as bronchial asthma, allergic rhinitis, and atopic dermatitis.[1-6] Among all these agents, pollen grains and fungal spores are the most predominant allergens in air. A detailed information on their daily, seasonal, and annual variations in the atmosphere is of paramount importance in effective diagnosis and therapeutic management of these ailments.

Pollen grains are among the earliest known allergens and are at present the major source of morbidity among atopic subjects.[7] Respiratory system is the direct target organ of airborne pollens taken in by inhalation. This results in immediate hypersensitivity disorders in genetically predisposed individuals and late hypersensitivity in others, causing clinical manifestations of allergic rhinitis, allergic alveolitis, asthma, atopic dermatitis, etc. John Bostock[8] was the first to suspect pollens as the cause of hay fever (allergic rhinitis). Later, Blackley[9] established that grasses are the important cause of hay fever in the UK. After more than 40 years, Scheppegrell[10] from the USA felt the need for field exploration and aerial surveys to record aeroallergens from the atmosphere. Subsequent studies from all over the world established pollen grains as the major causative agent for respiratory allergic disorders.[5,6,11-17]

Although pollen grains have been widely studied as aeroallergens throughout the world, far less is known about the fungal aerosols, which are present in much higher concentration than the pollen grains in the air. Early reports on fungal allergy attributed the symptoms to fungal spores prevailing in the patients' home or occupational exposure to them.[18-21] Fienburg[22] reported that outside air was an equally significant source of fungal spores and correlated it with the patients' symptoms. This gave impetus to the study of environmental conditions affecting prevalence of molds—indoors and outdoors, all over the world. Since then, several investigators from different geographical locations have investigated the role of fungal spores in allergic diseases.[16,23-29]

SOURCE OF AEROALLERGENS

Pollen Allergens

Plant spores, in a broader sense, are produced in all the divisions of the plant kingdom, but only those formed by the flowering plants, known as pollen grains, are the major component of air spora. Wind-pollinated (anemophilous) taxa are the chief source of inhalant pollen allergens including grasses, weeds/cultigens, and trees. The flowers of these taxa possess a set of adaptive characteristics such as reduction in size and number of floral appendages, lack of nectar, and small, smooth, dry, simple, and buoyant pollen grains. The amount of pollen production is also high in such species.[30]

The airborne allergenic pollen grains are traditionally grouped together as grasses, weeds, or tree pollen.

This is done merely because of convenience as they follow a generalized pattern of flowering in different seasons in the year. However, exceptions to generalized flowering pattern do occur. For example, *Prosopis juliflora* erratically flowers almost throughout the year, but with two peak pollination periods, i.e., in March–April and September–November. However, difference in the flowering pattern of the taxa is not uncommon for many species in India as reported by Singh and coworkers.[31,32]

Fungal Allergens

There are more than 80,000 species of fungi, which have an elaborate mechanism for spore dispersal and dissemination. The spore size facilitates their suspension in the atmosphere for a long time, leading to sensitization, when inhaled by the population.

In outdoor environments, the sources of fungal spores include cereal crops, decaying vegetables, and organic wastes on which fungi thrive. While in indoor environments, the sources are damp walls, dustbins, window pans, mattresses, leaking pipes, and humidifiers. Most studies on fungi as aeroallergens have been limited to the fungi imperfecti (Deuteromycetes) with little information on allergenicity of the members of other fungal groups. The literature is still insufficient regarding the development of allergic asthma by inhaled fungal spores,[33] and there is very little information available on the characterization of antigenic fractions of common fungal allergens.

MONITORING AIRBORNE ALLERGENS

For effective and efficient diagnosis and treatment of respiratory allergies caused by aeroallergens, information on diurnal, seasonal, and annual variations, and the type and concentration of airborne pollen and fungal spores is a prerequisite. Aerobiological sampling is therefore carried out to achieve this aim through various sampling devices currently used for bioparticulates.[34]

The recognition of aeroallergens is divided into two phases: (1) collection of material and (2) sample analysis.[35]

Different methods employed to achieve the objectives generally exploit the following basic regimes of collection:

- Fall out on a fixed surface through gravitational force
- Impaction on rapidly moving surface
- Impaction through suction of air
- Filtration
- Immunochemical assays.

And for the analysis of data, three procedures are followed:

1. Immunochemical assay for bulk reservoirs
2. Microscopic enumeration of individual particles
3. Tally of colonies produced in culture or semisolid media.

SAMPLING DEVICES

The various sampling devices and their principles of working have been enumerated as follows:

Gravimetric Samplers

This is based on the principle that bioparticulates settle down on a surface due to gravitational force. The Durham's gravity-sampling device consists of two horizontal disks with a diameter of 22.1 cm and 8.1 cm, respectively. The upper disk protects the slide from rain and sun. Nevertheless, this method presents certain disadvantages and has been discontinued in many parts of the world. It does not give diurnal variation and is dependent on wind velocity and favors large pollen grains. In spite of these drawbacks, it is economic, simple, independent of power, and still used in the Indian subcontinent by several workers. The slides are exposed daily, at a fixed hour, coated with adhesive glycerin jelly. After exposure, the slides are mounted in a drop of molten glycerin jelly, for various allergen types trapped. The results are expressed as number/unit area.

Impaction Samplers

In the impaction sampler, particles are sampled passively from air on adhesive-coated stationary or rotating rods.

Rotorod Sampler

The Rotorod sampler developed by Perkins[36] was the first such device to receive wide attention. Adhesive-coated clear lucite rods of 1–3 mm width are used as the collection surface. Collection efficiencies vary with the speed of travel and vary inversely with the width of the sampling area. This is a lightweight, portable, and DC-operated sampler. It has an arm that holds two cubical rods coated with silicone grease. The exposure time can be increased or decreased as required. The rods are mounted on a grooved slide in basic fuschin stain and scanned under microscope. For both, pollen and fungal spores, particles recovered are counted microscopically by transmitted light, and the results are easily expressed as "particles recovered/unit volume of the air sampled."

Suction Samplers

The method requires suction of certain volume of air according to a known velocity and for a chosen duration on a trapping. There are several instruments currently in use. The Hirst spore trap[37] is the most commonly used sampler. Trapping of bioparticles is done on slides coated with glycerin jelly, and slides are replaced each day with fresh slides.

Burkard 7-day Sampler

The Hirst spore trap was modified to Burkard trap in which slides were replaced with a drum, which can rotate and run continuously for 7 days with a definite speed (Fig. 4.1). Burkard continuous 7-day sampler uses a glycerin-coated tape mounted on a rotating drum. The drum is connected to a timer and rotates at a constant speed. The tape is changed every 7 days. Exposed tape is cut in seven strips corresponding to 7 days and mounted on a slide. This is a very good sampler to study diurnal or seasonal trends for fungal and pollen allergens.

Burkard Personal Slide Sampler

Burkard personal slide sampler is compact, battery operated, 10 cm in height, and 8 cm in diameter (Fig. 4.2A). It has a rectangular orifice at the top and a slit on the side to insert the microslide coated with glycerin jelly. The sampler takes in 10 L/minute air, particles got impacted on the slide in the form of a streak. It is mounted in glycerin and scanned. The exposed slides or trap is scanned for different pollen/spore traps and counts are expressed as number per cubic meter.

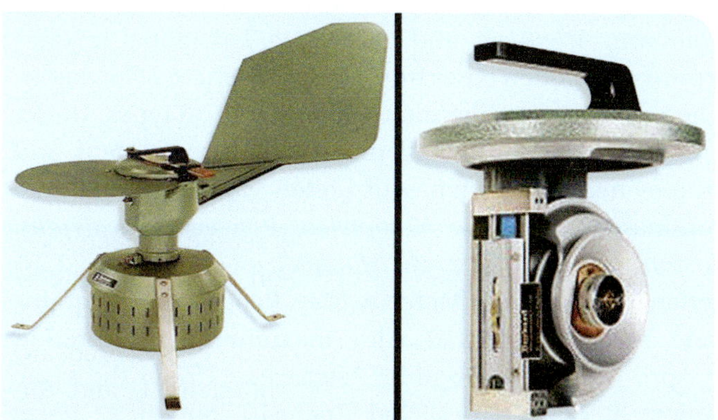

Fig. 4.1: Burkard 7-day volumetric sampler.

Burkard Petri Plate Sampler

Burkard petri plate sampler is similar to the above sampler except that it has a stage to hold a petri plate containing nutrient agar media instead of slide. These two samplers are appropriate for spot sampling (Fig. 4.2B).

Andersen Sampler

The best device for estimating culturable spores in indoor and outdoor environments is the Andersen six-stage/two-stage sampler. It utilizes petri plates containing nutrient media kept under sieves of different pore sizes, each having 400 pores. Circular orifice takes up air at the rate of 28.3 L/min and passes it through the sieves kept in the order of decreasing pore size. Finally, air passes out after impacting on the last petri plate. Exposed petri plates are incubated at 28–30°C to allow the colonies to grow, and later on the number and types of colonies are counted.

Filtration Devices

Filters of definite pore size offer volumetric potential especially appropriate for smaller aerosol classes and where ambient velocities are low. Bioparticulates are

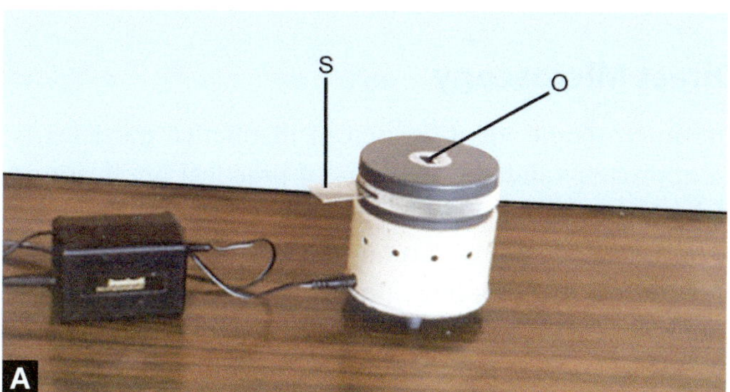

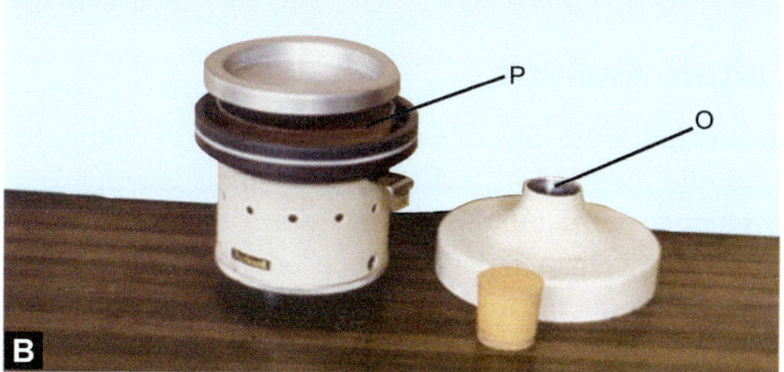

Figs. 4.2A and B: (A) Burkard single petri plate sampler; (B) Burkard slide sampler.

sucked through a filter and impinge on the media in a holder. Both media and holder are relatively inexpensive. But these are not widely used as in the morning air, as they may not faithfully align with the prevailing air stream.

The cultured samples may be examined microscopically after clearing the filters with immersion oil and other compatible fluids. Specific stains may be applied first. Alternatively, filters exposed with aseptic precautions may be collected on liquid culture media for colony growth, and colony-forming units can be identified.

Immunochemical Assays

Recently described immunochemical assays for airborne allergens relied on large (e.g., 20 cm × 25 cm) fiberglass filters exposed for 24 hour period in a high-volume (hi vol) sampler. They are rated for continuous operation and adapted to receive filter support. High volume devices are developed to study total suspended particles, and devices are operated traditionally with filters' surface directed upwards.

ANALYSIS OF SAMPLES

Regardless of their method of collection, samples of mixed biologic aerosols are analyzed by one of these following techniques.

Direct Microscopy

The microscopic identification of distinctive particles is an approach validated by years of practical applications of both gravimetric and volumetric samplers. A variety of particles, including certain basidiospores, ascospores, and spores of rust, smuts, downy mildew, and primitive green plants, are recognizable, which fail to grow on most laboratory media. Therefore, it is a most dependable way to identify most of the pollen and fungal spores.

Culture Analysis

This includes the tally of colonies produced in culture or semisolid media. This technique of analysis is employed to identify the culturable fungal spores on the basis of their colony characteristics, which otherwise cannot be identified under the microscope.

The culture plates, after exposure, are incubated at appropriate temperature, and impacted spores are allowed to grow for a couple of days till colonies start forming. Each colony represents one spore and considered a colony-forming unit.

Immunoassay

Immunochemical analysis following descending elution offers an analytic approach to dust without potential or defined form (e.g., dander, seed pomace, arthropod effluvia). If micronic aerosols do carry pollen allergens, these fractions are also accessible to immunoassay in bulk samples obtained by filtration. Procedure is based on inhibition by RAST and ELISA.

AEROBIOLOGICAL SURVEYS IN INDIA

Pollen Aerobiology

In India, the first systematic atmospheric survey was started in Calcutta by Cunningham[38] more than a century ago. After a prolonged gap, Kasliwal and his colleagues undertook such studies in Jaipur,[39] however, Shivpuri and his students did extensive studies in Delhi.[13] Since then researchers, all over India, have conducted exhaustive studies on airborne pollen types and their concentration. An "All India Coordinated Project on Aeroallergens and Human Health" sponsored by the Ministry of Environment and Forests, Govt. of India, has been successfully completed by AB Singh and his collaborators.[40] Important pollen and fungal allergens from 18 different places have been identified, quantified, and characterized for their allergenic properties. This provides the most scientific and up-to-date information on aeroallergens of India.

In Delhi, surveys have been conducted from time to time by Singh & Shivpuri,[41] Singh & Babu,[42] and Malik et al.[43] The dominant pollen types recorded are grasses, Cheno/Amaranth, *Ailanthus, Ricinus, Morus, Xanthium, Cannabis, Artemisia*, and *Holoptelea*. Lakhanpal & Nair[44] reported 30 pollen types from the atmosphere of Lucknow, whereas, Mittre & Khandelwal[45] reported 36 types. Under the All India coordinated project on aeroallergens and human health,[40] 43 types of pollen were recorded. The dominant types were *Holoptelea*, Poaceae, *Eucalyptus, Casuarina, Putranjiva*, etc. *Holoptelea* contributed 22.2% pollen to the air from March to May. Poaceae pollen grains were recorded (11.8%) with maximum concentration in April to June followed by Asteraceae. Under the same project at Solan (Himachal Pradesh), out of 22 types of pollen recorded, pollen of the family Poaceae and

Asteraceae were recorded in high concentration. The peak pollen season of Asteraceae was from March to October with maximum concentration in April. Poaceae pollen grains were recorded in high concentration in September. *Cassia, Quercus, Pinus,* and *Cedrus* were also important contributors to the pollen load.[40]

From Central India, surveys carried out at Bombay, Gwalior, Nagpur, Bhopal, and Kolhapur revealed that the dominant pollen types were from Poaceae, Asteraceae, and Apocynaceae families, *Rosa, Cicer, Ricinus, Ailanthus, Holoptelea,* Cheno/Amaranth, and Cyperus.[46,47] Grass pollen in India has been reviewed by Chaturvedi et al.[48] and has observed that highest percentage was reported from Aurangabad (80.64%) followed by Bhavnagar (70.26%) and Raipur (66.73%), all in Central India. Aerobiological surveys carried out at Mumbai, Pune, and Kolhapur revealed *Cicer, Ricinus communis, Holoptelea,* Cheno/Amaranth, *Argemone, Cocos nucifera,* and *Hibiscus* as the dominant pollen types.[49,50]

A recent survey[40] at Pune revealed *Parthenium* to be the highest contributor to the pollen load with two peak seasons, i.e., from September to November and January to April. *Cocos* and *Cassia* were observed throughout the year. *Cocos* pollen grains were recorded in high concentration in April to May and November to December.

At Aurangabad, *Datura alba* was prevalent in air from August to October with 8.2% annual concentration. *Cleome* contributed 6.8% pollen in June to August. Other important contributors were *Alternanthera, Typha, Bougainvillea,* etc.[40]

In Eastern India, Chanda and his students took up the work in the 1970s to assess the pollen types of Calcutta. Chanda and Sarkar[51] observed that grass pollen grains were the major contributors (39%) to the total pollen load in air. The other dominant pollen types being *Azadirachta, Caesalpinia pulcherrima, Carica papaya, Mangifera indica, Amaranthus, Chenopodium, Xanthium,* and *Argemone.*[52] From the Eastern Himalayas, Gupta and Chanda[16] and Singh and Devi[53] recorded the dominant tree pollen types as *Acer, Alnus nepalensis, Betula, Bucklandia populnea, Eucalyptus,* and *Pinus.* A recent survey[40] in West Bengal revealed, 59 types of pollen in air, and their maximum concentration was recorded in May. *Trema orientalis* pollen was in high concentration from May to July. Pollen types of families Asteraceae and Chenopodiaceae were maximum in June, and other important pollen types were from Asteraceae, *Pongamia, Areca catechu, Xanthium,* and *Cocos.* At Gauhati, Poaceae, Cheno/Amaranth, Asteraceae, *Putranjiva, Mangifera,* and *Eucalyptus* were the dominant types of pollen.[40]

From Southern India, studies carried out earlier at various places such as Visakhapatnam, Bangalore, Trivandrum, Kodaikanal, and Chennai revealed that *Casuarina, Parthenium, Spathodea,* Cheno/Amaranth, *Cocos,* and *Eucalyptus* were dominant pollen types. However, at Visakhapatnam, 24 pollen types were recorded, and Poaceae, *Peltophorum, Cocos, Casuarina,* Cyperaceae, and *Eucalyptus* were the dominant types.[40,54-58] The aerobiological survey at Trivandrum revealed 15 pollen types, and the dominant were Poaceae, Cheno/Amaranth, *Aporosa,* etc.[40] At Chennai, 38 pollen types belonging to 24 genera were identified. Pollen types from Poaceae were the most abundant types and contributed 19.4% to the total pollen load from June to August. Pollen types of *Acalypha* were recorded in highest concentration in the month of August, which is followed by the pollen of *Casuarina* in the month of January and March.[40]

Pollen calendars are very useful for clinicians as well as allergic patients to establish chronologic correlation between the concentration of pollen in air and seasonal allergic symptoms. Keeping this in mind, pollen calendars have been prepared for different geographical locations of the world.[14,28,59-61] Based on the aerobiological data obtained from India, pollen/flowering calendars have been prepared for Calcutta, Sambalpur, Gulbarga (now known as Kalaburagi) Imphal, and Kodaikanal by different workers.[53,57,62,63] The Center for Biochemical Technology (Council for Scientific and Industrial Research) now Institute of Genomics and Integrative Biology, had published a book on pollen calendars of 12 different states of India and is still very popular among allergists and clinical practitioners.[31] Important pollen seasons for grasses, weeds, and trees prevalent in India are provided in the book. A recent book by Singh and Khandelwal[32] with plant pictures, their local and scientific names, concentration, and season and pollen morphology, etc., provides a good tool for the selection of appropriate allergens for testing and immunotherapy.

Fungal Aerobiology

Fungi are ubiquitous in nature and are reported to be prevalent from different parts of the world, both in the indoor and outdoor environments. Airborne survey of fungal allergens has been reported from different parts of India.

Outdoor Environments

From Delhi and Dehradun, *Alternaria* is reported to be very high followed by *Cladosporium* in the studies concluded using the gravitational method.[64,65] At Solan and Lucknow, 17 and 40 types of fungal spores, respectively, were recorded from ambient air. Aspergilli-Penicilli followed by *Cladosporium, Helminthosporium, Epicoccum,* and *Drechslera* are the dominant types.[40]

Studies carried out at Gaya, Gauhati, Calcutta, Gorakhpur, and Imphal[40] revealed Aspergilli-Penicilli, *Cladosporium,* ascospores, rust and smuts spores, *Nigrospora, Periconia, Ganoderma,* and *Rhizopus* as the major types from East India.

From Western India, Deuteromycetes contributed 70% of the total fungal air spora. A recent survey has reported 18 spore types at Aurangabad and 22 at Pune. *Cladosporium,* Aspergilli-Penicilli, *Curvularia, Rhizopus,* and *Helminthosporium* were the abundant types.[40]

The dominant forms in Visakhapatnam, among 34 types, were Aspergilli-Penicilli, *Cladosporium, Curvularia,* Basidiospores, and Uredospores. In Chennai, 50 types were identified and, apart from the common genus, *Perconia, Curvularia,* and *Ganoderma* are the dominant types. In Trivandrum, *Tetraploa* was another dominant fungal spore prevalent in the air among other common types.[40]

In central India, surveys were conducted at Gwalior, Aurangabad, and Nagpur, and 15, 18, and 25 fungal types were recorded, respectively. Prominent types were Aspergilli-Penicilli, *Cladosporium, Helminthosporium, Curvularia, Drechslera, Pyricularia, Syncephalastrum,* and *Uredospores.*[40]

Indoor Environment

Besides the outdoor environment, indoor and work environments are also greatly influenced by fungi, especially occupational sites employing organic raw materials, e.g., granary, poultry, flour mills, bakery, and sugar factory.[2,66,67] A survey conducted at working environments of bakery, poultry, sugar factory, and libraries in Delhi revealed Aspergilli-Penicilli and smuts spores as significant contributors in indoor air.[68-70] Fungal spora and their seasonality at some of these work environments have been worked out in detail by our group and is described briefly here.[71]

Bakery

Altogether, 74 types belonging to 33 genera were isolated from the bakery environment in Delhi by Singh and Singh.[34] *Aspergillus flavus* was the predominant type in the storage (34.9%) and packing sections (20.2%) of the bakery. Highest concentration was recorded during summer months from June to September. *Cladosporium* concentration was less inside than just outside the bakery. It was significantly high in concentration from October to February. In the case of spore catch, Aepergilli/Penicilli were the dominant (69.2%) type with maximum concentration in October. Smut spores were the second highest contributor in the packing section (28.5%) from February to April.

Poultry

In the poultry environment, 130 fungal forms were isolated from the air survey. Predominant fungi observed particularly in the shed area and in the poultry air are *Candida albicans, Scopulariopsis brevicaulis, Penicillium nigricans,* and *Penicillium frequentans.* In the hatchery section, Aspergilli/Penicilli spores were abundant. As far as the seasonality of these fungi is concerned, *Candida* did not have a definite season. *Cladosporium* showed a seasonal prevalence from November to February. *A. flavus* had seasonal exacerbation from July to October.

Granary

Aspergillus contributed a maximum of 68.9% followed by *Cladosporium* in granary. Colony forming units of *A. flavus* had two distinct seasons from September to November and May to August, whereas, *Cladosporium* was prevalent in winter months. Other important contributors to the granary environment were *Rhizopus, Curvularia, Aspergillus versicolor, Aspergillus fumigatus,* and *Epicoccum nigrum. Aspergillus* alone contributed 74.7% inside the grain storage. The spores of *Alternaria* were observed in each month with seasonal exacerbation in summer from March to June.

Sugar Industry

Cladosporium was recorded in high concentration (60%) in both the cane cutting and bagasse storage regions of the sugar industry, almost parallel to outside concentration and was prevalent from November to March. This period also coincides with the main crushing season of the sugar industry. Other major contributors were *A. fumigatus, Epicoccum, Saccharomyces,* and smut spores. *Epicoccum* was characteristic for the month of November to May. Other fungi like *Aspergillus niger, A. versicolor, and A. flavus* did not show a definite seasonality.

Several epidemiological studies have correlated symptoms of allergic patients to fungal spores concentration in their houses (Roby and Sneller, 1979; Anderson and Korsgaard, 1986; Martin et al., 1987; Waegemaekers et al., 1989). Epidemiological survey conducted by Singh and coworkers (Singh, 1994) revealed 40% workers having respiratory problems in bakery, 59% in poultry, 40.5% in granary and 42.5% in sugar industry. The prevalence is 4–5 times higher in Delhi than what was estimated about 34 decades ago for general population.[72]

CLINICALLY IMPORTANT ALLERGENS

Pollen Allergens

Pollen types causing allergy are quite variable in different ecozones, which makes it very important to identify pollinosis-causing species from every region and prepare extracts from them for diagnosis and immunotherapy for the benefit of allergy sufferers.

Based on clinico-immunological studies with pollen antigens, important allergenic pollen of India have been identified. The work on pollen allergy was initiated in the 1950s by Shivpuri in Delhi. Subsequently, Kasliwal and his colleagues reported important pollen allergens of Jaipur.[73] Shivpuri & Parkash[74] observed *P. juliflora* as a major cause of pollinosis with 12% of patients showing a positive skin reaction. Later, important pollen types causing allergy were identified for Delhi by Shivpuri and his colleagues, some of them are *Ageratum, Ailanthus, Amaranthus, Anogeissus pendula, Artemisia, Cassia siamea, Cenchrus, Chenopodium, Cynodon, Ipomoea fistulosa, Paspalum distichum,* and *Poa annua.*[75] Singh et al.[76] recorded a positive skin reaction in 16.9% of patients to *Pinus roxburghii* from the foothills of Himalayas.

From Northern India, the important allergens identified are *P. juliflora, R. communis, Morus, Mallotus, Alnus, Quercus, Cedrus, Argemone,* etc. from studies carried out by Agnihotri & Singh[6,17,77] Reported, *Amaranthus, Chenopodium, Holoptelea,* and grasses are important offending allergens from this region (Table 4.1).

Tiwari[78] and Chaubal & Gadve[79] identified the important pollen types causing allergy from Central India. They are *Argemone, Brassica, Cannabis, Asphodelus, Parthenium, Cassia, Azadirachta,* and grasses. Under AICP project, *Morus* and *Trewia nudiflora* are recently added to the list of allergens.[40]

From Eastern India, Chanda et al.[80] carried out studies in Calcutta and reported that allergenically significant pollen types were *Lantana, Cucurbita maxima, Cassia fistula, C. nucifera,* and *Calophyllum inophyllum.* High sensitivity to *C. nucifera* has also been recorded by Karmakar et al.[81] Recent studies based on clinical and immunologic parameters reported *Phoenix, R. communis,* and *Aegle marmelos* as causative agents of allergy in this region.[40]

Acharya et al.[82] and Agashe & Anand[83] have reported *Cassia, Ageratum, Salvadora, Ricinus, Albizia lebbeck,* and *Artemisia scoparia* as important aeroallergens of South India. Subbarao et al.[84] recorded allergenicity to *Parthenium hysterophorus* pollen extracts in 34% of allergic rhinitis and 12% of bronchial asthma patients from Bangalore. Agashe & Soucenadin[85] recorded high skin reactivity to *Casuarina equisetifolia* in patients from Bangalore.

Clinical studies undertaken recently by various medical centers under AICP on Aeroallergens and Human Health[40] revealed the important allergenic pollen and fungi for various regions in India. Skin test reactivity from different centers is presented in Table 4.2. Altogether, 35 pollen and 30 fungal antigens were tested on atopic population. In Chandigarh, skin sensitivity was maximum against *Rumex acetosa* and *Ailanthus excelsa* (17.6%) followed by *T. nudiflora* (9.7%) and *Argemone mexicana* (9.5%), and 9.3% of the atopic persons showed sensitivity against *Cedrus deodara.* In Delhi, 12.6% of the atopic population were positive against *Amaranthus spinosus*, 8.46% to *Populus deltoides*, and 7.46% against *Dodonaea viscosa* and *Bauhinia variegata.* In Calcutta, 28.8% of the patients were sensitive against *Solanum sisymbriifolium* while, *Crotalaria juncea* (21.1%) and 18.18% each against *R. communis* and *I. fistulosa.* In Trivandrum, maximum skin reactivity was recorded against *Mallotus philippensis* (12.1%) followed by *P. juliflora* (6.3%).

Fungal Allergens

Like pollinosis, fungal allergy is also well established. The significant fungal types causing allergy have been identified on the basis of skin tests performed on symptomatic patients.

Agarwal and Shivpuri[86] performed intradermal skin tests on 1292 patients in Delhi using 27 fungal extracts. They found 19 fungal extracts to be of allergenic

Table 4.1: Common allergenic plants of different seasons in India.

Spring	*Autumn*	*Winter*
February–April	*September–October*	*November–January*
Grasses		
Cynodon dactylon	*Bothriochloa pertusa*	*Cynodon dactylon*
Dichanthium annulatum	*Cenchrus ciliaris*	*Eragrostis tenella*
Imperata cylindrica	*Heteropogon contortus*	*Phalaris minor*
Paspalum distichum	*Pennisetum typhoides*	*Poa annua*
Poa annua	*Sorghum vulgare*	–
Polypogon monspeliensis	–	–
Weeds		
Cannabis sativa	*Amaranthus spinosus*	*Ageratum conyzoides*
Chenopodium murale	*Artemisia scoparia*	*Argemone mexicana*
Parthenium -	*Cassia occidentalis*	*Chenopodium album*
-hysterophorus	*Ricinus communis*	*Asphodelus tenuifolius*
Plantago major	*Xanthium strumarium*	*Ricinus communis*
Suaeda fruticosa	–	–
Trees		
Ailanthus excelsa	*Anogeissus pendula*	*Cassia siamea*
Holoptelea integrifolia	*Eucalyptus* sp.	*Salvadora persica*
Prosopis juliflora	*P. juliflora*	*Mallotus philippensis*
Putranjiva roxburghii	*Cedrus deodara*	*Cedrus deodara*

Table 4.2: Skin test results from different medical centers in India.

Name of allergen	*Kolkata*	*Chandigarh*	*Delhi*	*Trivandrum*
Pollen Antigen				
Aegle marmelos	15.6	–	2.98	–
Ailanthus excelsa	–	17.6	–	–
Alnus nitida	–	4.8	3.5	–
Amaranthus spinosus	15.4	3.2	–	–
Argemone mexicana	–	9.5	4.26	4.8
Bauhinia variegata	17.8	–	7.46	–
Betula utilis	–	–	4.98	–
Borassus flabellifer	9.7	–	–	–
Carica papaya	7.07	–	4.48	–
Caryota urens	4.11	1.5	1.5	–
Cassia fistula	5.88	4.8	–	3.0
Cassia glauca	–	5.9	1.75	
Cocos nucifera	11.5	–	6.98	3.2
Casuarina equisetifolia	9.2	–	6.47	–
Callitris		4.8	2.3	–
Cedrus deodara	8.0	9.3	7.1	4.8
Celtis australis	–	–	3.48	–
Crotalaria juncea	21.05	6.4	–	–
Cycas circinalis	15.4	–	–	–
Dodonaea viscosa	4.34	4.3	7.46	1.5

(Contd...)

(Contd...)

Name of allergen	*Kolkata*	*Chandigarh*	*Delhi*	*Trivandrum*
Delonix regia	10.78	1.5	1.16	3.1
Holoptelea integrifolia	–	2.4	6.59	–
Ipomoea fistulosa	21.1	–	4.97	–
Mallotus philippensis	8.25	5.9	1.39	12.1
Phoenix sylvestris	8.0	–	–	3.1
Plantago ovata	10.8	3.2	4.48	–
Podocarpus	1.96	5.9	–	–
Populus deltoides	3.4	3.2	8.46	–
Prosopis juliflora	15.7	4.3	6.98	6.3
Quercus incana	–	4.8	5.81	–
Quercus dilatata	–	–	4.48	–
Ricinus communis	18.18	3.6	5.26	4.8
Rumex acetosa	–	17.6	–	–
Solanum sisymbriifolium	28.8	–	6.96	–
Trewia nudiflora	12.9	9.7	1.75	–
Fungal Antigens				
Alternaria alternata	–	3.5	1.1	–
A. candidus	4.9	–	5.4	–
A. clavatus	–	–	4.48	–
A. flavus	5.46	5.22	1.75	–
A. fumigatus	4.9	2.61	–	–
Aspergillus japonicus	3.12	4.76	3.51	1.6
A. nidulans	9.8	3.22	–	–
A. ochraceous	4.0	1.2	2.2	–
A. oryzae	4.9	–	5.47	–
A. sydowii	6.08	3.57	–	–
A. terreus	7.69	5.95	3.48	–
A. versicolor	10.99	–	2.2	–
Cladosporium cladosporioides	5.1	4.76	–	1.6
Cladosporium herbarum	3.65	–	4.48	–
Chaetomium	–		2.0	–
Curvularia pallescens	8.0	1.74	–	–
Epicoccum nigrum	10.0	3.57	–	–
Fomes pectinatus	7.14	4.76	–	–
Fusarium roseum	6.86	1.74	1.75	–
Ganoderma lucidum	6.86	2.6	6.2	1.6
Neurospora implicata	10.5	3.22	3.51	–
Neurospora sitophila	3.1	2.6	3.51	–
Paecilomyces variotii	9.1	3.22	4.17	–
Sphacelotheca cruenta	14.3	3.22	6.94	–
Sporotrichum pruinosum	6.67	6.45	5.55	–
Rhizopus nigricans	5.88	1.74	–	–
Uromyces aloes	1.23	6.45	5.56	–
Ustilago cynodontis	4.87	3.2	–	–
Ustilago scitaminea	2.7	9.68	2.8	–
Ustilago tritici	1.98	–	2.98	–

significance. Some of these are *Alternaria brassicae, Curvularia, Candida, Monilia, Phoma, Acrothecium, Helminthosporium, Mucor,* and *Aspergillus tamarii.* Shivpuri[29] further performed skin tests on 300 patients and observed besides the abovementioned fungi, *Cladosporium herbarum, A. niger,* and *A. fumigatus* were also important allergens.

Acharya[82] investigated on 300 nasobronchial allergy patients in Andhra Pradesh, important allergenic fungi were *A. flavus, Helminthosporium, Neurospora, Candida, Cladosporium,* etc. From Bangalore, *Mucor mucedo, Fusarium solani, Curvularia, Nigrospora,* etc., are observed to be important allergens.[83]

Clinical studies at various places in India under AICP on aeroallergens and human health[40] reported *A. ochraceus, A. japonicus, Cladosporium, Alternaria alternata, A. versicolor, Uromyces,* and *Ustilago* are major allergenic fungi (Table 4.2). Information on *A. ochraceus, A. japonicus, Uromyces, Ustilago, Neurospora sitophila,* and *Sporotrichum* has been obtained for the first time in India with respect to their allergenic properties and constitute important fungal allergens of India.

MOLECULAR APPROACH TO ALLERGENS CHARACTERIZATION

Pollen extracts are complex mixtures of several proteins, lectins, complex carbohydrates, lipids, nucleic acids, enzymes, etc. Every time an extract is prepared, there is considerable variation in their content within a company, besides intercompany variability. These great differences result in unreliable prick test results, prevent comparison of skin tests world over, and in generating dose–response data. Also, their use in therapeutics makes them necessary to have an international standard.

The need for standardization of allergenic extracts has been recognized since the advent of immunotherapy.[87] The early attempts toward standardization was based on consistency in crude w/v ratio or estimation of Protein Nitrogen Unit content of the extract. But it was found to be a poor indicator of allergen content.

The standardization of allergenic extracts can be done by biological standardization. The concept of biologic equivalence test was established by the Northern Society of Allergology and adopted by European investigators.[88] One HEP unit was defined as a positive skin prick test, which gave a wheal diameter equivalent to that given by a prick with 1 mg/mL concentration of histamine hydrochloride. Later on, Dirksen et al.[89] designated 1 HEP as the concentration of extract that gives a wheal diameter equivalent to 1 mg/mL of histamine hydrochloride.

Pollen and fungal extracts are also studied for their immunochemical properties, mainly protein and glycoproteinic fractions.

Pollen Allergens

Several pollen allergens are characterized for their protein profile. A number of fractions were identified in these antigens and most of the fractions are found to be acidic. Further allergenic fractions are also identified by RAST or Western blotting. Some of the well-characterized antigens *are P. juliflora,*[90] *R. communis, Holoptelea integrifolia,*[91,92] *Phoenix sylvestris,*[93] *I. fistulosa,*[94] *Madhuca indica,*[95] and *C. deodara.*[17]

Many pollen allergens are characterized under AICP on aeroallergens and human health.[40] They are *Mallotus philippensis, Quercus incana, C. nucifera, Celtis, Betula,* etc. (Table 4.3). All these pollen antigens are identified for the first time and are characterized for their antigenic and allergenic properties.

The protein profile as fractionated on sodium dodecyl sulfate-polyacrylamide gel electrophoresis (SDS-PAGE) showed considerable heterogeneity with the number of bands varying from 8 in *Broussonetia papyrifera* to 23 in *Caryota urens.* All 38 pollen antigenic extracts and 21 fungal extracts were characterized (Table 4.3) by using SDS-PAGE and isoelectric focusing (IEF). The profile of some of the antigens is described later.

Aegle marmelos

A total of 15 fractions was fractionated on SDS-PAGE. Their molecular weight ranged from 14.3 to 116 kD. Of these, most distinct protein bands were of 14.3, 21, 25.7, 37, 60, and 85 kD. While by electrofocusing, 11 fractions were detected in the acidic region (3.5–6.2 pI).

Alnus nitida

There were 21 proteins fractionated by SDS-PAGE. Their molecular weights ranged from 12.5 to 11.6 kD. Sixteen bands were identified by IEF within the pI range of 3.5–6.0. Among these 4.2, 5.2, and 5.3 pI bands were prominent.

Table 4.3: SDS-PAGE and isoelectric focusing (IEF) characterization of pollen antigens.

	SDS-PAGE		*IEF*	
Antigen	*Total No. of bands*	*MW range*	*Total No. of bands*	*pI range*
Aegle marmelos	15	14.3–116.0	11	3.5–6.2
Ailanthus excelsa	14	14.5–128.0	9	3.5–5.6
Alnus nitida	21	12.5–116.5	16	3.65–6.0
Argemone mexicana	17	12.2–125.0		
Amaranthus spinosus	14	12.2–124.0	17	3.5–8.95
Betula utilis	17	11.7–109.0	22	3.1–8.5
Borassus flabellifer	10	14.3–90.0	9	3.5–5.85
Broussonetia papyrifera	8	11.8–118.0	16	3.2–8.15
Carica papaya	6	17.0–43.0	6	3.75–4.9
Cassia fistula	13	12.2–134.0	9	3.6–5.3
Cassia sophera	10	13.0–131.0	12	3.7–6.2
Casuarina equisetifolia	13	13.5–126.5	16	3.9–8.2
Cedrus deodara	17	12.3–116.0	20	4.3–9.4
Ceiba pentandra	15	12.4–128.0	8	3.5–5.65
Celtis australis	11	14.3–95.0	12	3.45–9.4
Cocos nucifera	22	10.2–135.0	12	3.55–5.9
Dodonaea viscosa	18	14.0–111.0	13	3.2–6.1
Elaeis guineensis	7	11.7–140.0	12	3.7–5.85
Ipomoea biloba	9	12.2–60.0	19	3.95–8.3
Ipomoea fistulosa	19	14.3–116.0	12	3.57–8.55
Juglans regia	15	12.0–126.0	19	4.75–9.12
Mallotus philippensis	25	11.9–140.0	28	3.6–9.3
Pecan nut	17	11.7–140.0	17	4.1–9.3
Peltophorum pterocarpum	10	13.2–138.0	15	3.5–8.8
Phoenix sylvestris	10	14.2–125.5	13	4.1–9.3
Pinus patula	12	12.2–125.0	5	4.4–8.25
Populus deltoides	24	13.0–120.0	13	3.8–6.6
Plantago ovata	4	12.2–118.0	8	3.7–4.9
Punica granatum	10	16.5–112.0	21	3.9–9.3
Quercus dilatata	17	14.3–120.0	17	3.9–8.2
Quercus incana	16	14.3–120.0	22	3.9–9.35
Rumex setorum	22	14.3–118.0	16	3.95–6.7
Syzygium cumini	15	11.6–113.0	15	3.7–5.85
Solanum sisymbriifolium	8	13.5–115.0	19	3.57–7.3
Trewia nudiflora	10	11.5–119.0	16	3.5–5.95

Amaranthus spinosus

A total of 14 proteins were detected in the molecular weight range of 12.2–124 kD. Proteins of 113 and 122 kD were most distinct. On IEF, 17 proteins were fractionated in the pI range of 3.5–8.95. Two proteins were localized in the alkaline region (7.4 and 8.95). Rest of the proteins were with acidic pI. Proteins of 4.3, 4.65, 5.1, 5.2, and 9.85 pI were prominent among all.

Betula utilis

Antigenic extract fractionated on SDS-PAGE revealed 17 protein fractions ranging in molecular weights of 11.7 to

109 kD. Protein bands of 17.8 and 14 kD were the most distinct bands. Twenty-two proteins were identified by IEF in the pI range of 3.1–8.1. Two of the proteins were in the basic region.

Borassus flabellifer

Borassus antigen was fractionated in 10 protein bands between 14.3 and 90 kD. Among these 90.81, 56.8, 41, and 43.2 kD bands were the more prominent than others. While there were nine protein fractions identified in the acidic pI region (3.5–5.85), 3.5, 5.25, 5.3, 5.75 pI proteins are prominent among all.

Carica papaya

Antigen revealed only six protein bands by SDS-PAGE as well as IEF. Molecular weights of the proteins were between 17.0 and 43 kD, and pI was 3.75–4.9.

Ceiba pentandra

There were 15 bands between 10.4 and 128 kD molecular weight, when antigens was fractionated on SDS-PAGE. A band of 29 kD was the most intensely stained band. Only eight *protein* bands were identified on the IEF fractionation in the pI range of 3.5–5.65.

Ipomea biloba

Antigen was fractionated on SDS-PAGE and nine bands were detected. The molecular weights of these fractions varied from 12.2 to 60 kD, and 14.3, 23, 50, and 60 kD bands were distinct. As much as nine proteins were fractionated by IEF in the pI range of 3.95–8.3. Two of the proteins were localized in the alkaline region.

Plantago ovata

Plantago antigen was fractionated in only four bands on SDS-PAGE (12.2–118 kD) with 12.2, 22, and 33.5 kD the prominent ones. On IEF eight bands were detected in the low-pI range (pI 3.7–4.9) and most of the bands were clear and well stained, though 3.7, 3.95, 4.1, 4.4, and 4.6 pI fractions were prominent than others.

Populus deltoides

Twenty-four proteins were fractionated on SDS-PAGE with molecular weights ranging from 13.0 to 120 kD. Proteins of 15.2 and 56.0 kD were more prominent than others. By IEF, 13 proteins were identified in the pI range of 3.8–5.6. No bands were in the basic region. Proteins of 5.3 and 5.7 pI were prominent.

Quercus incana

Sixteen protein fractions were detected on SDS-PAGE. These proteins had the molecular weights ranging from 14.3 to 120 kD. A total of 22 protein bands were detected in the pI range of 3.9–9.35.

Solanum sisymbriifolium

Antigenic extracts of *S. sisymbriifolium* when fractionated on SDS-PAGE revealed eight bands in the molecular weights ranging from 13.5 to 115 kD; while on IEF 11 proteins could be detected in the acidic region (4.0–5.9).

Fungal Allergens

The most common fungal components that become airborne are conidia/spores. The fungal types that have been found dominant, all over the world, have a large species and strain. Besides, fungi have the tendency to undergo mutation under slight stress conditions. Some of them are so prone to change that it is impossible to maintain similar culture, that may yield similar antigenic components.[96] It has been reported by many workers that the prevalence of shared antigenic and allergenic components among closely related or even unrelated genera of fungi exists.[97–99] Due to these reasons, a very few fungi are studied in detail with a view to characterize the allergen content. The difficulty also arises because of the high number of allergenic components in the crude extracts.[33] Some of the allergens studied for molecular heterogeneity are *Cladosporium*, *Aspergillus*, *Drechslera Candida*, and Basidiomycetes.[10,20,96,100–105]

Many fungal allergens have been recently characterized in India. They are *Aspergillus ochraceus, Fomes, Ganoderma, Epicoccum, Fusarium, A. flavus*, and some others.[7,105–110] Further, under the All India coordinated project (AICP) many fungal allergens were characterized, such as *Paecilomyces, Uromyces, Ustilago tritici*, etc. IgE-binding fractions of some of these are identified and described in Table 4.4.

Aspergillus clavatus

Thirteen bands could be detected in the antigenic extract of *A. clavatus*, which lied in between 11.5 and 176 kD

Table 4.4: SDS-PAGE and IEF characterization of fungal antigens.

Antigen	*SDS-PAGE*		*IEF*	
	Total no. of bands	MW range	Total no. of bands	pI range
Alternaria alternata	8	13.8–145.5	–	–
Aspergillus fumigatus	22	24.0–134.0	11	3.9–6.0
A. japonicus	–	–	11	3.73–7.9
A. ochraceus	9	13.8–125.0	–	–
A. versicolor	4	20.0–130.0	2	4.55–4.76
A. sydowii	22	12.2–138.0	15	3.5–6.6
A. clavatus	13	11.5–176.0	8	2.1–6.7
A. candidus	9	12.4–166.0	2	4.7–5.1
C. herbarum	17	13.5–135.0	–	–
Curvularia lunata	–	–	4	3.8–4.8
Epicoccum nigrum	9	16.4–185.0	–	–
Fusarium roseum	14	13.5–139.0	–	–
Helminthosporium oryzae	19	12.2–138.0	7	3.9–5.9
Neurospora implicata	–	–	10	3.65–6.25
Paecilomyces variotii	7	12.0–138.0	14	3.7–6.2
Sphacelotheca cruenta	6	12.2–121.0	9	4.1–5.85
Sporotrichum pruinosum	20	12.5–128.0	–	–
Uromyces aloe	4	14.0–114.0	16	3.05–6.95
Ustilago cynodontis	10	12.2–130.5	9	4.1–6.35
Ustilago tritici	5	14.2–172.0	12	4.3–6.35
Ustilago scitaminea	13	12.2–126.5	15	3.65–6.4

molecular weights. A protein of 20 kD was most prominent. Only eight proteins were detected on IEF. All were in the acidic pI range (2.1-6.7).

Helminthosporium

Nineteen protein fractions were detected in the molecular weight range of 12.2-138 kD. Only seven fractions were detected on IEF. They were in the acidic pI range from 3.9 to 5.09. A protein of 3.9 pI was most distinct.

Sphacelotheca cruenta

Only six proteins were identified in the crude extract with molecular weights ranging from 12.2 to 128 KD. Bands of 12.2 and 121 kD were distinct among all the proteins.

Sporotrichum pruinosum

A total of 20 protein fractions could be detected in SDS-PAGE. Their molecular weights ranged from 12.5 to 128 KD.

Ustilago tritici

Antigenic extract was fractionated on SDS-PAGE and only five proteins were detected in the molecular weight range of 14.2-172 kD. On IEF, six proteins were detected in the pI range of 4.1-6.7. All the proteins were acidic.

Ustilago cynodontis

Only two proteins were fractionated on SDS-PAGE. Their molecular weights were 17 and 170 kD. A band of 17 kD was more prominent. Whereas, eight protein fractions were detected on IEF. All of them were acidic and were in the pI range of 3.5–6.7.

Uromyces aloe

Antigenic extract revealed four proteins only in the molecular weight range of 14–114 kD and 14 kD protein was most distinct. Sixteen fractions could be detected on IEF. All the proteins were in the acidic range of 3.4–6.7.

FUTURE TRENDS IN ALLERGEN RESEARCH

Since mid-1980, a fast growth has seen in the information on allergy. A large number of major allergens have been isolated, purified, and their amino acid sequencing and epitope mapping have been done. The allergenic epitopes have also been analyzed using human T cells.[111,112]

Molecular cloning of pollen allergens, which is underway, will further facilitate the production of defined allergens in virtually unlimited quantities. This is essential for the development of the following:

1. Highly discriminating diagnostic assays of allergens.
2. International standards of major allergens for use in immunotherapy.
3. Derivatives of allergens that may serve as effective therapeutic modalities.
4. Aid in the establishment of the structure of pollen allergens that interact with the components of immunosystem, such as IgE, IgG, T-cell receptors, V gene products, and major histocompatibility molecules.

The knowledge of epitopes in aeroallergens would lead not only to immunotherapy vaccines but also serve as a tool for the investigation of the cellular humoral mechanism in type I hypersensitivity.

RECOMMENDATIONS

Important pollen and fungal allergens vary in concentration and prevalence from place to place, so it is advisable to measure their concentration and establish relationship with the patient symptoms.

The remedial action depends on the actual problem and condition prevailing in different occupational sites, and following preventive measures are, in general, recommended.

Pollen Allergens

1. All the allergenically significant trees need to be deleted from the list of "Recommended tree plantation" in the Gazette of India.
2. Ornamental, insects-/bird-pollinated, and medicinally important trees or others, which can help in controlling pollution, should be encouraged in various tree plantation and afforestation programs.
3. The existing allergenically significant trees need to be replaced with nonallergenic trees in a phased manner.
4. On medical ground, citizens should have the right to cut or demand the removal of allergy-causing tree (s) in close vicinity. However, these should be replaced with some nonallergenic tree (s).
5. A genuine beginning needs to be made by sensitizing tree lovers/horticulturists/foresters/botanists and others associated with tree plantation and afforestation programs, so that the share of allergenically significant plants could be minimized in the near future. The earlier it is done, the better for allergy patients.

Fungal Allergens

1. It is important to isolate and identify important airborne fungi that cause allergic disorders.
2. Knowledge of the life history of these fungi is essential in identifying their source and environmental conditions that help in getting airborne in significant concentration.
3. "Prevention is better than cure", therefore it is suggested that the substrate on which microorganisms build up their numbers should be removed from the work place.
4. Reduction of moisture inside the work place.
5. Air quality can be enhanced by the periodic maintenance of air treatment plant, fumigation, application of antifungal agents, etc.
6. Personal filter masks of the pore size sufficient to stop the entry of respirable size microbes may be beneficial at the work place.
7. Environmental factors like air pollution and smoking also can aggravate the existing symptoms. These should be controlled.

Allergy has been known for more than a century now but the subject has suffered due to lack of knowledge about basic mechanisms involved in allergic diseases and poor diagnostic procedures. The rapid development in the field of immunology and clinical diagnosis in the pool of knowledge are of direct significance to allergy practitioners. The detailed information on indigenous pollen and fungal allergens will be very useful in the diagnosis and management of allergic patients in the country.

REFERENCES

1. Kang B, Velody D, Homburger H, Yuninger JW. Analysis of indoor environment and atopic allergy in urban population with bronchial asthma. J Allergy Clin Immunol. 1979;63: 80-9.
2. Lacey J, Crook, B. Fungal and actimomycetes spores as pollutants of workplace and occupational allergens. Ann Occup Hyg. 1988;32:515-33.
3. Aalberse RC, Bessot JC, Bjorksten B. Dust mite allergens and asthma- A worldwide problem. J Allergy Clin Immunol. 1989;83:416-27.
4. Burge H. Bioaerosols: prevalence and health effects in the indoor environments. J Allergy Clin Immunol. 1990;86:687-701.
5. Singh AB, Singh, A. Pollen allergy—A global scenario. In: Agashe SN, ed. Recent Trends in Aerobiology, Allergy and Immunology. New Delhi, India: Oxford IBH;1994.
6. Singh AB, Mathur C. An aerobiological perspective in allergy and asthma. Asia Pac Allergy. 2012;2:210-22.
7. Kjellman NIM. Prediction and prevention of allergy in infants and children. Allergy Clin Immunol News. 1993;5:131-4.
8. Bostock J. Case of a periodical affection of the eyes and chest. Med Chirugical Trans. 1819;10:161.
9. Blackley CH. Hay fever: experimental researches on the cause and treatment of catarrhus aestivus. Dawson 1959 (First printed by Bailliere, Tindall & Cox, London), 1873.
10. Aukrust L, Ass K. The diagnosis of allergy to *Cladosporium herbarum*. Difference between extracts and the efficacy of radioallergosorbent test (RAST). Allergy. 1978;33:24-9.
11. Fienberg SM. Mold allergy. Its importance in asthma and hay fever. Wisconsin Med J. 1935;34:254-62.
12. Naranjo P. Etiological agents of respiratory allergy in tropical countries of central and south America. J Allergy. 1958;29:363-74.
13. Shivpuri DN, Vishwanathan R, Dua LK. Studies on pollen allergy in Delhi area I—Pollination calendar. Ind J Med Res. 1960;48:15-20.
14. Leuschner RM. Investigation on airborne pollen in Basel and Davos (Switzerland) in connection with pollinosis. Grana (Abst). 1974;14:40.
15. Lewis WH. Pollen allergy. In: Korenblat PE, Wedner HJ, eds. Allergy: Theory and Practice. Orlando, Grune and Startton; 1984:353-69.
16. Gupta S, Chanda S. Aeropalynological survey in subtropical Eastern Himalayas, Kurseong. Grana. 1989;28:219-21.
17. Rawat A, Singh A, Singh AB, et al. Clinical immunological evaluation of Cedrus deodara pollen: a new allergen from India. Allergy. 2000;55:1-7.
18. Benton HS. Asthma due to a mould *Aspergillus fumigatus*. J Amer Med Ass. 1930;95:189-96.
19. Hopkins JG, Benham RW, Keston BM. Asthma due to a fungus- *Alternaria*. J Amer Med Ass. 1930;94:6.
20. Barkai-Golan R, Frank M, Kanotoorm D, et al. Atmospheric fungi in the desert town of Arad and in the coastal plain of Israel. Ann Allergy. 1977;28:270-4.
21. Crook B, Lacey J. Environment of airborne microorganism in work environment. Environ Tech Lett. 1988;9:515-20.
22. Fienberg SM. Mold allergy. Its importance in Asthma and Hay fever. Wisconsin Med J. 1935;34:254-62.
23. Fienberg SM. Probability of allergic reactions in fungus sensitive individuals: preliminary experiments. J Allergy. 1944;15:271.
24. Durham OC. The volumetric incidence of atmospheric allergens. IV. A proposed standard method of gravity sampling, counting & volumetric interpolation of results. J Allergy. 1946;17:79.
25. Nilsby I. Allergy to molds in Sweden. A botanical and clinical study. Acta Allergol. 1949;2:57-67.
26. Hyde HA, Williams DA. Allergy to mold spores in Britain. Brit Med J. 1956;1:886.
27. Prince HE, Morrow MB. A logical approach to mold allergy. Ann Allergy. 1969;12:253.
28. Nilsson S, Praglowski J, Nilsson N. Atlas of airborne pollen grains and spores in Northern Europe. Stockholm, Sweden: Almquist and Wiksell International; 1977.
29. Shivpuri DN. Clinically important pollen, fungal and insect allergens for nasobronchial allergy patients in India. Asp Allergy Appl Immunol. 1980;XIII:19-23.
30. Singh AB, Malik P. Pollen aerobiology and allergy: an integrated approach. Indian J Aerobiol. 1992;5:1-19.
31. Singh BP, Singh AB, Gangal SV. Calendars of different states, India. Delhi, India: CSIR Centre for Biochemicals; 1992.
32. Singh AB, Khandelwal A. An atlas of allergenically significant plants of India 2015. Mumbai, India: Himalaya Publishing.
33. Salvaggio J, Aukrust L. Mold-induced asthma. J. Allergy Clin Immunol. 1981;68:327-46.
34. Singh AB, Singh A. Fungi as allergenic agents. In: Rai B, Arora DK, Dubey K, Sharma PD, eds. Fungal Ecology and Biotechnology. 1993:195-208.
35. Solomon WR. Sampling airborne allergens. Ann Allergy. 1984;52(3):140-9.
36. Perkins WA. The rotorod sampler. The second semiannual report. Stanford University, US: Aerosl Lab. CML Standford University;186:66, 1957.
37. Hirst JM. An automatic volumetric spore trap. Ann Appl Biol. 1952;39:252-63.
38. Cunningham DO. Microscopic examinations of air. Calcutta, India: Govt. Press; 1873.
39. Kasliwal RM, Sethi JP, Soagi IC. Studies in atmospheric pollen: a daily census on pollen at Jaipur 1957-58. Ind J Med Res. 1959;47:515-21.
40. All India Coordinated Project on Aeroallergens and Human Health. New Delhi, India: Ministry of Environment and Forests; 1998.
41. Singh K, Shivpuri DN. Studies on yet unknown allergenic pollen of Delhi state metropolitan: botanical aspects. Ind J Med Res. 1971;59:1392-410.

42. Singh AB, Babu CR. Pollen types in the atmosphere of Delhi. Phytomorphology. 1980;30:180-9.
43. Malik P, Singh AB, Babu CR, Gangal SV. Atmospheric concentration of pollen grains at human height. Grana. 1991;30:129-36.
44. Lakhanpal RN, Nair PKK. Survey of atmospheric pollen at Lucknow. J Sci Inds Res. 1958;17C:80-7.
45. Mittre V, Khandelwal A. Airborne pollen grains and fungal spores at Lucknow during 1969–1970. Paleobotanist. 1973;22:177-85.
46. Chaubal PD, Kotmire SY. Aerobiological studies at Kolhapur. Acta Bot Ind. 1982;10:100-20.
47. Jain AK, Mishra R. Airborne pollen grain, fungal spores and other biocomponents at Gwalior. Ind J Aerobiol. 1988;1:30-4.
48. Chaturvedi M, Datta K, Nair PKK. Incidence of grass pollen in Indian environment. Ind J Aerobiol. 1992;5:20-4.
49. Tilak, ST. Aeropalynology in Maharashtra. MVM Patrika. 1974;9:125-31.
50. Deshpande SU, Chitaley DD. Pollen calendar of Nagpur, India. Rev Paleobot Palynol. 1976;22:253-62.
51. Chanda S, Sarkar PK. Pollen grains as a causative agent of respiratory allergy with reference to aeropalynology of Greater Calcutta. Trans Bose Res Inst. 1972;35:61-7.
52. Mandal S, Chanda SC. Incidence of airborne pollen in Kalyani, West Bengal with reference to meteorological parameters. Asp Allergy Appl Immunol. 1980;13.
53. Singh N, Devi KK. Aerobiology and allergic human diseases in Manipur.II. Airborne pollen grains of Imphal, Imphal District. *Ind J Aerobiol.* 1992;Special volume:49-60.
54. Reddi KM, Ramanujam CJK. An aerobiological study of Hyderabad (AP). Asian J Pl Sci. 1989;1:7-21.
55. Gopi TV, Kumar RP, Ravindran P, Nair PKK. Comparative analysis of airspora of two urban localities in Kerala. Ind J Aerobiol. 1990;3:39-44.
56. Atluri JB, Narayan Rao KVV, Ramachandraiah M. Site-to-site variation in airborne pollen grains at Visakhapatnam. Ind J Aerobiol. 1992; Special volume:29-38.
57. Maribhat M, Rajasab AJ. Flowering calendar of potentially allergenic pollen producing plants of Gulbarga. Ind J Aerobiol. 1992;Special Vol:89-95.
58. Satheesh R, Rao GR, Nair PKK. The airborne pollen incidence in relation to season and vegetation at Kodaikanal. Ind J Aeobiol. 1992;Special volume:37-42.
59. Nilsson S, Palmberg-Gotthard J. Pollen calendar for Huddinge (Sweden) 1977-1981. Grana. 1982;21:183-5.
60. Cadman A, Airspora of Johannesburg and Pretoria, South Africa, 1987/1988.I. Pollen Calendars. Grana. 1990;29: 313-7.
61. Emberlin J, Norris-Hill J, Bryant RH. A tree pollen calendar for London. Grana. 1990;29:301-9.
62. Chanda S. Atmospheric pollen flora of Greater Calcutta and Falta. Asp Allergy Appl Immunol. 1973;6:74-87.
63. Pande S, Das AP, Chanda S. Flowering calendar of Angiosperms in Sambalpur district, Orissa (India). Ind J Aerobiol. 1992;Special volume:67-88.
64. Agarwal MK. Studies on the Allergenic Fungal Spores of Delhi Atmosphere. [PhD thesis]. Delhi, India: University of Delhi; 1970.
65. Sandhu DK, Shivpuri DN, Sandhu RS. Studies on the airborne fungal spores in Delhi. Their role in respiratory allergy. Ann Allergy. 1964/1981;22:374.
66. Horejski M, Sach J, Tomsikova A, Med A. A syndrome resembling farmers' lung in workers inhaling spores of Aspergilli and Penicilli moulds. Thorax. 1960;15:212-7.
67. Roby RR, Sneller MR. Incidence of fungal spores at the homes of allergic patients in an agricultural community. II Correlation of skin test with mould frequency. Ann Allergy. 1979;43:286-8.
68. Singh A, Singh AB, Bhatnagar AK, Gangal SV. Prevalence of Aspergilli in bakery environment. Ind J Aerobiol. 1990;3: 15-21.
69. Singh A. Aerobiological and immunological studies on fungal spores of different occupational sites. [PhD thesis]. Delhi, India: University of Delhi; 1993.
70. Pandit T. Aerobiological and clinico-immunological studies of fungi of certain occupational sites. [PhD thesis]. Delhi, India: University of Delhi; 1994.
71. Singh AB. FTR, Ministry of Environment and forests, New Delhi. 1994.
72. Vishwanathan R. Definition, incidence, etiology and natural history of asthma. Ind J Chest Dis. 1964;6:108-24.
73. Kasliwal RM, Solomon SK. Correlation of respiratory allergy cases with atmosphere pollen concentrations and meteorological factors. J Ass Phys. 1958;6:180-95.
74. Shivpuri DN, Parkash D. A study in allergy to Prosopis juliflora (Kabuli keekar). Ann Allergy. 1967;25:643-8.
75. Shivpuri DN, Singh AB, Babu CR. New allergenic pollens of Delhi state, India and their clinical significance. Ann Allergy. 1979;42:49-52.
76. Singh BP, Singh AB, Parkash D. Skin reactivity to airborne pollen and fungal antigens in patients of Nasobronchial Allergy of Hill Regions (India). In: Chandra N, ed. Atmospheric Bio Pollution. Karad: Environmental Publication; 1987:125-34.
77. Agnihotri MS, Singh AB. Observations in pollinosis in Lucknow with special reference to offending factors. Asp Allergy Appl Immunol. 1971;5:135-41.
78. Tiwari UC. Studies in pollen allergy in Bhopal area. A preliminary report. Asp Allergy Appl Immunol. 1978;10:65-72.
79. Chaubal PD, Gadve SB. Study of aeropalynology and pollen allergy in Kolhapur (Part I). MVH Patrika. 1979; 14:43-8.
80. Chanda S, Mandal S, Lahiri SC. Occurrence of allergenic pollen in the atmosphere of Calcutta—Another cause for organic environmental pollution. Sci Cult. 1978;44:175-7.
81. Karmakar PR, Das A, Chatterjee BP. Placebo-controlled Immunotherapy with *Cocos nucifera* pollen extract. Int Arch Allergy Appl Immunol. 1994;103:194-201.
82. Acharya PJ. Skin test response to some inhalant allergens in patients of nasobronchial allergy from Andhra Pradesh. Asp Allergy App Immunol. 1980;XIII:14-8.

83. Agashe SN, Anand P. Immediate type hypersensitivity to common pollen & molds in Bangalore city. Asp Allergy App Immunol. 1982;15:49-52.
84. Subbarao M, Prakash O, Subbarao PV. Reaginic allergy to parthenium pollen: evaluation by skin test and RAST. Clin Allergy. 1985;15:449-54.
85. Agashe SN, Soucenadin S. Pollen productivity in some allergenically significant plants in Bangalore. Ind J Aerobiol. 1992;(Special Vol):63-7.
86. Agarwal MK, Shivpuri DN. Fungal spores- Their role in respiratory allergy. Adv Pollen Spore Res. 1974;1:78-128.
87. Noon L. Prophylactic inoculation against hay fever. Lancet. 1911 (Reprinted in Ann Allergy. 18:287-91).
88. Ass K. Some variables in skin testing standardization of clinical (Biological) methods, Workshop No. 4. Allergy. 1980;36:250-2.
89. Dirksen A, Malling HJ, Mosbech H, Soborg M, Biering I. HEP versus PNU standardization of allergen extracts in skin prick testing. Allergy. 1985;40:620-4.
90. Thakur IS. Fractionation and analysis of allergenicity of allergens from *Prosopis juliflora* pollen. Int Arch Allergy Appl Immunol. 1989;90(2):124-9.
91. Malik P, Singh AB, Gangal SV, Babu CR. Comparison of antigenic and allergenic components of *Holoptelea integrifolia* pollen collected from different source materials. Allergy. 1991;46:284-91.
92. Singh AB, Malik P, Parkash D, Gangal SV. Identification of specific IgE-binding Castor Bean (Ricinus communis) pollen obtained from different source materials. Grana. 1993;32:376-80.
93. Chakraborty P, Chowdhry I, Bhatacharya S, Gupta S, Sengupta DN, Chanda A. Clinicoimmunologic studies on *Phoenix sylvestris rox.* pollen: an aeroallergen from Calcutta, India. Allergy. 2001;54:985-9.
94. Mondal AK, Pauri S, Biswas SR, Mandal S. Identification of allergenic proteins of *Ipomea fistulosa* partial characterization and sensitivity test. Grana. 1997;36:301-5.
95. Boral D, Roy I, Bhattacharya K. Aerobiology, allergenicity and biochemistry of Madhuca indica gmel. Pollen. Ann Agric Environ. 1989;6:87-90.
96. Aukrust L. Allergens in Cladosporium herbarum. In: Oehling A, ed. Advances in Allergology and Immunology. Oxford: Pergamon Press; 1980.
97. Agarwal MK, Jones RT, Yunginger JW. Shared allergenic and antigenic determinants in *Alternaria and Stemphylium* extracts. J Allergy Clin Immunol. 1982;70:437-44.
98. O'Neil CE, Reed MA, Huges JM, Butcher BT. *Fusarium solani*: evidence for common antigenic/allergenic determinants with other fungi imperfecti. Clin Allergy. 1987;17:127-33.
99. O'Neil CE, Horner WE, Reed MA, Lopez M, Lehrer SB. Evaluation of Basidiomycete and Deuteromycete (fungi imperfecti) extracts for shared allergenic determinants. Clin Exp Allergy. 1990;20:533-8.
100. Yunginger JW, Jones R, Gleich GB. Studies on *Alternaria* allergens. III Isolation of a major allergenic fraction (Alt-1). J Allergy Clin Immunol. 1976;58:405-13.
101. Kim SJ, Chapras SO. Characterization of antigens from *Aspergillus fumigatus.* II Fractionation and electrophoretic immunologic and biologic activity. Am Rev Res Dis. 1978;118:547-52.
102. Horner WE, Ibanez MD, Liengswangwong V, Salvaggio JE, Lehrer SB. Charaterization of allergens from spores of the oyster mushroom- *Pleurotus ostreatus.* J Allergy Clin. Immunol. 1988;82:978-86.
103. Ibanez MD, Horner WE, Liengswangwong V, Sastre J, Lehrer SB. Identification and analysis of basidiospores allergens from puffballs. J Allergy Clin Immunol. 1988;82:787-95.
104. Yang M, Olsen E, Dolonich J, Sehon AH, Mohapatra SS. Immunologic characterization of a recombinant Kentucky bluegrass (Poa pratensis) allergenic peptide. J Allergy Clin Immunol. 1991;87:1096.
105. Kurup VA, Ramasamy M, Paul AG, Fink JN. Isolation and characterization of relevant *Aspergillus fumigatus* antigens with IgG and IgE-binding activity. Int Arch Allergy Immunol. 1988;86:176-82.
106. Dixit BA, Lewis WH, James H. The allergens of *Epicoccum nigrum* Lnk. J Allergy Clin Immunol. 1992;90:11-20.
107. Verma J, Gangal SV. *Fusarium solani.* Immunological characterization of allergens. Int Arch Allergy Appl Immunol. 1994;104:175-83.
108. Singh A, Prakassh D, Singh AB. Sensitization to different species of *Aspergillus* in bakery workers and general population. Asian Pac J Allergy Immunol. 1998;16:5-15.
109. Gupta, SK, Pariera BMJ, Singh AB. Fomes pectinatis: an aeroallergen in India. Asian Pac J Allergy Immunol. 1999;17:1-17.
110. Gupta S, Pariera BMJ, Singh AB. *Ganoderma lucidum*: partial characterization of spore and whole body extract. J Invest Allergol Clin Immunol. 2000.
111. Perez M, Ishioka GY, Walker LE, Chestnut ER. scDNA cloning and immunological characterization of the rye grass allergen Lol p I. J Biol Chem. 1990;265:16210-15.
112. Rogers BL, Morgenstern JP, Griffith IJ, et al. Complete sequence of the allergen Amb a II: recombinant expression and reactivity with T cells from ragweed allergic patients. J Immunol. 1991;147:2547-52.

CHAPTER 5

Cross-reactivity for the Practicing Clinician

Harshveer Singh Malhi

INTRODUCTION

Type I hypersensitivity reactions are mediated by IgE antibodies specific to particular allergens. Patients presenting with symptoms of allergies are often sensitized to multiple allergens. This can result from cosensitization or cross-reactivity. *Cosensitization* is a phenomenon when the patient reacts simultaneously to more than one allergen. However, in *cross-reactivity*, IgE specific to a particular allergen binds with another allergen having sequential and structural homology. Therefore, a person allergic to one species may show allergic symptoms due to the presence and exposure to a cross-reactive allergen.[1] In general, cross-reactivity seems to occur when two allergens have a sequence identity of more than 70%. Cross-reactivity rarely happens when there is a sequence identity of <50%.[2]

It is important to differentiate cross-reactivity from cosensitization. In cosensitization, a person is sensitized to more than one allergen. These sensitizations are associated with structurally unrelated allergen groups.[3] This difference manifests as a difference in the prevalence of these two entities.

MECHANISM OF CROSS-REACTIVITY

In allergic reactions, the allergen is responsible for the cross-linking of IgE antibodies present on sensitized cells. The IgE antibodies do not bind with the entire allergen, but recognize particular structures on the surface of these allergens, called epitopes.[4] The ability to identify epitopes can help the antibodies to distinguish between closely related antigens, as each of them can have different epitopes.[5] At the same time, an IgE antibody may not be able to distinguish between different antigens if they share the same or similar epitopes.[4,5] This phenomenon is described as the cross-reactivity of IgE antibodies.

Cross-reactivity can arise due to the[6]

- Presence of "shared epitopes on multivalent antigens." Herein, the binding affinity of the IgE antibodies to the epitopes should remain the same.
- Presence of "conformational similarity of epitopes." Herein, the binding affinity of IgE antibodies would be lesser.

One example for IgE cross-reactivity is the presence of so-called panallergens, which are widespread in our environment and can be found among the different allergen sources. Panallergens are defined as "homologous molecules that originate from a multitude of organisms and cause IgE cross-reactivity between evolutionary unrelated species."[7]

TYPES OF CROSS-REACTIVITY

Cross-reactivity can be divided into three types:[1]

- Clinical: as evidenced by patient's symptoms
- Taxonomic: as observed in species that are either closely related or are distant due to the shared sequences
- Biochemical: as evidenced by the presence of epitopes in different allergens that are either identical or similar.

IMPORTANCE OF CROSS-REACTIVITY FOR THE PRACTICING ALLERGIST

Cross-reactivity is a concern because it has an influence on both allergy diagnosis and therapy. Sensitization to a plant that is not present in the patient's environment may result from exposure while traveling in another geographical location or can result from cross-reactivity with local plants. The inclusion of such pollen in immunotherapy depends on factors such as whether such addition can provide a sufficient immunological coverage. Use of cross-reactive allergens in the same immunotherapy formulation will be associated with an increase in the allergen dose administered and thereby can cause side effects.[6]

In patient management, it is of utmost importance to apply the knowledge of syndromes of cross-reactivity between inhaled allergens and food allergens. The decision on a therapeutic strategy for patients allergic to certain aeroallergens proposing avoidance of foods that possess potentially cross-reactive epitopes to these inhalant allergens should be individualized based on the risk stratification for the particular patient and with respect to the clinical cross-reactivity.[8]

CROSS-REACTIVITY AMONG POLLENS

India, a tropical country, is inhabited by a large number of plant species, which flower for most part of the year.[1]

Cross-reactivity of Tree Pollen Allergens

Studies carried out in various countries suggest cross-reactivity among various tree pollens.[1] The allergenic tree pollens are mainly derived from the families Betulaceae, Cupressaceae, Fabaceae, Fagaceae, Moraceae, Oleaceae, Pinaceae, Salicaceae subfamily: Populus, Salicaceae subfamily: Salix, Sapindaceae subfamily: Acer, and Ulmaceae. Cross-reactivity is known to exist between members of the same family; for example, silver birch (*Betula verrucosa*), European alder (*Alnus glutinosa*), hazelnut (*Corylus avellana*), and hornbeam (*Carpinus betulus*) belong to the family of Betulaceae and strongly cross-react among themselves. The Betulaceae are also known to cross-react with the family Fagaceae, which includes the trees oak and beech.[9] Among the other trees of importance in India,

- Mesquite (*Prosopis spp.*) belonging to the family Fabaceae cross-reacts with other members of the family including locust (*Robinia pseudoacacia*).[9]
- *Holoptelea integrifolia* (Indian elm) has demonstrated cross-reactivity with *Parietaria judaica*.[10]

Cross-reactivity among Grass Pollen

Grass pollens are important sensitizers in the Indian patients.[1] The allergenic grass pollens belong to the following subfamilies:[9]

- Chloridoideae
- Panicoideae
- Pooideae.

Bermuda grass (*Cynodon dactylon*) from the subfamily Chloridoideae cross-reacts with other members of Chloridoideae (such as love grass) but has limited cross-reactivity to the Pooideae grasses.[9] Similarly, grasses from the Panicoideae (Bahia, corn, and Johnson) cross-react among themselves but have limited cross-reactivity with Pooideae grasses.[9] The Pooideae grasses are known to strongly cross-react with each other. The examples of the Pooideae grasses are Kentucky bluegrass (*Poa pratensis*), ryegrass (*Lolium perenne*), timothy grass (*Phleum pratense*), and others (Flowchart 5.1).[9]

Cross-reactivity among Weed Pollen

The common allergenic weeds belong to the families Amaranthaceae (including subfamily Chenopodiaceae), Asteraceae, Plantaginaceae, Polygonaceae, and Urticaceae.[9,11]

FLOWCHART 5.1: Cross-reactivity among grasses.

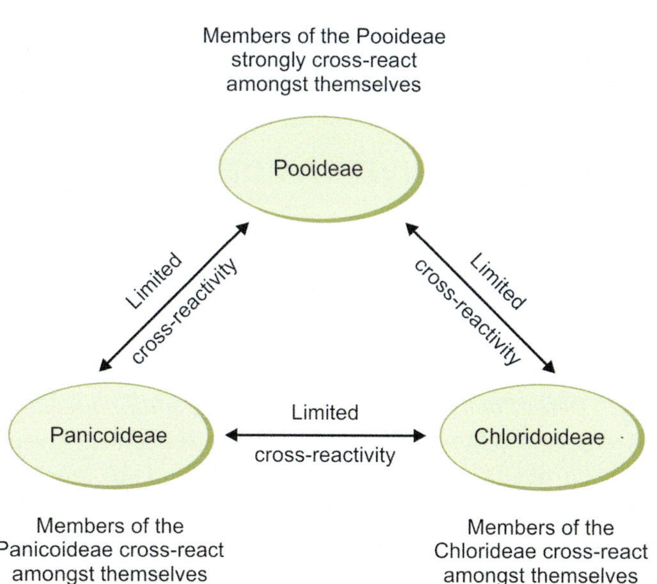

Amaranthus sp. and *Chenopodium* sp. cross-react within their genus.[9] Strong cross-allergenicity has been observed between *Artemisia* species, and it is recommended that multiple species should not be used and a single sp., e.g., *Artemisia vulgaris*, may be used as a representative.[9] Among the different families, cross-reactivity has been observed between ragweed (*Ambrosia artemisiifolia*) and feverfew (*Parthenium hysterophorus*).[9]

CROSS-REACTIVITY AMONG FUNGAL ALLERGENS

The most frequent allergenic fungi include *Alternaria alternata*, *Aspergillus fumigatus*, *Candida albicans*, *Cladosporium herbarum*, and *Penicillium notatum*. Among the patients allergic to fungal allergens, patients sensitized to *Alternaria* and *Candida* exhibit a high tendency towards monosensitization, whereas sensitizations to *Aspergillus*, *Cladosporium*, and *Penicillium* has been associated with sensitizations to other fungal allergens. The majority of the fungal allergens (except the species-specific major allergens) (e.g., A. fumigatus Asp f 1, Alt a 1, and a few others) are cross-reactive and represent or belong to different protein families.[12] Cross-reactivity in fungi can be observed between different species of one genus; for example, cross-reactivity and shared allergenicity of allergenic components are reported among the Aspergillus species *As. fumigatus*, *As. flavus*, *As. citrinum*, *As. versicolor*, and *As. niger*,[13,14] within one fungal phylum, between different fungal phyla, or in even with nonfungal allergens of different species.[15]

CROSS-REACTIVITY AMONG ARTHROPODS

Cross-reactivity among Mites

Dust mites are important sources of indoor allergens. Cross-reactivity has been reported among the house dust mite (*Dermatophagoides farinae* and *Dermatophagoides pteronyssinus*). Limited cross-reactivity has been observed between the *Dermatophagoides* species and the storage mites (such as *Acarus siro*, *Blomia tropicalis*, *Glycyphagus domesticus*, *Lepidoglyphus destructor*, and *Tyrophagus putrescentiae*).[16,17]

Table 5.1: Cross-reactivity among arthropods.

Species	*Cross-reactivity*
House dust mites (*D. pteronyssinus*, *D. farinae*)	Dermatophagoides species cross-react, but also have significant unique allergens
Storage mites (*Ac siro*, *Bl. tropicalis*, *G. domesticus*, *L. destructor*, and *T. putrescentiae*)	Storage mites have limited cross-reactivity with house dust mites
American cockroach (*Pe. americana*)	Limited cross-reactive allergens
German cockroach (*B. germanica*)	Among the cockroach species

Cross-reactivity among Insects

Allergens from insects, such as mosquitoes and cockroaches play an important role in the occurrence of respiratory diseases. Cross-reactivity in mosquitoes is not common, and allergenic components are mostly species specific.[1] In the cockroaches, *Blattella germanica* and *Periplaneta americana*, the only cross-reactive allergen is the group 1 allergen and the others are unique allergens.[1,18] Tropomyosin, an allergen, is found in cockroach and also among other insects, mites, crustaceans, mollusks, and parasites (Table 5.1).

CROSS-REACTIVITY AMONG ANIMAL DANDER

Sensitization to furry animals such as cat, dog, and other indoor animals is a known risk factor for respiratory allergic diseases.[19] Data from studies in young children have shown an association of sensitization to cat, dog, and horse dander.[20] This association can result from cosensitization or cross-reactivity. Cross-reactivity among the animal species can result from the presence of cross-reactive allergens belonging to the same protein family such as albumins and lipocalins.[21]

CROSS-REACTIVITY AMONG FOOD

Cross-reactivity also exists among food allergens. This has implications on the diagnosis and management of food allergies.[22]

Milk

Cow's milk protein allergy is among the most common food allergies. Cross-reactivity of cow's milk proteins is present in the milk of other mammals such as milk from goats, sheep, and buffalo. Milk from nonbovid mammals (mare, donkey, and camel) shows lesser cross-reactivity to cow's milk and may be tolerated by some patients (Flowchart 5.2).[22,23]

Egg

Cross-reactivity has been reported between egg proteins from different species such as chicken, duck, and goose.[22] Therefore, in egg-allergic patients, avoidance of eggs from other birds would be recommended until tolerance is proven.

Fish

Parvalbumins are responsible for extensive cross-reactivity between fish proteins from different fish families. However, the intensity and likelihood of clinical reactivity can vary. It is estimated that approximately 50% of the fish-allergic patients will react to at least one other fish species.[22] Hence, in patients with fish allergy, avoidance of other fishes should be practiced until tolerance is proven.

Shellfish

Allergy to shellfish (crustaceans and mollusks) is an important and increasing health issue in both children and adults. Cross-reactivity between shellfish species is mostly associated with the major allergen tropomyosin. Tropomyosins have a high degree of molecular homology among the different species of shellfish, which thereby translates to significant degrees of IgE cross-reactivity.[22,24]

Meat

Cross-reactivity has been documented among meat from different mammals and also among poultry meat with other birds.[22]

FLOWCHART 5.2: Cross-reactivity of cow's milk.

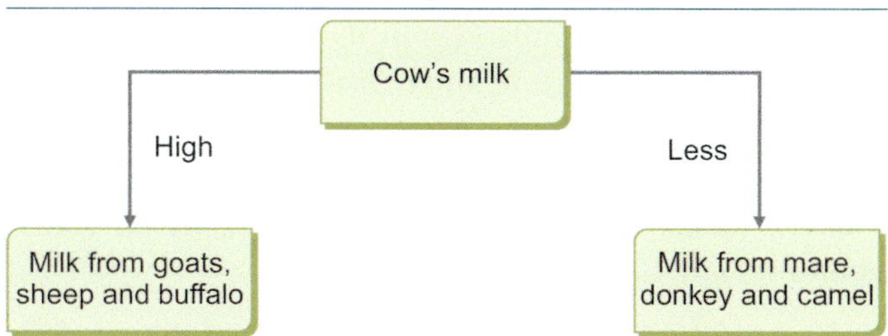

Cereals

The cereals wheat, rye, and barley demonstrate high cross-reactivity, which results from several cross-reactive proteins.[25]

Nuts and Legumes

Cross-reactivity between different nuts is frequently seen. It has been documented that 28–49% of peanut-allergic patients clinically react to another nut. Among the hard-shelled nuts, clinical cross-reactivity to more than one species is seen in one of three patients and is most common in the nuts belonging to the same taxonomic family.[22]

As with nuts, cross-reactivity is also commonly seen among the legumes. The clinical relevance would be based on the consumption in diet and also on the culprit legume.[22]

Cross-reactivity patterns among the nuts and legumes can be ascribed to the presence of homologous storage proteins such as albumins, globulins, lipid-transfer protein, oleosins, and PR-10 (pathogenesis-related (PR) proteins of class-10).[22]

Cross-Reactivity between Aeroallergens and Food Allergens

Cross-reactivity between aeroallergens and food can present with clinical symptoms spanning from oral allergy syndrome to anaphylaxis.[8] Oral allergy syndrome is the manifestation of allergic reactions localized to the oral mucosa after the consumption of certain food items that are known to be cross-reactive to aeroallergens. The usual symptoms are a sudden occurrence of pruritus, stinging pain, and vascular edema involving the oropharyngeal space. Less commonly, ear itching and throat tightness may be observed.[26]

Allergens having cross-reactivity with foods are present among the pollen allergens (trees, grasses, and weeds), fungal allergens, and animal-origin allergens.[8,24,26]

Cross-reactivity between Pollen Allergens and Food Allergens

Patients allergic to pollen often develop symptoms upon the intake of plant-derived foods, which results from cross-reactive epitopes shared by these particular pollen and food allergens.[8] These reactions are known as pollen-food syndromes and typically involve fruits and vegetables that are eaten raw.[8] The pollen-food syndrome is usually induced by allergens that are heat labile and susceptible to digestion, and thus, they are unable to induce sensitization via the gastrointestinal tract. However, these allergens can provoke reactions in patients who have been sensitized to cross-reactive aeroallergens via the respiratory tract. Furthermore, such reactions are observed mainly in adults in contrast to the common food allergy, which mainly affects young children (Flowchart 5.3).[8]

Cross-reactivity between Fungal Allergens and Food Allergens

Fungal allergens such as *Al. alternata* are known to cross-react with allergens present in spinach and mushroom.[2,8] These reactions can present within the range of oral allergy syndrome and anaphylaxis. Cases of severe reactions in fungal allergen-sensitized patients have been reported in the literature after the consumption of cross-reactive fungal allergens in food (e.g., pancakes).[27]

Cross-reactivity between Mite Allergens and Food Allergens

Tropomyosin (a panallergen) has been documented in many invertebrate species including crustaceans, mollusks, cockroaches, and mites. Many patients sensitized to shrimp show positive skin prick tests to house dust mites with or without clinical relevance (Flowchart 5.4).[8,24]

FLOWCHART 5.3: Examples of cross-reactive pollen and food allergens.

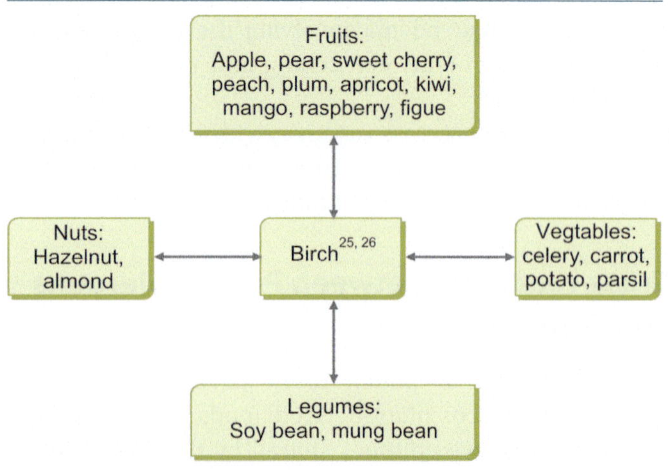

FLOWCHART 5.4: Presence of cross-reacting tropomyosin in different allergens.

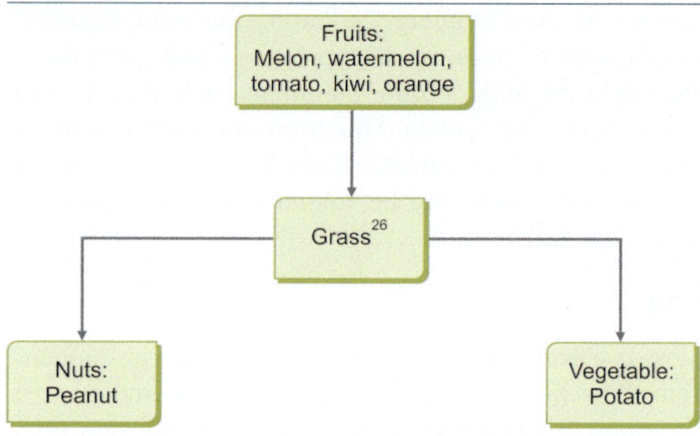

Cross-reactivity between Dander and Food Allergens

Examples of cross-reactivity between food and animal allergens include reactions to pork consumption in cat-allergic patients and reactions to egg in bird aeroallergen-sensitized patients.[2,8]

Cross-Reactivity of Latex with Aeroallergens and Food Allergens

Latex can cause adverse reactions that can be categorized as immunological and nonimmunological. Among the immunological reactions, latex can cause both type I IgE-mediated and type IV cell-mediated reactions. The latex proteins responsible for the type I or allergic reactions are known to cross-react with both aeroallergens and food allergens.[28]

Latex cross-reacts with the following aeroallergens—ragweed (Ambrosia sp.), mugwort (*Ar. vulgaris*), Kentucky bluegrass (*Po. pratensis*), timothy grass (*Ph. pratense*), oilseed rape pollens (*Brassica napus*), and weeping fig (*Ficus benjamina*). Due to similarities in their sequences, cross-reactivity with *As. fumigatus* and *C. herbarum* might occur.[29]

Latex has been documented to have cross-reacting IgE antibodies against a number of food allergens such as fruits, seeds, vegetables, herbs, legumes, wheat germ agglutinin, and breadfruit.[29]

CROSS-REACTIVITY AND THE PRINCIPLE OF HOMOLOGOUS ALLERGENS

The European Medicines Agency has published guidelines on the acceptance of the principle of homologous group of allergens as suggested by Lorenz et al.[30,31] Allergens can be grouped as homologous if they have[30]

- Comparable physicochemical and biological properties of the source material
- Cross-reactivity/structural homology of the allergens
- Identical formulation of the finished product
- Identical production process of the allergen extract and of the finished product.

As seen above, cross-reactivity is an important component used to define the homologous allergens.

Homologous groups have been defined for the house dust mites and the pollen allergens. The homologous group of house dust mites consists of the two Dermatophagoides species (*D. pteronyssinus* and *D. farinae*). In pollen, homologous groups have been defined for tree pollen, grass pollen, and weed pollen. Homologous groups have not been defined for the other aeroallergen groups (animal dander and molds/fungi), insect venom, and food allergens.[30-32]

The "Guidelines for practice of allergen immunotherapy in India: 2017—An update" have endorsed that the principles of homologous groups can guide the clinician on the strategy of monoallergen immunotherapy or mixing of allergens.[32] For the AIT treatment of polyallergic patients, no standardized guideline is in place.[31] Nevertheless, the recommendations given in a recent practice-based review was adopted in which the authors state that if the patient is allergic to allergens within a homologous group, "the use of a single course of AIT with a mixture of allergens that mimics natural exposure is recommended" (e.g., a mixture of *D. pteronyssinus* and *D. farinae* or a mixture of Pooideae grasses). A mixture of these particular species would provide the most appropriate exposure for obtaining an optimal response to allergen immunotherapy as the patient would develop sensitization to cross-reactive and species-specific allergens.[33]

If the decision is made to treat for two clinically relevant nonhomologous allergens, it would be preferable to administer them as separate AIT formulations and not mix them together.[30,33]

SUMMARY

The concept of cross-reactivity has evolved significantly over the past few decades. Knowledge about cross-reactivity patterns among aeroallergens, food allergens, and between aero and food allergens can result in appropriate management of allergic diseases.

REFERENCES

1. Singh BP, Sinha S, Arora N. Cross reactive allergens: status and their clinical implications. Indian J Allergy Asthma Immunol. 2008;22:105-18.
2. Ferreira F, Hawranek T, Gruber P, et al. Allergic cross-reactivity: From gene to the clinic. Allergy. 2004;59:243-67.
3. Migueres M, Dávila I, Frati F, et al. Types of sensitization to aeroallergens: definitions, prevalences and impact on the diagnosis and treatment of allergic respiratory disease. Clin Transl Allergy. 2014;4:16.
4. Yagami T. Allergies to cross-reactive plant proteins. Int Arch Allergy Immunol. 2002;128:271-9.
5. Schroeder HW Jr, Cavacini L. Structure and function of immunoglobulins. J Allergy Clin Immunol. 2010;125:S41-52.
6. Weber RW. Cross-reactivity of plant and animal allergens. Clin Rev Allergy Immunol. 2001;21:153-202.
7. Hauser M, Roulias A, Ferreira F, Egger M. Panallergens and their impact on the allergic patient. Allergy Asthma Clin Immunol. 2010;6:1.
8. Popescu F. Cross-reactivity between aeroallergens and food allergens. World J Methodol. 2015;5:31-50.
9. Sharma J, Singh V. Holoptelea Integrifolia: an overview. Eur J Appl Sci. 2012;4:42-6.
10. Singh AB, Khandelwal A. Cross reactive pollen allergens. In: An Atlas of Allergenically Significant Plants of India. 1st ed; 2016.
11. Weber RW. Guidelines for using pollen cross-reactivity in formulating allergen immunotherapy. J Allergy Clin Immunol. 2008;122:219-21.
12. Crameri R, Zeller S, Glaser AG, Vilhelmsson M, Rhyner C. Cross-reactivity among fungal allergens: a clinically relevant phenomenon? Mycoses. 2009;52:99-106.
13. Chou H, Lin WL, Tam MF, Wang SR, Han SH, Shen HD. Alkaline serine proteinase is a major allergen of Aspergillus flavus, a prevalent airborne Aspergillus species in the Taipei area. Int Arch Allergy Immunol. 1999;119: 282-90.
14. Verma J, Sridhara S, Singh BP, Gangal SV. Studies on shared antigenic/allergenic components among fungi. Allergy. 1995;50:811-6.
15. Simon-Nobbe B, Denk U, Pöll V, et al. The spectrum of fungal allergy. Int Arch Allergy Immunol. 2008;145:58-86.

16. Thomas WR, Smith W. House-dust-mite allergens. Allergy. 1998;53:821-32.
17. van Hage-Hamsten M, Johansson SG, Johansson E, Wiren A. Lack of allergenic cross-reactivity between storage mites and Dermatophagoides pteronyssinus. Clin Allergy. 1987;17:23-31.
18. Özdemir Ö. Cockroach allergy, respiratory allergic diseases and its immunotherapy. Int J Immunol Immunother.2014;1:1-5.
19. Bjerg A, Winberg A, Berthold M, et al. A population-based study of animal component sensitization, asthma, and rhinitis in schoolchildren. Pediatr Allergy Immunol. 2015;26:557-63.
20. Nilsson OB, Binnmyr J, Zoltowska A, et al. Characterization of the dog lipocalin allergen Can f 6: the role in cross-reactivity with cat and horse. Allergy. 2012;67:751-7.
21. Konradsen JR, Fujisawa T, van Hage M, Hedlin G. Allergy to furry animals: new insights, diagnostic approaches, and challenges. J Allergy Clin Immunol. 2015;135:616-25.
22. García BE, Lizaso MT. Cross-reactivity syndromes in food allergy. J Investig Allergol Clin Immunol. 2011;21: 162-70.
23. Martorell-Aragonés A, Echeverría-Zudaire L, Alonso-Lebrero E, et al. Position document: IgE-mediated cow's milk allergy. Allergol Immunopathol (Madr). 2015;43:507-26.
24. Faber MA, Pascal M, El Kharbouchi O, et al. Shellfish allergens: tropomyosin and beyond. Allergy. 2017;72: 842-8.
25. Matricardi PM, Kleine-Tebbe J, Hoffmann HJ, et al. EAACI molecular allergology user's guide. Pediatr Allergy Immunol. 2016;27:1-250.
26. Kondo Y, Urisu A. Oral allergy syndrome. Allergol Int. 2009;58:485-91.
27. Bennett AT, Collins KA. An unusual case of anaphylaxis. Mold in pancake mix. Am J Forensic Med Pathol. 2001;22:292-5.
28. Kahn SL, Podjasek JO, Dimitropoulos VA, Brown CW Jr. Natural rubber latex allergy. Dis Mon. 2016;62:5-17.
29. Turjanmaa K, Mäkinen-Kiljunen S. Latex allergy: prevalence, risk factors, and cross-reactivity. Methods. 2002;27:10-4. Review. Erratum in: Methods. 2003;30:106.
30. Committee for Medicinal Products for Human Use (CHMP). Guideline on allergen products: production and quality issues. EMEA/CHMP/BWP/304831/2007. http://www.ema.europa.eu/docs/en_GB/document_library/Scientific_guideline/2009/0 9/WC500003333.pdf. Accessed April 4, 2018.
31. Lorenz AR, Lüttkopf D, May S, et al. The principle of homologous groups in regulatory affairs of allergen products—A proposal. Int Arch Allergy Immunol. 2008;148:1-17.
32. Gaur SN, Kumar R, Singh AB, et al. Guidelines for practice of allergen immunotherapy in India: 2017-An update. Indian J Allergy Asthma Immunol. 2017;3-33.
33. Demoly P, Passalacqua G, Pfaar O, et al. Management of the polyallergic patient with allergy immunotherapy: a practice-based approach. Allergy Asthma Clin Immunol. 2016;12:2.

CHAPTER 6

Role of Aerobiological Monitoring in the Practice of Allergy

Shripad N Agashe, Jacob N Abraham

Aerobiology involves the study of airborne particles of plant and animal origin. These bio-particles get into the atmosphere after their release from the source. Pollen grains are bio-particles and are nature's gift to mankind. They are responsible for pollination, fertilization, fruit and seed setting, and multiplication of plants. However, if the pollen grains do not succeed in pollination, they float in the air for some time before settling down on the ground. Some of the pollens while airborne come in contact with human beings and produce allergic manifestations.

Basically, there are three ways in which pollen grains come in contact with humans. On that basis, they are classified as inhalants, ingestants, and contactants. Pollen grains enter through the nose or mouth along with the air a person breathes. They come into contact with the exposed part of human skin, eyes, and nose. In sensitive individuals, they produce allergic symptoms such as sneezing; itching of eyes, nose, and skin; breathlessness; watering of eyes; and running nose.

The primary objective of aerobiological studies is to monitor the occurrence of airborne pollen and fungal spores and their relative representation in the atmosphere. The air samples collected from the pollen traps or air-sampling devices are scanned microscopically, and the various trapped pollen grains and fungal spores are identified. The atmosphere consists of several hundred types of pollen grains and fungal spores. In applied aerobiology, only those having significance in allergy are concentrated on.

The general public, allergy patients, and medical doctors should be made aware of the occurrence of allergenically significant atmospheric pollen and fungal spores. Aerobiologists all over India have to take efforts in this direction. Such an attempt has been successfully made by us in the Aerobiology and Allergy Laboratory of the Department of Botany, Bangalore University, since 1982. For the first time in India and perhaps among developing nations, the results of weekly monitoring of pollen and fungal spores were compiled in the laboratory and published in the daily newspaper, *The Times of India*, Bangalore edition. From 1995 to 2003, our weekly monitoring results were published every Tuesday in the science supplement of the newspaper under the caption "Bangalore Pollen and Mould Watch."

A cursory glance at the *Pollen Watch* presented in the form of a pie diagram in the newspaper indicated the occurrence of significant allergenic pollen along with their relative abundance or percentage frequencies in the Bengaluru air. Such dissemination of pollen information to the mass media is of utmost use to patients suffering from pollen allergy and should be taken up by all aerobiology laboratories. It took us several years—1982 onwards—to develop the modalities and acquire the knowhow to report the results through the mass media. Patients of pollen allergy can take precautionary measures once they know the occurrence and abundance of their allergic pollen in the atmosphere through the newspaper announcements.

More than 100 different pollen types have been recorded from the Bengaluru atmosphere over the past 30 years. Of these, about six types are allergenically important, namely, *Parthenium hysterophorus*, grass, *Casuarina equisetifolia*, amaranth-chenopod, *Cocos nucifera*, and *Holoptelea integrifolia*.[1-6]

How mass media announcements of atmospheric pollen help allergy patients can be explained with the example of *H. integrifolia* pollen. There are not too many trees of *H. integrifolia* in Bengaluru. Yet, there is a significant amount of its pollen occurring regularly in the air during February and March. The onset of flowering, peak in flowering, and fruit and seed setting of *Holoptelea* take place in a matter of 2–3 weeks, either in late February or in March. The presence of *Holoptelea* pollen in the air perfectly coincides with the flowering–fruiting phenomena of the tree. If the allergenicity of *Holoptelea* pollen is proved in a patient, and as the period of occurrence of pollen in the air is known, the patient can take precautionary measures. The patient can avoid getting into contact with the pollen by staying indoors as far as possible. However, a far more pragmatic and better approach would be to take their preseasonal or coseasonal immunotherapy shots with the offending pollen antigens and lead a fairly allergy-free life.

REFERENCES

1. Agashe SN, Abraham JN. Pollen calendar of Bangalore city. Part I. Indian J Aerobiol. 1988;1:35-8.
2. Agashe SN, Abraham JN. Pollen calendar of Bangalore city. Part II. J Palynol. 1990–1991;1990–1991:297-304.
3. Agashe SN, Mathew B. Seasonal periodicity pf predominant pollen in the Bangalore atmosphere. Indian J Aerobiol. 1998;11:16-8.
4. Agash SN, Anuradha HG, Scinthia, JDM. Atmospheric pollen scenario in Bangalore during the past 15 years (1982–1997). Indian J Aerobiol. 1999;12:30-2.
5. Mridula PA. *Aeropalynological Survey of Rajajinagar, Bangalore for Studies on Pollen Allergy* [MPhil dissertation], Tiruchirapalli, Tamil Nadu: Bharathidasan University; 2007.
6. Mridula PA, Mahesh PA, Abraham JN, et al. *Dolichandrone platycalyx*: new entomophilous Pollen—a report on pollen sensitization in allergic individuals. Am J Rhinol Allergy. 2011;25:e34-8.

CHAPTER 7

Significance of Pollen Calendar in Management of Allergy

Asha Khandelwal, Rajendra Prasad

INTRODUCTION

The importance of aerobiological researches in the diagnosis of respiratory diseases has been well documented. Airborne particles of biological origin are a matter of concern to both aerobiologists and allergists. Airborne dust and its particles, which include pollen grains and fungal spores, animal danders, mites, and other allergens in indoor air, are the major sources of allergic reaction. They enter into the respiratory tract of a human being and trigger a hypersensitive reaction, which is manifested in the form of allergic rhinitis, bronchial asthma, atopic dermatitis and eczema, and gastrointestinal and autoimmune diseases. Asthma, eczema, and hay fever (allergic rhinitis) are the commonly known allergic diseases, though frequent sneezing, rhinorrhea, cough, breathlessness, and dermatitis are also classified under this group. A housewife may suffer from a bout of sneeze accompanied by itchy nose, headache, and cough with difficult breathing (asthma) during or immediately after cooking or dusting of the house. A man may develop nasal symptoms (rhinitis) or breathlessness (asthma) during or immediately after lawn mowing. There are certain environmental factors that can aggravate the symptoms of allergic rhinitis. In our modern lifestyle, tightly sealed houses, wall-to-wall carpeting, and air-conditioning provide an optional environment for certain allergens to grow and proliferate.

Pollen grains are important aeroallergens that are extensively studied for the diagnosis of respiratory allergies. The rapid industrialization and urbanization have increased the risk of allergic disorders. The uninhibited planting of exotic trees has also contributed much to the pollen load of the atmosphere. Airborne pollen grains are produced in enormous numbers and are generally in the size range of 20–40 μ. During a certain period of the year, when many plants are flowering and shedding their pollen, the air contains a huge amount of diverse mixture of pollen in the form of atmospheric plankton. The allergic sufferers know that the allergy is seasonal depending upon prevailing weather conditions, so that some days will be worse than the others. Illustrative pollen calendars provide instant information on airborne pollen allergens and their precise seasons, namely, beginning, peak, and end of the season. This kind of information is of paramount importance in effective diagnosis and therapeutic management of disease. To adapt an avoidance strategy toward plant allergen, it is very essential to identify the plant and know its flowering period. Unfortunately, most of the allergenic plants are difficult to be identified by the patients and physicians as it is a specialized job of a taxonomist/palynologist. Hence, an attempt has been made to provide aerobiological and phonological details of some of the allergenic plants such as *Argemone mexicana* (Satyanashi), *Amaranthus spinosus* (Katevali chauli), *Holoptelea integrifolia* (Chilbil), *Prosopis juliflora* (Kabuli keekar), *Ricinus communis* (Arandi), *Parthenium hysterophorus* (Congress grass), and *Putranjiva roxburghii* (Putranjva).

AEROBIOLOGICAL STUDIES

Aerobiology has been used as a discipline and a tool for other disciplines such as medicine (allergology—both human and animal diseases, immunology, and occupational hygiene), agriculture (plant pathology, pest management, arthropod dispersal), forestry and gene ecology, meteorology, climatology, biometeorology, microbiology, biodeterioration, indoor air quality, air pollution, industrial aerobiology, cultural heritage, and palaeobotany. *Aerobiology* embodies the study of various biological particulates present in the atmosphere. These aerobiopollutants occur in varying concentrations depending upon the climatic factors, height from the ground level, location (outdoor and indoor), altitude, and proximity to the source.

Aerobiological investigations are broadly distinguished as outdoor or extramural aerobiology and indoor or intramural aerobiology. The study of aerobioparticles in closed system such as buildings, hospitals, libraries, and museums is known as *indoor aerobiology*; whereas *outdoor aerobiology* is concerned with the survey of biological materials in open spaces such as crop fields and forests.

Pollen and Pollen Allergy

Allergy is defined as a hypersensitive reaction in the body of a person from a substance that normally does not cause any harm to normal persons. The aeroallergens include several microorganic entities, such as pollen, spore, bacteria, virus, small insect animal fluff, plant fragments, and other microscopic particles of biological origin, which may spark off allergic reactions in people who may show sensitivity to these things. The symptoms induced by pollen grains, such as sneezing, runny nose, nasal congestion, itching of the nose, and red itchy eyes, are termed as *pollinosis, pollen allergy,* or *hay fever*. Interestingly, there is no role of either hay or fever in hay fever. This is typically caused by an allergy to pollen of grasses, trees, or weeds. It is one of the most common chronic diseases.

The signs and symptoms of pollen allergy are as follows:

- Sneezing, the most common, may be accompanied by a runny or clogged nose.
- Itching eyes, nose, and throat.
- Allergic shiners (dark circles under the eyes caused by restricted blood flow near the sinuses).
- Allergic salute (in a child, persistent upward rubbing of the nose that causes a crease mark on the nose).
- Conjunctivitis (an inflammation of the membrane that lines the eyelids, causing red-rimmed eyes).

Aeropalynology is the study of airborne pollen grains and spores of plants. Pollen grains, the male reproductive units of the flowering plants, are microscopic. The individual grain usually consists of a single cell, which is enclosed within an inner wall called intine and an outer wall called exine. The exine is extraordinarily resistant to chemical reagents. These are easily observable and form useful diagnostic criteria for pollen grains and spores. The variation in pollen morphological characters helps academicians in the classification of plant taxa and assessment of their phylogenetic relationship.

Hay fever-causing pollen grains are small and light enough to be carried by the air, and so most of the offenders are wind-pollinated plants, such as grasses and trees with catkin-like flowers. They are disseminated by various agencies, such as wind, water, insects, and animals. Although many kinds of pollen can provoke symptoms if an allergic person is exposed to them; in practice, it is pollen from trees and grasses that causes asthmatics the most problems. Unlike brightly colored and sweet-smelling flowers, which attract insects to pollinate them, some of the trees and most of the grasses rely on the wind to carry their pollen to other members of their species. The flowers of wind-pollinated plants are generally inconspicuous, and most of the allergenic plants are difficult to be identified by the patients and physicians, as it is a specialized job of a plant taxonomist. The amount of pollen production is also high in wind-pollinated plants. For example, *H. integrifolia* produces 6,000–15,000 pollens per anther of a flower. Therefore, the figure of pollen production by a *Holoptelea* tree remains uncountable. It was suggested that roadside plantation of *H. integrifolia* should be discouraged because of its pollen allergenicity.[1]

Entomophilous pollen grains are generally caught in low frequency but sometimes have high allergenic potentiality. The aerial incidences of such pollen grains are due to either proximity of the sampler to the source or favorable high wind velocity. Sometimes pollen grains are attached to the body of insects and get detached during flight schedule of insects and thus become airborne. Some plants that are normally pollinated by insects have pollen sufficiently small to become airborne and cause hay fever. Many such species, both anemophilous and entomophilous, have been caught from the air in Lucknow.

Proteins and glycoproteins of pollen grains are responsible for the manifestation of allergic reaction. Antibodies are proteinaceous molecules produced in response to a foreign body, which is termed as antigen. The allergens (such as pollen and fungal spores) when taken up from the air either through inhalation or via food cause hypersensitive reactions with antibody, causing allergy. The allergic reaction starts when pollen or some other allergen is inhaled for the first time. The immune system responds by producing Y-shaped antibodies called immunoglobulin E (IgE), which attach themselves to mast cells lining the lungs, throat, and nose. On the second-time exposure to pollen, they bind to the preinduced IgE molecules on the mast cells. These mast cells react by producing histamines and other chemicals giving common symptoms of allergic reactions, such as frequent sneezing, skin rashes, wheezing, and asthmatic breathing.

Air Monitoring

Efficient and reliable monitoring is a prerequisite for any kind of aerobiological surveys. Airborne particles of biological origin are a matter of major concern to aerobiologists, in general, and allergists, in particular, for correct diagnosis and treatment of allergic disorders. In recent studies, three internationally recognized and recommended apparatuses, namely, Andersen two-stage sampler, Burkard personal sampler, and Rotorod impaction sampler received in All India Coordinated Project entitled "Aeroallergens and Human Health: Aerobiological Studies" coordinated by Dr AB Singh, Institute of Genomics and Integrative Biology, Delhi, were employed for recording the qualitative and quantitative abundance of aerobiota in different places of Lucknow city and around. This methodology has advanced the knowledge of aerobiota in two ways: first, by adding a few more new taxa in the list and second, by exhibiting the amount of recorded taxa in a definite volume of air at a particular time. The data, thus, generated have proved to be more meaningful than those of the earlier records obtained at Lucknow and from some other parts of the country based upon the quantitative estimates only. By using these volumetric air samplers, both the quantitative and qualitative incidences of aerobiota have been recorded, which have, undoubtedly, enhanced the ambit of aerobiology in general and pollen allergy in particular (Fig. 7.1).

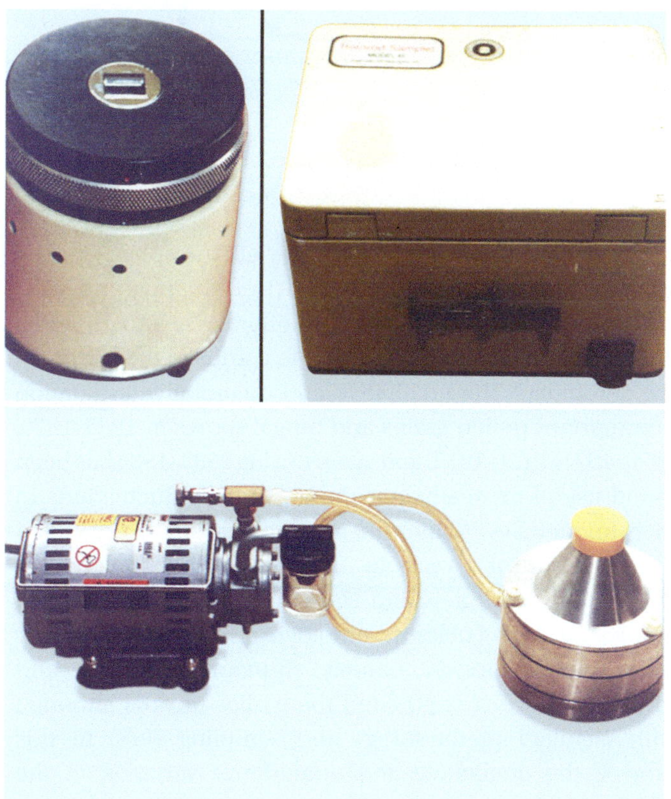

Fig. 7.1: Air samplers.

Identification and Counting of Pollen Grains

The prerequisite of aerobiological studies is collection of polleniferous material and preparation of pollen reference slides. For that purpose, the first step is frequent field trips to collect the botanical details of various plants of the study area. A list of all flowering plants in relation to their mode of pollination, frequency, distribution, habit and habitat, and phenology is prepared. The plants collected are preserved in the form of herbarium, and anthers are stored in small vials containing acetic acid. Reference pollen slides are prepared by the method suggested by Wodehouse[2] in which fresh pollen is treated with alcohol, stained with safranin, and mounted in glycerine jelly. The permanent reference slides prepared are also prepared simultaneously by the acetolysis technique.[3] The identification of atmospheric pollen grains is done by comparing them with the corresponding pollen in the reference collection. The shape, size, kind, and distribution of apertures and various patterns of ornamentation of pollen grains are the chief characters employed for the identification of atmospheric pollen grains. To facilitate the identification of the atmospheric pollen grains, the comprehensive study of pollen morphology of anemophilous and the common entomophilous plant species distributed in the Lucknow district are thoroughly studied. A workable pollen key of common plants was prepared for ready references.[4] The counting of pollen from an exposed slide is accomplished by examining a slide under microscope in narrow horizontal traverses across the width of slide until the entire surface of the slide has been covered. It is possible to identify most of the atmospheric pollen to specific, generic, or familial rank. Reference to the flowering periods too sometimes helps in specific identification. Because of the great degree of similarity, the pollen grains are grouped together under the natural order Poaceae, Amaranthaceae, Asteraceae, Brassicaceae, Chenopodiaceae, etc. The daily counts of atmospheric pollen grains are recorded on tally sheets having date, time, and duration of exposure. The monthly and annual charts were then prepared from data on these tally sheets, where the number of pollen grains is shown along the vertical axis, and dates and months along the horizontal axis (Fig. 7.2).

The daily pollen concentrations are highly dependent on the meteorological conditions. The dry, warm, and sunny weather is favorable for high pollen concentrations. On the contrary, cloudy and rainy weather will cause low pollen concentration as the release of pollen will be minimized, and also a washout of pollen in the air windy and turbulent conditions will cause large dispersion of pollen and low concentration. The pollen calendar shows

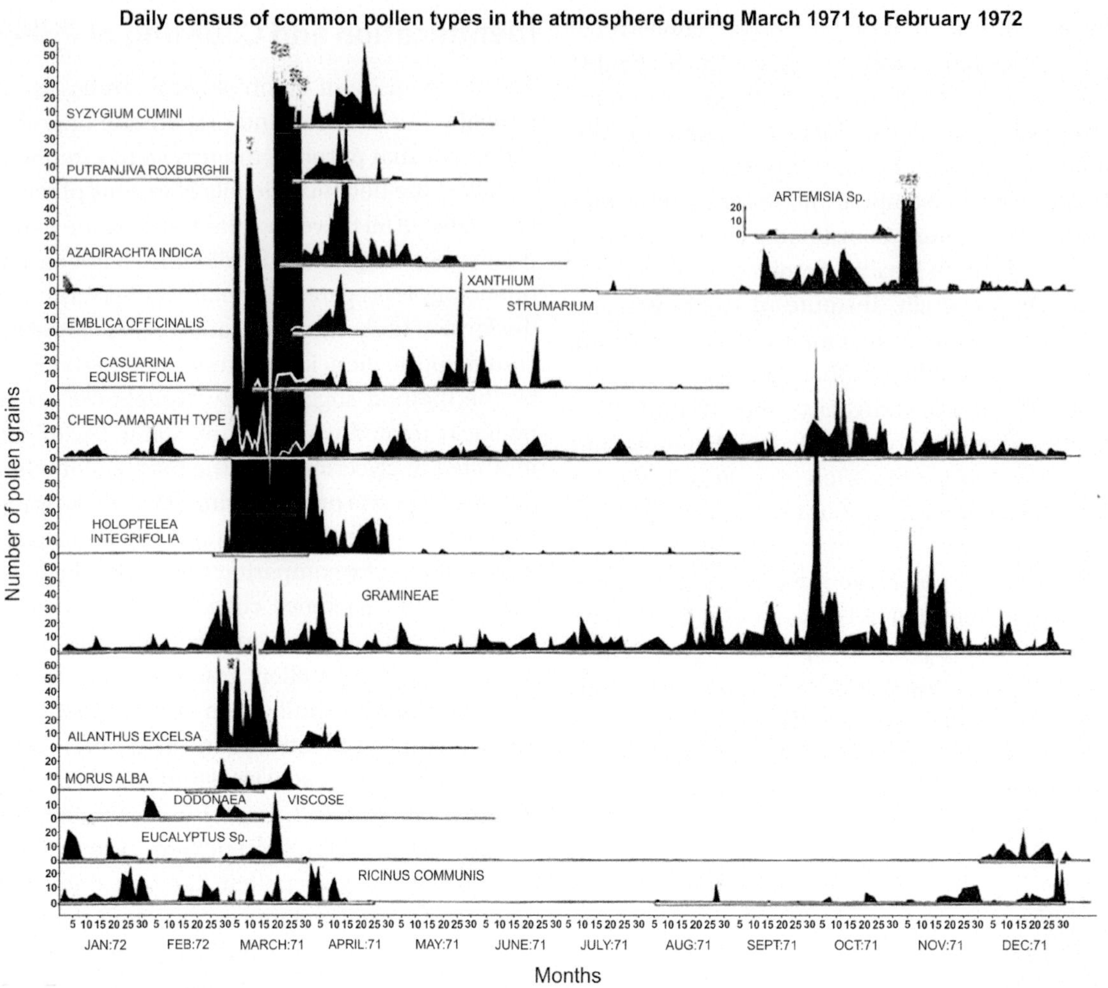

Fig. 7.2: Annual pollen calendar during March 1971–February 1972 exhibiting dominant plant taxa.

the distribution of important pollen types through the year. It shall be emphasized that the yearly pollen variations can be large concerning short length and strength of pollen seasons. It may differ from year to year depending on the weather and on biological factors.

Pollen Calendars

The pollen spore calendars are useful in identifying allergies against particular airborne pollen and fungal spore types. However, the limitation of pollen calendar is the occurrence of year-to-year variation in both the number and the time of appearance of each type of pollen grains and fungal spores. Several pollen calendars have been prepared in the past six decades from Lucknow by different workers. Birbal Sahni Institute of Palaeobotany (BSIP), Lucknow, has generated an important dataset to identify the specific aeroallergen at both regional and local scales. The survey of atmospheric pollen grains at BSIP was earlier carried out by Lakhanpal and Nair.[5] In 1969, the analysis of aeromycoflora was incorporated along with pollen studies in order to complete the picture of the aerobiota.[1] The qualitative and quantitative evaluation of important pollen grains and fungal spores in 1969–1970, 1970–1971, 1971–1972, and again during 1983–1986 has been found useful for ready assessment of daily fluctuations in their frequencies.[4,6] Later on, aerobiological data generated over a period of 4 years in All India Coordinated Project entitled "Aeroallergens and Human Health: Aerobiological Studies" at BSIP, Lucknow, employing three internationally recognized samplers, namely, Burkard, Rotorod, and Andersen, have strengthened the earlier records although with changed methodology and sampling sites. In this project, the qualitative and quantitative variation in the number and composition of airspora has been recorded from both urban and suburban areas of Lucknow. However, the pollen grains of family Poaceae were found dominant almost from all the investigated sites. Codominance was recorded by pollen grains of families Chenopodiaceae/Amaranthaceae. Overall, three following periods were recognized:

- Spring and early summer (February–May)—when arboreal pollen grains charge the atmosphere.
- Late summer and rainy seasons (June–September)—when pollen grains of grasses and weeds abound.
- Late rainy season and winter (October–January)—when pollen grains of both wild and cultivated grasses predominate.

Overall, the emphasis has been laid for continuous periodical monitoring at different sites in a given area in order to provide specific zonal data to local clinicians/allergists.[7,8] Besides BSIP, a 2-year (1980–1981) survey of airborne pollen was carried out in the National Botanical Research Institute, Lucknow.[9] Thus, The palynological dataset obtained in the last five decades is being successfully utilized as a "ready reckoner" for periodic biopollutant predictions required for the treatment of allergic disorders in general and allergic rhinitis in particular.

Aeroallergenic Pollen Grains of Lucknow

The first systematic aerobiological work in India was pioneered in Calcutta by Cunningham.[10] Later on, two important centers SMS Medical College at Jaipur and Vallabhbhai Patel Chest Institute at Delhi initiated the aerobiological investigation with a particular emphasis on clinical relevance of airborne pollen. Now the aerobiological studies have their own national network at many centers in the states such as Kolkata, Bengaluru, Gwalior, Chennai, Hyderabad, Imphal, Gorakhpur, Pune, Aurangabad, Delhi, Nagpur, and Lucknow.

The clinical investigation carried out so far in King George Medical University, Lucknow, has proved the allergenicity of many pollen grains present in the air of Lucknow.[4,11] Some of the proved aeroallergens are *Alstonia scholaris, Ailanthus excelsa* (Urru), *A. mexicana* (Satyanashi), *A. spinosus* (Katevali chauli), *Azadirachta indica, Cannabis sativa, Chenopodium album, Cynodon dactylon, Cyperus rotundus, H. integrifolia* (Chilbil), *Morus alba* (Shahtoot), *P. juliflora* (Kabuli keekar), *R. communis* (Arandi), *Xanthium strumarium* (Chhota gokhru), *P. hysterophorus* (Congress grass), and *P. roxburghii* (Putranjva). Again, during the period 1995–1999, the allergy tests were performed on 108 patients of bronchial asthma.[12] In this investigation, 32 pollen allergens were employed for skin testing such as *Cyperus, Cynodon, Lawsonia, Eucalyptus, Holoptelea, Brassica, Melia, Xanthium, Putranjiva, Prosopis, Zea mays, Amaranthus, Parthenium, Azadirachta, Gynandropsis, Rumex, Chenopodium murale, Cenchrus, Ageratum, Ricinus, Cassia, Imperata, Adhatoda, Ailanthus, Sorghum, Morus, C. album, Cannabis, Argemone, Typha, Pennisetum,* and *Dodonaea.* The skin sensitivity to these pollen antigens varied from zero to 18.5%. High incidence of positive skin reactions (2+ to 4+) was shown by *Cyperus, Cynodon, Lawsonia, Eucalyptus, Holoptelea, Brassica,* and *Melia,* whereas *Typha, Pennisetum,* and *Dodonaea* did not show markedly positive skin reactions. Besides the role of intact pollen grains, microaerosols originating from the same or different taxa contributing toward total allergenic load are yet to be thoroughly studied.

Pollen Forecast

A reliable pollen forecast has a great significance for pollen allergic individuals as they can take steps to avoid exposure or premedicate as necessary. The forecast is performed by the meteorologist in collaboration with the aerobiological who is counting the pollen. The pollen forecast gives the average concentration for the following day and is expressed in three levels (few, moderate, and high). Prediction of pollen concentrations needs profound knowledge of the production of pollen, potentially of pollen available at a given time, as well as details regarding its release, dispersion, and deposition. The process is primarily based on the measured pollen concentration and the weather forecast with a special focus on the maximum temperature, sunshine coverage, and precipitation. There is considerable interest in the ability to predict the onset and severity of the pollen season and to predict the pollen count for the following days. Katelaris et al.[13] developed a model to forecast the next day's pollen count after examination of a number of variables. This model uses the predicted maximum temperature and the previous day's total pollen count as the input variables for a computer-generated program.[14,15]

Aerobiological and Phenological Details of Common Allergenic Plants

Plant details pertaining to their family, local name, habit, distribution, phenology, pollen incidence in the air of Lucknow and other parts of the country, pollination period, pollen morphology, and allergenic significance are listed here.

Amaranthus spinosus Linn.

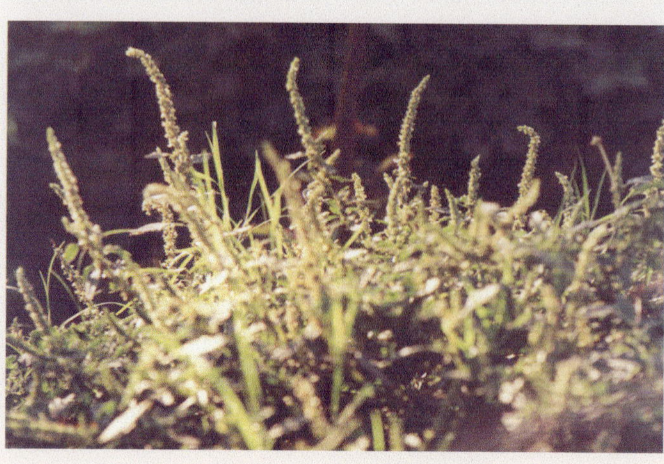

Family	*Amaranthaceae*
Local name	Kantevali chulai
Distribution and phenology	Common in open, waste places becoming gregarious at some spots. An erect, spinous herb or undershrub. Spines, sharp, straight. Leaves ovate or lanceolate, spine tipped. Flowers green, unisexual, in dense clusters. Male flowers with five stamens.
Flowering period and mode of pollination	Throughout the year/anemophilous
Pollen peak and percentage in annual pollen calendars of Lucknow	March–April, 6.7–12.5%
Aerial incidence in other parts of the country	Agra, Aurangabad, Balrampur, Bengaluru, Bikaner, Calicut, Delhi, Gulbarga, Gwalior, Imphal, Jaipur, Jabalpur, Kanpur, Mumbai, Secunderabad, Trivandrum, Visakhapatnam
Pollen morphology	Pollen grains panporate, spheroidal, 30 µ. Pores circular, 1.5 µ, 40–45 in no. Exine 2.5 µ thick, sexine thicker than nexine, granulate, tegillate. (Generally palynologists count such pollen under amaranth/chenopod type.)
Allergenic significance	Allergenic

Argemone mexicana Linn.

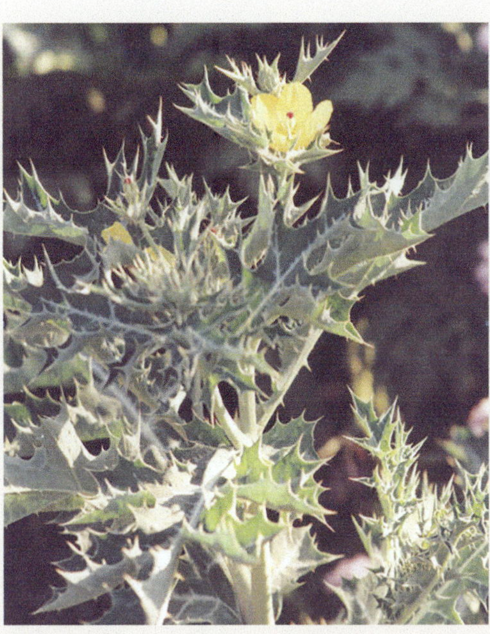

Family	*Papaveraceae*
Local name	Satyanashi, Peeli kateli
Distribution and phenology	Common in waste places, fallow fields, and along roadside. A robust herb. Leaves glaucous, prickly, sinuate-pinnatifid. Flowers yellow.
Flowering period and mode of pollination	October–April, anemophilous
Pollen peak and percentage in annual pollen calendars of Lucknow	February, 0.13–0.58%
Aerial incidence in other parts of the country	Agra, Bengaluru, Balrampur, Bhopal, Bikaner, Delhi, Gorakhpur, Gulbarga, Gwalior, Hyderabad, Jabalpur, Kanpur, Kolkata, Mysore, Nagpur, Waltair
Pollen morphology	Pollen grains (3-4 colpate), prolate spheroidal, 39 × 38 µ. Colpi long, broad, margins thickened, apices obtuse. Exine 3 µ, sexine as thick as nexine, finely reticulate, tegillate.
Allergenic significance	Significantly allergenic

Azadirachta indica A. Juss.

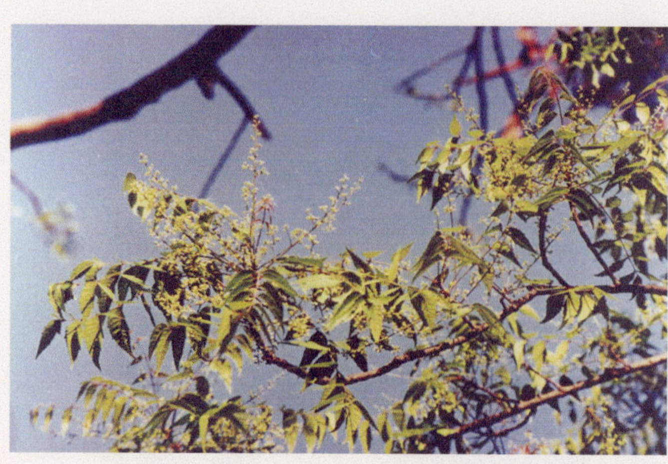

Family	*Meliaceae*
Local name	Neem
Distribution and phenology	A common roadside large tree. Leaves 20–30 cm long, crowded near the end of the branches, pinnate. Flowers white, scented.
Flowering period and mode of pollination	March–May, anemophilous/entomophilous
Pollen peak and percentage in annual pollen calendars of Lucknow	April, 0.78–3.6%
Aerial incidence in other parts of the country	Agra, Aurangabad, Bhopal, Balrampur, Calicut, Delhi, Gulbarga, Gwalior, Hyderabad, Imphal, Jaipur, Jabalpur, Kanpur, Kolhapur, Kolkata, Mysuru, Pune, Tirupati, Mumbai, Nagpur, Secunderabad, Tiruchirapalli
Pollen morphology	Pollen grains 4–5 zonocolporate, subprolate 60–65 × 48–50 μ. Colpi long and margins thickened. Os lalongate. Exine 3.8 μ thick, Sexine as thick as nexine, faintly reticulate, tegillate.
Allergenic significance	Highly allergenic

Brassica campestris Linn. var. *sarson* Prain

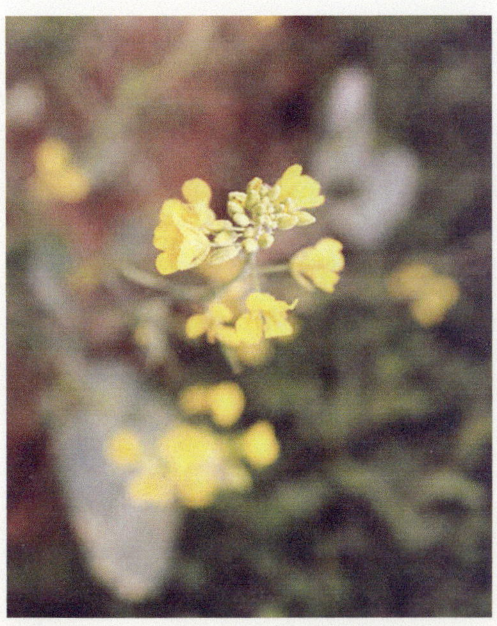

Family	*Brassicaceae*
Local name	Peeli Sarson
Distribution and phenology	An erect, annual herb. Lower leaves large lyrately pinnatifid, upper smaller. Flower bright yellow in corymbs elongating into racemes. Seeds yellow.
Flowering period and mode of pollination	January–March, anemophilous/entomophilous
Pollen peak and percentage in annual pollen calendars of Lucknow	February, 0.72–1.5%
Aerial incidence in other parts of the country	Agra, Aurangabad, Balrampur, Delhi, Gorakhpur, Imphal, Kanpur, Kolkata, Modinagar, Nagpur, Secunderabad
Pollen morphology	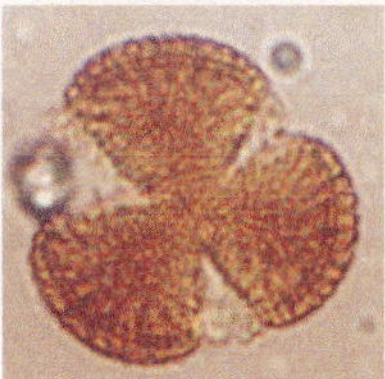 Pollen grains 3-colpate, subprolate, 34 × 30 μ. Colpi broad. Exine 2.5 μ thick, retipilate, nontegillate. (Generally palynologists count such pollen under Brassicaceae.)
Allergenic significance	Highly allergenic

Cannabis sativa Linn.

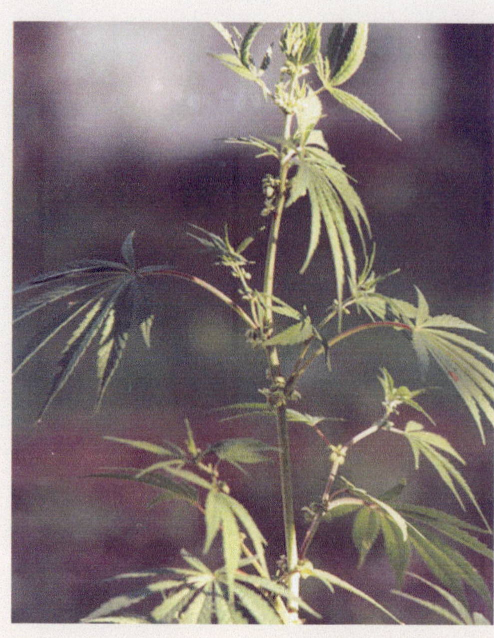

Family	*Cannabaceae*
Local name	Bhang
Distribution and phenology	Common in waste grounds, often becoming gregarious along the edges of fields and irrigation channels of gardens. A herbaceous or shrubby, smelling, annual plant. Leaves 3–8 foliate, long-petioled; lobes lanceolate. Flowers dioecious. Male plants flowers in axillary short panicle cymes. Female plants flower crowded with leafy bracts.
Flowering period and mode of pollination	All throughout the year mainly in February–April, anemophilous
Pollen peak and percentage in annual pollen calendars of Lucknow	March, 0.19–1.27%
Pollen morphology	Pollen grains 3–5 porate, spheroidal, 20–50 µ. Pores circular, 3 µ, annulate. Globally distributed. Exine 1.4 µ thick, sexine as thick as nexine, finely. Granulate, tegillate.
Allergenic significance	Allergenic

Chenopodium album Linn.

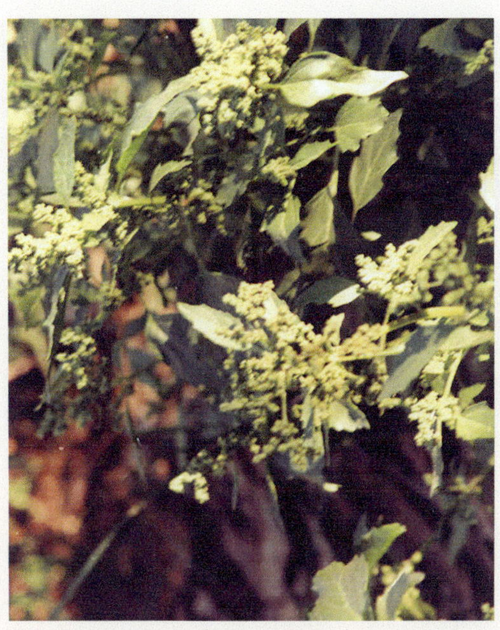

Family	*Chenopodiaceae*
Local name	Bathua
Distribution and phenology	A common weed of wheat crop, on soils of ancient buildings and cultivated grounds. An erect herb coated with white, mealy, granular pubescences. Leaves variable in size, entire, toothed, or lobed. Flowers in terminal and axillary clusters.
Flowering period and mode of pollination	October–March/anemophilous
Pollen peak and percentage in annual pollen calendars of Lucknow	February, 6.75–12.56%
Aerial incidence in other parts of the country	Aurangabad, Bengaluru, Bombay, Delhi, Gaya, Gorakhpur, Gulbarga, Gwalior, Hyderabad, Imphal, Jabalpur, Jaipur, Kanpur, Kolkata, Nagpur, Pune, Shillong, Tirupati
Pollen morphology	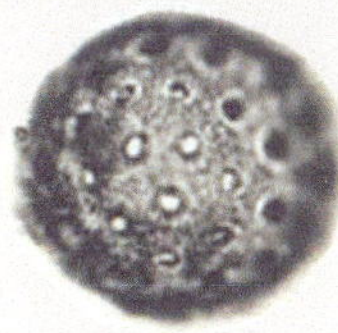 Pollen grains panporate, spheroidal, 18–30 μ. Exine 2 μ thick, sexine and nexine almost equally thick, granulate, tegillate. (Generally palynologists count such pollen under Chenopodiaceae.)
Allergenic significance	Significantly allergenic

Cynodon dactylon Pers.

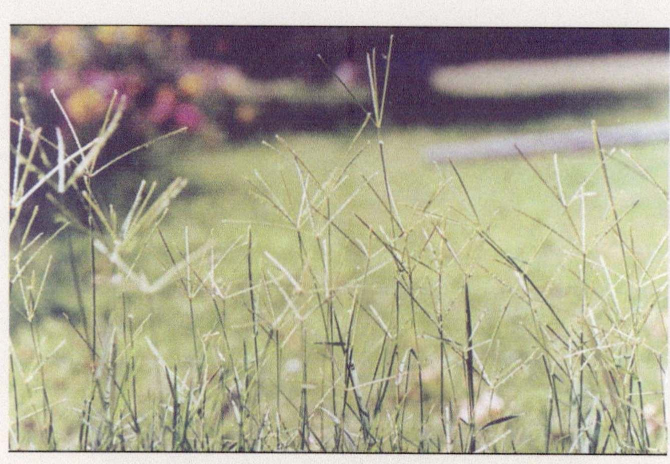

Family	*Poaceae*
Local name	Doob
Distribution and phenology	A perennial grass with an extensively creeping base. Common and abundant, forming a carpet in lawns. Leaves linear, acuminate, spikes 4–5 digitate, arcuate spreading, green or purplish.
Flowering period and mode of pollination	Abundant throughout the year but mainly during July–December, anemophilous
Pollen peak and percentage in annual pollen calendars of Lucknow	August/September/October, 15.1–34.6%
Aerial incidence in other parts of the country	Reported from all over the country
Pollen morphology	Pollen grains monoporate, spheroidal, 30.5 μ. Pores annulate. Exine 2 μm, sexine slightly thicker than nexine, faintly granulate, tegillate. (Generally palynologists count such pollen under Poaceae.)
Allergenic significance	Allergenic

Cyperus rotundus Linn.

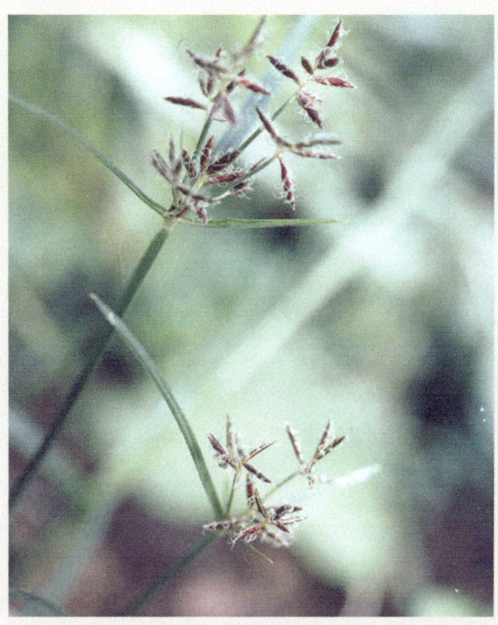

Family	*Cyperaceae*
Local name	Motha ghas
Distribution and phenology	Plants are very common on the margins of the pond and banks of the rivers and marshy places.
Flowering period and mode of pollination	Throughout the year mainly after rains
Pollen peak and percentage in annual pollen calendars of Lucknow	Insignificant, 0.58–1.9%
Aerial incidence in other parts of the country	Bengaluru, Delhi, Gulbarga, Imphal, Jabalpur, Jaipur, Kanpur, Kolkata, Meerut, Nagpur, Pune, Tiruchirapalli, Waltair
Pollen morphology	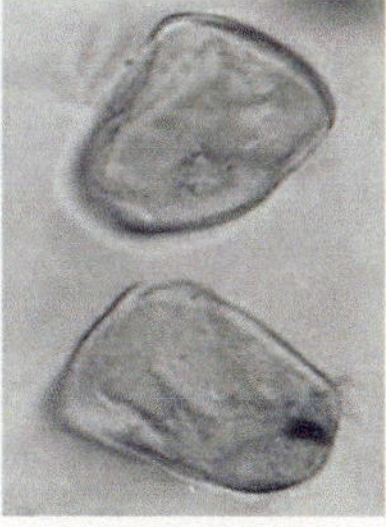 Pollen grains pear shaped, 45 × 35 μ, 1-ulceroidate and with 3 longitudinal culpoid streaks on the lateral sides. Exine 1.5 μ thick, sexine slightly thicker than nexine, granulate. (Generally palynologists count such pollen under Cyperaceae.)
Allergenic significance	Allergenic

Eucalyptus citriodora Hook.

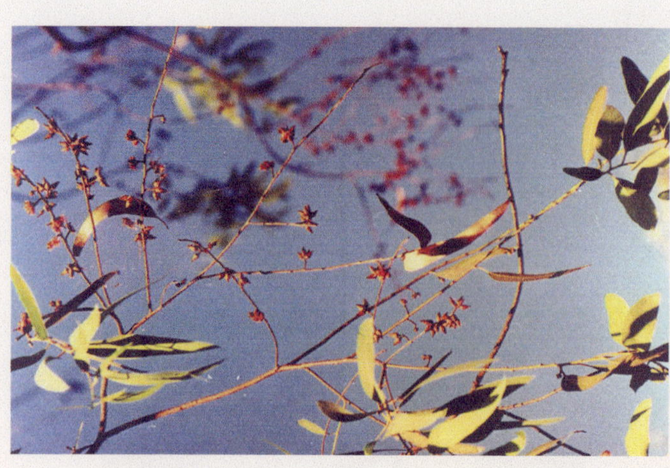

Family	*Myrtaceae*
Local name	Eucalyptus
Distribution and phenology	Commonly planted as roadside tree. A tall, handsome tree. Bark shining, whitish or reddish-gray. Leaves lanceolate, 15–20 cm long, scented. Flowers in white, small, in 3 or many short panicles. Stamens 30–35, inflexed in bud.
Flowering period and mode of pollination	December–May, anemophilous/entomophilous
Pollen peak and percentage in annual pollen calendars of Lucknow	January, 0.26–3.2%
Aerial incidence in other parts of the country	Balrampur, Berhampur, Calicut, Delhi, Gulbarga, Gwalior, Imphal, Jabalpur, Kodaikanal, Meerut, Nagpur, Thoubal, Tiruchirapalli, Trivandrum, Visakhapatnam
Pollen morphology	Pollen grains 3-colporate, parasyncolpate triangular in polar view, oblate, 11 × 18 μ. Exine 1.4 μ thick, psilate. (Generally palynologists count such pollen under Myrtaceae.)
Allergenic significance	Allergenic

Holoptelea integrifolia Planch.

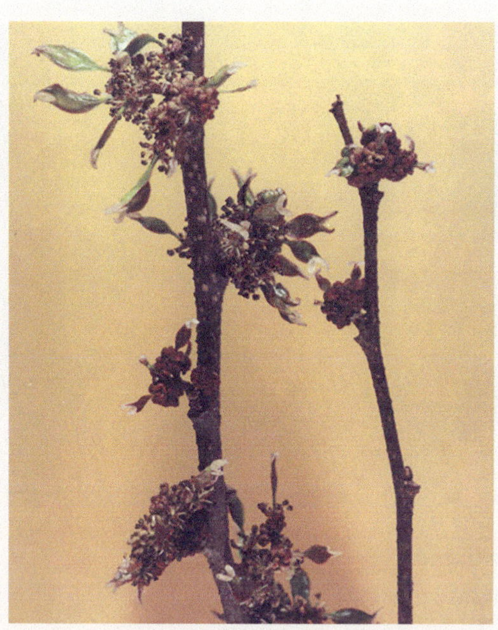

Family	*Ulmaceae*
Local name	Chilbil
Distribution and phenology	Roadside tree. A large, deciduous tree, bark gray. Leaves broad, ovoid, acuminate, subcoriaceous. Flowers green, in numerous fascicles on the leafless branches.
Flowering period and mode of pollination	February–March, anemophilous
Pollen peak and percentage in annual pollen calendars of Lucknow	First week of March, 13.0–39.7%
Aerial incidence in other parts of the country	Aurangabad, Bengaluru, Delhi, Gwalior, Hyderabad Jabalpur, Jaipur, Kanpur, Mumbai, Secunderabad, Visakhapatnam
Pollen morphology	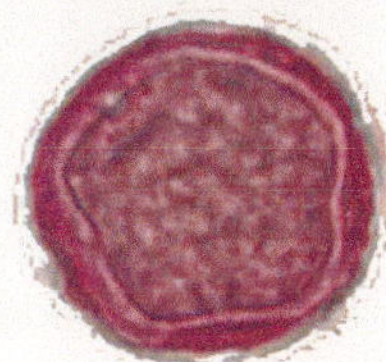 Grains 4–6 porate, spheroidal, to suboblate, 22 × 27 μ to 27 × 33 μ (average 27.1 × 33.1 μ), pores more or less circular with a diameter of about 2.3–3.7 μ. Exine about 1.5 μm thick, sexine with small irregular ridges separated by small spaces, sexine thicker than nexine.
Allergenic significance	Allergenic

Parthenium hysterophorus Linn.

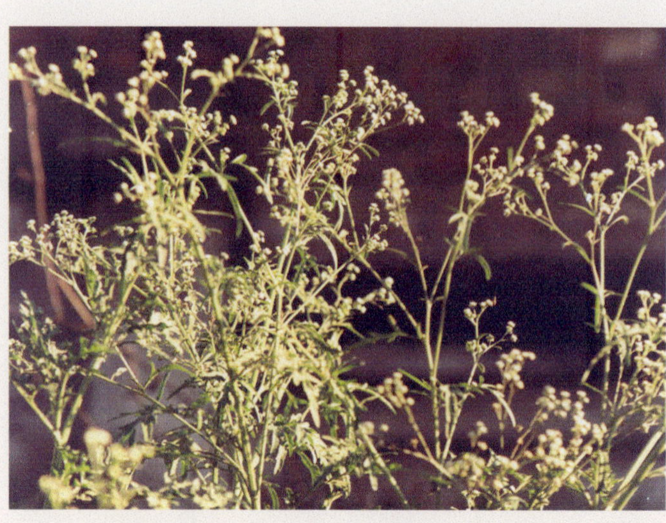

Family	*Asteraceae*
Local name	Congress grass
Distribution and phenology	Common in waste places along roadside and near habitation, often gregarious. A scabrous, erect herb with greenish yellow flowers.
Flowering period and mode of pollination	Almost all throughout the year, anemophilous/entomophilous.
Pollen peak and percentage in annual pollen calendars of Lucknow	September–October, 0.40–1.40%
Aerial incidence in other parts of the country	Agra, Aurangabad, Bengaluru, Bombay, Delhi, Gulberga, Hyderabad, Jabalpur, Kanpur, Kashmir, Kolhapur, Mysore, Nagpur, Pune, Secunderabad, Thoubal, Waltair
Pollen morphology	Pollen grains 3-colporate, oblate spheroidal, 16.6–19.8 µ amb spheroidal. Exine (spinules included) 4.4 µ thick, spinulose. (Generally palynologists count such pollen under Asteraceae.)
Allergenic significance	Highly allergenic

Prosopis juliflora (Sw.) Dc.

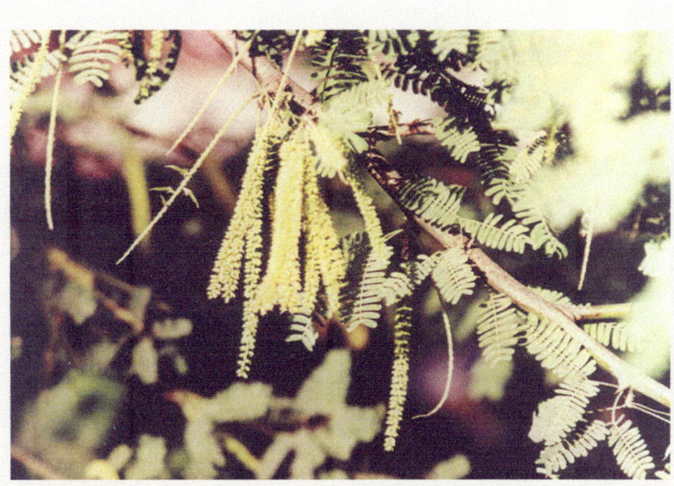

Family	*Mimosaceae*
Local name	Kabuli Kikar
Distribution and phenology	A small or moderate-sized, drought-resistant tree with drooping branches and spreading crown. Pinnae usually 4. Leaflets 17–20 pairs, obliquely oblong. Flowers cream colored or yellow in hanging spikes. Stamens are 10, free, having 4–4.5 mm long filaments and glandular anthers.
Flowering period and mode of pollination	April–September, anemophilous/entomophilous
Pollen peak and percentage in annual pollen calendars of Lucknow	May, 0.47%
Aerial incidence in other parts of the country	Aurangabad, Agra, Bengaluru, Bhopal, Bikaner, Delhi, Gwalior, Hyderabad, Jaipur, Kolkata, Kolhapur, Mumbai, Mysuru, Pune, Tirupati, Visakhapatnam, Waltair
Pollen morphology	Pollen grains 3-colporoidate, subspheroidal, 30–32 × 27–28 μ. Colpi long. Exine 2 μ thick, sexine thicker than nexine, exine punctate-scrobiculate forming islands of various sizes.
Allergenic significance	Significantly allergenic

Ricinus communis Linn.

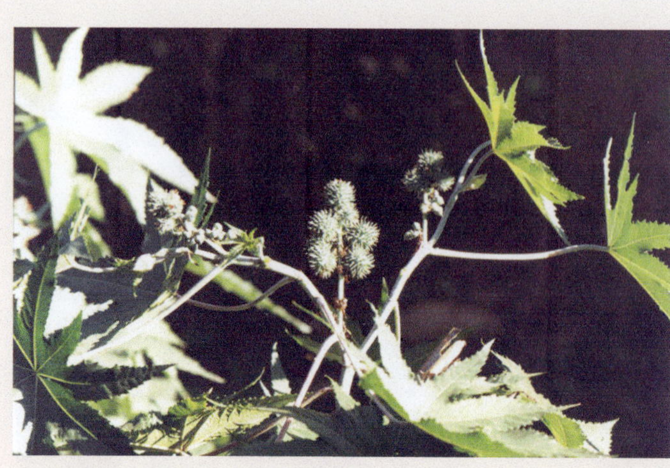

Family	*Euphorbiaceae*
Local name	Arand, Arandi
Distribution and phenology	Cultivated as well as growing in wastelands. An evergreen shrub or small tree. Leaves palmately lobed, peltate. Flowers greenish white or reddish, monoecious in branching terminal raceme. Male flowers occupying the upper portion, stamens numerous, female flowers with spathaceous calyx.
Flowering period and mode of pollination	Greater part of the year mainly in October–June, anemophilous/entomophilous.
Pollen peak and percentage in annual pollen calendars of Lucknow	December, 2.2–9.46%
Aerial incidence in other parts of the country	Agra, Berhampur, Bikaner, Delhi, Gwalior, Imphal, Jabalpur, Nagpur, Secunderabad, Thoubal, Tiruchirapalli, Visakhapatnam
Pollen morphology	Pollen grains 3 colporate, 28–30 × 26–23 μ. Colpi thin and long. Os la-longate. Exine 2.2 μ thick, sexine as thick as nexine, finely reticulate
Allergenic significance	Allergenic

CONCLUSION

- Overall, aerobiologists should encourage closer collaboration among themselves and with the scientists involved in clinical studies in order to achieve more meaningful results. Regional and global aerobiological network and integrated and coordinated national programs need to be strengthened.
- Future priorities of aerobiology in relation to clinical studies should include standardization of methods and procedures.
- The database generated on aerobiological and clinical studies has provided the proof of allergenicity of several plants growing in the neighborhood of human settlements. Despite the availability of data regarding allergy-causing plants, several allergenically significant trees are still being planted by various agencies. The plantation of such allergenic trees should be discouraged.
- Most of the advanced countries have devised an efficient integration of aerobiology with the early warning system for forecasting plant and human diseases by using mass media such as newspaper, television, radio, and electronic media. A similar pattern of warning and prediction system should be evolved in our country, which might contribute toward a more direct and immediate benefit to allergic patients.

REFERENCES

1. Vishnu-Mittre, Khandelwal A. Air-borne pollen grains and fungal spores at Lucknow during 1969–1970. Palaeobotanist. 1973;22:177-85.
2. Wodehouse RP. Pollen Grains. New York: McGraw-Hill Book Company; 1935.
3. Erdtman G. An Introduction to Pollen Analysis. Waltham, MA: Chronica Botanica Co; 1943.
4. Khandelwal A. Studies in Atmospheric Pollen Grains and Fungal Spores at Lucknow [PhD thesis]. Lucknow, India: Lucknow University, 1974.
5. Lakhanpal RN, Nair PKK. Survey of atmospheric pollen at Lucknow. J Sci Ind Res. 1958;17:80-7.
6. Khandelwal A. Pollen and spore rain in Lucknow city during 1983–1986. In: Agarwal OP, Dhawan S, eds. Proceedings International Conference Biodeterioration of Cultural Property. Lucknow: N.R.L.C.; 1991;387-96.
7. Khandelwal A. Survey of aerospora by Rotorod sampler: qualitative and quantitative assessment. Aerobiologia. 2001;17:77-83.
8. Khandelwal A. Long-term monitoring of air-borne pollen and fungal spores and their allergenic significance. Palaeobotanist. 2002;51:153-9.
9. Chaturvedi M, Datta K, Nair PKK. A fresh survey of airborne pollen at Lucknow. J Palyn. 1987-88;23–24:117-43.
10. Cunningham DD. Microscopic Examination of Air. Calcutta, India: Government Press; 1873.
11. Agnihotri MS, Singh AB. Observations on pollinosis in Lucknow with special reference to offending factors. Aspects Allergy Appl Immunol. 1971;5:135-41.
12. Prasad R, Kumar R, Verma SK, Pandey US. A study of skin sensitivity to various allergens by intradermal test in patients of Bronchial asthma. Indian J Allergy Asthma Immunol. 2001;15:17-21.
13. Katelaris CH, Burke TV, Byth K. Is it possible to predict the next day's pollen count? Indian J Aerobiol. 2006;19: 31-6.
14. Khandelwal A, Vishnu-Mittre. Palynology of Holoptelea integrifolia Planch. Palaeobotanist. 1975;22:127-32.
15. Anonymous AICP. Aeroallergens and Human Health: Aerobiological Studies (42/14/94-RE). Vol 2. New Delhi, India: Ministry of Environment and Forest; 1994–1998.

CHAPTER 8

Allergen Preparation and Standardization: An Overview

AB Singh, Chandni Mathur

INTRODUCTION

Allergy is defined as an exaggerated response of the adaptive immune system typified by immunoglobulin E (IgE) responses against the offending substance called "allergen[1]." The immunologic basis of allergic diseases is observed in two phases: sensitization and development of memory T- and B-cell responses along with IgE production.[2] Allergy manifests in the form of various conditions, such as anaphylaxis, urticaria, angioedema, allergic rhinoconjunctivitis, allergic asthma, serum sickness, allergic vasculitis, hypersensitivity pneumonitis, atopic dermatitis (eczema), contact dermatitis, and granulomatous reactions, as well as the colorful spectrum of food- or drug-induced hypersensitivity reactions.[2]

Asthma, allergic rhinitis, atopic dermatitis, and inhalant sensitization have been appropriately referred to as the first wave of the epidemic of the 21st century.[3,4] During the past 60 years, there has been a rise in the epidemic prevalence of allergic disorders, which is expected to reach up to 4 billion in the 2050s.[5]

Allergic reactions are initiated by certain types of antigens, referred to as allergens, which have been broadly categorized into four classes: inhalants (pollen, fungi, dust), ingestants (food, drugs), contactants (latex, plant trichomes), and injectants (drugs/insects).

Allergen immunotherapy (AIT) has been used to treat allergic diseases since the early 1900s.[6] Allergen-specific immunotherapy (also known as allergy shots) identified as disease-modifying intervention for allergic diseases involves subcutaneous administration of gradually increasing quantities of the patients, relevant allergens until a dose is reached that is effective in inducing immunologic tolerance to the allergens.[7] Instead of subcutaneous, sublingual AIT has also been introduced recently.

The term "allergen extracts" refers to solutions of proteins or glycol proteins extracted from source material not yet incorporated into a therapeutic AIT extract.[8] Vials of AIT extracts are prepared individually (specifically customized) using saline buffers for each patient to reduce the risk of allergen cross-contamination, anaphylactic side effects, and sensitization to unknown allergens in extracts. Major allergens responsible for allergy in extracts can be modified chemically or enzymatically in order to reduce their allergenic potential while still retaining the immunogenicity for achieving the same tolerance as a natural counterpart.

The collection of raw materials for allergen preparation should be performed by qualified personnel, and appropriate measures should be taken to ensure correct characterization and quality check of source materials. For AIT-trained personnel including, but not limited to, registered nurses, medical assistants, or physicians' assistants must be employed, who strictly follow allergen extract preparation guidelines.

The AIT efficacy and precision of diagnostic allergy skin testing are entirely dependent on the quality of the allergen extracts used.[8] Standardized allergen preparations have been recommended for use in diagnostic kits and immunotherapy as is evident by different position papers published.[8-10] The advantage of standardized extracts is that the biologic activity is more consistent, and therefore, the risk of an adverse reaction caused by extract potency variability should be diminished.

ALLERGEN PREPARATION

Allergen source materials are prerequisite and are broadly classified into the following categories:

Pollen allergens: The natural sources of inhalant allergens from plants are the pollens. The collection may be performed by vacuuming or drying flower heads followed by grinding using a sterile mortar and pestle. The crucial step of cleaning is done by passing through sieves of different mesh sizes and storing in sealed containers at −20°C. The pollen samples are subjected to pollen purity checking for actual pollen content. As recommended, samples with pollen content 90% or more and plant/floral parts less than 10% of the same species are accepted for extraction of antigens. In no case, fungal spores and other pollen and dust particles together should exceed more than 2%. Pollens may show a large variation in quantitative composition depending on the season and location of growth. So, to achieve a relatively constant composition, harvests from different years and collection sites should be pooled. An important point is to perform pollen collection during beginning and peak of flowering and that too in brown paper bags to avoid fungal contamination. Defatting using diethyl ether is done for selected pollens to get rid of the lipid matter. Extract manufacturing procedures may vary, including buffer composition, extraction temperature, and time; also, the incorporation of stabilizers influence the final quality of the extract. Preferably, physiological buffers such as sodium carbonate (pH 9.6), phosphate-buffered saline (PBS) (pH 7.2), ammonium bicarbonate (pH 8.0), and tris-buffered saline (TBS) (pH 7.5) are used. Pollen grains contain certain proteolytic enzymes that may degrade rapidly the allergenic content in the sample. To overcome this, protease inhibitors such as phenyl methyl sulfonyl fluoride (PMSF; 1 mM) and chelating agents such as ethylene diamine tetra acetate (EDTA; 5 mM) are added during extraction.

Fungal allergens: The primary inoculum should be obtained from fungal culture banks such as Indian Agriculture Research Institute, Delhi; Institute of Microbial Technology, Chandigarh; and National Chemical Laboratory, Pune. Fungi are cultured under controlled conditions of temperature and growth media composition. Usually Sabouraud's broth with/without yeast extract is preferred. The mycelia mat or surface growth consisting of "mycelia-spore mass" is used for the extraction of antigens instead of culture filtrate, which mostly contain mycelia antigens. Owing to the difficulties in maintaining a constant composition of fungal cultures, it is recommended that extracts be derived from several independent cultures of the same species.[11]

Insect allergens: The optimal source for insect allergens is dependent on the natural route of exposure: inhalation, injectant (bite/sting), contactant, and ingestant (accumulation of feces, vomitus, and debris in house dust). Where whole insects or insect debris is inhaled, the whole insect body is selected as an allergen source. However, for biting or stinging insects, saliva or venom, respectively, is the proper allergen source. In some cases, mixed species of cockroach, mosquitoes, houseflies, moths, and ants are used for antigen extraction. Live insects are stored in deep freezers, lyophilized, and crushed to be further used for antigen preparation.[11]

Dust mites: Two mite species, namely, *Dermatophagoides pteronyssinus* and *Dermatophagoides farinae*, are common indoor allergens in India. However, recent surveys on dust mites have reported Acarus, Glycyphagus, Blumea, etc., as allergenically important. It is worthwhile to mention that mites collected in different culture phases show variable allergenic reactivity.[12] Mites are highly difficult to be grown in bulk. The specific conditions required are low temperature (26°C), high humidity, and specific media such as sprouting gram powder, dog meals, and human scales. Extracts based on the whole mite culture include material from mite bodies, eggs, larvae, and fecal particles as well as mite decomposition material. Separation of mites from the growth medium is a tedious task.[11]

Food allergens: Protein-rich food items of family Leguminosae such as pulses, peanut, soybean, and cereals are procured from local markets for antigen preparation in saline buffers which can be further stored. In the case of fresh dairy products such as milk, egg, and fresh vegetables and fruits, direct prick-to-prick method is preferred.

Miscellaneous allergens: Other miscellaneous allergenic materials include vegetable and farm dusts and danders collected from source materials. Pigeon feathers and droppings also serve as the antigenic source for some hypersensitive patients.

EXTRACTION OF ALLERGENS

Antigen Extraction

Since allergens and antibodies are proteinaceous in nature, utmost focus needs to be toward preventing protein denaturation during allergen extraction procedure and further storage. Allergen extraction mimics physiological conditions present in the human airways (i.e., pH and ionic strength). Elevated temperature, high ionic strength, and organic solvents need to be avoided.[11]

In general, various steps involved in antigen preparation from various raw material (s) are described in detail. It is to be ensured that autoclaved lab ware, approximate pH, and cold temperature conditions during mixing or transferring of suspension need to be ensured for efficient preparation.

1. *Grinding*: It is necessary to crush the solid source material to fine powder to increase the surface area for efficient extraction. The solid source material can be crushed to fine powder using a sterile pestle and mortar or using a blender or a juicer (for juicy fruits).
2. *Defatting*: It is done to obtain a clear supernatant of proteinaceous antigenic substances, free from lipid oily layer and nonspecific irritants such as resins, waxes, and pigments. Fresh solvent ether, toluene, or acetone in excess amount (3–4 times) is added to the material to be defatted in a conical flask with manual shaking and kept at 4°C. The upper oily layer is decanted and process is continued until no color is visible. The solid suspension needs to be cleared through filtration. The material thus obtained is desiccated or air-dried inside laminar hood for 24–48 hours and stored in plastic containers at –20°C till further processing for antigen extraction.
3. *Extraction*: A defined amount of defatted dried material powder is suspended in weight-by-volume (w/v) alkaline buffer (pH 8.0) in an Erlenmeyer flask. Protease inhibitors such as 5 mM EDTA and 1 mM PMSF are added to the mixture and are subjected to continuous stirring on a magnetic stirrer at 4°C for 8–20 hours as the case may be. For liquid samples, volume-by-volume (v/v) measurements are estimated. As for 1:50 extraction, 50 mL of saline buffer is added to 1 mL of the liquid sample. Preferably extracting solutions are alkaline (pH 8.0) buffer saline or ammonium bicarbonate solution.
4. *Clarification*: The antigen extract solution is then subjected to centrifugation at 10,000 grams for 20 minutes and kept at 4°C for separating the soluble ingredients. The supernatant is retained and the solid suspension is discarded.
5. *Dialysis*: Low-molecular-weight, i.e., below 5,000 Da, nonantigenic materials such as resins and pigments should be removed from the extract by dialysis. Any substance excluded from the final product should be proved to be nonallergenic.[11] For dialysis, the extract supernatant is filled in a clipped cellophane tubing of defined size and immersed in buffered saline, which is subjected to magnetic steering at low temperature. Change of the dialysis tube at defined intervals will ensure efficient removal of unwanted substances. For some substances (e.g., house dust, mustard, potato, spinach, beets, coffee, pepper) give nearly universally positive reactions unless dialyzed.
6. *Sterilization*: The supernatant obtained after centrifugation or dialysis is filtered through a sterile 0.45-μm membrane filter fitted in a sterile Millipore filter assembly and further transferred aseptically to sterile labeled antigenic glass vials. The entire process of sterilization is carried out inside laminar hood. It is better to prepare small aliquots for which can be stored at 4°C or lyophilized for further storage to avoid repeated freezing and thawing.
7. *Lyophilization*: The prepared antigenic extracts in small aliquots are lyophilized in a lyophilizer chamber and finally stored at –20/–70°C for future use to enhance its shelf-life.
8. *Sterility testing*: Microbial assays for identifying bacterial and fungal contamination, if any, in antigenic extracts, should be carried out using suitable media.

ALLERGEN STANDARDIZATION

The two important factors for consideration during allergen standardization are: (1) selection of a reference extract, and (2) selection of an assay or protocol to compare the manufactured extracts with the selected reference extracts.[8]

In the United States, the Food and Drug Administration (FDA) and Center for Biologics Evaluation and Research (CBER)—a division of allergenic products and parasitology, regulate the licensing of allergenic extracts for clinical use.[13-16]

While more specifically for AIT, allergen extract preparation guidelines have been established by two entities: the US Pharmacopeia (USP) and American Academy of Allergy, Asthma, and Immunology/American College of Allergy, Asthma, and Immunology/Joint Council of Allergy, Asthma, and Immunology Joint Task Force. The allergy immunotherapy practice parameter's (AIPP) third update included the previously proposed, but now formally adopted, guidelines and the USP chapter 797 guidelines.

The US-licensed extracts are supplied as aqueous, glycerinated, lyophilized, and acetone- and alum-precipitated formulations. The list of commonly used allergens that have been standardized includes extracts for cat hair, cat pelt, *D. pteronyssinus*, *D farinae*, short ragweed, Bermuda grass, Kentucky bluegrass, perennial rye grass, orchard grass, timothy grass, meadow fescue, red top, sweet vernal grass, and Hymenoptera venoms (yellow jacket, honeybee, wasp, yellow hornet, and white-faced hornet).

The potency of allergen extracts is assessed by using quantitative skin tests and stated in terms of bioequivalent allergy units (BAU). The quantitative test is called the intradermal dilution for 50 mL sum of erythema (ID50EAL). Standardized extracts with a wide range of biological potencies are available as 10,000 and 100,000 BAU for grasses; 5,000 and 10,000 BAU for cat allergens; 5,000, 10,000, and 30,000 AU for dust mites; and 100,000 AU or 1:10 and 1:20 wt/vol for short ragweed, with the, 'Amb a 1' concentration listed in FDA units on the label of the weight/volume extracts.[8] A point to mention is that allergy unit (AU) is bioequivalent to BAU. For standardized allergen extracts, the potency of the manufacturer's extract is recognized by comparing the extract with the CBER's reference control using an in vitro enzyme-linked immunosorbent assay (ELISA).[17] The acceptable range for a 10,000- or 100,000-BAU/AU extract is based on a statistical test for equivalence at CBER/FDA. Based on dose–response studies using US-licensed allergen extracts, the probable effective dose ranges for standardized US-licensed allergenic extracts have been estimated from clinical trials primarily conducted in Europe.[8]

In the case of nonstandardized extracts, maintenance doses are much more difficult to calculate. This is because nonstandardized extracts' w/v or protein nitrogen unit (PNU) labeling does not essentially correlate with biological potency. This concept is supported by data provided from one of the leading extract manufacturers (ALK-Abelló Denmark), highlighting that the major allergen content in Bermuda grass extracts ranged from 141 to 422 g/mL of Cyn d 1.[18]

The AIPP third update provides new dosing recommendations for Bermuda grass, imported fire ant, and nonstandardized extracts distinguishing between pollen (0.5 mL of a 1:100 or 1:200 vol/vol) and mold/fungi or cockroach (highest tolerated dose) extracts.[18]

In Europe, manufacturers report allergen extract potency as units based on an in-house reference standard (IHRS), making it difficult to understand the exact doses used. One of the European allergen extract manufacturers uses IHRSs that are based on titrated skin prick testing of allergic patients. Consequently, in vitro test (ELISA inhibition) compares the potency of commercial batches with the in-house reference, and the potency is assigned as arbitrary units, which is not printed on packed vials. Quantifying the major allergen is not an acceptable criterion for standardization worldwide as the techniques, monoclonal antibodies used in ELISA, and the patient natural exposure are variable and cannot be compared. Consequently, in 2001 European Union sponsored a study "CREATE"—Certified References for Allergens and Test Evaluation. Under this program, manufacturers have implemented protocols that have overall IgE-binding potencies as their focus and supports the introduction of major allergen-based standardization for effective immunotherapy. The objectives of CREATE was to produce purified recombinant allergens and compare these with their natural counterparts to serve as the gold standard. Nine recombinant molecules representing eight major allergens were produced: rBet v 1, rPhl p 1, rPhl p 5a and rPhl p 5b, rOle e 1, rDer p 1, rDer p 2, rDer f 1, and rDer f 2. Recombinant allergens were compared with purified natural allergens for physicochemical (identity, purity, folding, aggregation state, solubility, and stability) to serve as Certified Reference Materials. Immunological parameters (IgE-binding potency, biological activity, and dose–response behavior in ELISA) were also assessed.[19] Two of the recombinant allergens—rBet v 1 and rPhl p 5a—have qualified to be good reference materials for use in immunotherapy clinical trials.

In India, the Drug Controller of India and the respective nodal agencies regulate the allergen manufacture for diagnostic and therapeutic purposes. Till date, the emphasis is on good manufacture practice to be followed by allergen units. Allergen potency is expressed as w/v (weight/volume), protein estimation (PNU in μg/mL) and sodium dodecyl sulfate poly acrylamide gel electrophoresis protein profile is followed for maintaining/comparing the quality of antigens in different batches. Coordinated and ambitious efforts are required by allergists/immunologists and commercial manufacturers to upgrade the quality control of allergen extracts following the standard of the World Health Organization and the International Union of Immunological Societies protocols.[20] In fact, the need to develop allergen certification center in the country such as FDA and CBER has been realized much earlier. In recent times, few of the government-funded (Ministry of Health and Family Welfare) research institutes such as the National Institute of Biologicals and Indian Pharmacopoeia Commission have been recognized for the quality control of commercial allergen extracts and dissemination information on allergen preparation and standardization of allergen extracts that are classified as drugs.

During the past two decades, research projects were pursued to characterize the allergen extracts from diverse sources at the Institute of Genomics and Integrative Biology and VP Chest Institute, Delhi. Indian flora is very rich and diverse in different parts of the country; hence, a large number of pollens are predominant at different times in the atmosphere.[21] About 30 species of fungi have been recorded from "air spora" responsible for type I hypersensitivity. Additionally several allergens from insects, mites, animal epithelia, etc., also contribute in inducing and aggravating respiratory allergy diseases in predisposed individuals. The task of characterizing allergens in our country is comparatively difficult than in Europe and the United States, where only few allergens are prevalent.

ALLERGEN STANDARDIZATION: NEW TRENDS

Allergens as natural extracts are complex mixtures of major and minor allergens. Allergens are proteinaceous in nature and exhibit genetic variations/sequence polymorphisms, which results in different isoforms. This heterogeneity affects the IgE-binding capacity and imparts signature peptide sequences to each allergen isoform.[22] Currently used methods for major allergen determination include single radial immunodiffusion, rocket immunoelectrophoresis, and ELISA. The quantitative aspects of these techniques are dependent on monoclonal antibodies as reagents, which are prone to degradation with time, unsuitable for concomitant quantification of several allergens, and able to identify single epitopes and/or single isoallergens only.

The basophil histamine release test that relies on the same principle as the skin test has also been recommended to demonstrate qualitative differences in biological activity or the composition of allergen preparations, which is undetectable by IgE inhibition assays. The limiting factor is that it is technically demanding and difficult to perform and also offers less precision.

Besides the routine use of monoclonal and polyclonal antibodies for quantifying the potency of allergenic extract, other advanced physiochemical methods such as mass spectrometry (MS) have been used for allergen standardization. Using advanced MS techniques for allergen extract characterization and standardization offers advantages as various allergens of the extract can be studied simultaneously. High-resolution and accurate mass MS detects peptides with high selectivity and mass accuracy (<3 parts per million) and is able to recognize single amino acid substitution on the allergen surface.

Two reference materials (rBet v 1 and rPhl p 5a) and relevant ELISAs are under validation for future establishment as international references under the guidance of the European Directorate for the Quality of Medicine after extensive biological and biochemical investigation. Currently, these two reference materials are under further validation by the BSP090 project. IgE or IgG recognition could be affected even by a single amino acid substitution on the surface of the allergens.

REFERENCES

1. Cookson W. The alliance of genes and environment in asthma and allergy. Nature. 1999;402:B5-B11.
2. European Academy of Allergy and Clinical Immunology, EAACI. The underlying mechanism of allergy. In: Akdis and Agache, eds. Global Atlas of Allergy. 2014;39-43.
3. Holgate ST. The epidemic of allergy and asthma. Nature. 1999;402:B2-B4.
4. Prescott S, Allen KJ. Food allergy: riding the second wave of the allergy epidemic. Pediatr Allergy Immunol. 2011;22:155-60.
5. Lötvall J, Pawankar R, Wallace DV, et al. American Academy of Allergy, Asthma & Immunology (AAAAI), the American College of Allergy, Asthma & Immunology (ACAAI), the European Academy of Allergy and Clinical Immunology (EAACI), and the Word Allergy Organisation (WAO). We call for iCAALL: International Collaboration in Asthma, Allergy and Immunology. World Allergy Organ J. 2012;5:39-40.
6. Jutel M, Agache I, Bonini S, et al. International consensus on allergy immunotherapy. J Allergy Clin Immunol. 2015;136:556-68.
7. Moote W, Kim H. Allergen-specific immunotherapy. Allergy, Asthma Clin Immunol. 2011;7:S5.
8. Cox L, Nelson H, Lockey R, et al. Allergen immunotherapy: a practice parameter third update. J Allergy Clin Immunol. 2011;127:S1-55.
9. Nelson HS. The use of standardized extracts in allergen immunotherapy. J Allergy Clin Immunol. 2000;106:41-5.
10. Anonymous. Position statement. The use of standardized allergen extracts. American Academy of Allergy, Asthma and Immunology (AAAAI). J Allergy Clin Immunol. 1997;99:583-6.
11. Larsen JN, Dreborg S. Standardization of allergen extracts. Methods Mol Med. 2008;138:133-45.
12. Eraso E, Martinez J, Garcia-ortega P, et al. Influence of mite growth culture phases on the biological standardization

of allergenic extracts. J Investig Allergol Clin Immunol. 1998;8:201-06.
13. Lowenstein H. Overview: biological standardization. Arb paul Ehrlich Inst Bundesamt Sera Impfstoffe Frankf A M. 2003;94:67-9.
14. Esch RE, White W. Standardization: dreams, myths and reality. Arb paul Ehrlich Inst Bundesamt Sera Impfstoffe Frankf A M. 1997;91:134-6.
15. Lin Y, Miller CA. Standardization of allergenic extracts: an update on CBER's standardization program. Arb paul Ehrlich Inst Bundesamt Sera Impfstoffe Frankf A M. 1997;9:127-30.
16. Turkeltaub PC. Biological standardization. Arb paul Ehrlich Inst Bundesamt Sera Impfstoffe Frankf A M. 1997;91:145-56.
17. Slater JE. Standardized allergen vaccines in the United States. Clin Allergy Immunol. 2008;21:273-81.
18. Cox L, Esch RE, Corbett M, Hankin C, Nelson M, Plunkett G. Allergen immunotherapy practice in the United States: guidelines, measures, and outcomes. Ann Allergy Asthma Immunol. 2011;107:289-99.
19. Van Ree R, Chapman MD, Ferreira F, et al. The CREATE project: development of certified reference materials for allergenic products and validation of methods for their quantification. Allergy. 2008;63:310-26.
20. Gaur SN, Singh BP, Singh AB, et al. Guidelines for practice of allergen immunotherapy in India. Indian J Allergy Asthma Immunol. 2009;23:1-21.
21. Singh AB, Kumar P. Aeroallergens in clinical practice of allergy in India. An overview. Ann Agric Environ Med. 2003;10:131-6.
22. Seppälä U, Dauly C, Robinson S, et al. Absolute quantification of allergens from complex mixtures: a new sensitive tool for standardization of allergen extracts for specific immunotherapy. J Proteome Res. 2011;10: 2113-22.

CHAPTER 9

Diagnosis of Allergy: Clinical

Rajendra Prasad, Nikhil Gupta

INTRODUCTION

Allergy encompasses a wide range of immunological reactions that generally have adverse consequences involving one or many organ systems of the body. The term "allergy" was coined by Clemens von Pirquet in 1906[1] to describe the ability of animals and humans to develop altered responses to foreign substances after repeated exposure. The substance that causes an altered response is called an allergen. The term "atopy" was coined in 1923 by Coca and Cooke[2] to describe the genetic susceptibility to develop clinical allergy against the common allergen encountered in the environment. However, isolation of IgE from the serum of allergy patients by Ishizaka and Ishizaka in 1966[3] was the important landmark in the medical history in the development of allergy research. The prevalence of allergic diseases is rising dramatically in both developed and developing countries. These diseases include bronchial asthma, rhinitis, anaphylaxis, drug, food, insect allergy, eczema, urticaria, and angioedema; it is estimated that almost one in the two people in the developed world exhibits an allergic response to some common environmental factor.[4,5] In India, approximately 20–30% of the population is reported to have one or other type of allergic disorder.[6-10] Two studies conducted in Bombay[11-12] concluded that the prevalence of atopy in the Indian population is as high as 25.3%. Although almost any tissue in the body may be affected by allergy, yet it has a predilection for the respiratory tissue and the skin. The most common manifestations of allergic diseases are rhinitis, bronchial asthma, urticaria, and eczema. The respiratory allergic diseases include allergic rhinitis (seasonal and perennial) and bronchial asthma.

Misuse of the term allergy has led to a variety of unexplained phenomenon being labeled as allergic disease. Allergic diseases are probably among the most misdiagnosed and mismanaged disease entities of the modern era. The mainstay of diagnosis in allergic disorder is based on the accurate clinical history supplemented by various diagnostic tests (skin test, detection of allergen-specific IgE in serum, and challenge test). The history of allergic patients differs from a usual medical history in at least one respect. In allergy, diagnosis is often apparent, hence the history is not directed primarily at establishing the ultimate diagnosis, but rather at discovering the underlying causes.

CLINICAL DIAGNOSIS

The clinical diagnosis includes the diagnosis based on the clinical history and the physical examination of the individual patient.

Clinical History

The value and importance of an adequate and careful history as an aid in the diagnosis of disease is well known. The history of allergic patients differs from the usual medical history. In the average medical condition, the purpose of history is to aid in making the diagnosis by suggesting the site of trouble, giving necessary clue for further investigation relating to exact diagnosis. In allergy, on the other hand, the diagnosis is often apparent. The allergic history therefore is not directed primarily at establishing the ultimate diagnosis, but rather at discovering the underlying cause. Thus, it can be said that an allergic history is an etiological history rather than a diagnostic history. The purpose of history taking in allergic patients has the following two objectives:

1. To determine whether the patient has an allergic disease.
2. To ascertain the factors, which contribute to the development of symptoms in an individual.

It should also be borne in mind that skin tests, which are the most commonly employed laboratory procedure for the diagnosis of allergic diseases, are not completely diagnostic. They are merely confirmatory. The skin test must be correlated with clinical history for correct diagnosis. Since an allergy workup involves a complete medical evaluation, together with additional specialized history, a good amount of time is needed for a new patient. Besides, the doctor should be vigilant enough and have a sound knowledge of botany and aerobiology of grass, trees, weeds, pollens, as well as fungal spores, so that an accurate history of allergens can be elicited.[13] The clinical history taking consists of the following:

- *General information* about individual patient like name, age, sex, marital status, and occupation.
- *Chief complaints* sneezing, rhinorrhea, nasal congestion, difficulty in breathing, cough, expectoration, sore throat, postnasal drip, headache, rashes, etc.
- *Present illness*
    1. *Duration of illness* (including age of onset)—usually the onset of allergic diseases dates back to childhood.
    2. *Nature of onset and severity*—this includes nature of onset, frequency and duration of attacks, changes in nature, frequency, or duration of attacks.
    3. *Symptoms at onset*

       Seasonal rhinitis—sneezing, rhinorrhea, itching of nose, eyes, ears, palate, lacrimation, ocular itching and redness, headache, sore throat, postnasal drip, pain over paranasal sinuses, loss of smell and taste, and recurrent epistaxis. These symptoms are seasonal and usually occur at the change of the season.

       Perennial rhinitis—same as seasonal, but with chronic nasal blockage, sneezing, and catarrh are more common; sinusitis or otitis media may be associated. Symptoms are present round the year.

       Bronchial asthma—breathlessness, wheezing, cough usually nonproductive, and chest tightness with nocturnal worsening of symptoms. With the help of history, asthma can be classified according to the severity and thereby helps in the stepwise management of the disease. On the basis of clinical history, asthma is classified as shown in Table 9.1.
    4. *When symptoms occur*
        a. Season—if the symptoms are perennial, i.e., all the time in a year, then house dust mites, animal dander, mold spores, and cockroaches are common allergens. When symptoms are present in a particular season or during the change of season, pollens are the most common allergens.
        b. Time of day and location—it is important to learn when and where the attacks occur, e.g., if attacks occur only in daytime and at workplace, occupational contacts are likely suspect. If attacks occur only in night, then articles found in bedroom are under suspicion or asthma is poorly controlled. If attacks occur at playtime, grasses or weeds in or near the playground are important. A housewife may report asthma only during house cleaning that clearly indicates

Table 9.1: Classification of asthma severity.

	Daytime symptoms	*Nighttime symptoms*
Severe persistent	Continuous Limited physical activity	Frequent
Moderate persistent	Daily Attacks affect activity Use of inhaled short-acting β_2-agonist daily	>1 time a week
Mild persistent	≥1 time a week but <1 time a day	>2 times a month
Intermittent	<1 time a week Asymptotic between attacks	≤2 times a month

house dust/dust mites could be the likely allergen.

5. *Precipitating or predisposing factors*
History of exposure to various precipitating factors like inhalants (house dust/dust mites, cotton dust, wheat dust, old paper dust, rice dust, flower, plants, animal dander, and hair), ingestants (foods, drugs), contactants (oil, soap, cosmetics, perfumes, silk, chemical varnish, polyethylene fibers, etc.), insects (cockroach), psychological factors (marriage, marital relation, tension, worry, financial and social depression), and physical agents (cold, heat, sunlight, rains).
6. *Impact of illness*
The number of lost days from work or school, social adjustments, limitation of activities, presence of nocturnal symptoms, frequency of unscheduled physician visits, emergency room visits, or hospitalization, fatigue, sleep disturbances, and learning and attention problems.

- *Past history*
Past history taken with respect to diseases of infancy and childhood, pointing toward any atopic illness, other past illness, vaccination and serum therapy, any operation especially of nose, throat, and prior history of drug or food allergies and intolerances. Review of various previous treatments and their response.
- *Family history*
Family history is an important part of history in patients of various allergic disorders. Genetics is an important component of atopy, and children not only inherit a tendency to atopy from their parents but also are likely to develop the same allergic disorder. The predisposition to respond to environmental allergens occurs in about 13% of the children when neither parents is atopic, in 30% if one parent or sibling is atopic, and in about 50% if both parents are affected. Hence, the history of various allergic disorders must be sought in family members. The association between family history and adult onset of the disease is less striking.
- *Personal history*
Personal history regarding present job, past occupation, job at onset of symptom, hobbies, diet, home condition, etc., may point toward the offending agent responsible for the allergic condition of the patient. Exposure to active or passive smoking is also important.
- *Occupational history*
Occupations and exposure to allergens or irritants at work.
- *Environmental history*
A thorough environmental history relevant to symptoms is important, which may not be detected by any tests. History of use of detergents, carpets, air conditioners, and source of specific allergens irritants at home.

Physical Examination

A complete physical examination is mandatory. Specific attention should be directed to areas where atopic diseases are manifested—nasopharynx, skin, eyes, ears, chest, and gastrointestinal tract.

Allergic Rhinitis

The classic picture of allergic nose is seen as enlarged moist, pale turbinate with glistening, clear serous, or watery discharge. A swollen, pale nasal mucous membrane is quite characteristic but some patients may have erythematous mucosa. Other common findings include the following:

- Allergic shiners—dark discoloration in the orbital-palpebral grooves beneath the lower eyelids.
- Allergic salute—common in children, involves using the palm of a hand in upward thrust of the nose, thereby relieving itching and opening of nasal airway.
- Allergic or adenoid facies—mouth breathing, gaping expression, allergic shiners, and dental malocclusion.
- Dennie's line—a wrinkle just beneath the lower lids, present from early infancy and is associated with atopic dermatitis and allergic rhinitis.
- Abnormalities of oral cavity—high-arched palate, overriding maxillary incisors, hypertrophic lymphoid follicle on posterior pharyngeal wall, and postnasal drip.
- Geographic tongue—characterized by sharply outlined bald patches on the tongue.

Bronchial Asthma

Acute attack—tachypnea, tachycardia, use of accessory muscles of respiration, suprasternal retractions, pursed lip expiration, vesicular breathing with prolonged expiration with rhonchi/wheeze, or diminished breath sounds.

Peripheral signs of marked severity—accentuation of above findings with cyanosis, pulsus-paradoxus, miosis, papilledema, changes in sensorium, severe hyperinflation, marked reduction in respiratory excursions, and silent chest. During remission, chest examination may reveal no physical sign.

After the principal organ is examined, the entire skin, conjunctiva, and middle ear should be examined carefully for important physical findings along with a complete and thorough physical examination of other systems.

In conclusion, the diagnosis of specific allergy is based mainly on the clinical history supplemented by various diagnostic tests. Hence, an adequate and careful history taking and physical examination is of much importance for the diagnosis and treatment of allergic diseases.

REFERENCES

1. von Pirquet C. Allergic Munch Med., Wochenschr 1906; 30.
2. Coca AF, Cooke RA. On the classification of the phenomenon of hypersensitiveness. J Immunol. 1923;8:163-82.
3. Ishizaka K, Ishizaka T. Identification of IgE antibodies as a carrier of reaginic activity. J Immunol. 1967;99:1187-98.
4. Holgate ST. Allergic disorders—science, medicine & the future. BMJ. 2000;320:231-4.
5. Beasley R, Keil U, von Mutius E, Pearce N. Worldwide variation in prevalence of symptoms of asthma, allergic rhinoconjuntivitis, and atopic eczema: ISAAC. Lancet. 1998;351:1225-32.
6. Anonymous. All India Coordinated Project on Aeroallergens and Human Health Report. New Delhi, India: Ministry of Environment and Forests; 2000.
7. Chhabra SK, Gupta CK, Chhabra P, Rajpal S. Prevalence of bronchial asthma in schoolchildren in Delhi. J Asthma. 1998;35:291-6.
8. Prasad R, Kumar R. Allergy situation in India: what is being done. Indian J Chest Dis Allied Sci. 2013;55:7-8.
9. Jindal SK, Aggarwal AN, Gupta D, et al. Indian study on epidemiology of asthma, respiratory symptoms and chronic bronchitis in adults (INSEARCH). Int J Tuberc Lung Dis. 2012;16:1270-7.
10. Kumar R, Kumari D, Srivastava P, et al. Identification of IgE mediated food allergy and allergens in older children and adults with asthma and allergic rhinitis. Indian J Chest Dis Allied Sci. 2010;52:217-24.
11. Shaikh WA. Allergies in India: an analysis of 1619 patients attending an allergic clinic in Bombay. Int Rev Allergol Clin Immunol. 1997;3:101-4.
12. Shaikh WA. Allergies and asthma in India: an analysis of 2467 patients seen over a 6-year period. Ind J Clin Pract. 1998;8:23-6.
13. Prasad R, Jain VK. Diagnosis of allergic diseases: clinical. In: Prasad R. Advances in Allergy and Asthma. Lucknow. Shivam Publication. 2000;48-53.

CHAPTER 10

Diagnosis of Allergic Diseases In Vivo: Skin Tests

VK Jain, Shubhra Jain, Abhimanyu Garg

INTRODUCTION

Allergy and Allergic disorders are common medical problems prevalent globally and commonly reported to the practicing clinicians. Allergy is an allergen-specific hypersensitivity and immunologically mediated disorder that can affect any organ, commonly skin and mucous membrane. Allergic diseases (IgE mediated) are caused by exposure to various allergens and a usual practice to establish a diagnosis by re-exposure to the allergens. In clinical practice, the diagnosis of specific allergy is based on clinical history, physical examination, and confirmed by various diagnostic tests, i.e., skin, provocative, and immunological. In 1865, Charles Harrison Blackley first time used skin test as a diagnostic tool for allergy, using whole pollen grains on himself by placing allergen on abraded skin.[1] Von Pirquet in 1908 introduced cutaneous test for tuberculosis and became the chief impetus for subsequent allergy testing.[2] Schloss used scratch test by rubbing small, blood-free scratched skin in children for diagnosis of food allergy.[2] Scratch method has been used in the past extensively and later fallen out due to poor reproducibility, residual pigmented/depigmented areas, and patient's discomfort. Schick and Cooke later used intracutaneous diagnostic test.[3] Prick/puncture test was introduced in the early 1950s by Thomas lewis who suggested the puncture technique as an alternative.[4] The value of quantitative aspects of various proteins detecting sensitization by the method of prick/puncture technique was suggested and later widely accepted globally.[5] Skin test, a diagnostic application, is easy to perform, rapid, reliable, cost-effective, practical, and sensitive means of presence of allergen-specific IgE-mediated antibodies.[6-15] The skin test can be performed at any age with less reaction in elderly and small children. The advantage is to test different allergens simultaneously in clinical practice compared to a direct target organ provocative test, which is more of research value.

PATHOPHYSIOLOGY OF SKIN REACTION

The IgE-mediated skin allergic response presents in two forms, i.e., immediate reaction (IR) and late-phase reaction (LPR). IR is presented as wheal and flare dependent on both the proinflammatory and the neurogenic mediators. It is induced by mast cell degranulation after allergen challenge and release of histamine and tryptase, and the reaction begins about 5 minutes after allergen injection and peaks after 30 minutes. LPR starting after 3–4 hours, peaks at 6–12 hours, and resolves in 24–48 hours. It is also IgE mediated and represented by an erythematous inflammatory reaction.[16,17]

BASIC PRINCIPLE

The basic principle of skin testing is to introduce a minimal amount of standardized allergen extract into the epidermis or dermis. These are often prepared with phenol to preserve the allergens and glycerin to prevent drops of allergen extracts from running across the skin. The various types of sterile lancets and specialized needles have been made to improve the reproducibility of the test.[18] The wheal (raised itchy area) and flare (erythema) reactions depend on the degree of sensitivity, number of mast cells, site of the body, age, gender, race, circadian rhythm, pathological conditions, concentration, quality, potency of allergen extract, seasonal variations, prior use of antihistaminic, antidepressant, anti-inflammatory drugs, and so on.[6-15,19-30] In general buffer, saline is used as negative and histamine as positive control. Interindividual variation in the skin response to histamine is quite variable, with greater response in atopic than nonatopic individuals. Skin test should not be performed in patients having eczema, leukoderma, dermographism, severe dermatitis, or any chronic skin ailment. In case of doubtful skin, reaction test should be repeated. In case of history of high sensitivity, test should be performed with more diluted allergen extracts. Skin tests are to be performed by trained medical personnels in the presence of the physician with basic facility to manage adverse reactions including anaphylaxis. Suppression of endogenous cortisol may affect LPRs (skin and pulmonary) without change in early-phase responses.[31] The response of prick and intracutaneous tests is not affected during menstrual phase.[32]

First-generation antiallergic drugs and tranquilizers should be stopped at least 3 days before the test and second-generation antihistamines for at least 7 days.[33-35] H1 and H2 blockers[36,37] should be discontinued 24 hours prior testing and ketotifen/tricyclic antidepressants[38] should be avoided for at least 2 weeks. Bronchodilators and oral prostaglandin D2 inhibitors, e.g., indomethacin,[39] given several hours before testing may increase the wheal area by 17%, whereas cysteinyl leukotriene antagonist (montelukast, zafirlukast)[39,40] has negligible effects. Adrenaline[41] and steroids[42-44] do not affect sensitivity of the skin test.

Prior to skin test, written informed consent with complete clinical history, examination, and investigations must be taken and recorded. During and after allergy test, symptom evaluation and clinical examination are done and managed accordingly. The testing room should be properly equipped to manage anaphylaxis with appropriate medications. The procedure and interpretation of skin test reaction should be done by the trained doctor or technician/nurse to ensure better accuracy and reproducibility. The late-phase cutaneous response (Arthus reactions) should be read between 16 and 24 hours after testing. The practice parameter guidelines of skin tests related to methodology, devices, interpretation, drug effects, quality and quantity of allergen extract, and so on should be followed as reported (Table 10.1).[10-15,45-49]

Table 10.1: Suppressant effects of drugs on immediate skin tests.[10,14]

Drugs	*Withholding period (days)*	*Comments*
Antihistaminics first generation		
Chlorpheniramine	4	Withholding period is variable in individuals due to difference in metabolism Four days for first generation and 7 days for second generation is recommended as a general advice before skin test
Pheniramine	4	
Clemastine	5	
Cyproheptadine	9	
Dexchlorpheniramine	4	
Diphenhydramine, trimeprazine	2	
Dimenhydramine	2	
Hydroxyzine	5	
Doxylamine	2	
Promethazine	3	
Tripelennamine	3	
Brompheniramine	5	
Antihistaminics second generation		
Azelastine nasal	2	
Cetirizine	4	
Levocetirizine	4	
Fexofenadine	2	
Loratadine	7	
Desloratadine	4	
Levocabastine nasal	0	
Levocabastine ophthal	0	
Tricyclic antidepressants and tranquilizers		
Desipramine	2	
Imipramine	10	
Doxepin	6	
Doxepin topical	11	
H2 antagonists		
Ranitidine	1	Minimal suppression effect on skin test
Famotidine	1	
Cimetidine	1	
Neuroleptics		
Chlorpromazine		Withholding period not established due to variable antihistaminic effects of drugs in individuals May be up to 2 weeks
Clozapine		
Fluphenazine		
Olanzapine		
Pericyazine		
Quetiapine		
Risperidone		
Zuclopenthixol		
Antiemetics		
Prochlorperazine		Weak antihistamine

OBJECTIVES OF SKIN TEST

Diagnostic

- To know immediate hypersensitivity caused by various allergens.
- To know specific allergen causing allergy (pollen, dusts, fungi, insects, foods, drugs, and so forth).
- To know sensitization in atopic individual.
- To know antigen-specific IgE antibodies in allergic diseases.

Therapeutic

- For avoidance of specific allergen exposure as preventive measure.
- For allergen-specific immunotherapy (SIT).

Prognostic

- To know outcomes/results of allergen SIT.
- To know newer allergens causing allergy in a patient by retesting.
- To know status of SIT whether declining or increasing in order by repeat skin test.

DISEASE INDICATIONS

- Rhinitis/rhinoconjunctivitis/rhinosinusitis/allergic conjunctivitis
- Asthma
- Atopic dermatitis
- Food allergy
- Suspected latex allergy
- ABPA
- Eosinophilic esophagitis/gastroenteritis
- Drug allergy
- Venom allergy.

IN VIVO TEST

1. Skin/dermal test
2. Provocative/mucosal challenge test—bronchial, nasal, conjunctival; double-blind placebo-food challenge test.

TYPES OF SKIN/DERMAL TESTS

- Skin prick/puncture test (SPT)[6,12-19,56]
- Intradermal (ID)/intracutaneous test
- Patch test
- Scratch test (not in practice).

Prick Test

Prick/puncture test is common and widely used in clinical practice to detect IgE-mediated sensitization and is of biological relevance. The test was first described by Lewis and Grant in 1924.[4] Later, it became popular and widespread after modified by Pepys in 1970.[48] Prick test may be performed at any age as young as 1 month. It is done on volar aspect of the forearm/outer upper arm resting on tabletop in a comfortable position and occasionally on the back. Marking is done with a tip pen or grease pen. The individual prick tests are done at a distance of 2–3 cm to avoid false-positive reactions.[12,50] It is advisable to site the test more than 5 cm at wrist and 3 cm from antecubital fossa.[10,14] The skin is cleaned with nondetergent soap water first, then with 70% alcohol swab, and then the skin is allowed to dry. In a simple prick test, a small drop of allergen extract (1:10/20 w/v) in 50% glycerinated buffered saline is placed on the skin, and a prick lancet needle is passed vertically through the drop puncturing the skin slightly and quickly. Skin prick sites of various allergens should be marked by numbers for better identification.[14] For modified prick test, the blood lancet/small needle tip is allowed to penetrate the skin at 45–60° angle horizontally and gently lifted to create a small break superficially in the epidermis. The skin should not be pricked too deeply and escaped blood should be avoided. Another technique is to use multiwell tray dip then prick test. Hypodermic needles are currently not recommended as they increase the risk of bleeding. Multiple use of same lancet device is also not recommended as it may result in the carryover of allergen to avoid false-positive test and always use separate lancet or needle for each allergen test. A standardized stable allergen extracts for testing should be used for better results (Fig. 10.1).

It is estimated that, in a prick, 3-µmL allergen extract is injected. Buffer saline is used as a negative control and histamine phosphate 1:100 (histamine 10 mg/mL) as a positive control. Histamine-positive control should be read after 10–15 minutes and allergens at 15–20 minutes after performing the test.[14] Reaction of the test should be compared with both the positive and the negative controls. Wheal and erythema (flare) both should be recorded and compared with positive and negative control. If the test is left for more than 20 minutes to read, it may diminish or lose the test reaction and may require repeat testing. The patient should be monitored for at least 30 minutes after the completion of test. Preferably,

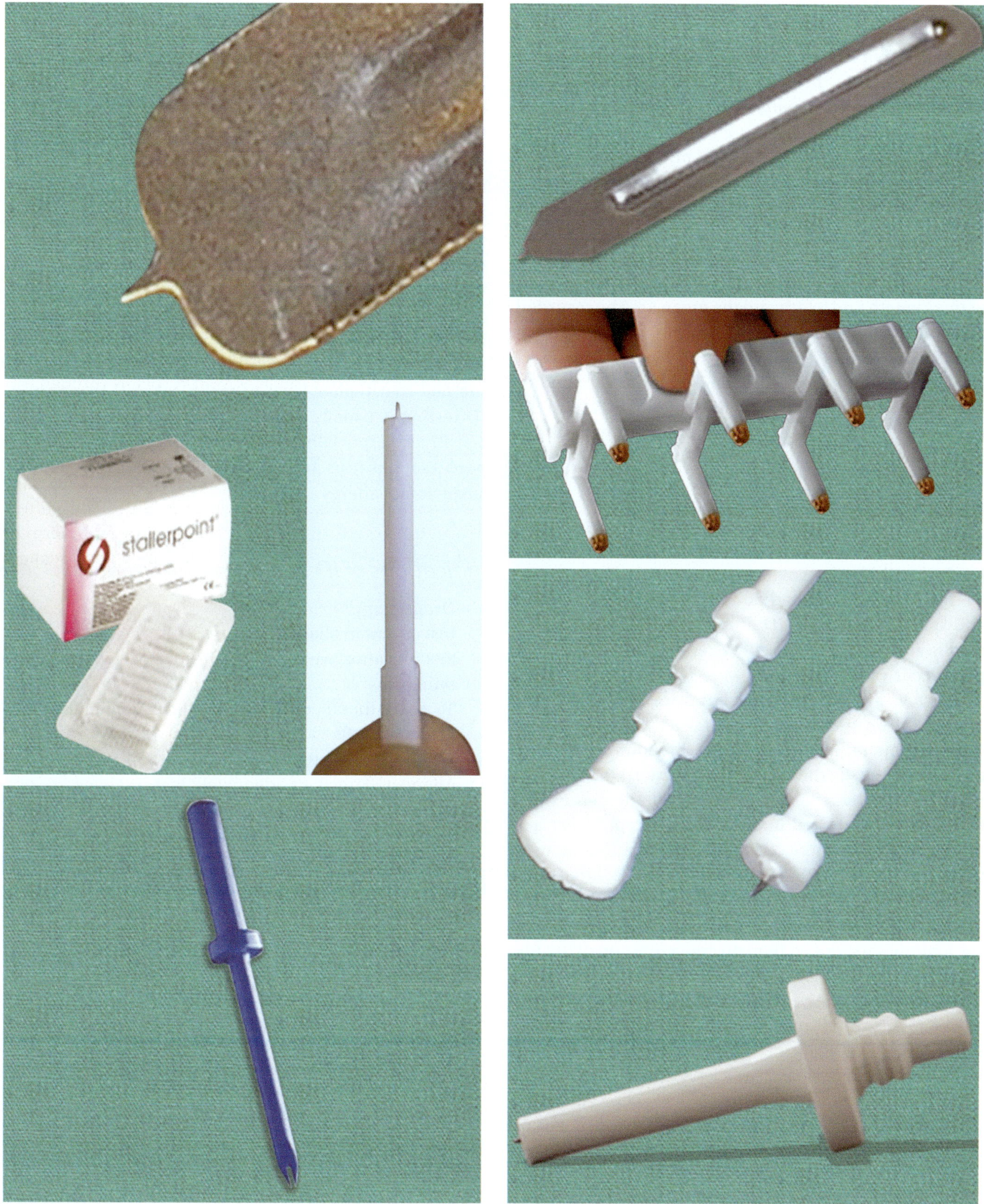

Fig. 10.1: Various lancets used in skin prick test (SPT).[43]

the test results are recorded by a transparent adhesive tape. The positive control should optimally show a wheal of 3 mm or more, and the negative control should show no reaction. In prick test, a wheal diameter of 3 mm or more of the negative control is the most reliable cutoff point for differentiating between sensitized and nonsensitized individuals. A true 3 mm wheal represents 10 times as much specific IgE compared to 2 mm wheal.[50] A prick test with a reaction of at least 3 mm diameter more than the diluents control is required as a proof for allergen-specific IgE.[51-53] The size of the skin reaction of both the wheal and the erythema should be measured with its length and width and the mean area be recorded. The global guideline does not support the use of grading of the skin response; however, the size of wheal and erythema should be recorded. The Indian guidelines recommend a grading system both for SPT and ID. Grading is done according to the criteria mentioned in the following[11,15,46]:

Intradermal Test (Intracutaneous)

The ID test is much more sensitive (10,000 times more) but less specific than skin prick test. Tested allergen is 10–100 fold more diluted and used presently in limited and specific situations. ID produces more false-positive results and has higher risk of systemic reaction although they occur rarely.[12] ID tests were widely used in North America as an alternative to skin prick test.[6] The test is performed on the upper arm or volar surface of both the forearms rather than back for it allows application of tourniquet if the systemic reaction occurs. For most of the allergens, 0.01–0.02 mL of allergen extract (1:500 w/v) is injected intradermally except insect and mite allergens, where 1:5,000 concentration is used in sterilized disposable tuberculin syringe fitted with 26- to 30-gauge fine needle producing ID bleb of about 3 mm in diameter. The size of reaction is less dependent on the amount introduced than on concentration of the test solution.[19] A wheal reaction less than 5 mm in diameter is regarded as negative. Buffer saline 0.1 mg/mL is used as negative control and histamine phosphate in buffer saline 1:10,000 (100 μg/mL) as positive control. The skin is cleaned with nondetergent soap water first, then with 70% alcohol swab, and then the skin is allowed to dry. If the alcohol is causing irritation, then the skin can be cleaned with nondetergent gentle soap and swabbed with distilled water. The individual test sites are 5 cm apart. The tests are read after 15–20 minutes, and grading is done according to modified criteria of Shivpuri and Agarwal (Table 10.2).[54] Patients should be monitored for 30 minutes after testing. The LPRs are read between 6th and 12th hours of testing. Preadministration of drugs, such as calcineurin inhibitors and misoprostol, may cause complete inhibition, while prednisolone and azelastine cause partial inhibition of late-phase cutaneous response. Routine use of large number of allergens for ID test should not be taken unless there is a definite clinical history of exposures, occupations, environmental, and living conditions. In experienced hands, the ID skin test is slightly more reproducible than the skin prick test, but this advantage is offset while the fact that higher level of technical skill is required. ID testing is usually reserved for venom and antibiotic sensitivity especially penicillin allergy testing when percutaneous tests are negative but there is high clinical suspicion of allergy.

Indications of ID Test in Special Situations

- Drug allergy[10-15,45,52]
- Insect venom allergies
- SPT negative with positive history of exposure and symptoms
- To assess therapeutic success of immunotherapy
- To detect LPRs
- When allergen preparation of SPT is not available
- Allergen extracts of adequately high potency are not available (Table 10.3).

Table 10.2: Grading of intradermal test

Grade	*Wheal (mm)*
Negative	Same as buffer saline control
+/–	<1+
1+	>Twice the size of negative control, but >6 mm
2+	3 times the size of negative control
3+	4 times the size of negative control with one to two pseudopodia
4+	>4 times the size of negative control with >2 pseudopodia

Table 10.3: Comparative status of skin prick test versus intradermal test.[55,56]

	Skin prick test	*Intradermal test*
	Small drop (1:10/20 w/v)	0.1–0.2 mL (1:500 w/v)
Safety	More	Less
Reproducibility	Less	More
Speed	More	Less (20–40 tests at one sitting)
Feasibility/ simplicity	Simple to perform	Needs skill to perform
Pain	Less	More
Sensitivity	Less	More
Specificity	More	Less
Safety	More	Less
False-negative reactions	More	Less
False-positive reactions	Less	More
Interpretation of positive and negative reactions	More	Less
Influence of age	More suited in children and young people	More suited in old age
Testing in infants	More than 1 month	Not preferred
Influence of higher reactive skin	Suitable in highly reactive skin/ dermatographia	Not suitable in highly reactive skin or in dematographia
Ideal order of testing	Suggestive by h/o of allergy	Begin with antigens, which have negative SPT with positive h/o

FACTORS INFLUENCING SKIN TEST RESULTS

Skin test results are affected by a particular technique and the site used, age, sex, race, amount/concentration of allergen, and previous treatment with drugs.[10,14,19-35]

- *Quality of allergen extract*: Skin test reactions may be affected by poor quality and unstandardized allergen extracts and may give false-negative reaction. Allergen extract should be used only if their potency, composition, and stability have been properly documented. Preservatives used in allergen extracts may also be irritative and may affect the quality of wheal and flare reaction and may give a false-positive reaction.
- *Surface area of body*: The surface area of various parts of body may affect the results of skin tests. The mid-back and upper back are more reactive than the lower back, and the back as a whole is more reactive than the forearm. The antecubital fossa of arm is more reactive, whereas the wrist of the forearm is the least reactive. The ulnar side of the arm is more sensitive than the radial side. It is recommended that the test should not be placed in areas 5 cm from the wrist or 3 cm from the antecubital fossae.
- *Age*: Skin reactivity may vary with age; infants react more with a larger erythematous flare and smaller wheal. Skin test wheal increases in size from infancy to adulthood and often declines with progressing age after 50 years.
- *Gender*: There is no gender variation is terms of skin test reactivity. However, a recent study has demonstrated optimal response to allergens tested at midcycle of menstruation.[32]

REFERENCES

1. Blackley CH. Experimental Researches on the Cause and Nature of Catarrhus Aestivus (Hay Fever or Hay Asthma). London, UK: Bailliere, Tindall, Cox; 1873. Quoted from: Connell JT. Aleergic rhinitis. In: Weiss EB, Segal MS, eds. Bronchial Asthma. Mechanisms and Therapeutics. Boston, MA: Little, Brown and Co.; 1976:481-9.
2. Feinberg SM. Allergy in Practice. 2nd ed. Chicago, IL: Year Book Medical Publishers; 1946.
3. Indrajana T, Spieksma STH, Voorhorst R. Comparative study of the intracutaneous, scratch and prick test in allergy. Ann Allergy. 1971;12:639-50.
4. Lewis T, Grant R. Vascular reaction of the skin to injury. Part II. The liberation of a histamine-like substance to injured skin, the underlying cause of factitious urticaria and of wheals produced by burning and observations upon the nervous control of certain skin reactions. Heart. 1924;209:1924.
5. Squire JR. The relationship between horse dandruff and horse serum antigens in asthma. Clin Sci. 1950;9:127-50.
6. Kay AB. Principles and practice of diagnosis and treatment of allergic disease. In: Kay AB, ed. Text Book of Allergy and Allergic Diseases. Vol 2: Blackwell Science ltd. 1997:1271.

7. Kathuria PC. Methods of Allergy Tests & Role of Immunotherapy in Allergic Diseases, Recent Advances. J IMA College of general practitioners. 1982 Vol 1; 9.
8. Nelson HS. Diagnostic procedure in allergy skin testing. Ann Allergy. 1983;51:411.
9. Pepys J. Skin testing. Br J Hospital Med. 1975;14:412.
10. Bernstein L, Li JT, Bernstein D, et al. Allergic diagnostic testing: an updated practice parameter. Ann Allergy Asthma Immunol. 2008;100:S1-148.
11. Gaur SN, Singh BP, Singh AB, Vijayen VK, Agarwal MK. Guidelines for practice of allergen immunotherapy in India. Ind J Allergy Asthma Appl Immunol. 2009;23: 1-20.
12. Bousquet J, Heinzerling L, Bachert C, et al. Position paper. Practical guide to skin prick tests in allergy to aeroallergens. Allergy. 2012;67:18-24.
13. Heinzerling L, Mari A, Bergmann KC, et al. The skin prick test-European standerds. Clin Transl Allergy. 2013;3:3.
14. Smith W. A Manual on Skin Prick testing for the diagnosis of allergic disease. Endorsed by Australasian Society of Clinical Immunology and Allergy (ASCIA Council). 2016.
15. Gaur SN, Singh BP, Singh AB, Vijayen VK, Agarwal MK. Guidelines for practice of allergen immunotherapy in India-A 2016 update. Ind J Allergy Asthma Appl Immunol. 2017;31:3-33.
16. Solely Go, Gleish GJ, Jordon RE, Schroeter AL. The late phase of immediate wheal and flair skin reaction: its dependence upon IgE antibodies. J Clin Invest. 1976;58:408-20.
17. Van Arsdel PP Jr, Larson EB. Diagnostic tests for patients with suspected allergic disease: utility and limitations. Ann Intern Med. 1989;110:304-12.
18. Holgersson M, Stahlenheim G, Dreborg S. The precision of the skin test with Phazet, the Osterballe needle and the bifurcated needle. Allergy. 1985;40:64.
19. Dreborg S. Position paper on skin tests in type-I hypersensitivity. Allergy. 1989;44:1-59.
20. Van-Niekerk CH, Prinsloo AE. Effect of skin pigmentation on the response to intradermal histamine. Int Arch Allergy Appl Immunol. 1985;76:73.
21. Vichyanond P, Nelson HS. Circadian variation of skin reactivity and allergy skin tests. J Allergy Clin Immunol. 1989;83:1101.
22. Haahtela T, Jokela H. Influence of Pollen season on immediate skin test reactivity to common allergens. Allergy. 1980;35:15.
23. Oppenheimer JJ, Nelson HS. Seasonal variation in immediate skin test reactions. Ann Allergy. 1993;71:227-9.
24. Uehara M. Reduced histamine reaction in atopic dermatitis. Arch Dermator. 1982;118:244.
25. Long WF, Taylor RJ, Wanger CJ, et al. Skin test suppression by antihistamines and the development of sub sensitivity. J Allergy Clin Immunol. 1985;76:113-7.
26. Philips MJ, Meyrick Thomas RH, Moodley I, Davies RJ. A comparison of the in vivo effects of ketotifen, clemastine, chlorpheniramine and sodium cromoglycate on histamine and allergen induced wheals in human skin. Br J Clin Pharmacol. 1983;15:277-86.
27. Wolfe HI, Fontana VJ. The effect of tranquilizers on the immediate skin wheal reaction. J Allergy. 1964;35:71.
28. Slott R, Jweiman B. A control study of the effect of conticosteriods on immediate skin test reactivity. J Allergy Clin Immunol. 1974;54:229-34.
29. Chipps BE, Sobotka AK, Sanders JP, et al. Effect of theophylline and terbutaline on immediate skin test. J Allergy Clin Immunol. 1980;65:61-4.
30. Menardo JL, Bousquet J, Rodiere M, et al. Skin test reactivity in infancy. J Allergy Clin Immunol. 1985;75:646-51.
31. Herrscher RF, Ksper C, Sullivan TJ. Endogenous cortisol regulates immunoglobulin E-dependent late phase reactions. J Clin Invest. 1992;90:596-603.
32. Kirmaz C, Yuksel H, Mete N, et al. Is the menstrual cycle affecting the skin prick test reactivity? Asain Pac J Allergy Immunol. 2004;22:197-203.
33. Cook TJ, MacQueen DM, Wittig JH, et al. Degree and duration of skin test suppression and side effect with antihistamines. J Allergy Clin Immunol. 1973;51:71-7.
34. Almind M, Diekson A, Neilsen NH, Svendsen UG. Duration of the inhibitory activity on histamine-indused skin wheals of sedative and non-sedative histamines. Allergy. 1988;43:593-6.
35. Simons FE, Simons KJ. Clinical pharmacology of new histamine H1 receptor antagonists. Clin Pharmakinet. 1999;36:329-52.
36. Milller J, Nelson HS. Suppression of immediate skin tests by ranitidine. J Allergy Clin Immunol. 1989;84:895-9.
37. Harvey RP, Schocket AL. The effect of H1 and H2 blockade on cutaneous histamine response in man. J Allergy Clin Immunnol. 1980;65:136-9.
38. Rao KS, Menon PK, Hillman BC, et al. Duration of suppressive effect of tricyclic antidepressants on histamine induced wheal and flair reactions in human skin. J Allergy Clin Imunol. 1988;82:752-7.
39. Saarinen JV, Harvima RJ, Horrsemanheimo M, Harvima IT. Modulation of immediate allergic wheal reaction in the skin by drugs inhibiting the effects of leucotrine C4 and prostaglandine D2. Eur J Clin Pharmacol. 2001;57:1-4.
40. Hill SL III, Krouse JH. The effect s of montelukast on intradermal wheal and flare. Otolaryngol Head Neck Surg. 2003;129;199-203.
41. Agarwal MK, Gaur SN, Chaudhary S. Effects of prior medication on intradermal test response in patients with respiratory allergies. J Asthma. 1988;25:275-9.
42. Slot RI, Zeiwman B. A controlled study of effect of coerticosteriods on immediate skin test reactivity. J Allergy Clin Immunol. 1974;54:229-35.
43. Des Roches A, Paradis L, Bougeard YH, et al. Long term oral corticosteroid therapy does not alter the result of immediate type allergy skin prick tests. J Allergy Clin Immunol. 1996;98:522-7.

44. Olson R, Kaprik MH, Sheilaski S, et al. Skin reactivity to codein and histamine during prolonged corticosteroid therapy. J Allergy Clin Immunol. 1990;86:153-9.
45. Mailing HJ. Methods of skin prick testing. Allergy. 1993; 48:55-6.
46. Agarwal MK, Jhamb S. Immunodiagnosis of type I respiratory allergic disorders. Cardiothorasic J. 1995;1:36.
47. Kausar MA, Vijayan VK, Bansal SK, et al. Mosquitoes as a source of inhalant allergens: clinicoimmunologic and biochemical studies. J Allergy Clin Immunol. 2007;120: 1219-21.
48. Pepys J. Skin testing. Br J Hosp Med. 1975;412.
49. Pastorello EA. Skin tests for IgE mediated allergy EAACI. Position papers 14,1993;14:48-57.
50. Nelson HS, Knoetzer J, Butcher B. Effect of distance between sites and region of the body on results of skin prick test. J Allergy Clin Immunol. 1996;97:596-601.
51. Johnston SL, Clough JB, Opattemore PK, et al. Longitudnal changes in skin prick test reactivity over two years in a population of school children with Test reading is done after 15 minutes respiratory symptoms. Clin Exp Allergy. 1992;22:948.
52. The American Academy Of Allergy, Asthma and Immunoloy (AAAAI) and American College of Allergy, Asthma and Immunology (ACAAI). Allergy diagnostic testing: an updated practice parameter. Ann Allergy Asthma Immnuol. 2008;100:S1-148.
53. McCann WA, Ownby DR. The reproducibility of allergy skin test screening and interpretation by board certified/ board eligible allergists. Ann Allergy Asthma Immunol. 2002;89:368-71.
54. Shivpuri DN, Aggarwal MK. Studies on the allergic fungal spores of the Delhi India Metropolitan area. J Allergy. 1969;44:204.
55. Shivpuri DN. Comparative evaluation of the sensitivity of common methods of diagnostic antigen tests in patients of respiratory allergy. Ind J Chest Dis. 1969;4:102.
56. Demoly P, Michel F, Bousquet J. In vivo methods for allergy skin tests, technique and interpretation. Textbook of allergy principles & practice. In: Middleton, Reed, Ellis, et al, ed. Allergy, Principals and Practice. Vol 1, 5th ed. St Louis, MO: Mosby Co; 1998:530-9.

CHAPTER 11

Laboratory Diagnosis of Type I Allergic Respiratory Disorders: An Extract-based to Molecular-based Approach

MK Agarwal, Shashi Chawla

INTRODUCTION

Hypersensitivity encompasses a wide range of immunological reactions involving one or many organs of the body. The manifestations of Type I hypersensitivity, mediated by immunoglobulin E (IgE), are triggered by some foreign substances referred to as allergens. The allergens are usually harmless to the general populations and affect only genetically predisposed individuals. Depending on the route of exposure, allergens are classified as (1) inhalants, (2) ingestants, (3) contactants, and (4) injectants.

Type I allergic disorders affect almost all the organs of the body; the most frequently affected being the upper and lower respiratory tracts, gastrointestinal tract, and skin. Type I allergic disorders of the respiratory tract are allergic rhinitis and/or bronchial asthma. Various causative and triggering factors for these disorders include allergens, air pollutants, infections, climatic conditions, and emotional factors. Of these, inhalants play the most important role and include airborne bioparticles derived from plants (pollen, fungal spores), dusts (house dust mite), animals (danders), insects (emanations and detritus), etc.

DIAGNOSIS OF TYPE I RESPIRATORY ALLERGIC DISORDERS

The management of respiratory allergic diseases includes allergen avoidance, pharmacotherapy, and immunotherapy. Hence, the identification of causative allergens is the key prerequisite for their avoidance by the patients and for immunotherapy. Presently, various in vivo and in vitro tests are used for the diagnosis of causative allergen(s). However, the molecular or component-resolved allergy diagnosis is gaining importance over classical diagnostic procedures. Before the performance of these tests, the clinician should make a provisional diagnosis based on the patients' personal and family history, physical examination, spirometry, and various other laboratory investigations.

Extract-based Allergy Diagnosis: In Vivo Tests

Skin testing is the most commonly used in vivo procedure in routine clinical practice of respiratory allergic diseases. Both intradermal tests and skin prick tests (SPTs) are convenient, simple, clinically relevant, reproducible, and easy to perform, with low cost and high sensitivity.[1] They are considered to be the gold standard for the diagnosis of respiratory allergic disorders.[2] Other in vivo tests include mucosal challenge tests, such as bronchial challenge, nasal provocation, and conjunctival tests. All these tests have been discussed elsewhere in the book. Besides, a number of in vitro tests (discussed below) may also be used for quantifying the circulating total or allergen-specific IgE antibodies in the sera of patients.[3,4]

Extract-based Allergy Diagnosis: In Vitro Tests

Even though skin test is regarded as the gold standard for determining the patient's clinical sensitivity to specific allergens, it has some limitations. Skin tests cannot be performed on patients who are (1) not in a position to discontinue medications such as antihistamines, (2) have dermographism, (3) suffering from widespread leukoderma, and (4) suffering from severe cardiac disease. In such cases, serological diagnosis is recommended wherein various in vitro tests are used to detect the presence of circulating total and allergen-specific IgE antibodies and their quantification.

TOTAL IGE QUANTIFICATION

Serum concentration of the IgE antibodies increases slowly with age and reaches adult levels at approximately 5–7 years. Elevated IgE levels (<20 IU/mL) in serum at birth or during infancy have been found to correlate with the development of allergy in future life.[5] The upper limit of IgE levels in normal healthy subjects has been reported to be 120 and 200 IU/mL.[6,7] However, in the Indian population, this limit has been reported to be higher.[8-11] Even though the mean IgE level in individuals with allergic disorders is higher, a few allergic individuals may have normal or low IgE levels. Increased levels of serum IgE have also been observed in other clinical conditions (Box 11.1). Thus, raised level of IgE alone does not serve as a diagnostic criterion for allergy and should be supported with a positive clinical history.

Quantification of total IgE levels[5,12] may be accomplished by (1) competitive displacement radioimmunoassay, (2) two-site immunoradiometric assay, and (3) two-site enzyme immunoassay.

Competitive Displacement Radioimmunoassay

Antihuman IgE antibodies are coupled to a solid phase (plastic tubes, paper, sepharose particles, etc.). A known amount of radiolabeled IgE antibodies and test serum sample is incubated with the solid-phase antihuman IgE complex. After washing, the radioactivity bound is measured using a gamma counter. Simultaneously, different concentrations of standard IgE samples are also used in the assay to obtain the standard curve. Increasing amounts of IgE antibodies in the sample (standard/test serum) compete with radiolabeled IgEs for binding to the antihuman IgE antibodies in the solid phase resulting in a dose-related decrease in radioactive counts. This decrease is expressed as percentage of the counts obtained with a negative control, i.e., buffered saline. The tubes containing standard IgE samples exhibit dose-related decrease in the counts. A standard curve is plotted, and the amount of IgE in test samples is calculated. The results are expressed in international units (IU).

BOX 11.1: Clinical conditions associated with increased serum immunoglobulin E (IgE) levels.

- Parasitic infestations (*Ascaris*, *Toxocara*, etc.)
- Hyperimmunoglobulin E syndrome
- Bronchopulmonary aspergillosis
- IgE myeloma
- Smoking
- Pulmonary hemosiderosis
- Some T-cell immunodeficiency states
- Hodgkin's disease
- Wiskott–Aldrich syndrome
- Bullous pemphigoid
- Graft-versus-host reaction after bone marrow transplantation

Two-Site Immunoradiometric Assay

Total IgE levels are measured by incubating increasing amounts of standard IgE samples with a fixed amount of solid phase–anti-IgE complex. Simultaneously, a fixed volume of test serum is also incubated with the same amount of solid phase–anti-IgE complex. The IgE antibodies (present in the standard serum or in the patient's serum) bind to the solid phase–anti-IgE complex resulting in the formation of solid phase–anti-IgE–IgE complex (SP–anti-IgE–IgE complex). After incubation for a fixed time, the unbound serum components are removed by washing. This is followed by addition of a fixed amount of radiolabeled anti-IgE antibodies to the SP–anti-IgE–IgE complex (Fig. 11.1). After incubation, the solid-phase samples are washed, and the radioactivity bound is measured. A dose-related increase in the radioactive counts with an increasing amount of standard IgE is obtained. A standard curve is plotted, and the amount of IgE in test sera is calculated from the standard curve based on the radioactive counts obtained with the test sera.

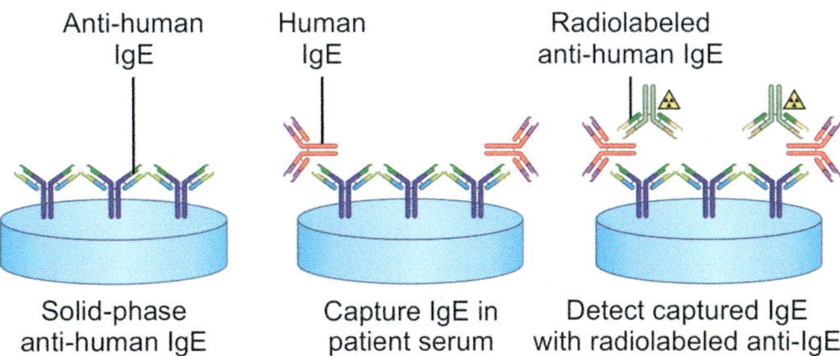

Fig. 11.1: Two-site immunoradiometric assay.

Source: https://biology-forums.com/index.php?action=gallery;sa=view;id=31637.

Table 11.1: A list of enzyme substrate detection systems.

Enzyme	*Substrate*	*Type of substrate*	*Color after stopping*	*Absorbance at (nm)*
Alkaline phosphate (AP)	*para*-Nitrophenyl phosphate (pNPP)	Chromogenic	Yellow	405
	VisiGlo	Chemiluminescent	Emits light	425
	4-Methylumbelliferyl phosphate (MUP)	Fluorogenic	Emits fluorescence	360
Horseradish peroxidase (HRP)	2,2′-Azino-di-ethylbenzothiazoline sulfonic (ABTS) acid	Chromogenic	Green	415
	Tetramethyl benzidine (TMB)/H_2O_2	Chromogenic	Yellow	450
	LumiGLO	Chemiluminescent	Emits light	425
	10-Acetyl-3,7-dihydroxyphenoxazine (ADHP)	Fluorogenic	Emits fluorescence	570
β-Galactosidase	*O*-Nitrophenyl-β-D-galactopyranoside (ONPG)	Chromogenic	Yellow	420

Two-Site Enzyme Immunoassay

The procedure for this assay is the same as that for the two-site immunoradiometric assay except that radiolabeled antihuman IgE is substituted by an enzyme-labeled reagent. Therefore, after the last washing of the solid phase, a suitable substrate is added and tubes are incubated at 37°C. The reaction is stopped after 30 minutes by adding a stopping reagent. The color developed is measured using a colorimeter. Selection of the substrate depends on the enzyme tagged to antihuman IgE, e.g., *p*-nitrophenyl phosphate for alkaline phosphatase tagged to anti-IgE and tetramethyl benzidine/H_2O_2 for horseradish peroxidase-labeled antihuman IgE. Development of the color depends on the selection of the substrate which, in turn, depends on the enzyme used. Table 11.1 displays the list of enzymes used, their substrates, and the color developed after stopping the enzyme reaction during the test.

ALLERGEN-SPECIFIC IGE ESTIMATION

IgE antibodies specific to the causative allergens are found in the sera of patients. These allergen-specific IgE antibodies can be detected using two types of methods: Individual test for each allergen [allergosorbent tests—radioallergosorbent test (RAST) and enzyme-linked immunosorbent assay (ELISA)] or a single test for multiple allergens [such as multiple allergen simultaneous test (MAST)]. The latter type includes tests such as MAST chemiluminescent assay (CLA) and MAST-immunoblot assay. These methods compare very well.

Allergosorbent Test (RAST/ELISA)

The allergosorbent test is a two-site immunometric assay. In the first stage of the assay, the test serum specimen for specific IgE antibodies is incubated with a solid-phase allergen (SPA). During this incubation, specific IgE antibodies bind to the allergen. In the second stage, nonbound serum components are removed by washing, and the SPA is incubated with enzyme or radiolabeled anti-IgE antibodies. This leads to the formation of allergen–IgE–anti-IgE antibodies complex. After 16–18 hours, the SPA is washed thoroughly, and the enzyme or radioactivity is measured.

Various materials used as solid phases include filter paper discs, microcrystalline cellulose particles, agarose beads, and polystyrene wells. Similarly, a variety of tracers are used for detecting the complex formed on SPA, e.g., I^{125}-labeled and enzyme-labeled anti-IgEs are used in RAST and ELISA, respectively (Figs. 11.2 and 11.3). In ELISA, a suitable substrate is required for monitoring the enzyme activity (details given in total IgE estimation). ELISA is preferred over RAST as it does not require a radioactive isotope.[13]

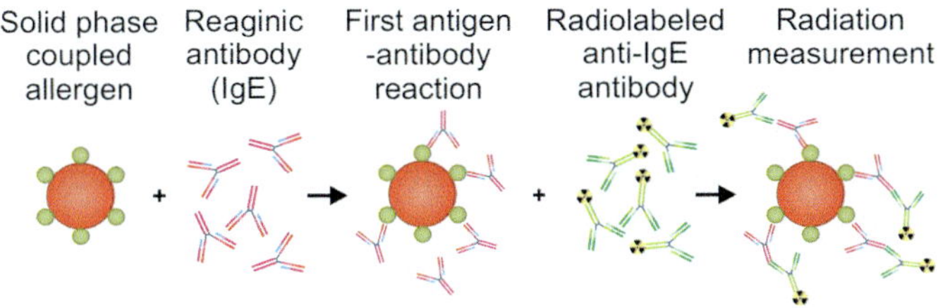

Fig. 11.2: Radioallergosorbent test.

Source: https://www.intechopen.com/books/allergen/allergen-based-diagnostic-novel-and-old-methodologies-with-new-approaches.

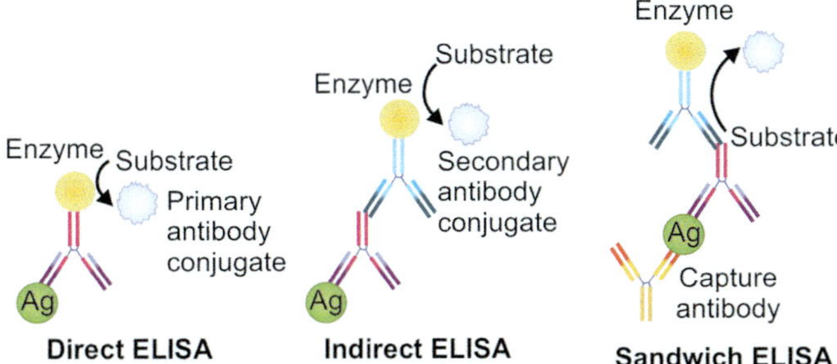

Fig. 11.3: Different types of ELISA. Direct ELISA mostly used for antigen detection; indirect ELISA mainly used for antibody detection; sandwich ELISA used for total IgE detection.

Source: https://www.intechopen.com/books/allergen/allergen-based-diagnostic-novel-and-old-methodologies-with-new-approaches.

One of the major limitations of this technique is nonavailability of a uniform quantitative scoring system. Different researchers have devised their own criteria to score and report results. Usually, RAST results are expressed in terms of RAST ratios[14] calculated as follows:

$$\text{RAST ratio} = \frac{\text{CPM with patient's serum}}{\text{CPM with normal human serum}}$$

The allergosorbent test kits are available for most of the allergens including pollen of grasses, weeds and trees, animal epithelia, foods, molds, dusts, insect venoms, some drugs, etc. Since allergens vary from place to place both quantitatively and qualitatively, it is important to have SPAs prepared from local allergens.

Multiple Allergen Simultaneous Test

In RAST and ELISA, each allergen has to be tested separately; it is time-consuming and needs a considerable amount of serum. However, MAST is an immunological diagnostic test capable of measuring multiple allergens simultaneously with small amount of serum. MAST can be subdivided based on the agent used for labeling anti-IgE. The first method developed was MAST-RIA. This method had advantages over RAST, as it offered miniaturized RAST-type testing for a panel of allergens and simultaneous estimation of total IgE. It showed good correlation with RAST results as well as skin testing. One year later, a better version called MAST CLA was developed, and MAST-RIA was withdrawn from the market. MAST CLA required neither radioactive elements nor an expensive device and could also test multiple allergens simultaneously. It needed a shorter testing time and used easy-to-keep reagents. The more recently developed MAST-immunoblot method reduces the testing time from 48 to 3 hours.

MAST Chemiluminescent Assay

In this test, chemiluminescent reagent is used for the detection of allergen-specific and anti-IgE complex, which is known as MAST CLA.[15] In this test, allergens immobilized in the solid phase of a specialized reaction container (Fig. 11.4) are incubated with serum so that allergen-specific IgE antibodies, if present in the serum, get bound to the allergen (s). The solid phase or screening panel has extracts of house dust mite, cat and dog dander, mold spores, tree, grass, and weed pollen, and can be adapted to include locally implicated aeroallergens. Addition of enzyme-labeled antihuman IgE forms a complex of allergen-specific IgE and enzyme-labeled anti-IgE. To detect the formation of this complex, luminescent reagent (luminol, hydrogen peroxide) is dispensed. The degree of luminescence is measured using a specialized luminometer. These assays are often modified as the manufacturers improve allergens or change reagents to optimize the test performance, affecting the diagnostic efficiency of those assays.

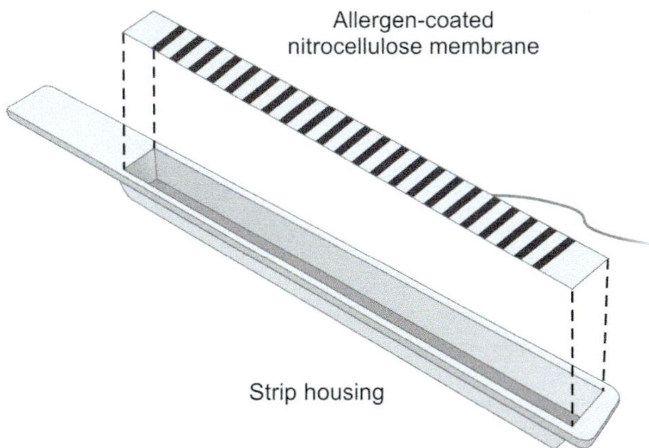

Fig. 11.4: Specialized reaction container for housing a multiple allergen-coated nitrocellulose strip.

Like other non-isotopic immunoassays, CLAs are becoming an increasingly attractive alternative to radiolabels in new immunoassay methods. MAST CLA is relatively a low-cost and a highly sensitive and specific test. It requires no standard curve or volume-dependent pipetting steps, incorporates both positive and negative controls for each sample, and quantifies allergen-specific IgE at picomolar concentrations. Also, its results correlate well with SPTs. However, the main drawback is that it has no clear cutoff levels and requires a lengthy testing time. It frequently shows concurrent positive results for multiple allergens, thereby making it difficult to interpret the results as multiple allergens and multiple allergic reactions, cross-reactivity, or false positives. In such cases, it does not indicate which individual allergens are implicated but rather whether there is respiratory allergy.

MAST-Immunoblot Assay

Immunoblotting or Western blotting is a technique used for analysis of individual proteins in a protein mixture. In this technique, the component s of a protein mixture (in this case, allergen extract) are separated on a gel by size, charge, or other differences under the influence of current. The separated protein bands (allergenic components) are then transferred to a carrier membrane (e.g., nitrocellulose). This process is called *blotting* (Fig. 11.5).

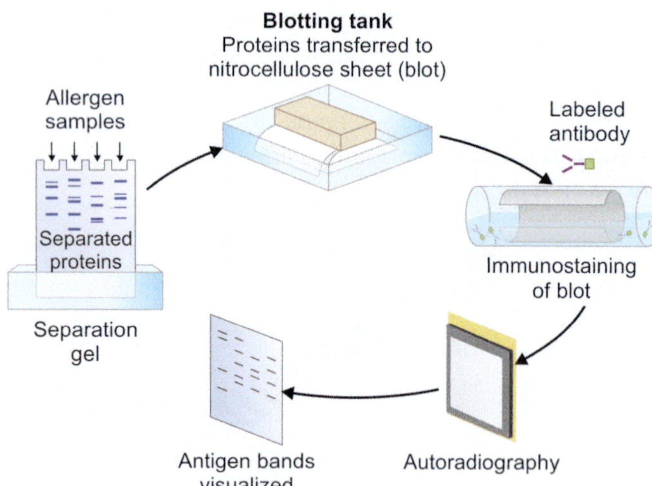

Fig. 11.5: Technique of Western blotting: separation of allergen on a sodium dodecyl sulfate-polyacrylamide gel electrophoresis (SDS-PAGE). Transfer (blotting) of separated components to a nitrocellulose membrane. Incubation of blot with the serum samples and then with a radiolabeled secondary antibody. Detection of IgE antibodies by autoradiography.

Source: https://www.intechopen.com/books/allergen/allergen-based-diagnostic-novel-and-old-methodologies-with-new-approaches.

The proteins adhere to the membrane in the same pattern as they are separated on the gel. The blotted proteins on this immunoblot are then detected by applying primary antibodies (here patient's serum containing IgE), which are then recognized by a secondary antibody (anti-IgE) conjugated with enzymes or fluorescent or radioactive labels. The blot is then analyzed by using different imaging systems such as color reaction, luminescence, and autoradiography.

Immunoblot method entails various advantages over other immunosorbent assays such as ELISA and MAST.[16] The described method of stripping allows for the identification of specific allergenic component(s) after enzymatic digestion of an allergenic extract, their size, biochemical nature, etc. It is used to identify cross-reacting peptides. It is also possible to (semi-) quantify the proteins of interest. Similarly, the protein content of the samples can be compared.

Nowadays, MAST-immunoblot kits are available, which contain test strips coated with parallel lines of components of different allergens separated by electrophoresis. Each line has the cross-reactive carbohydrate determinant marker, total IgE, and separated components of a specific allergen. In the first reaction step, the test strips are incubated with a patient's serum. If a specimen contains IgE for a specific allergen, it would bind to that allergen. To detect the bound IgE, a second incubation is performed using an enzyme-labeled monoclonal antihuman IgE (i.e., enzyme conjugate). A color reaction develops. The test strips are then scanned to identify the bands, to measure their intensity, and to automatically sort the bands into classes from 0 to 6. Classes 1–6 are considered positive results.

LEUKOCYTE HISTAMINE RELEASE TEST

Leukocyte histamine release test is another valuable tool for in vitro diagnosis of allergy and is used mostly for research purposes. Leukocytes are isolated from the peripheral blood of a patient and incubated with varying concentrations of an allergen extract at 37°C overnight. During incubation, allergen binds to the allergen-specific IgE on the basophils resulting in the release of histamine in the supernatant. The histamine released can be determined by various methods: (1) chemical methods, (2) enzymatic isotopic assay, and (3) radioimmunoassay. The results obtained can be expressed as either (1) the concentration of allergen required to release 30% or 50% of total cellular histamine (cell sensitivity) or (2) the maximum histamine release obtained with a given amount of allergen (cell reactivity). A positive (anti-IgE) and a negative (PBS) control are also used.[17] The test can be simplified by eliminating the process of leukocyte preparation and using the heparinized whole blood. The use of leukocyte histamine release is confirmed for the diagnosis of allergy to house mite, cow's milk, and birch pollen.[18-20]

TRYPTASE ESTIMATION

One of the mediators released by mast cells is tryptase. In patients with allergic rhinitis, nasal fluid can be tested for the level of mast cell tryptase. The method involves incubation of nasal fluid in the coated tubes, washing followed by second incubation with the radiolabeled antibody. The tubes are washed, and the bound radioactivity is measured using a gamma counter. The tryptase levels are calculated from the curve obtained with the standards. Levels of mast cell tryptase are significantly higher in patients with allergy than in controls and patients with other non-mast-cell-related nasal diseases.[21]

MOLECULAR-BASED ALLERGY DIAGNOSIS

Recombinant Allergens

Most of the allergy diagnostic assays and treatment are performed with crude allergen extracts. These extracts are easy to prepare, contain multiple allergenic proteins, and are easily available. However, there are many disadvantages with these extracts:[22,23]

- Crude extracts are the mixtures of allergenic and nonallergenic components.
- Allergen content varies from batch to batch.
- Purification, characterization, and standardization of crude allergen extracts involve time-consuming protein chemistry techniques such as gel chromatography, isoelectric focusing, affinity chromatography, and the preparation and use of monoclonal antibodies.
- Important allergens may be absent from these extracts as the important allergenic components may be lost during extraction due to instability of proteins, protease activities in the extracts, etc.
- They may contain contamination from other sources eliciting false-positive tests in some patients.

Many of these problems can be overcome with the use of genetically engineered recombinant allergens. The first report on the successful use of recombinant allergens for the diagnosis of allergy appeared in 1991.[23] A recombinant allergen is a biotechnologically produced allergen molecule originally identified and characterized from a crude allergen extract. Most of the existing recombinant allergens are expressed in *Escherichia coli*, yeast, and insect cells. They are usually comparable with their natural counterparts (proteins) in structural features and immunological properties.[24] In many cases, a three-dimensional structure of these allergens has been determined, and their B-cell and T-cell epitopes have been mapped. These studies have revealed that allergens have diverse biologic functions (they may be enzymes, enzyme inhibitors, lipocalins, or structural proteins).[25] However, as a rule, none of these functions is related to the ability of the allergen to generate IgE antibody responses. Recombinant allergens mostly have IgE antibody-binding capacity comparable to that of the natural allergen and generally show good reactivity in an in vivo as well as in vitro diagnostic tests. To date, many different allergen components from various allergen sources such as mites, pollens, animal dander, insects, and foods have been cloned, sequenced, and expressed as recombinant proteins.

The advantages of recombinant allergens are as follows:[22,26]

- They are highly pure proteins of defined quality.
- Each batch has the same amount of allergen with reproducible quality.
- Their allergenic potential can be modified. For diagnosis, allergens mimicking the wild-type allergens can be made, whereas for immunotherapy, safe hypoallergens can be produced.
- Use of recombinant allergens not only points to the causative allergen but also helps in the identification of actual protein component(s) eliciting the allergic symptoms.
- Their use also helps in discriminating genuine sensitization from cross-reactivity.

Single recombinant allergen tests offer new opportunities to determine whether a patient is a good candidate for SIT, and for suggesting the optimal therapy. If the patient is allergic to the maj or allergen component of birch pollen like Bet v 1, he/she is likely to respond well to immunotherapy with a common extract, as it contains a high amount of this component. On the other hand, if the patient is sensitized to, another component, e.g., Bet v 2 or Bet v 4 in birch pollen, immunotherapy with extracts having a high amount of Bet v 1 will probably not be effective enough. There are even concerns that immunotherapy with allergenic components to which the patient is not sensitized may, in fact, induce new sensitization.

Also, several studies have shown extensive cross-reactivities among the relevant allergens, indicating that the number of epitopes needed for diagnosis and specific immunotherapy is less diverse than originally anticipated and might be soon covered by recombinant molecules.[27]

Despite the abovementioned benefits, there are some disadvantages associated with recombinant allergens. They are as follows:

1. Establishing the process for production of recombinant allergens may be expensive but easy to produce again and again.
2. Difficult in acceptance as the products are new.
3. Panel of allergens for certain sources are not yet complete.

COMPONENT-RESOLVED DIAGNOSIS: A NEW APPROACH IN ALLERGY DIAGNOSTICS

Cocktails of recombinant allergens can be formulated with predetermined and uniform allergen levels, which could replace natural allergens and result in the development of innovative, patient-based tests for allergy diagnosis. Recently, recombinant allergens have been developed for microarray-based multi-allergen tests, which provide component-resolved diagnosis (CRD) of the patient's sensitization profile. In this test, a small amount of patient's serum is added to a microarray immune solid-phase allergen chip containing >150 purified allergens (Figs. 11.6 and 11.7). The chip has been shown to be superior to allergen extract testing. With CRD, the total antibody reactivity profile of an allergic patient may be identified, along with the disease-eliciting allergens and potential cross-reactivity interactions.[28] CRD has the potential to revolutionize allergy diagnostics. In the future, diagnoses based on detailed individual reactivity profiles at a molecular level may enable specific immunotherapy with the exact proteins that the individual has become sensitized to, and much better and more precise advice on allergen avoidance.

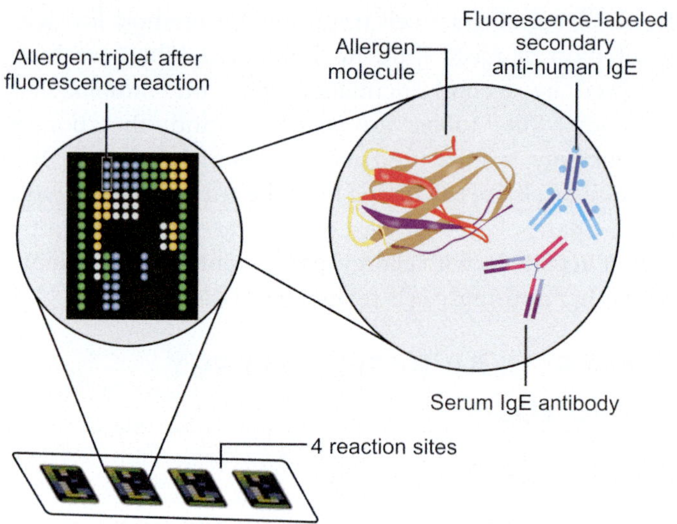

Fig. 11.6: Immune solid-phase allergen chip (ISAC) assay. The recombinant allergens on the chip are recognized by sIgE from serum samples; a secondary antibody fluorescent-labeled interacts with IgE. Fluorescence is measured by using a biochip, and the results are analyzed using a specialized software.

Source: https://www.intechopen.com/books/allergen/allergen-based-diagnostic-novel-and-old-methodologies-with-new-approaches.

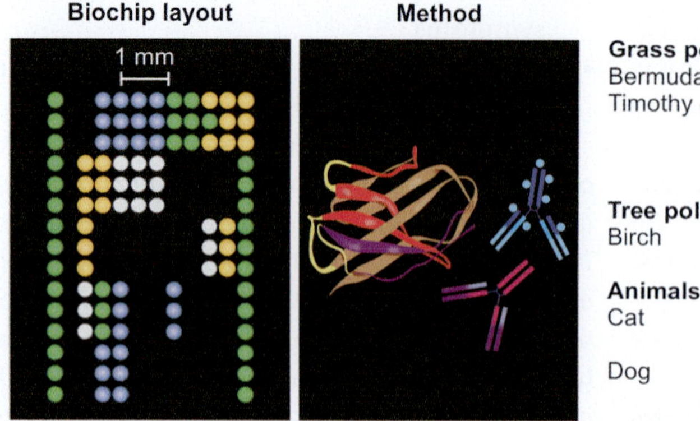

Result

Grass pollen		
Bermuda grass	nCyn d 1	1 ISU
Timothy grass	rPhi p 1	1.8 ISU
	rPhi p 5	1.1 ISU
	rPhi p 6	0.9 ISU
Tree pollen		
Birch	rBet v 1	27 ISU
Animals		
Cat	rFel d 1	5.5 ISU
	rFel d 4	1.5 ISU
Dog	rCan f 1	5.5 ISU

Fig. 11.7: An immune solid-phase allergen chip (ISAC) biochip layout. Results are reported in arbitrary units named ISAC-standardized units (ISU).

Source: https://www.intechopen.com/books/allergen/allergen-based-diagnostic-novel-and-old-methodologies-with-new-approaches.

Moreover, recombinant protein technology and peptide chemistry have been used to construct isoallergens, allergen mutants, allergoids, T- and B-cell peptides, hypoallergens, and mimotopes with reduced allergenicity but enhanced immunogenicity for developing prophylactic allergen vaccines.[29]

Comparative Evaluation of Various In Vivo and In Vitro Diagnostic Tests

None of the test procedures employed for the identification of causative allergens in patients with respiratory allergic disorders correlates perfectly with clinical assessment of disease severity. Since skin testing is the oldest and most commonly used technique for identifying causative allergens in the patients, the efficiency of other techniques has been evaluated, considering it as the gold standard procedure.

The correlation between skin tests and BPTs varies widely, and depends on the factors such as the criteria employed for grading skin and bronchial provocation responses, the concentration and the quality of allergen extracts used, and the type of allergen. Good correlation has been obtained between markedly positive skin responses and BPTs with fungi, insects, dusts, animal danders, and other allergen extracts.[30,31] Various factors responsible for cases with a positive skin test and a negative BPT are as follows:

- A false-positive skin test due to hyper-reactivity of the skin, the presence of nonspecific irritants, or the improper performance or grading of the test.
- The presence of immunologic defect and absence of bronchial reactivity.
- Inadequate challenge while performing BPTs.

By contrast, patients eliciting negative skin test but positive challenge test responses are rare. This discordance between the two tests may be attributed to (1) the false-negative skin test due to improper performance or a stringent criterion followed for grading serum test positivity and/or (2) the liberal criteria used for evaluating the bronchial reactivity.

A number of studies have compared the results of RAST experiments with those of skin tests and correlations ranging from 20% to 89% have been reported.[32-34] In our experience, correlations varied in different groups of allergens as well as from allergens to allergens in the same group. RAST positivities using SPAs of the extracts of 20 insects, 42 fungi, 3 animal danders, and 4 dusts were 80% with insects, 47.7% with male American cockroach (*Periplaneta americana*), 90% with mosquito (*Anopheles stephensi*), 75% with fungi, 50% with *Paecilomyces* to 87% with *Aspergillus tamarii*, 60% with dusts, and 51% with animal danders.[35-46] In general, correlations obtained with insects and fungal allergen extracts were better compared to the results with dander and dust extracts. Further, RAST positivity increased with an increase in the intensity of skin reactions. It varied from 12% to 79.5% in insects; 35% to 92% in fungi, and 7% to 100% with animal danders in 1+ to 4+ cutaneous reactors, respectively. Some cases exhibiting positive skin reactions showed negative RASTs. The possible reasons may be the following:

1. Interference by allergen-specific IgG and IgG4 antibodies.
2. Low levels of allergen-specific IgE.
3. Low levels of specific allergens in the crude extract used for preparing SPAs.
4. Biochemical nature of allergen extract.
5. Inappropriate representation of allergenic component on the SPAs used in RASTs.
6. Activation of a nonspecific mediator system resulting in false-positive skin response.
7. Liberal criteria used for grading skin tests.
8. Strict criteria used for evaluating RASTs.

On the other hand, the percentage of cases with negative skin test responses and a positive RAST is very low. In different groups of allergens it varies, e.g., 4.5% in fungi, 7.6% in dusts, and 10% in insects.[39,41,44,46] The most plausible explanation for positive RAST in cases with negative skin tests is that a skin test can be false negative due to the influence of drugs and improper performance or grading of the test.

Even though the specificity and sensitivity of RAST are quite high, reproducibility is acceptable and the shelf life of reagents is quite long; the biggest drawback is the high health hazard. Hence, ELISA is preferred over RAST. Its correlation with skin tests, specificity, sensitivity, and reproducibility are almost the same as those for RAST. The only limitation in ELISA is low shelf life of its reagents.

Studies on the comparison of MAST CLA and MAST-immunoblot with skin tests as well as RAST have shown good agreement for a variety of allergens.[47-49] However, a comparison of MAST CLA and MAST-immunoblot with ImmunoCAP has revealed a higher agreement rate between ImmunoCAP and MAST-CLA results compared with MAST-CLA and MAST-immunoblot results.[50]

The diagnostic efficiency of all the in vivo and in vitro tests depends on the quality of allergen extracts used.

The biopotency of most of the commercially available allergens varies from batch to batch and manufacturer to manufacturer, and only a limited number of standardized extracts are available. Thus, the sensitivity and specificity of each diagnostic test may differ. To overcome this difficulty, the same batch of allergen extract should be used for various diagnostic tests. Further, all these methods also have their own merits and limitations (Table 11.2). Therefore, a combination of an in vivo and an in vitro test should be employed for proper diagnosis of patients with respiratory allergic disorders.

Allergen extracts contain a number of different potential allergenic components. A specific RAST or ELISA can test only a few of the potential allergens that can bind

Table 11.2: Merits and limitations of various in vivo and in vitro tests.

Test	*Merits*	*Limitations*
Skin test	Immediate results	Allergens lose potency in dilute solution
	Broad selection of allergens	Influenced by some drugs
	Relatively inexpensive	Risk of systemic reactions
	Higher degree of sensitivity	Cannot be used in patients with dermographism
Provocation tests	Precise identification of allergen	Time-consuming
		Risk of systemic reaction
		Influenced by different drugs
Total immunoglobulin E (IgE) estimation	Safe and convenient	Expensive
	No influence of drugs	Does not identify the causative allergens
		Overlap in values between normal and allergic subjects
Allergosorbent test	Safe, convenient	Limited selection of allergens
	Not influenced by drugs	Semiquantitative
	Solid-phase allergens stable	Expensive
	Good correlation with clinical symptoms, skin reactions by end-point dilution, bronchial challenge, and in vitro leukocyte histamine release	Less sensitive
		Allergen-specific immunoglobulin G (IgG) may interfere
MAST CLA	Simultaneous testing of a large number of allergens	No fixed cutoff point for a positive result
	Simple, convenient, and safe	Variable specificity and sensitivity
	Long-term reagent stability	Cannot differentiate between cross-reactivity and false positivity of the test
	Limited amount of serum requirement	Longer laboratory time
MAST-immunoblot*	Shorter laboratory time	
	Can differentiate between cross-reactivity and false positivity of the test	
Leukocyte histamine release test	High sensitivity	Cumbersome and time-consuming
	Requires small amount of allergen	Low specificity
	No interference by allergen-specific IgG	Requires large volume of fresh blood from patients/donors

*MAST-immunoblot is a recent technique. Its limitations are yet to be reported.

to the solid phase. Some patients who may be sensitized only to a minor allergenic component in a particular allergen may exhibit a negative allergosorbent test, while they may be still highly allergic to that allergen.

For this reason, a new range of recombinant allergens have been developed to measure the specific components. These proteins can occur in diverse unrelated allergens such as birch pollen and apple flesh or latex and avocado. If the specific allergen is then identified on blood test, the person can be advised exactly what allergens to avoid. These recombinant allergen tests are, however, very expensive. This screening is very useful for people who suffer from multiple allergies and helps to identify to which group(s) of allergens they are cross-reacting. It can predict the severity of future reactions and whether they would benefit from immunotherapy.

REFERENCES

1. Klein GL. Diagnosing allergic asthma. In: Gershwin ME, Albertson TE, eds. Current Clinical Practice: Bronchial Asthma: A Guide for Practical Understanding and Treatment. 5th ed. Totowa, NJ: Humana Press Inc.; 2006:31-44.
2. Pawankar R, Canonica G, Holgate S, Lockey R. WAO White Book on Allergy, 2011-2012. Milwaukee, MI: World Allergy Organization; 2012.
3. Diaz RC, Meyers AD. Diagnostic allergy testing. http://emedicine.medscape.com/article/2068676-overview. 2016.
4. Rusznak C, Davies RJ. Diagnosing allergy. British Med J. 1998;316:686.
5. Owen JA, Punt J, Stranford SA, Jones PP. Kuby Immunology, 7th ed. New York: W.H. Freeman; 2013.
6. Marsh DG, Bias WB, Ishizaka K. Genetic control of basal serum immunoglobulin E level and its effect on specific reaginic sensitivity. Proc Natl Acad Sci USA. 1974;71: 3588-93.
7. Platts-Mills TAE. Type I or immediate hypersensitivity; hay fever and asthma. In: Lachman PJ, Peter DK, eds. Clinical Aspects of Immunology, 4th ed. Oxford: Blackwell Scientific Publications; 1982:579.
8. Mital OP, Kaiyar SK, Prasad R. Serum IgE estimation in cases of respiratory allergy. Asp Allergy Appl Immunol. 1978;XI:92-100.
9. Menon MPS, Kapoo A. Serum IgE levels in healthy and allergic respiratory disorders. J Ass Phys Ind. 1975;23:629-34.
10. Saha K, Kulpati DD, Padmini R. Serum immunoglobulin including IgE in patients of bronchial asthma with relation to the spectrum of the disease. Asp Allergy Appl Immunol. 1975;VIII:105-18.
11. Sharma S, Kathuria PC, Gupta CK, Nordling K, Ghosh B, Singh AB. Total serum immunoglobulin E levels in a case-control study in asthmatic/allergic patients, their family members, and healthy subjects from India. Clin Exp Allergy. 2006;36:1019-27.
12. Augustin R. Techniques for the study and assay of regains in allergic subjects. In: Weir DM, ed. Handbook of Experimental Immunology, Vol 3, Application of Immunological Methods. Oxford: Blackwell Scientific Publications; 1978:45.1-64.
13. Adolphson CR, Gieich GJ, Yunginger JW. Standardization of allergens. In: Rose NR, Friedman H, Fahey JL, eds. Manual of Clinical Laboratory Immunology. Washington, DC: American Society for Immunology; 1986:632-59.
14. Chaudhry S, Jhamb S, Chauhan UPS, et al. Shared and specific allergenic and antigenic components in the two sexes of American cockroach—Periplaneta americana. Clin Exp Allergy. 1990;20:59-65.
15. Brown CR, Higgins KW, Frazer K, et al. Simultaneous determination of total lgE and allergen-specific IgE in serum by the MAST chemiluminescent assay system. Clin Chem. 1985;31:1500-5.
16. Park DS, Cho JH, Lee KE, et al. Detection rate of allergen-specific IgE by multiple antigen simultaneous test-immunoblot assay. Korean J Lab Med. 2004;24:131-8.
17. Platt-Mills TAE. Laboratory evaluation of allergy. In: Kay AB, Goetxl EJ, eds. Current Perspectives in Allergy. New York: Churchill Livingstone; 1982:25-39.
18. Wegner F, Kochamp R, Rutschke A, et al. Superiority of the histamine release test above case history, prick test, and radioallergosorbent test in predicting bronchial reagibility to the house dust mite in asthmatic children. Klin Wochenschr. 1993;61:43-7.
19. Prahl P, Krasilnikof F, Norn S. Basophil histamine release in children with adverse reactions to cow milk. Comparison with RAST and skin prick test. Allergy. 1988;43:442-8.
20. Valenta R, Sperr WR, Ferreira F, et al. Induction of specific histamine release from basophils with purified natural and recombinant birch pollen allergens. J Allergy Clin Immunol. 1993;91:88-97.
21. Rasp G, Hochstrasser K. Tryptase in nasal fluid is a useful marker of allergic rhinitis. Allergy. 1993;48:72-4.
22. Curin M, Garib V, Valenta R. Single recombinant and purified major allergens and peptides: How they are made and how they change allergy diagnosis and treatment. Ann Allergy Asthma Immunol. 2017;119:201-9.
23. Valenta R, Duchene M, Vttala S, et al. Recombinant allergens for immunoblot diagnosis of tree-pollen allergy. J Allregy Clin Immunol. 1991;88:889-94.
24. Cromwell O, Häfner D, Nandy A. Recombinant allergens for specific immunotherapy. J Allergy Clin Immunol. 2011;127:865-72.
25. Chapman MD, Smith AM, Vailes LD, et al. Recombinant allergens for diagnosis and therapy of allergic disease. J Allergy Clin Immunol. 2000;106:409-18.
26. Tscheppe A, Breiteneder H. Recombinant allergens in structural biology, diagnosis, and immunotherapy. Int Arch Allergy Immunol. 2017;172:187-202.
27. Valenta R, Vrtala S, Laffer S, et al. Recombinant allergens. Allergy. 1998;53:552-61.
28. Treudler R, Simon JC. Overview of component resolved diagnostics. Curr Allergy Asthma Rep. 2013;13:110-7.

29. Ramos JD, Valmonte GR, de Guia RM. Recombinant proteins and peptides as diagnostic and therapeutic reagents for arthropod allergies. Protein Pept Lett. 2007;14:992-1002.
30. Bryant DH, Burns MW, Lazarus L. The correlation between skin tests, bronchial provocation tests and the serum level of IgE specific for common allergens in patients with asthma. Clin Exp Allergy. 1975;5:145-57.
31. Vanto T, Viander M, Koivikko A. Skin prick test in the diagnosis of dog dander allergy: a comparison of different extracts with clinical history, provocation tests and RAST. Clin Allergy. 1980;10:121-32.
32. Ahlstedt S, Eriksson N, Lindgren S, Roth A. Specific IgE determination by RAST compared with skin and provocation tests in allergy diagnosis with birch pollen, timothy pollen and dog epithelium allergens. Clin Allergy. 1974;4:131-40.
33. Pascual HC, Reddy PM, Nagaya H, et al. Agreement between radioallergosorbent test and skin test. Ann Allergy. 1977;39:325-7.
34. Bar-sela S, Shalit M, Kalbfleisch JH, Fink JN. The relative vaue of skin tests and radioallergosorbent test in the diagnosis of bee sting hypersensitivity. J Allergy Clin Immunol. 1983;72:690-4.
35. Chaudhry S. Clinico-Immunologic Studies on the Significance of Insects as Inhalant Allergens in Respiratory Allergic Disorders [PhD thesis]. New Delhi, India: University of Delhi; 1998.
36. Agarwal MK, Sethi S, Jhamb S, Bansal S. Current concepts in the etiologic significance of insects in respiratory allergy. In: Proceedings of CME International Symposium on "Recent advances in Allergy and Immunology";1988:30-6.
37. Gupta S, Jain S, Chaudhry S, Agarwal MK. Role of insects as inhalant allergens in bronchial asthma with special reference to the clinical characteristics of patients. Clin Exp Allergy. 1990;20:519-24.
38. Agarwal MK, Chaudhry S, Jhamb S, et al. Etiologic significance of mosquito (Anopheles stephensi) in respiratory allergy in India. Ann Allergy. 1991;67:598-602.
39. Jhamb S. Studies on the Allergen Specific Immune Response in Type I Hypersensitivity of Respiratory System Including Observations on the Etiologic Role of Influenza Virus [PhD thesis]. New Delhi, India: University of Delhi; 1992.
40. Jhamb S, Jain SK, Chhabra SK, et al. Insects as inhalant allergens in India: Studies on allergenic and antigenic properties, their aerosolization and heterogeneous immune response in patients. Indian J Allergy Appl Immunol. 1992;6:7-14.
41. Aggarwal S. Clinico-Immunologic Studies on Yet Unknown Allergenic Fungal Spores of Delhi Metropolitan Area [PhD thesis]. New Delhi, India: University of Delhi; 1992.
42. Nigam A. Clinico-Immunologic Studies on the Role of Fungi in the Etiology of Nasobronchial Allergy [MD. thesis]. New Delhi, India: University of Delhi; 1992.
43. Sharma AK. Clinico-immunologic Study on the Role of Aspergillus Infection in Asthmatic and Non-asthmatic Chronic Respiratory Diseases [MD. thesis]. New Delhi, India: University of Delhi; 1993.
44. Singh P. Clinico-immunologic and Immunochemical Studies on the Allergenic and Antigenic Properties of Fungal Allergens of Delhi Area [PhD thesis]. New Delhi, India: University of Delhi; 1996.
45. Gupta S, Bidani RK, Jhamb S, Agarwal MK. Role of animal danders as inhalant allergens in bronchial asthma in India. J Asthma. 1996;33:339-48.
46. Wadhawan A. The Etiologic Significance of Various Dusts and Related Arthropods as Inhalant Allergens in Patients with Bronchial Asthma [MD thesis]. New Delhi, India: University of Delhi; 1995.
47. Scolozzi R, Boccafogli A, Vicentini L, et al. Correlation of MAST chemiluminescent assay (CLA) with RAST and skin prick tests for diagnosis of inhalant allergic disease. Ann Allergy. 1989;62:193a-193b.
48. Agata H, Yomo A, Hanashiro Y, et al. Comparison of the MAST chemiluminescent assay system with RAST and skin tests in allergic children. Ann Allergy. 1993;70:153-7.
49. Finnerty JP, Summerell S, Holgate ST. Relationship between skin prick tests, the multiple allergosorbent test and symptoms of allergic disease. Clin Exp Allergy. 1989;19:51-6.
50. Ihm YK, Kang So-Y, Kim MH, Lee WI. Chemiluminescent assay versus immunoblotting for detection of positive reaction to allergens. Science. 2012;43:91-5.

CHAPTER 12

Patch Test

Mahesh Goyal, Aditya Goyal, Srishti Sareen

INTRODUCTION

A patch test is a diagnostic procedure that is used for identifying a specific substance that comes in contact with the skin and causes inflammation. The test basically relies on the allergen being absorbed in sufficient quantity to induce a reproducible inflammation of the skin at the site where it is applied. History of patch tests dates back to 1847 when Staedtler made the use of a blotting paper to test idiosyncratic reaction. A German dermatologist named Josef Jadassohn founded the technique following this in 1869. Then in 1911, a Swiss dermatologist Bruno Bloch explained the mechanism of patch testing. Later in 1960, Scandinavian dermatologists developed a standardization protocol for patch tests. During the twentieth century, Sulzberger[1] highlighted the patch test a one of the important advances in clinical dermatology.

Patch testing holds its importance today as being the only legible and scientific method to discover the causative agent of contact allergic dermatitis. Apart from this, the patch test has other dermal and nondermal indications as well. It is used in the diagnosis of irritant contact dermatitis and airborne allergic dermatitis. Its nondermal indications include detection of food allergies such as cow milk allergy; it is used to confirm the role of inhalants such as house dust mites in atopic dermatitis and also to see the late-phase reaction in cases of type I allergies.

A good patch test should indicate contact sensitization, produce no false-positive reaction, be done with a pure allergen in the right concentration, have low risk of active sensitization, have minimum irritant reaction, be easy to apply, be stable and easy to read, and should be suitable for the patient.

MATERIALS AND METHODS

Patch testing involves the use of different standardized kits containing antigens either in the form of prefilled syringes or as dried strips. The kits also contain Finn chambers, aluminum disks, a hypoallergic micropore tape, and filter papers. In India, we use the Indian standard battery; whereas in the United States, thin-layer rapid-use epicutaneous (TRUE) test kit is in practice. These kits contain antigens whose concentrations have been standardized on the basis of extensive field tests. The commonly used vehicle for the test is petroleum jelly because of its neutral properties, but ethanol, acetone, and water may also be used.

Many different series like European based series,[2] Japanese series, TRUE test kit, Indian standard battery, and North American series are used for patch testing across the world.

TRUE Test Kit

During the fourth quarter of the last century, Fischer and Malbach did a lot of work on the technique of patch testing and evaluated the concept of patch testing. They also introduced the TRUE test kit, an innovative patch test kit (Fig. 12.1).

It stands for thin-layer rapid-use epicutaneous test patch. It includes a set of many allergens along with other testing materials. It is a commercially available ready-to-use test kit, which uses polyester patches coated with allergens in a hydrophilic vehicle. It meets almost all prerequisites of the most suitable test method due to the least possible time-consumed and has been widely used for basic standard patch testing by dermatologists and allergists. Easy application is an advantage of this kit, but it may have lower sensitivity and limited availability of allergens than other standard series.[3]

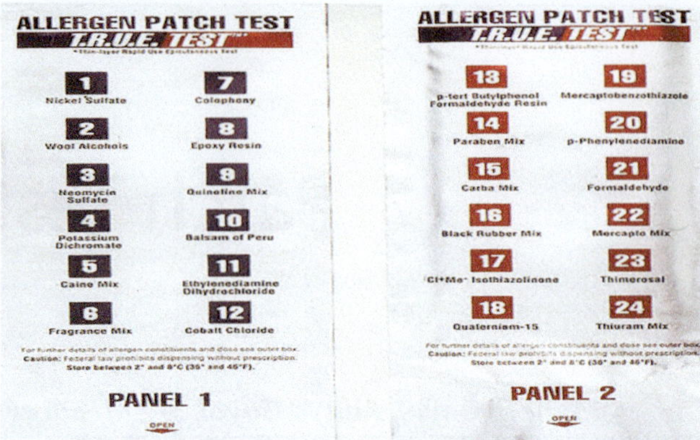

Fig. 12.1: TRUE test kit.

Indian Standard Battery Kit (Table 12.1)

It is used by most centers in India. It contains many ready-to-use chemical antigens in prefilled syringes. The Indian standard battery contains a few plant allergens in dried strip form. It has been approved by the "Contact and Occupational Dermatomes Forum of India." It also contains Finn chambers made of aluminum or plastic with a diameter of 10–15 mm and a volume of 15–100 μL.[4] The Finn chamber is currently the most commonly used test unit. It consists of stiff aluminum and has a diameter of 10 mm and a depth of 0.5 mm. The particular advantage of this chamber is its tight opposition to skin, thus localizing reaction only to the test site. Hypoallergic hypodermic allergic tape is used to fix these Finn chambers on the skin. This contact should be firm otherwise a leakage of even minute amounts of allergen can cause diffuse reaction and may mix with adjacent allergens causing false results. Occasionally, metal salts such as mercury, cobalt, and nickel interact with aluminum. In this situation, plastic-coated Finn chambers can be used (Fig. 12.2).

Small number of substances account for the majority of contact allergies. Authorities of patch test recommend that a mix of allergens can be used to find out the causative allergen, and testing of these 20–25 mixes detects approximately 70–80% of allergic contact sensitivity. There are certain special allergens such as plastics, fragrances, cosmetics, and sunscreens. The prevalence is more common in engineering workers, hair-dying industry, bakery workers, and dentistry. Nonstandard substances may be used but for these utmost care is required.

To find out a nonirritant concentration, most chemicals may be tested with three concentrations, i.e., 10%, 1%, and 0.1% in aqueous or petroleum base. However, a positive reaction should not be accepted as allergic unless at least 20 controls are negative.

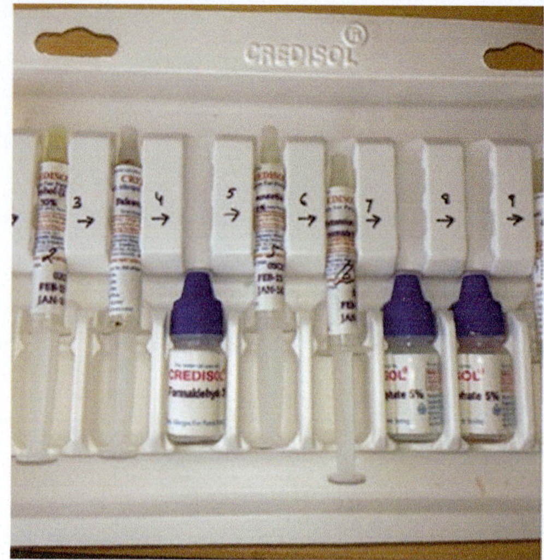

Fig. 12.2: Plastic-coated Finn chambers

The allergens must be stored properly so that they are protected from environmental influence and external contamination. Polypropylene syringes are usually used to keep petroleum base allergens, and these should be kept in cool, dark places preferably in refrigerator. Allergens should be protected from heat, light, UV rays, contaminated air, humidity, and microbial contamination.

An atopic patch test (APT) can be done in patients having atopic diathesis. Its application is similar to that of a patch test, and the allergens tested are similar to those in skin prick test. The patch is applied for 48 hours, and then readings are taken twice at 48 and 72 hours, respectively.[5]

Table 12.1: List of allergens included in the Indian standard battery kit.

S. no.	*Allergen*	*Commonly found in*
1.	Negative control	Microcrystalline cellulose
2.	Potassium dichromate	Cement, tannin, textile dye, metallurgy, photo
3.	Neomycin sulfate	Antibiotic in topical creams, ointments, and drops
4.	Cobalt chloride	Glass paints, jewelry, zipper, tools, dyes
5.	Benzocaine	Topical anesthetic in ointments
6.	Phenylenediamine	Hair dyes, fur dyes, developers, oil, grease, etc.
7.	Parabens	Food preservatives, baked food, dairy food, glues

(Contd...)

(Contd...)

S. no.	Allergen	Commonly found in
8.	Nickel sulfate	Alloys, earrings, watches, buttons, zippers, battery
9.	Colophony	Ink, papers, adhesives, polish, wax, cosmetics
10.	Gentamicin	Topical antibiotic
11.	Mercapto mix	Rubber products such as shoes, gloves, elastic of garments, condoms, medical devices, renal dialysis, and swimming costumes
12.	Epoxy resin	Adhesives, insulations, laminations, paint ink
13.	Fragrance mix	Cosmetics, soap, perfumes tooth paste, food items
14.	Mercaptobenzothiazole	Rubber products
15.	Nitrofurazone	Topical antibiotics, sprays
16.	Chlorocresol	Pharmacy products
17.	Wool alcohol	Cosmetics, moisturizers, topical drugs, textile
18.	Balsam of Peru	Drinks, pastries, cakes, wine,
19.	Thiuram mix	Rubber products
20.	Chinoforms	Topical medicines
21.	Ethylene dihydrochloride	Stabilizer in topical preparations
22.	Black rubber mix	Rubber products
23.	Formaldehyde resin	Shoes, plywood, automobiles, deodorants
24.	Quaternium	Cosmetics, joint cements, metal work
25.	Formaldehyde	
26.	Kathon Cg	
27.	Chrysanthemum	
28.	Propylene glycol	
29.	Parthenium	
30.	Xanthium	

Some of the common allergens that cause contact allergic dermatitis are Balsam of Peru, benzocaine, chrome, nickel, cobalt, epoxy resin, parabens, formaldehyde, fragrances, urea, and neomycin. Airborne contact dermatitis due to *Parthenium hysterophorus* is a very common entity in Indian subcontinent. Parthenium dermatitis is distressing dermatitis caused by the airborne allergen of the Compositae weed *P. hysterophorus*.[6]

PREPARATION

Allergens for the patch test are selected on the basis of a variety of factors, namely occupation, age, sex, site of dermatitis, habits, duration of disease, visit to workplace, and a detailed history of the allergen obtained from the patient by asking him to bring the causative allergen with him if possible. The common sites for application are the upper back (it has maximum primed T lymphocytes so best suited for the reaction), the lower back, and the lateral aspect of the upper arm, forearm, thigh, or abdomen.

Before applying a patch on the patient, some points to rule out false negatives and positives should be kept in mind. Oral steroids should be withdrawn at least 5–7 days before the test; patient should be asked not to apply any topical steroid on the area of skin to be tested.[7] It is better to stop oral antihistamines 3–5 days before patch testing as they have minimal, if any, effect on the mechanism of delayed hypersensitivity.

Skin should not be exposed to sunlight for prolonged duration before the test; skin should be healthy and intact without major abrasions; and if the patient has hairy skin, it should be properly shaved.

PROCEDURE

To begin, first mark at the top of the patch test unit from 1 to 10 or 11 to 20 and so on for an efficient reading later on. Then, remove the protective foil and place the test unit on the table with aluminum chambers facing up. Put 2–3 mm length of allergen ointment from the syringe in the center of the chambers. For liquid allergens, pick a piece of filter paper and wet it with a drop of allergen and then place it on the aluminum chamber. Once the unit is ready for application, clean the upper back of the patient gently with ethyl alcohol or spirit. Care should be taken not to rub excessively on the site of application of the patch. After disinfecting the site of application, mark the skin for each punch (usually 24) with a pen for later identification. Thereafter, apply the patch test unit on the back of the patient as shown in the photograph here (Fig. 12.3). The patches must remain in place for about 48 hours, during which they must remain dry. In case of severe itching or pain, patient should be asked to remove the patch and inform the doctor immediately.

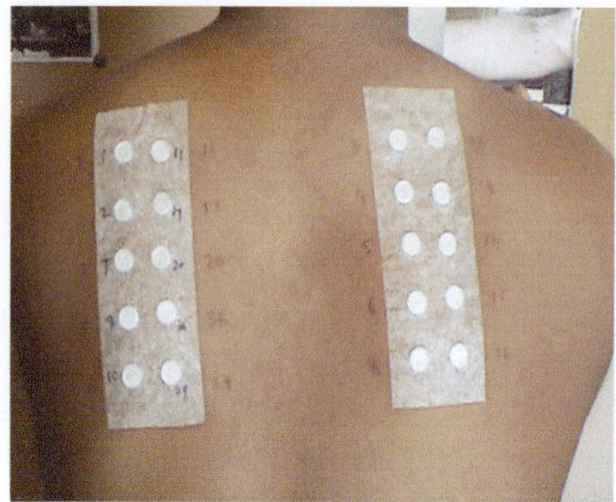

Fig. 12.3: Patch test unit on the back of the patient.

The patient should be instructed not to take bath, wash, or wet the back during this period; to avoid tight underclothes; not to exercise or indulge in any other activity that may cause sweating; to avoid any friction or rubbing; to avoid lying on the back; and to avoid exposure to direct sunlight and UV light. The patch test must be left for 2 days and 2 nights (48 hours) for effective results after which the patient is asked to report to the doctor.

Mechanism: A patch test basically relies on the type IV hypersensitivity reaction. The patient becomes allergic after sensitization to the allergen. The antigen-presenting cells in the skin called the dendritic cells and the Langerhans cells eat up the substance and break it into smaller pieces. Then the substance is attached to the surfaces of these cells, and then they move in the lymphatic system and lymph nodes and present the substance to the CD4+ cells or helper T cells. These helper cells then recognize the substance as dangerous and proliferate in response to the antigen. On re-exposure of the antigen, the T cells release cytokines, thus inducing a cascade of skin inflammation, itching, and rash of contact dermatitis.

READING AND RESULTS

A patch test is read after removing it from the site of application after 48 hours. The surface of the skin should be first cleaned with saline. The patch test is read in two steps. The first reading is done after 1 hour of removing the patch and cleaning it with saline. The second reading is done after 24–48 hours of the first reading.

Certain allergens such as neomycin and *p*-phenylenediamine often produce slow reaction after application that appears on days 4–7. This may occur with other allergens as well.[8] Thus, it is almost imperative to take a second reading on days 4–7 because 50% error is likely if only one reading is taken on day 2.[9] By the time of the second reading, immediate irritant reaction subsides and true reaction of the slowest allergen fully develops.

The results of a patch test are graded as follows (Fig. 12.4):

Appearance	*Interpretation*
No reaction	Negative (–)
Pink area	Equivocal reaction/ uncertain reaction
Slightly elevated pink or red papules	Weak positive (+)
Papulovesicular reaction	Strong positive (++)
Blister/ulcer formation	Extreme positive (+++)

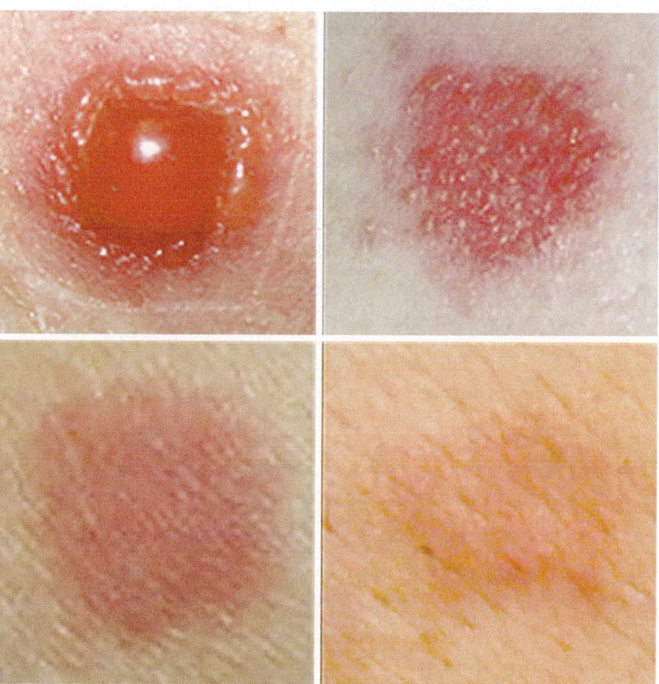

Fig. 12.4: Positive patch test results: From left to right: +++ reaction (extremely positive); ++ reaction (strongly positive, note the microvesicles); + reaction; +/– reaction (equivocal).

Certain factors may affect the final results of the patch test such as the use of excessive high or low concentrations of the allergen, patch placed on inflamed or injured skin, results examined too early or too late, failure to seal the patch tightly, steroid taken orally or applied topically, rubbing or sweating at or around the test site, or development of angry back.

False-negative reaction: In this, the patch test is negative despite the patient being sensitive to the allergen. Various causes include the use of small substances, low concentrations, loose contact of the Finn chambers, early removal, and application of local steroid at the site of testing.

Refractory state: It sometimes occurs after a very severe allergic dermatitis.

ADVERSE REACTIONS

- *Active sensitization*: A negative reaction is followed by a late positive reaction after 10–20 days.
- *Angry back*: Sometimes, the results are inconclusive and misleading, with multiple concomitant positive reactions to the diagnostic patch test for allergic contact dermatitis (Fig. 12.5). In this, a single repeated challenge reveals some of them to be nonreproducible.[10] Nearly all test areas become red and itchy. It is a false-positive result also called as angry back or excited skin syndrome or crazy back or status eczematicus based on the red fiery appearance. It is most likely to occur while the dermatitis is in its highly active phase. A detailed retake of history is important, and a retest should be done after 6–8 weeks with patches placed widely apart.
- *Flare of dermatitis*: Usually not a serious event and helps to validate the positive reaction.
- *Adhesive tape reaction*: A rare reaction seen with the use of current acrylate-based adhesive tapes.
- *Koebner phenomenon*: It can be seen in patients with active psoriasis and lichen planus.[11]
- *Persistent positive reaction*: It is seen more often with gold.

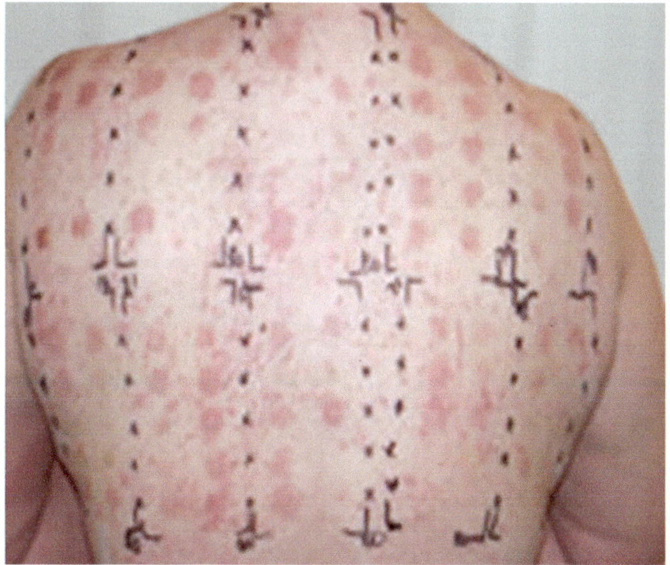

Fig. 12.5: Angry back

- *Pigmentary alteration*: This includes post-inflammatory hyper and hypopigmentation.
- *Pressure effect*: Imprint caused by pressure from the chamber or when testing a solid material.
- *Bacterial and viral infections*: Though rare, certain patients may develop such infections, while testing to plant substances.
- *Necrosis/scar/keloid*: Risk of testing to unknown caustic substances that burn a hole in the skin.[12]
- *Sarcoidal reaction*: It has been described with metals including palladium.
- *Anaphylactoid*: It is extremely rare but a potential risk with bacitracin, neomycin and contact urticaria.

PHOTOPATCH TEST

Some chemicals tend to produce an allergic reaction only when exposed to light (UV Type A light). Photopatch test is a gold standard test in the diagnosis of photosensitive patients. Two identical sets of allergens are applied on the back of the patient. After 48 hours, the patch is removed and one set is exposed to UVA light and then examined as usual. A positive photopatch test is recorded when an allergic reaction appears only on the light-exposed site. Fragrance mix is found to be the most common contact and photo-contact allergen amongst all tested antigens in the photopatch test.[13]

The main advantages of the patch test are that it is a no-pain procedure, it can be performed in any age group of patients, and there are no systemic reactions. There are also a few disadvantages: the results are less reproducible, it is a time-consuming procedure, the rate of false positive and false negatives are high, the standardization of allergens is difficult, and there is a shortage of good kits for testing.

RELEVANCE

Clinical relevance of a positive reaction in patch test is definite when:

- Allergen is found in the patient's environment.
- Allergen is found in the patch test.
- Dermatitis corresponds to the point of contact with allergen.
- Dermatitis improves upon isolation of the allergen or recurred with rechallenge (provocative test).

The relevance is probable when the criterion is the same as above, but there is no ability to obtain follow-up information on the improvement of status or rechallenge.

REFERENCES

1. Sulzberger MB, Wise F. The contact or patch test in dermatology: its uses, advantages and limitations. Arch Derm Syphilol. 1931;23:519-31.
2. Lachapelle JM, Ale SI, Freeman S, et al. Proposal for a revised international standard series of patch tests. Contact Dermatitis. 1997;36:121-3.
3. Fischer TI, Maibach HI. The thin layer rapid use epicutaneous test (TRUE-test), a new patch test method with high accuracy. Br J Dermatol. 1985;112:63-8.
4. Fischer T, Maibach H. Finn chamber patch test technique. Contact Dermatitis. 1984;11:137-40.
5. Krupa Shankar DS, Chakravarthi M. Atopic patch testing. Indian J Dermatol Venereol Leprol. 2008;74:467-70.
6. Lakshmi C, Srinivas C. Parthenium the terminator: an update. Indian Dermatol Online J. 2012;3:89-100.
7. Sukanto H, Nater JP, Bleumink E. Influence of topically applied corticosteroids on patch test reactions. Contact Dermatitis. 1981;7:180-5.
8. Macfarlane AW, Curley RK, Graham RM, et al. Delayed patch test reactions at days 7 and 9. Contact Dermatitis. 1989;20:127-32.
9. Rietschel RL, Adams RM, Maibach HI, et al. The case for patch test readings beyond day 2. Notes from the lost and found department. J Am Acad Dermatol. 1988;18:42-5.
10. Bruynzeel DP, Maibach HI. Excited skin syndrome (angry back). Arch Dermatol. 1986;122:323-8.
11. Weiss G, Shemer A, Trau H. The Koebner phenomenon: Review of the literature. J Eur Acad Dermatol Venereol. 2002;16:241-8.
12. Thijs L, Deraedt K, Goossens A. Granuloma possibly induced by palladium after ear piercing. Dermatitis. 2008;19:E26-9.
13. Jindal N, Sharma NL, Mahajan VK, et al. Evaluation of photopatch test allergens for Indian patients of photodermatitis: preliminary results. Indian J Dermatol Venereol Leprol. 2011;77:148-55.

CHAPTER 13

Provocation Tests in Diagnosis of Allergy

Suresh Koolwal, Roopam Sehajpal

INTRODUCTION

Allergy is a multifactorial disorder, consisting of genetic inheritance of atopic tendency and exposure to environmental factors. The basic background is atopic tendency, in a person, who when exposed to certain environmental agents, develops clinical features of allergy.

In addition to a detailed clinical history and examination, there are various ways to precisely detect these environmental agents responsible for allergy.

These are as follows:

- In vivo tests like skin prick testing
- In vitro tests, e.g., ELISA, RAST (radioallergosorbent test), and immunoCAP system
- Provocation tests.

All the above tests are indirect methods[1,2] of detection of allergens and are not very specific except provocative tests, which involve direct testing[3] with the suspected allergens. These tests are done by deliberately exposing the airways, nasal mucosa, conjunctiva, and GIT to the suspected allergen/chemical/physical stimuli and watching the development of typical signs and symptoms of allergy. The provocative tests are not usually required and are not done in routine clinical practice, and they are more of academic and research value. However, in the following situations they can be of use to establish the cause of allergy and aid in guiding further treatment:

- Occupational asthma—to establish the temporal relation between exposure and precipitation of symptoms.
- In cases with equivocal results from skin prick tests, provocation tests can help to uncover the particular agent in the environment.
- Planning immunotherapy.
- Demonstration of bronchial hyper-responsiveness (BHR) in suspected asthmatic, where atypical symptoms are present, and spirometry is normal.
- To convince a patient about the cause of his problem when he refuses to believe and avoid exposure.
- Guide to adjustment of inhaled corticosteroid therapy.
- BHR testing for management of chronic cough.
- Identifying new causes of asthma.
- In epidemiology, to describe asthma phenotype.
- Medicolegal purposes.

PRINCIPLES OF PROVOCATION TESTS[4]

When an atopic individual is exposed to some antigen, the antigen is taken up by the allergen-presenting cells (APCs) like dendritic cells, basophils, and macrophages in the airways and nasal mucosa. Within the APC, the allergen is digested to peptides and interacts with the major histocompatibility complex (MHC) (class 2 HLA) and migrates to the surface of the APC. Upon interaction with T-cell receptors, the Th2 cell activation takes place, producing IgE with the help of B cells, IL4, and CD23. These IgE antibodies attach to mast cells, eosinophils, platelets, and basophils by affinity receptors. This is called primary sensitization.[5]

When these individuals are exposed to the same allergen naturally or deliberately, as in provocative tests, the Ag–Ab reaction takes place on the cell surface releasing mediators, which act on end organs producing clinical features of allergies like bronchial asthma, allergic rhinitis, conjunctivitis, etc.

As histamine is one of the chemical mediators responsible for causing bronchoconstriction, it can be used as an agent for the diagnosis of BHR in an atopic individual as a nonspecific provocation agent.[6] Other chemical agents and physical stimuli induce clinical features through actions on neurological receptors and by releasing chemical mediators.

Provocation tests can be bronchial, nasal, oral, and conjunctival challenge tests.

PROVOCATION TESTS: BRONCHIAL[7]

1. *Nonspecific methods*
   i. Chemical: Using agents either causing smooth muscle contraction by acting on β_2 receptors and through cholinergic agonist action, e.g., histamine, methacholine, adenosine, mannitol, LTC4, LTD4, etc., or indirectly acting via the release of chemical mediators like leukotrienes, prostaglandin, etc.
   ii. Physical: Indirectly acting by releasing leukotrienes, e.g., cold air, exercise, hyperventilation, hyper- or hypotonic saline, etc.
2. *Specific tests*
   i. By using agents cause immune-mediated bronchoconstriction, inflammation, and hyper-responsiveness in specific subsets of atopic individuals, e.g., allergens like pollens, molds, dust, animal dander, and low-molecular-weight compounds like isocyanates.
   ii. Agents like nonsteroidal anti-inflammatory drugs (NSAIDs), aspirin, food additives, etc., which cause bronchoconstriction nonimmunologically.

Methacholine Provocation Test[8]

Bronchial hyper-responsiveness, which is commonly seen in asthma, can be detected by the methacholine provocation test (MPT).

An inhalational challenge is given with methacholine, a cholinergic agent that evokes constriction in both central and peripheral airways. Aerosolized methacholine is delivered in increasing doses, at concentrations ranging from 0.1 to 25 mg/mL.

When FEV_1 falls by 20% of the baseline value, the test is stopped and the concentration of methacholine is noted, and this dose is called PC20.

If PC20 is less than 8 mg/mL, the test is considered to be positive for bronchial hyper-responsiveness and is diagnostic for bronchial asthma.

The severity of airway obstruction is directly proportional to the dose of methacholine in asthmatic patients, whereas a plateau is reached after a certain dose in normal individuals and in chronic obstructive pulmonary disease (COPD).

The MPT is not only more sensitive and specific for diagnosis of asthma when compared with peak expiratory flow rate and exercise testing,[9] it can be used for a wide spectrum of age groups ranging from 6 years to elderly patients.[10]

The bronchospasm caused by methacholine is fully reversible within 1 hour or within a few minutes after salbutamol inhalation, and it is not necessary to monitor pulse, BP, and SpO_2 during the test procedure. Rarely, at higher doses of 16–25 mg/dL, it can cause severe bronchial hyper-responsiveness. Test requires repeated deep breathing maneuvers, therefore some patients consider it a rather unpleasant experience.

Test Procedure

Pretest instructions include asking the patient to avoid medication and factors affecting the test results. A careful history is taken to determine any contraindications for the test. Methacholine solution should be stored in a refrigerator. Concentrations are prepared to obtain 'doubling doses' in the range of 0.03–25 mg/mL (Table 13.1).

Two techniques are used for the administration of each dose.

1. *Two-minute tidal breathing dosing protocol*:[11] It involves inhalation of aerosol from a nebulizer and a face mask. Aerosolized methacholine can also be administered by a hand-held squeeze bulb nebulizer.
2. *Five inspiratory capacity breath dosimeter protocol.*[8,12]

Two-minute Tidal Breathing Dosing Protocol

A baseline, good-quality spirometry is performed, and if FEV_1 is more than 70% of that predicted at baseline, then one can proceed with the test.

Patient is instructed to breathe quietly for 2 minutes (tidal breathing), and then nebulization is begun with timer set for 2 minutes.

First of all, the lowest dose of methacholine is administered, and FEV_1 is measured at 30 and 90 seconds after nebulization, and subsequently higher concentrations are administered (Fig. 13.1).

After each dose (at 5 minutes interval), highest FEV_1 is recorded. When FEV_1 falls >20% from the baseline, no further methacholine is given and PC20 is recorded.[9]

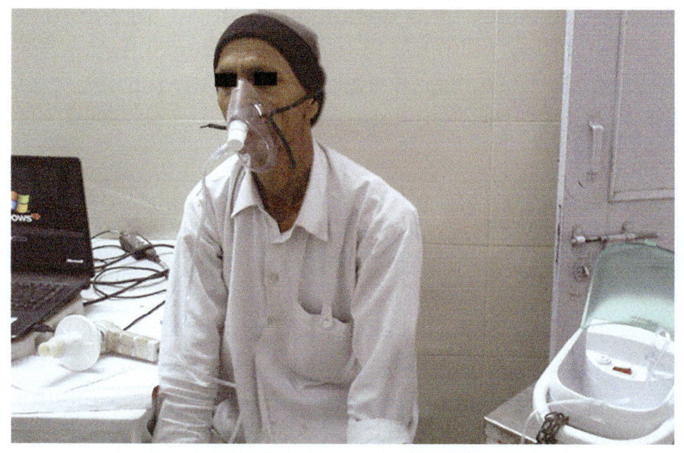

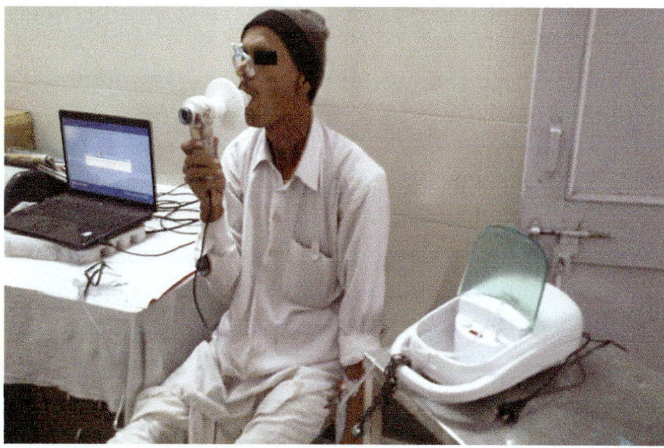

Fig. 13.1: Administration of methacholine by nebulization and subsequent measurement of FEV_1.

Table 13.1: Dilutions of methacholine are prepared 30 minutes before use and kept at room temperature.

Label strength	*Take*	*Add normal saline (mL)*	*Obtain dilution (mg/mL)*
Two-minute protocol, 100 mg	100 mg (vial)	6.25	A-16
	3 mL of dilution A	3	B-8
	3 mL of dilution B	3	C-4
	3 mL of dilution C	3	D-2
	3 mL of dilution D	3	E-1
	3 mL of dilution E	3	F-0.5
	3 mL of dilution F	3	G-0.25
	3 mL of dilution G	3	H-0.125
	3 mL of dilution H	3	I-0.0625
	3 mL of dilution I	3	J-0.031
Five-breath dosimeter protocol, 100 mg	100 mg (vial)	6.25	A-16
	3 mL of dilution A	9	B-4
	3 mL of dilution B	9	C-1
	3 mL of dilution C	9	D-0.25
	3 mL of dilution D	9	E-0.0625

Schedule obtained from Methapharm (Brantford, ON, Canada).

Patient is discharged after FEV_1 returns to >90%. Salbutamol nebulization is given if there are persistent symptoms.

Five Inspiratory Capacity-breath Dosimeter Protocol

The patient is asked to inhale increasing concentrations of methacholine at functional residual capacity from a dosimeter by slow and deep inhalations for 5 seconds. The breath is held at total lung capacity for 5 seconds each time. These steps are repeated for five inspiratory capacity breaths and should be performed in no longer than 2 minutes.

Interpretation of Results

PC20 < 1 mg/dL confirms the diagnosis of asthma. If PC20 is more than 16 mg/mL, it points against the diagnosis of bronchial asthma.[13]

Other factors need to be considered if PC20 is between 1 mg and 16 mg/mL.

1. PC20 between 1 mg and 8 mg/mL—asymptomatic patient:
   i. Mild intermittent asthma—poor recognition of symptoms by the patient.
   ii. The patient has not been exposed to environmental triggers or never exercises to get bronchospasm.
   iii. Subclinical asthma—where the patient is prone to develop asthma in the future.
2. PC20 between 1 mg and 8 mg/mL—symptomatic patient: Indicates high probability of asthma.

Negative MPT Test

A negative MPT result is commonly defined as no response to the highest concentration (usually 16 mg/mL) of methacholine.

Causes of False-positive Results

- Allergic rhinitis
- Smokers with COPD.[14]

False-negative Results

- Patients taking anti-inflammatory medication prior to test
- If the patient was asymptomatic for several weeks prior to the tests especially after allergy season is over.

MPT in Children

The *MPT* helps to establish the diagnosis of asthma in children of 2–8 years of age group. It also differentiates asthma from other airway diseases.[15]

Positive Test Response

1. Development of wheezing on auscultation after methacholine administration.
2. Fall in SpO_2 by 5% or more.
3. Increase in respiratory rate by 50% of the baseline.

In 96% of cases, the positive test occurs with PC20 of 0.4 mg/mL.[16]

Adenosine monophosphate is safer and is used in children in place of methacholine. Adenosine monophosphate acts by releasing mediators from mast cells. Used either by 5 dosimeter protocol or 2-minute tidal breathing methods in increasing concentrations of 3.125, 6.25, 12.50, 25, 50, 100, 200, and 400 mg/mL, and PC20 is measured.

Nonspecific Bronchial Provocation Tests with Other Agents[17]

1. Hypertonic saline (4.5%) inhalation[18]—at 30 seconds, 1 minute, 2 minutes, 4 minutes, 8 minutes—total 15.5 minutes. FEV_1 is measured 1 minute after the end of inhalation and a fall more than 15% is positive response-*PC15*.
2. Mannitol test[17]—This test was developed in Australia. It can be done in a field or a lab. This test helps to identify exercise-induced asthma and estimate its severity. It also helps to monitor response to steroids. It is more sensitive than histamine to identify persistent airway hyper-responsiveness in asthmatics well controlled on steroids.

   Mannitol being a hypertonic solution increases osmolarity and releases mediators from mast cells and sensory nerves. It is inhaled, at an interval of 2 minutes, from gelatin capsules in doubling concentrations starting from 5 mg to a maximum cumulative dose of 635 mg. FEV_1 is measured after 1 minute of each dose. PC15 is usually achieved at 64 mg. PC15 > 635 mg excludes asthma. Recovery occurs within 60 minutes, and this test is well tolerated by patients.

Provocative Exercise Test[19,20]

These tests are useful in the diagnosis of exercise-induced dyspnoea, when wheeze is absent and resting spirometry and PEFR is unremarkable. The patient is asked to do any of the following exercises:

- Free running
- Treadmill exercise
- Bicycle
- Swimming or brisk walking
- Duration—age less than 12 years—6 minutes.
  Age more than 12 years—8 minutes
  (must reach 40–60% of MVV (FEV_1 × 35) in first 2–3 minutes).

This induces bronchoconstriction at the end of exercise and is maximum at 5–10 minutes, thereafter FEV_1 is measured every 5 minutes up to 30 minutes.

A fall in FEV_1 by 10% minimum or preferably 15% or more is diagnostic of exercised-induced asthma.[16] About 40–70% asthmatics have exercise-induced dyspnea.

Specific Bronchial Provocation Tests[21]

Suspected antigen is deliberately delivered to airways by one of the following ways:

1. Aerosol generated by nebulizer and delivered to face mask or mouth piece and inhaled by tidal breathing for 2 minutes.
2. Aerosol generated by nebulizer delivered to mouthpiece and inhaled by 5 inspiratory capacity breathes.
3. Hand-operated nebulizer with aerosols generated by squeezing the bulb of nebulizer.

Increasing concentration of allergen in buffered normal saline is given, and FEV_1 is measured at 10 minutes intervals for half an hour, at 30 minutes interval for an hour and then hourly till 8 hours. The test is said to be positive if allergen causes sustained fall in FEV_1 below 80% of measured baseline FEV_1.

Various types of positive responses (i.e., 20% fall in FEV_1) can be observed:

- Immediate reaction in 10–30 minutes and recovery in 1 hour.
- Late reaction in 1–2 hours or after 4–8 hours.
- Dual reaction—Both immediate and late responses.
- Recurrent nocturnal asthma.
- Progressive-reaction within minutes and progression up to 7–8 hours.
- Square wave form—these reactions show with no recovery between early and late reactions.
- Prolonged—these are immediate reaction with slow recovery.

Advantage

True diagnosis is established for allergen avoidance and immunotherapy.

Disadvantages

- Specific provocation test is potentially dangerous because there is always a potential for triggering severe, life-threatening asthmatic attack.
- There is always a risk of late phase reaction so constant watch sometimes up to 24 hours is required.
- BHR may last for a longer period (3 months), resulting in frequent nocturnal asthma.
- Inconvenient to patient and medical personnel performing the test.
- Needs specialized laboratories and close supervision of an experienced physician and adequate resuscitative measures.
- Drugs, infections, and allergen exposure before the test can affect the results of the test (Boxes 13.1 and 13.2).

However, specific bronchial provocation tests (SBPTs) are still considered as a gold standard in diagnosis of occupational asthma,[22] where the test is done in a special chamber or an aerosol generator-regulating dose, concentration, particle size, and temperature of the suspected occupational powder gas or liquid, and also done by pouring dust from one tray to another, or by creating the atmosphere mimicking the exposure at work place. A worker is exposed to one substance at a time, at a dose much lower than exposure at work place for duration shorter than at work place. Immediate, late, or dual reaction can take place, resulting in a sustained fall in FEV_1 by more than 20%. Peak expiratory flow rate, forced expiratory flow (FEF 25–75%), FVC, and specific airway conductance (SGaw) can be used as surrogate markers of airway hyper-reactivity; measurement of FEV_1 remains the best physiologic index for the detection of changes in central and large airways. Reduction of SGaw by more than 35% is considered as a positive test.

BOX 13.1: Factors that reduce the provocation test response.

- Short-acting β_2 agonist/anticholinergics taken within 8 hours
- Long-acting β_2 agonists taken within 48 hours
- Antihistamines taken within 3 days
- Leukotriene modifiers used within 24 hours
- Steroids and mast cell stabilizers may affect the response up to 3 months. The results will be falsely improved
- Sustained release of theophylline should be withheld for at least 48 hours.

BOX 13.2: Factors that enhance the provocation test results.

- Viral infection in the recent past (3 – 6 weeks)
- Recent exposure to the relevant allergen (1 – 3 weeks)
- Exercise in cold and dry air
- Air pollution
- Recent exposure to some newer occupational agent (months)
- Cigarette smoking (hours).

BOX 13.3[7]: Contraindications to bronchial provocation tests.

Absolute

- Absence of emergency resuscitative facilities or experienced medical staff during test
- Severe airflow obstruction. FEV_1 less than 50% of predicted or less than 1 L
- Acute MI or stroke in past 3 months
- Uncontrolled hypertension (SBP > 200 or DBP > 100)
- Aortic aneurysm.

Relative

- Moderate airflow obstruction, FEV_1 < 60% or less than 1.5 L
- Inability to perform acceptable spirometry
- Pregnancy
- Use of cholinesterase inhibitors for myasthenia gravis.

In occupational asthma, while doing SBPT, for accurate results exact material, appropriate exposure levels, and the physical form in which the antigen is exposed should be known and used.

Nonspecific bronchial hyper-responsiveness along with a serial measurement of PEFR at 2-hour intervals while the patient is awake, over consecutive periods at work and away from work can establish definite diagnosis of occupational asthma.

Regular monitoring of FEV_1 at 15-minute intervals in the first hour, 30-minute intervals for the second hour, then hourly for up to 8 hours after the end of the exposure is required. In certain circumstances, monitoring may be required for 8–24 hours after the challenge.

Negative SBPT in laboratory does not always exclude the diagnosis of occupational asthma and a significant increase in responsiveness to histamine or methacholine is suggestive of prior sensitization (Box 13.3).

NASAL PROVOCATION TEST[23]

Nasal provocation test involves the administration of the suspected allergen directly into the nose, in order to determine nasal sensitivity of an allergen. Subjective nasal and extranasal symptoms reported by the patient along with the measurement of nasal airflow with active anterior rhinomanometry are used to measure the response.

Procedure

Allergen extract in buffered normal saline is sprayed into the nose using a spraying device. Within 10-15 minutes the response is watched. An allergen concentration of 1:10,000 w/v is given as the initial dose. If the clinical symptoms are negative and rhinomanometry at 15 minutes <20%, then the concentration of the allergen extract is reduced to 1:3,000 w/v. If the test is still negative then the concentration can be further reduced to 1:1,000 w/v after 15 minutes.

Test is positive if 2 of the following 3 reactions are seen:[24]

- More than five sneezes.
- More than 0.5 mL secretions.
- More than 50% fall is nasal peak flow.

Sensitivity—++++

Specificity—+++

If the patient remains asymptomatic even after receiving the 1:1,000 w/v extract or maximum allergen dose, the test is deduced to be true negative.[24]

Advantages

- Easy to perform.
- True diagnosis is reached.
- Correlates well with airway allergy.
- More convenient than bronchial provocation test (BPT).
- Simple, safe, sensitive, specific, and reproducible.

CONJUNCTIVAL PROVOCATION TESTS[25]

Allergen molecules in sterile physiological isotonic saline are instilled into the conjunctiva as droplets and the reaction is observed. The test is said to be positive if two of the following three reactions occur:

- Redness
- Itching
- Running eyes.

Advantages

- Simple and reproducible
- True diagnosis can be reached
- Minimal inconvenience
- In-office test.

ORAL PROVOCATIONS TESTS[26]

Food allergens are placed in GIT by oral route through tube as capsule or directly. Positive reaction is manifested by colic, vomiting, diarrhea, and meteorism.

FOOD PROVOCATION (CHALLENGE) TESTS

Diagnosis of food allergy is very challenging. Despite a careful history taking, the correlation between suspected food allergy and food allergy as confirmed by the challenge test is only 30–40%.

Skin prick test, food prick to skin prick test, patch test, specific IgE and elimination diets followed by food challenges are various ways by which food allergy can be diagnosed.

Food challenges can be done by the following three ways:[27]

1. *Open challenges*:
   They are usually done in office settings and can be performed when dealing with objective symptoms, especially in patients with oral allergy syndrome and children below 3 years of age. These tests are prone to bias.
2. *Single-blind challenges*:
   They are less prone to patient bias as only the health personnel know, without the knowledge of the patient, which dose is active and which is placebo.
3. *Double-blind placebo-controlled food challenge (DBPCFC):*[28]
   Neither the patient, nor the health personnel know, which dose is active and which is a placebo. Hence, reduces both patient and observer bias. It is used as the gold standard for research purposes as well.

   It has to be noted that no universally accepted protocol has been agreed on these tests.

Indications of Test[29]

- For diagnosis of food allergy in patients of any age with an unwanted reaction to a food
- To determine the tolerance levels and patient's sensitivity to a food
- In patients suffering from chronic symptoms that may be related to a food
- When the skin prick test is positive but the patient is not sure about the consumption of food previously
- A patient on an unsatisfactory elimination diet
- Assessment of cross-reactivity
- Scientific reasons in clinical trials.

Contraindications

- Patients with a clear history of anaphylaxis after consumption of a particular food
- Children with specific IgG levels
- Very high-risk patients suffering from diseases like angina pectoris, acute infections, or seasonal allergies
- Patients taking medications that may influence the results.

Methods

- Careful history and physical examination are important to form a basis of diagnosis of food allergy.
- Eliminate the food from diet for a period determined by the symptoms and disease pattern. This period may vary from 2 to 6 weeks. For additives, it should be at least 24 hours.
- Starting dose should be within a safe threshold, i.e., the lowest amount of the offending food that would elicit symptoms, like mild urticaria, erythema, and oral angioedema in the most sensitive persons.
- Dose may be doubled after each interval, allowing 15–60 minutes time between each dose the challenge should continue until 8–10 g of the dried food is ingested as a single dose, thus providing a total dose of 15–20 g.

When 8–10 g of dried food has been administered without any symptoms, the provocation test may be considered negative. Capsules can be used as a challenge vehicle, when using dried food. When using real food, not dried food, then about 60–100 g of wet food is used for challenge.

A positive reaction is usually obtained within 2 hours.

For small children, wet food like milk in increasing doses of 5 mL, 10 mL, 30 mL, 200 mL; or egg in increasing doses of 0.5 g, 2 g, 4 g, 10 g, 30 g; wheat in increasing doses 0.5 g, 2 g, 4 g, 10 g, 15 g, can be administered orally and reaction is observed within 10 minutes of ingesting food. Each dose is administered at intervals of 20–40 minutes.[30]

These tests should be performed by a trained health person with the availability of resuscitative measures, and a sufficient time of observation and follow-up is necessary.

Limitations

These do not correlate with airway allergies and are time-consuming.

Bronchial provocation test (BPT) reduces the possibility of over and underdiagnosis of asthma solely based on history and symptoms. Methacholine challenge testing is quiet safe and useful in establishing the diagnosis of asthma when conventional tests like spirometry provide equivocal results.[31] It is also a valuable tool in diagnosing occupational asthma.

REFERENCES

1. Anderson SD, Brannan JD. Methods for indirect challenge tests, including exercise, eucapnic voluntary hyperpnea, and hypertonic aerosol. Clin Rev Allergy Immunol. 2003;24:27-54.
2. Joss GF, O'Connor B, Anderson SD, et al. Indirect airway challenges. Eur Respir J. 2003;21:1050-68.
3. Cockcroft DW. Direct challenge tests airway hyper-responsiveness in Asthma: its measurement and clinical significance. CHEST J. 2010;138:18S-24S.
4. Del Prete GF, De Carli M, D'Elios MM, et al. Allergen exposure induces the activation of allergen-specific Th2 cells in the airway mucosa of patients with allergic respiratory disorders. Eur J Immunol. 1993;23: 1445-9.
5. von Bubnoff D, Geiger E, Bieber T. Antigen-presenting cells in allergy. J Allergy Clin Immunol. 2001;108:329-39.
6. Popa V, Singleton J. Provocation dose and discriminant analysis in histamine bronchoprovocation: are the current predictive data satisfactory? Chest. 1988;94:466-75.
7. Spector SL. Bronchial provocation tests. In: Michel FB, Bousquet J, Godard P. eds. Highlights in Asthmology. Berlin, Heidelberg: Springer; 1987:421-30.
8. Crapo RO, Casaburi R, Coates AL, et al. Guidelines for methacholine and exercise challenge testing-1999. This official statement of the American Thoracic Society was adopted by the ATS Board of Directors, July 1999. Am J Respir Crit Care Med. 2000;161:309-29.
9. Goldstein MF, Veza BA, Dunsky EH, et al. Comparisons of peak diurnal expiratory flow variation, postbronchodilator FEV_1 responses, and methacholine inhalation challenges in the evaluation of suspected asthma. CHEST J. 2001; 119:1001-10.
10. Bowden JJ, DeKIlerk NH, Firth MJ, et al. Lung function, bronchial responsiveness, and asthma in a community cohort of 6 year-old children. Am J Respir Crit Care Med. 2004;169:600-10.
11. Juniper EF, Cockcroft DW, Hargreave FE. Tidal breathing method. Histamine and Methacholine Inhalation Tests: Laboratory Procedure and Standardization, 2nd ed. Lund, Sweden: Astra Draco AB; 1994.
12. Sterk PJ, Fabbri LM, Quanjer PH, et al. Airway responsiveness: standardized challenge testing with pharmacological, physical and sensitizing stimuli in adults. Statement of the European Respiratory Society. Eur Respir J. 1993;6:53-X3
13. Gilbert R, Auchincloss JH. Post-test probability of asthma following methacholine challenge. CHEST J. 1990;97: 562-5.
14. Tashkin DP, Altose MD, Bleecker ER, et al. The lung health study: airway responsiveness to inhaled methacholine in smokers with mild to moderate airflow limitation. The Lung Health Study Research Group. Am Rev Respir Dis. 1992;145:301-10.
15. Avital A, Springer C, Bar-Yishay E, Godfrey S. Adenosine, methacholine, and exercise challenges in children with asthma or paediatric chronic obstructive pulmonary disease. Thorax. 1995;50:511-6.
16. Schulze J, Smith H-J, Fuchs J, et al. Methacholine challenge in young children as evaluated by spirometry and impulse oscillometry. Resp Med. 2012;106:627-34.
17. Brannan JD, Anderson SD, Perry CP, et al. The safety and efficacy of inhaled dry powder mannitol as a bronchial provocation test for airway hyperresponsiveness: a phase 3 comparison study with hypertonic (4.5%) saline. Respir Res. 2005;6:144.
18. Smith CM, Anderson SD. Inhalational challenge using hypertonic saline in asthmatic subjects: a comparison with responses to hyperpnoea, methacholine and water. Eur Respir J. 1990;3:144-51.
19. Boulet LP, Morin D, Turcotte H. Variations of airway responsiveness to methacholine and exercise in asthmatic and normal subjects over a 12 months period. Clin Invest Med. 1990;13:60-6.
20. Wasserman K, Hansen JE, Sue DY, et al. Principles of exercise testing and interpretation. Philadelphia, PA: Lea & Febiger; 1994.
21. Chan-Yeung M, Kinsella M, Ostrow DN. Specific bronchoprovocation testing. Clin Rev Allergy Immunol. 1990;8:147-57.
22. Cartier A, Bernstein IL, Sherwood Burge P, et al. Guidelines for bronchoprovocation on the investigation of occupational asthma: report of the Subcommittee on Bronchoprovocation for Occupational Asthma. J Allergy Clin Immunol. 1989;84:823-9.
23. Schumacher MJ, Cota KA, Taussig LM. Pulmonary response to nasal-challenge testing of atopic subjects with stable asthma. J Allergy Clin Immunol. 1986;78:30-5.
24. Filiaci F, Lucarelli N. Behaviour on the nasal provocation test in patients affected by conjunctivitis and/or asthma of allergic origin. Rhinology. 1981;19:173-7.
25. Möller C, Björksten B, Nilsson G, Dreborg S. The precision of the conjunctival provocation test. Allergy. 1984;39:37-41.
26. Muraro MA. Diagnosis of food allergy: the Oral provocation test. Pediatr Allergy Immunol. 2001;12 Suppl. 14:31-6.
27. Bindslev-Jensen C, Ballmer-Weber BK, Bengtsson U, et al. Standardization of food challenges in patients with immediate reactions to foods-position paper from the European Academy of Allergology and Clinical Immunology. Allergy. 2004; 59:690-7.
28. Bock SA, Sampson HA, Atkins FM, et al. Doubte-blind placebo controlled food challenge as an office procedure; a manual. J Allergy Clin Immunol. 1988;82:986-97.
29. Sicherer SH. Food allergy: when and how to perform oral food challenges. Pediatr Allergy Immunol. 1999;10:226-34.
30. Niggemann B, Wahn U, Sampson HA, Niggemann B. Proposals for standardization of oral food challenge tests in infants and children. Pediatr Allergy Immunol. 1994;5: 11-13. doi:10.1111/j.1399-3038.1994.tb00212.
31. Martin RJ, Wanger JS, Irvin CG, Bucher Bartelson B, Cherniack RM, Asthma Clinical Research Network. Methacholine challenge testing: safety of low-starting FEV_1. Chest. 1997;112:53-6.

CHAPTER 14

Diagnosis in Allergy: Serology—Component-resolved Diagnosis

PC Kathuria

ALLERGY DIAGNOSIS AND TESTING

According to the World Allergy Organization (WAO), allergy is defined as a hypersensitivity reaction initiated by immunological mechanisms. These hypersensitivity reactions can be either antibody- or cell-mediated. Individuals are usually considered to have clinically significant allergy when they have both detectable allergen-specific IgE and have developed symptoms upon exposure to substances containing the specific allergen. *Sensitization* refers to the production of allergen-specific IgE only, unrelated to any associated clinical symptoms. Allergy tests should, therefore, always be interpreted in the context of the patient's clinical history, as a positive allergen-specific IgE test demonstrates sensitization and not necessarily clinical reactivity. The major limitations of allergen extracts for skin prick test and specific IgE are represented by (1) the content, because each extract is a heterogeneous mixture composed of major and minor allergenic proteins, and other biologically inactive components such as nonallergenic proteins, glycoproteins, and carbohydrates, (2) the production process, because some allergens may undergo partial degradation during the extraction, and (3) the cross-reactions, as different biological sources may contain cross-reactive allergens.[1,2]

ALLERGEN AND COMPONENT NOMENCLATURE

Allergen sources are numbered and referred according to the allergen group to which they belong to. The first letter in the allergen reference indicates the allergen group (e.g., t = tree pollen, f = food, g = grass pollen, etc.). The number indicates the sequence in which the allergen was identified. An x in the "code" refers to a mixture of allergens (e.g., f × 5, where f = food; × = mixture; 5 = number 5). Allergen components are referred by the allergen source's scientific name, usually an abbreviation of the Latin name and a number. The letters "r" or "n" that precede the allergen component name refer to the origin of the allergen component used in the assay, i.e., "recombinant" or "native." Thus, r Ara h2 denotes a recombinant *Arachis hypogaea* with allergen number 2 for peanut. All protein sources possess the potential to elicit an antibody response and cause allergic reactions. Allergen sources (e.g., cow's milk) contain several different proteins that we refer to as allergen components (e.g., whey and casein in the cow's milk). Each allergen component or protein consists of different epitopes to which antibodies are formed. These epitopes may be species-specific, thus only present in the specific allergen source. Alternatively, the epitopes presenting the allergen source may resemble epitopes present in other allergen sources, leading to cross-reacting antibodies between different allergen sources or species. These allergens are often referred to as pan-allergens. Patients with IgE antibodies to species-specific proteins are more likely to suffer from more severe and systemic reactions as opposed to patients with cross-reacting antibodies to panallergens. Allergen protein stability is another important aspect to be taken into consideration in multi-sensitized patients. Allergens that are stable to heat and pepsin digestion are more likely to cause severe clinical reactions, whereas heat- and digestion-labile proteins are more likely to be tolerated, or cause milder or only local reactions.[3,4]

ALLERGEN FROM PLANT COMPONENTS

Plant protein families are shared between species; the closer the species are related, the more similar the proteins can be. This increases the potential for IgE molecules directed against pollen allergen epitopes to bind to similar allergen epitopes in food. There are five main types of plant protein. These are storage proteins, nsLTP, PR-10, profilin proteins, and CCDs (cross-reactive carbohydrate determinants) (Table 14.1 and Figs. 14.1 A to D).[5]

Table 14.1: CRD in food allergy diagnosis/Laury Masthoff/EAACI, 2015 (Figs. 14.1 A to D).

Protein family	*Risk for systemic reactions?*	*Do I have to consider many different allergen sources?*
Storage proteins	*Yes.* Storage proteins are heat and digestion stable, which explains their ability to more often cause systemic reaction in addition to OAS.	*No.* Storage proteins are not cross-reactive, except for very closely related allergen sources (e.g., between legumes such as soy and peanut).
nsLTP	*Yes.* nsLTPs are heat and digestion stable which explains their ability to more often cause systemic reaction in addition to OAS.	*Yes.* Partly cross-reactive (the degree of structural similarity varies between nsLTPs in plant food and pollen).
PR-10	*Low.* Often cause only local symptoms such as OAS due to their sensitivity to heat and digestion, but a few cases with systemic reactions have been reported, e.g., for soy Gly m 4 and Celery Api g 1.	*Yes.* Partly cross-reactive (the degree of structural similarity varies between PR-10 in plant food and birch-related pollen).
Profilin	*Low.* Often have little clinical relevance in allergic diseases. However, profilins may cause local reactions in some patients allergic to plant foods including citrus fruits, banana, and tomato, and a few cases with systemic reactions have been reported, e.g., melon and lychee.	*Yes.* Highly cross-reactive (high degree of structural similarity between profilins in pollen, plant food, and latex).
CCD	*Very low.* Usually not associated with clinical reactions but may induce IgE antibody responses in some patients.	*Yes.* Highly cross-reactive (same CCD structure in pollen, plant food, and venoms).

CRD, component-resolved diagnosis; OAS, oral allergy syndrome; nsLTP, non-specific lipid transfer proteins; CCDs, cross-reactive carbohydrate determinants.

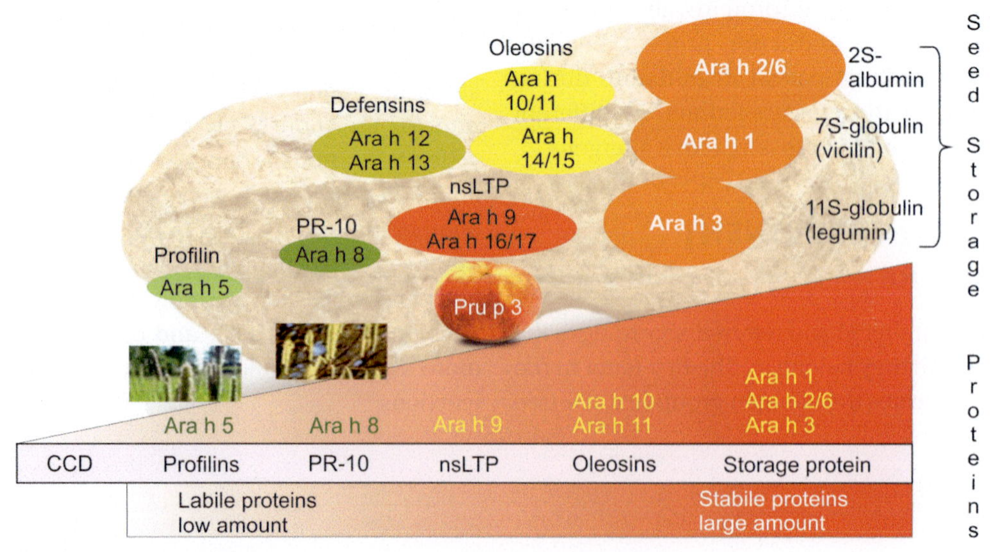

Fig. 14.1A: Peanut allergens.

Source: CRD in Food Allergy Diagnosis/Laury Masthoff/ EAACI 2015(7)

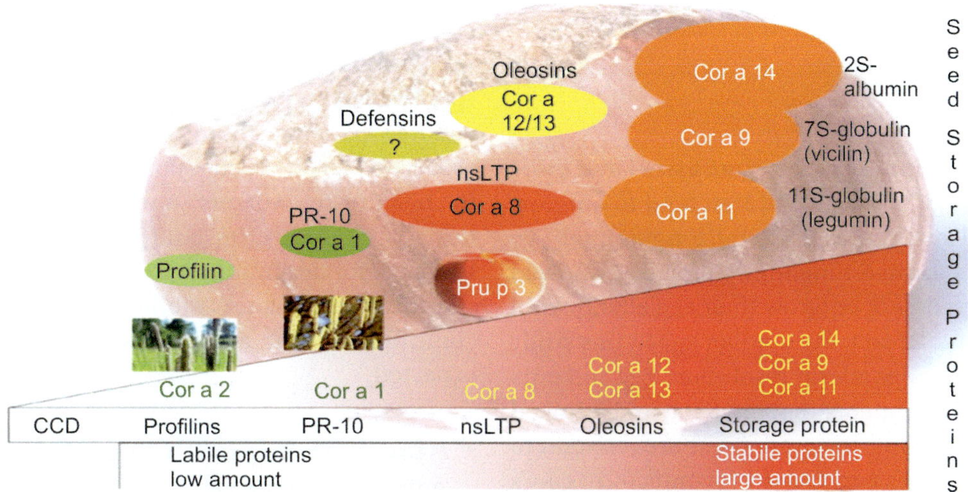

Fig. 14.1B: Hazelnut allergens.

Source: CRD in Food Allergy Diagnosis/Laury Masthoff/ EAACI 2015(7)

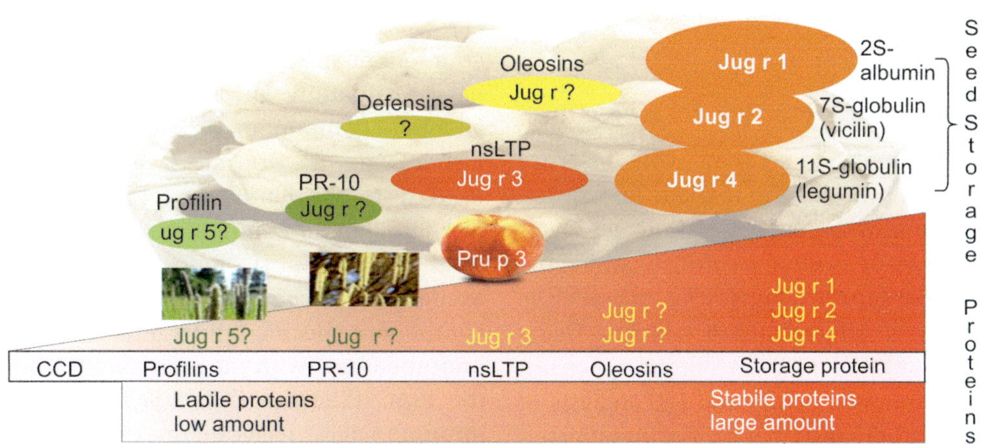

Fig. 14.1C: Walnut allergens.

Source: CRD in Food Allergy Diagnosis/Laury Masthoff/ EAACI 2015(7)

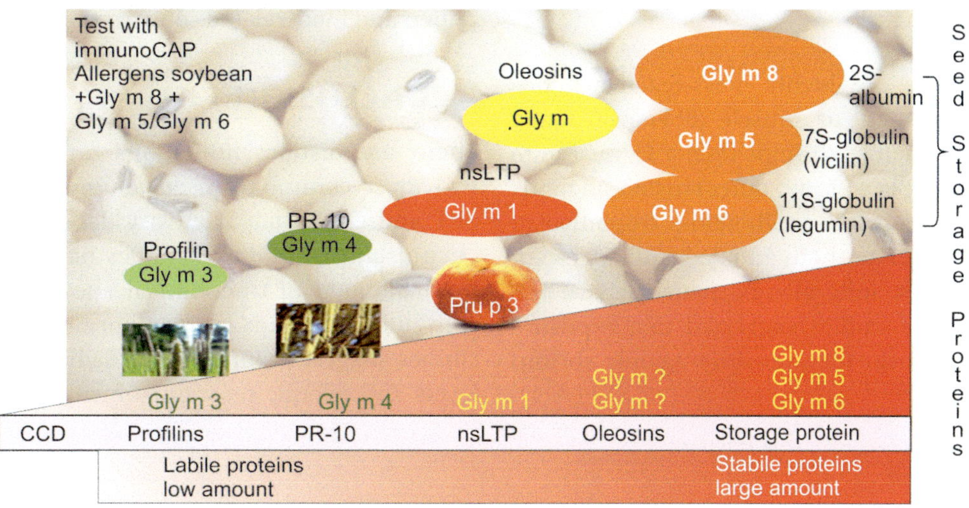

Fig. 14.1D: Soy allergens.

Source: CRD in Food Allergy Diagnosis/Laury Masthoff/ EAACI 2015(7)

ALLERGENS FROM NON-PLANT SOURCES

Egg and Milk

Dairy products such as milk and egg are associated more with pediatric allergy in which children tend to outgrow at a young age. However, in a recent longitudinal egg allergy study in the United Kingdom, Clark et al. showed that many children do not outgrow their egg allergy until well past 5 years old; in fact, the median age in this study was 10 years of age for egg allergy resolution. Egg and milk contain allergen components that are likely to be linked to more severe symptoms; these allergens are resistant to metabolic change [hen's egg, Gal d 1 (ovomucoid); cow's milk, Bos d 8 (casein)]. Therefore, patient groups negative to these tests have been observed to tolerate cooked forms of the allergen. Conversely, persistent allergy is associated with the same epitopes, which can again be used as risk markers.[6,7]

Parvalbumins

Cyp c 1 (carp, oily fish) and Gad c 1 (cod, white fish) are both major fish allergen proteins and markers for fish IgE sensitization. Parvalbumins are expressed in lower levels in certain fish species such as tuna, swordfish, and some mackerel, and this perhaps explains why fish-allergic patients can sometimes tolerate these species. Using ImmunoCAP Cyp c 1 and Gad c 1 gives a broad-spectrum coverage of the parvalbumins family and IgE analysis of fish. A negative result to both tests in a patient investigated for food allergy would inform the clinician of potential low risk of oral challenge and/or lead to further investigations for other possible culprit allergens.[6,7]

Tropomyosins

Tropomyosin proteins are highly cross-reactive actin-binding proteins located in muscle fibers of many invertebrate species such as shrimps (Pen a 1), dust mite (Der p10), cockroach (Bla g 7), and other crustacean foods such as crab, lobster, and mollusc. Therefore, tropomyosin is an allergen that can be both inhaled and ingested. About 10% of the dust mite allergic patients have IgE to tropomyosin. Some studies suggested that exposure to dust mite tropomyosin may sensitize against shrimp tropomyosin.[6,7]

Latex

IgE antibodies to Hev b 1 and Hev b 3 are considered specific markers for latex allergy, especially in multi-operated children/patients. IgE to Hev b 5 and Hev b 6 are mainly associated with occupational exposure to latex, e.g., in healthcare workers and food-handling personnel using latex gloves. Hev b 8 (profilin) and Hev b 6.02 can be used for examining cross-reactivity. If an exclusive sensitization to latex profilin (Hev b 8) occurs, then clinically relevant allergic symptoms are hardly to be expected.[6,7]

ALLERGEN COMPONENT ASSAY SYSTEMS

Many different in vitro immunoassays have been developed worldwide. In South Africa, two systems are mainly used for the measurement of allergen-specific components: (1) *Quantitative* measurement of *individual* allergen component-specific IgE: An immunoassay method is used to quantify IgE levels to a native or recombinant allergen component in IU/L. ImmunoCAP®(Thermo Fisher Scientific, Uppsala, Sweden) is the most frequently used test for identifying IgE to allergen components. Not all allergen components are available as individual tests, but the most clinically relevant components are available, (2) *Semiquantitative* measurement of allergen-component-specific IgE by means of a microarray-based immunoassay with a predefined test panel such as the ISAC® (Thermo Fisher Scientific, Uppsala, Sweden) immuno-solid-phase allergy chip with 112 components from 51 allergen sources. This is a semiquantitative assay (ISU units) which is best indicated in multisensitized patients with both food and inhalant allergies. The ISAC microarray will be able to identify cross-reactions between pollen and food-related sensitizations (Table 14.2).[5,8]

CONCLUSION

There are distinct limitations and advantages of the two most commonly used allergy diagnostic methods, SPT and s-IgE, that may vary depending on the testing circumstances. Multiple studies have demonstrated that the likelihood of true clinical allergy directly correlates with the SPT and allergen-specific IgE results. Some studies suggest a similar relationship with SPT and s-IgE levels and allergic reaction severity. Advances in allergy

Table 14.2: Fundamental features of clinically used allergen-specific IgE antibody assays.[8]

Name	*Company*	*Solid-phase matrix*	*Enzyme-labeled detection antibody*	*Substrate*	*Calibration system*	*Analytical sensitivity*
HYTEC-288	Hycor-Agilent	Paper disk	Alkaline phosphatase labeled anti-IgE	*p*-Nitrophenyl phosphate	Total IgE system	0.1 kUa/L
ImmunoCAP	Phadia	Cellulose sponge	β-Galactosidase labeled anti-IgE	4-Methylumbelliferyl β-D galactoside	Total IgE system	0.1 kUa/L
Immulite	Siemens	Biotinylated-allergen and avidin particle	Alkaline phosphatase-labeled anti-IgE	4-Methoxy-4-(3-phosphate phenyl)-spiro-1,2-dioxetane-3,2′-adamantine	Total IgE system	0.1 kUa/L
Immuno-solid-phase allergen chip (ISAC)	Phadia	Biochip	β-Galactosidase-labeled anti-IgE	4-Methylumbelliferyl β-D galactoside	Positive controls	Semiquantitative

laboratory testing through CRD have improved the prognostic and diagnostic accuracy of food evaluations, which may eliminate or significantly decrease the need for OFC in the future. Similar advances may improve the accuracy of aeroallergen diagnosis which, in turn, may guide clinicians to prescribe more specific allergen immunotherapy.

REFERENCES

1. Johansson S, Bieber T, Dahl R, et al. Revised nomenclature for allergy for global use: report of the nomenclature review committee for the world allergy organization, October 2003. J Allergy Clin Immunol. 2004;113:832-6.
2. Lack G. Epidemiologic risks for food allergy. J Allergy Clin Immunol. 2008;121:1331-6.
3. Host A, Andrae S, Charkin S, et al. Allergy testing in children: why, who, when and how? Allergy. 2003;58:559-69.
4. Wolthers OD. Component-resolved diagnostics inpaediatrics. ISRN Pediatr. 2012;Article ID 806920:1-6.
5. Allergy Education, Immunocap, A clinical reference guide to molecular allergy. March 2014.
6. Molecular Allergology / User's Guide EAACI 2016, paolo maria matricardi, jorg kleine-tebbe & others.
7. CRD In Food Allergy Diagnosis/Laury Masthoff/ EAACI 2015.
8. Cox L. Overview of serological-specific IgE antibody testing in children. Curr Allergy Asthma Rep. E. Christina, MD Ciaccio, Jay M, Portnoy MD, Section ed. Pediatric Allergy and Immunology. doi 10.1007/S11882-011-0226-3.

CHAPTER 15

Prevention of Allergy

VK Jain, Rajendra Prasad

INTRODUCTION

Allergy and allergic diseases pose a global public health problem to a large segment of the population and have increased to two- to threefold over the past 40 years and are affecting the quality of life. Worldwide, sensitization (IgE antibodies) to foreign proteins in the environment is present in up to 40% of the population.[1] The rise in prevalence of allergic diseases has continued in the industrialized world for more than 50 years. The rise is attributed to urbanization, industrialization, environmental pollution, tobacco smoke, changing lifestyle, and increasing awareness.[1-5] The consequent economic burden has been tremendous in terms of overall healthcare management, medical expenditure, and loss of productivity.[2-8] Sensitization rates to one or more common allergens among school children are currently approaching 40–50%.[1] Respiratory allergy is a common problem globally. Over the past 10 years, the general concept of the pathogenesis of respiratory allergy has markedly changed and evolved with greater emphasis on the link between the upper and lower respiratory airways (one airway, one disease). It is estimated that over 40% of the world population is atopic.[9] In the United States in 2012, 10.6% or 7.8 million children reported respiratory allergies in the past 12 months.[10]

In India, 20–30% of the population is reported to have one or the other allergic disorders.[11] Allergic diseases have been less common in Asia than the in Western World but is rapidly catching up.[8] The knowledge of natural history of development of allergy (sensitization) and allergic disorders in children has been described in several birth cohort studies.[9,11-16] The "Allergy March" is the progression from eczema and food hypersensitivity in infancy to rhinitis and asthma in later childhood with concomitant shift from food to inhalant sensitization.[12-16] Different phenotype characterizations of allergic diseases and pattern of sensitization are based on various prospective studies, and it is a prerequisite for future work on the prevention of allergic diseases.[17,18] Primary and secondary levels of prevention depend on early detection of clinical markers, especially in infancy.[19] Some of the cohort studies have reported sensitization as a predictor in young children for later development of allergic diseases.[16,20-29]

Allergic rhinitis or asthma is not confined to a specific target organ, but rather a disorder involving the entire respiratory tract. Bronchial asthma is one of the commonest respiratory allergic disorders and is usually associated with allergic rhinitis. Asthma is a chronic inflammatory disorder of airways, which affects about 10–15% of children and 5–7% of adults.[2-9] It affects health, quality of life, and economy. The disease is genetically determined and environmentally triggered.[12] Evidence-based guidelines have been recommended by the World Allergy Organization (WAO),[9] Canadian Asthma Consensus,[30] and by others for the prevention of allergy and allergic diseases.[31-34]

DEVELOPMENT OF ALLERGIC SENSITIZATION

Genes involved in the pathogenesis of allergy and asthma in general have not been identified with certainty, although potential candidate genes have been defined. Sensitization to aeroallergens is a major risk factor for the development of allergic rhinitis and asthma.[35,36] The risk of sensitization to allergens increases with age during childhood.[35-37] Sensitization to food allergens is common below 3 years of age and diminishes in later childhood.[32,38] Prevalence of aeroallergen sensitization is low as reported in various studies.[37-40] Increasing prevalence of asthma in children and young adults has been reported in Western and Asian countries.[1-9,17,41] Atopy is also an important risk factor for the development of allergy and allergic diseases.[9,14-19,42]

Genetics/Hereditary Factors

Individuals with a family history of atopy have an increased risk of developing IgE sensitization.[9,10,14-19,42] Atopic constitution is a major risk factor for the development of allergic diseases. The risk of developing allergic disease in a particular organ is related to the family history of that disease. The contribution of genetic factors to the development of IgE sensitization, and to the family history of an IgE-mediated disease, is 70–80%.

Adjuvant/Trigger Factors

These factors are environmental tobacco smoke (ETS), air pollutants (diesel particulates, SO_2, nitrogen dioxide), and recurrent respiratory viral infection, including biomass exposure and urbanization. Lifestyle, dietary habits, exercise, nutrition, and behavior changes may also contribute.[9,17,43-64]

Etiological Factors

These factors are mainly biological aeroallergen exposure from both the indoor and outdoor environments.[9,13,14,21-24,37-39,49-51,57-60,64,65] Allergens prevalent in the indoor environment are mainly house dust mites (HDMs), mold, insects, pet animals (cat, dog, and rabbit), hair, and dander. Outdoor allergens are mainly pollen, dust, and fungi. These factors will initiate the allergic sensitization, especially in genetically susceptible individuals, and will further develop the airway hyper-responsiveness, leading to the development of asthma or other allergic diseases. Exposure to these factors is important in early age in neonates and infants.

ETS in the Development of Allergic Sensitization

Passive smoking by the family members increases the risk of upper and lower respiratory tract infection causing bronchitis and pneumonia in infants and children.[6,7,43-50] Maternal smoking during and after pregnancy promotes sensitization and development of childhood asthma and also deteriorates fetal lung function and increases risk of wheezing. ETS causes wheezing in infants and aggravates asthma. Smoking during pregnancy also increases the IgE levels in neonates. Therefore, smoking avoidance by mother, family members, and caretakers is an important preventive measure against the development of allergic sensitization and further development of nasorespiratory allergic diseases in children.

Role of Early Childhood Infections in the Development of Allergy

Respiratory infections (pertussis and respiratory syncytial virus) in early childhood may enhance IgE sensitization and increase the risk of allergic diseases. A longitudinal multicentric allergy study[53] has suggested that repeated rhinitis and allergy infection of herpes type in early life (below 3 years) may stimulate the immature immune system toward the Th_1 phenotype and reduce the risk of bronchial hyperresponsiveness (BHR), wheeze, and asthma up to school age. Lower respiratory infection in early childhood increases the risk of wheeze up to the age of 7 years. Immunological programming is initiated very early in life. It is driven by exposure to ubiquitous, dietary, and inhalant allergens and modulated by microbial exposure and vaccines (hygiene hypothesis). Lack of microbial exposure particularly in early life may enhance the development of allergic diseases.[36-39,52,53,65]

SCREENING TESTS FOR PREDICTION OF ALLERGY/SENSITIZATION

No ideal test with sufficient accuracy to detect the risk of developing atopic allergy is available. The following tools are used to assess the risk of development of allergy and allergic disorders.

Cord Blood Tests

- Measurement of IgE level in the cord and capillary blood (fifth day) in neonates is popular; however, it is less sensitive (25%) but more specific (>90%).[9,54,56]
- Measurement of human leukocyte antigen haplotype, histamine release from basophils, and phosphodiesterase from lymphocytes of the cord blood is also reported by workers.
- Eosinophil and platelet counts in cord blood are also recommended to predict the development of respiratory allergy.

Genetic Markers

Autosomal recessive gene linked to *D11S97* on chromosome *11q13* is proposed to be atopic gene and preferentially active when inherited from the maternal side.[56] The other genes have also been described by the various workers with variable results.

CATEGORIES OF PREVENTION (FLOWCHART 15.1)

Prevention is the earliest part of intervention against the development of allergy and allergic diseases.[9,31-34] Prevention of allergic sensitization is the first step to prevent allergy. Prevention is preferred to symptomatic treatment. It can be made at three levels:

1. *Primary prevention* (*prevention of allergic sensitization*): It is the prevention of immunological sensitization (development of IgE antibodies). The aim is to avoid the risk factors before the development of allergic sensitization. This can be achieved by removal of all the adjuvant and causative factors during in utero life (antenatal care) and during early life (neonates and infants), especially below 3 years.
2. *Secondary prevention* (*prevention of development of allergic diseases and/or asthma*): The aim is early detection and cure before the symptoms of asthma appear. This can be achieved by removal of trigger (risk) and causative factors in infants, children, adolescents, and adults. Secondary prevention reduces the incidence of respiratory diseases such as rhinitis/asthma.
3. *Tertiary prevention* (*treatment of allergic diseases and asthma*): The aim is to control disease and minimize morbidity in children, adolescents, and adults. This can be achieved by avoidance of allergens, trigger factors, and use of pharmacotherapy (steroids/bronchodilators) and preventive therapy (immunotherapy, gene therapy, and anti-leukotrienes).

Flowchart 15.1: Categories of prevention.

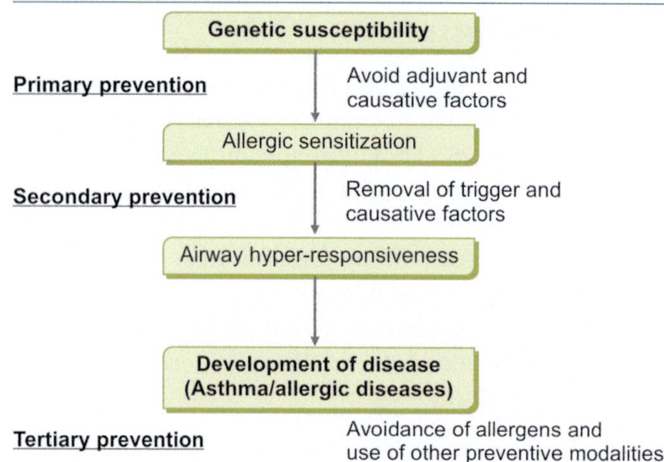

ROLE OF PREVENTIVE MEASURES IN ALLERGY

Environmental pollution control is an important preventive measure for the development of allergy.[9,31-34,43-53,66] It is essential to distinguish between causative (allergen exposure) and adjuvant/trigger (risk) factors such as tobacco smoke, air pollutants, infections (viral), and nutrition. It is also essential to know the different levels of pollutants to interfere with the development of allergy and allergic diseases. Environmental control is done by air conditioning, which in general is not easy and feasible. Change in lifestyle may minimize trigger exposure. The major influence is focused on infant-feeding practices, parental smoking habit, nutrition, air pollution, and recurrent airway infection, especially viral infection.

Prenatal Measures

- Avoidance of maternal smoking and exposure to tobacco smoke, environmental pollutants, and indoor and outdoor allergen exposure.
- Avoidance of allergic diet (milk, dairy products, eggs, etc.) during pregnancy—results are variable and not recommended.
- Australasian Society of Clinical Immunology and Allergy (ASCIA) recommended healthy balanced diet rich in fiber, vegetables, and fruits.
- Exclusion of any/highly allergenic foods is not recommended and has not shown any prevention.
- Up to three times, oily fish/week (rich in omega-3 fatty acids) have shown some preventive effects on eczema in early life.
- Moderate evidence of probiotics may help, but specific recommendation cannot be made.

Postnatal Measures

- All prenatal measures.
- No special diet to lactating mother.

Breastfeeding

Prolonged breastfeeding reduces the risk of allergy, especially in atopic infants. Delaying the weaning of high-risk infants appears to be beneficial. The WHO recommends breastfeeding up to 6 months and as long as mother and infant wish to continue it (ASCIA). Breastfeeding may prevent the development of allergy. Withholding of solid foods in children at risk may have (4–6 months) beneficial effect. All are having low evidence.[66]

Role of Hydrolyzed Formulae

Hydrolyzed formula is a modified cow's milk to reduce its antigenicity and renders it useful in milk protein allergy. It should be given during the first 6 months in infants having allergy to cow's milk, and this will further prevent primary protein sensitivity to atopic diseases. Evidence is not so conclusive to support the use of hydrolyzed formulae over breastfeeding.[31]

Role of Probiotics during and after Pregnancy

In a randomized controlled trial, Lactobacillus GG given during pregnancy to mothers with a family history of atopy and for 6 months to their infants resulted in a significant reduction in atopic dermatitis up to 2 years.

The WAO currently recommends that probiotic during pregnancy and lactation has low evidence in preventing respiratory allergy in children,[9] whereas ASCIA reported moderate evidence, but specific recommendation cannot be made.

Role of Antioxidants (Vitamins A, C, and E and Selenium) and Omega-3 Polyunsaturated Fatty Acids (PUFAs)

Various studies have shown variable results regarding the protection against the development of various allergic disorders and asthma.[9,31-34]

Outdoor Environmental Control

Avoiding exposure to outdoor allergens and air pollutants (SO_2, NO_2, O_3) is an important step in all categories of prevention of allergy and its diseases but impossible due to ubiquitous nature. Staying indoors during mid-day and afternoon, use of nasal filter/mask, and changing work place/occupation are recommended.

Indoor Environmental Control

Avoiding exposure to indoor allergens (HDMs, pet animals, dander, and mold) is required for the prevention of allergy/asthma. If removal of pets from house is not possible, frequent washing and bathing of pets will reduce the amount of dander and dried saliva on carpets, furniture, mattresses, and in the room. Regular cleaning of beds, bathrooms, kitchen, and basement with chlorine bleach is also essential. Cleaning of mattresses, carpets, and curtains also reduces the indoor environment pollution. HDMs control is also required. Wearing masks while cleaning the house is beneficial. Removal of allergens from indoor air is done by using mechanical and electrical filters. Avoidance of indoor irritants such as tobacco smoke, wood smoke, strong odor or perfume, and fresh paints is also required. Indoor humidity to be maintained is below 50%.

HDM Control

Avoidance of exposure to HDM during childhood has shown beneficial effects in the development of allergic disorders.[5,26,27,37,63-71] Control of HDM in a house can be done by placing the barriers, killing or removing the mites, or making the environment less suitable for mites and/or to moving the patient to the dust-free environment. Placing the barriers between the patient and the reservoirs of dust mite by encasing mattresses and pillows by air-tight plastic covers, expensive microporous covers are also used. Electric blankets on beds (which dry the mite environment) have also been used. Killing of mites can be achieved by weekly washing of beddings and pillows in hot water (>60°C), by using acaricides (benzyl benzoate, tannic acid), dry heating, and by using liquid nitrogen. Vacuum cleaners are used for removal of dead mites and dust, and high-efficiency particulate air filters are used for removal of air-borne mites. Less-suitable environment for mites can be achieved by avoiding sleeping or lying on upholstered furniture, reducing indoor humidity to <50%, air conditioning or mechanical ventilation, or by removal of carpets and dust collectors laid on concrete. Removal of the patients to an HDM-free environment is very effective, but it is practically inconvenient and expensive.

WAO GUIDELINES AND STRENGTH OF RECOMMENDATIONS

Primary Prevention

- Avoid smoking and exposure to ETS, particularly during pregnancy and early childhood (B).[9]
- Tobacco smoke should be removed from workplaces (B).
- Avoid damp housing conditions (C) and reduce indoor air pollutants (C).
- Breastfeed exclusively until 6 months (B). No special diet for lactating mother (A).

- Avoidance of solid foods in infants for at least 4 months of age seems to be effective for allergy prevention.
- Reduce exposure to inhalant allergens in young children at high risk (dust mites, cockroaches, and furred pets) (B).
- Eliminate sensitizing and highly irritating agents in occupational environments (C). If this is not possible, implement measures to prevent employee exposure.
- WHO recommends exclusively breastfeeding for 6 months in general, and avoidance of solid foods for at least 4 months seems to be effective for allergy prevention.

CONCLUSION

Allergy and allergic diseases are increasing worldwide and are genetically determined and environmentally triggered. The original hypothesis for allergy prevention was that allergic diseases could be avoided by preventing the onset of the "allergic sensitization." Environmental control, both indoor and outdoor, is an important step in the prevention of allergy. Primary preventive measures during antenatal and early life are important for preventing sensitization. Evidence-based guidelines are available for the prevention of allergy/sensitization.

REFERENCES

1. Pawankar R, Canonica GW, Holgate ST, Lockey RF. White book on allergy 2011 -2012 executive summary. Geneva: World Health Organization; 2012.
2. Peat JK, van den Berg RH, Green WF, et al. Changing Prevalence of Asthma in Australian children. BMJ. 1994;308:1591-6.
3. Aberg N, Hesselmar B, Aberg B, Eriksson B. Increase of asthma, allergic rhinitis and eczema in Swedish school children between 1979 and 1991. Clin Exp Allergy. 1995;25:815-9.
4. Strachan DP, Anderson HR, Limb ES, et al. National survey of asthma prevalence, severity and treatment in Great Britain. Arch Dis Child. 1994;94:895.
5. Wright AL, Holberg CJ, Martinez FD, et al. Epidemiology of physician-diagnosed allergic rhinitis in childhood. Pediatrics. 1994;94:895-901.
6. Weiss KB, Gergen PJ, Hodgson TA. An economic evaluation of asthma in the United States. New Engl J Med. 1992;24:297.
7. Zhong NS. A topic diseases in the Chinese community. Clin Exp Allergy. 1994;24:297.
8. Ann JW, Jennifer KP, Louise MT. Changing prevalence of allergies worldwide progress. Allergy Clin Immunol. 1995;3:167.
9. Johansson SGO, Haahtela T. WAO Guidelines for prevention of allergy and allergic asthma. Allergy Clin Immunol Int J World Allergy Org. 2004;16:176-85.
10. Summary Health Statistics for U.S. Children: National Health Interview Survey; 2012, Table 2.
11. Prasad R, Kumar R. Allergy situation in India: What is being done? Editorial. Indian J chest Dis Allied Sci. 2013; 55:7-8.
12. Illi S, Von Mutius E, Lau S, et al. The natural course of atopic dermatitis from birth to age 7 years and association with asthma. J Allergy Clin Immunol. 2004;113:925-31.
13. Kulig M, Bergmann R, Klettke U, et al. Natural course of sensitization to food and inhalant allergens during the first 6 years of life. J Allergy Clin Immunol. 1999;103:1173-9.
14. Rhodes HL, Sporik R, Thomas P, et al. Early life risk factors for adult asthma: a birth cohort study of subjects at risk. J Allergy Clin Immunol. 2001;108: 720-5.
15. Rhodes Hl, Sporik R, Thomas P, et al. A birth cohort study of subjects at risk of atopy: twenty two-year follow-up of wheeze and atopic status. Am J Respir Crit Care Med. 2002;15:165:176-80.
16. Gustafsson D, Sjoberg O, Foucard T. Development of allergies and asthma in infants and young children with atopic dermatitis—a prospective follow-up to 7 years of age. Allergy. 2000;55:240-5.
17. Halken S. Prevention of allergic disease in childhood: clinical and epidemiological aspects of primary and secondary allergy prevention. Pediatr Allergy Immunol. 2004;15:4-5, 9-32.
18. Holt PG, Sly PD. Prevention of allergic respiratory disease in infants: current aspects and future perspectives. Curr Opin Allergy Clin Immunol. 2007;7:547-55.
19. Holt PG, Jones CA. The development of the immune system during pregnancy and early life. Allergy. 2000;55:688-97.
20. Kulig M, Bergmann R, Niggemann B, et al. Prediction of sensitization to inhalant allergens in childhood: evaluating family history, atopic dermatitis and sensitization to food allergens. The MAS study group. Multicentre allergy study. Clin Exp Allergy. 1998;28: 1397-03.
21. Nickel R, Kulig M, Forster J, et al. Sensitization to hen's egg at the age of twelve months is predictive for allergic sensitization to common indoor and outdoor allergens at the age of three years. J Allergy Clin Immunol. 1997;99: 613-7.
22. Dean T, Venter C, Pereira B, et al. Patterns of sensitization to food and aeroallergens in the first 3 years of life. J Allergy Clin Immunol. 2007;120:1166-71.
23. Tariq SM, Matthews SM, Hakim EA, Arshad SH. Egg allergy in infancy predicts respiratory allergic disease by 4 years of age. Pediatr Allergy Immunol. 2000;11:162-7.
24. Gustafsson D, Sjoberg O, Foucard T. Sensitization to food and airborne allergens in children with atopic dermatitis followed up to 7 years of age. Pediatr Allergy Immunol. 2003;14:448-52.
25. Sigurs N, Hattevig G, Kjellman B, et al. Appearance of atopic disease in relation to serum IgE antibodies in children followed up from birth for 4 to 15 years. J Allergy Clin Immunol. 1994;94:757-63.

26. Lowe AJ, Abramson MJ, Hosking CS, et al. The temporal sequence of allergic sensitization and onset of infantile eczema. Clin Exp Allergy. 2007;37:536-42.
27. Lowe AJ, Hosking CS, Bennett CM, et al. Skin prick test can identify eczematous infants at risk of asthma and allergic rhinitis. Clin Exp Allergy. 2007;37:1624-31.
28. Arshad SH, Bateman B, Matthews SM. Primary prevention of asthma and atopy thorax. 2003;58:489-93.
29. Illi S, Von Mutius E, LauS, et al. The pattern of atopic sensitization is associated with the development of asthma in childhood. J Allergy Clin Immunol. 2001;108:709-14.
30. Warner JO. Can we prevent asthma? Allergy Clin Immunol Int-J World Allergy Org. 2004;16:186-91.
31. Becker, et al. Prevention stratagies for asthma—primary prevention. JAMC. 2005;173:s20-4.
32. Fleischer DM, Spergel JM, Assa'ad AH, Pongracic JA. Primary prevention of allergic disease through nutritional interventions. J Allergy Clinic Immunol Pract. 2013; 1:29-36.
33. Arshad SH. Primary prevention of asthma and allergy. J Allergy Clin Immunol. 2005;116:3-14.
34. Wonderen KEV, Mark LB, Mohrs J, et al. Prediction and treatment of asthma in preschool children at risk: study design and baseline data of a prospective cohort study in general practice (ARCADE). BMC Pulm Med. 2009;9: 132-466.
35. Illi S, Von Mutius E, Lau S, et al. Perennial allergen sensitization early in life and chronic asthma in children: a birth cohort study. Lancet. 2006;368:763-70.
36. Porsbjerg C, Von Linstow ML, Ulrik CS, et al. Risk factors for onset of asthma: a 12-year prospective follow-up study. Chest. 2006;129:309-16.
37. Silvestri M, Rossi Ga, Cozzani S, et al. Age dependent tendency to become sensitized to other classes of aeroallergens in atopic asthmatic children. Ann Allergy Asthma Immunol. 1999;83:335-40.
38. Kulig M, Bergmann R, Klettke U, et al. Natural course of sensitization to food and inhalant allergens during the first 6 years of life. J Allergy Clin Immunol. 1999;103:1173-9.
39. Douwes J, Van Strien R, Doekes G, et al. Does early indoor microbial exposure reduce the risk of asthma? The prevention and incidence of asthma and mite allergy birth cohort study. J Allergy Asthma Immunol. 2006;117:1067-73.
40. Arshad SH, Tariq SM, Matthews S, Hakim E. Sensitization to common allergens and its association with allergic disorders at age 4 years: a whole population birth cohort study. Pediatrics. 2001;108:E33.
41. Host A, Andrae S, Charkin S, et al. Allergy testing in children: why, who, when and how? Allergy. 2003;58:559-69.
42. Hess J, De Jongste JC. Epidemiological aspects of paediatric asthma. Clin Exp Allergy. 2004;34:680-8.
43. Stick SM, Burton PR, Gurrin L, et al. Effects of maternal smoking during pregnancy and a family history of asthma on respiratory function in newborn infants. Lancet. 1996;348:1060-4.
44. Cunningham J, Dockery DW, Speizer FE. Maternal smoking during pregnancy as a predictor of lung function in children. Am J Epidemiol. 1994;139:1139-52.
45. Cook DG, Strachan DP. Health effects of passive smoking: Parental smoking and prevalence of respiratory symptoms and asthma in school-age children. Thorax. 1997;52: 1081-94.
46. Dijkstra L, Houthuijs D, Brunekreef B, et al. Respiratory health effects of the indoor environment in a population of Dutch children. Am Rev Respir Dis. 1990;142:1172-8.
47. Strachan DP, Cook DG. Health effects of passive smoking: Parental smoking and childhood asthma: longitudinal and case-control studies. Thorax. 1998;53:204-12.
48. Soyseth V, Kongerud J, Boe J. Postnatal maternal smoking increases the prevalence of asthma but not of bronchial hyper responsiveness or atopy in their children. Chest. 1995;107:389-94.
49. Halken S, Høst A, Husby S, et al. Recurrent wheezing in relation to environmental risk factors in infancy. A prospective study of 276 infants. Allergy. 1991;46:507-14.
50. Halken S, Høst A, Nilsson L, Taudorf E. Passive smoking as a risk factor for development of obstructive respiratory disease and allergic sensitization. Allergy. 1995;50:97-105.
51. Duhme H, Weiland SK, Keil U. Epidemiological analysis of the relationship between environmental pollution and asthma. Toxicol Lett. 1998;102-3:307-16.
52. Illi S, Mutius E, Lau S. The role of early childhood infectious diseases in the development of asthma up to school age. Allergy Clin Immunol Int. 2001;13/3:99-106.
53. Sigurs N, Bajarnason R, Sigurbergsson F, et al. Asthma and immunoglobulin E antibodies after respiratory syncytial virus bronchiolitis: a prospective cohort study with matched controls. Pediatrics. 1995;95:500-5.
54. Croner S, Kjellman N-IM. Development of atopic disease in relation to family history and cord blood IgE levels. Eleven-year follow-up in 1654 children. Pediatr Allergy Immunol. 1990;1:14-20.
55. Odelram H, Kjellman N-IM, Bjorksten B. Predictors of atopy in newborn babies. Allergy. 1995;50:585-92.
56. Asher I, Dagli E, Holgate ST. Genetic and Environmental Influence. Allergy Clin Immunol Int. 2000;12:290-1.
57. Miyamoto T, Takafuji S. Environment and allergy. In: Ring J, Przybilla B, eds. New Trends in Allergy III. Berlin, Heidelberg: Springer; 1991:459-68.
58. Tunnicliffe WS, Burge OS, Ayres JG. Effect of nitrogen dioxide and sulphur dioxide on airway response to inhaled allergen in asthmatic patients. Lancet. 1994;344:1733-6.
59. Molfino NA, Wright SC, Katz I, et al. Effect of low concentrations of ozone on inhaled allergen responses in asthmatic subjects. Lancet. 1991;338:199-203.
60. Rusznak C, Devalia JL, Davies RJ. Airway response of asthmatic subjects to inhaled allergen after exposure to pollutants. Thorax. 1996;51:1105-8.
61. Ring J, Kramer U, Schafer T, et al. Environmental risk factors for respiratory and skin atopy: results from epidemiologic studies in former East and West Germany. Int Arch Allergy Immunol. 1999;118:403-7.

62. Schafer T, Vieluf D, Behrendt H, et al. Atopic eczema and other manifestations of atopy: results of a study in East and West Germany. Allergy. 1996;51:532-9.
63. Prasad KVN. Prevention of Allergy: Clinical Advances in Allergy and Asthma. In: Dr. Rajendera Prasad, ed. Shivam Publication. 2000:69-74.
64. Heidrum B, Karl-Heinz F, Ursula K, et al. The role of indoor and outdoor air pollution in allergic diseases. Prog Allergy Clin Immunol. 1995;3:83.
65. Govaere E, Van Gysel D, Massa G, et al. The influence of age and gender on sensitization to aeroallergens. Petiatr Allergy Immunol. 2007;18:671-8.
66. ASCIA guidelines for allergy prevention in infants 2016. www.allergy.org.au/patients/allergy-prevention.
67. Sporik R, Heymann PE, Femandez-Caldas E, Platts-Mills TAE. Indoor allergens and asthma. In: Tinkelman DG, Naspitz CK, eds. Childhood Asthma. Pathophysiology and Treatment. New York: Marcel Dekker; 1993:497-535.
68. Platts-Mills TAE, Thomas WR, Aalberse RC, et al. Dust mite allergens and asthma: report of a second international workshop. J Allergy Clin Immunol. 1992;89:1046-60.
69. Arruda LK, Rizzo MC, Chapman MD, et al. Exposure and sensitization to dust mite allergens among asthmatic children in Sao Paulo, Brazil. Clin Exp Allergy. 1991;21:433-9.
70. Denson-Lino JM, Wilies-Jacobo LH, Rosas A, et al. Effect of economic status on the use of house dust mite avoidance measures in asthmatic children. Ann Allergy. 1993;71: 130-2.
71. Ehnert B, Lau-Schadendorf S, Weber A, et al. Reducing domestic exposure to dust mite allergen reduces bronchial hyper reactivity in sensitive children with asthma. J Allergy Clin Immunol. 1992;90:135-8.

CHAPTER 16

Preventive Measures and Devices in Management of Inhalant Allergy Disorders

Komarla Nagendra Prasad

INTRODUCTION

Natural and man-made activities release tiny air particles in the environment. These particles range from millimeter to micrometers. Because of less weight, they easily float in the air and remain in the air for a prolonged period before they settle on the ground. There are two types of air pollutants. First, the particles of biological origin, which have property of an allergen to induce allergy in sensitized individuals. These biopollutants are mainly classified as pollen, fungal spores, insects, house dust mites, and animal danders. Second, the particles of nonbiological origin, such as organic pollutants, which are generated by mechanical activities including natural phenomenon such as wind erosion, and which promote the allergen to induce and aggravate the allergy inflammation, such as carbon monoxide, oxides of sulfur, nitrous oxide, and ozone.[1] Allergens are classified as inhalants, ingestants, contactants, and injectants.

These particles in the atmosphere are called "dust" which are dry pulverized particles of earth ranging from 0.2 to 10 µm. Most of the liquids produce aerosols which, on drying, form less than 1-µm size particles suspended in the air. Fumes are formed by gases and volatile vapors, which are less than 0.2 µm in size. Smoke is formed by incomplete combustion of material with characteristic appearance of tiny particles of carbon. These air pollutants do not cause allergy, but they act as a triggering factor for allergic diseases.

The species of angiosperms including trees, herbs, and shrubs release enormous quantities of pollen in the air during their flowering period. The species of fungi release spores during their life cycle, some of which cause allergic reactions and are IgE mediated. This chapter deals with the sources of bio- and non-bioparticles with relevance to allergenic reaction and effective prevention of these particles using simple mechanical barriers that is devised to eliminate or reduce these particles from the surrounding environment. Defense against allergy disorders is to prevent or avoid allergen exposure by use of preventive devices.

STRATEGY TO DECREASE OR ELIMINATE ALLERGY SYMPTOMS

Less sensitive patients develop symptoms on exposure to heavy allergen load, whereas high sensitive patients develop symptoms quickly on exposure to less allergen load in the environment.[2] Successful allergen avoidance strategy will decrease or eliminate symptoms, and effective preventive measure may not be necessary to eliminate total allergen exposure.

Indoor and outdoor air pollution is a major index of pollution load. 50% of indoor air is made out of outdoor air. Outdoor air pollutants are generated by motor vehicles and factories in urban areas and by spraying pesticides and herbicides in agriculture forms and animal danders in rural areas. Air pollution is also caused by electromagnetic radiation from transformers, radio, television, cellular phones, and radon from earth. Volatile organic substances such as benzene, xylene, and toluene are released from various furniture and building materials.[3]

Irrespective of indoor or outdoor, it is difficult to selectively control the specific aeroallergen, which is a cause for allergic disorder. Following allergy, preventive measures can be adopted to manage or reduce symptoms in case of specific aeroallergens.

POLLEN-PREVENTIVE MEASURES

The release of tree pollen is seasonal and restricted to summer or winter season, and some of the weeds release throughout the year and are influenced by regional effect of temperature and humidity.[4] The pollen is released in the air in two peaks—favoring temperature and humidity, which are in the early morning and late evening. Pollen allergen can be avoided by avoiding outdoor activity in the morning and evening with pollen peak of high counts. Outdoor activities are preferred in the late afternoon and after heavy rain with reduced pollen load. Windows should be closed and air conditioners should be used to minimize the exposure to pollens. After washing, clothes should be dried indoors to prevent the pollens from adhering to clothes. Pollen can be transported indoors by people and pets, who are frequent movers from outdoors to indoors. Grass pollens have high cross-reactivity and are small in size; thus, those who are sensitive to these pollens should avoid moving on lawns, spending time on lawns, and remain away from people who work in the fields as they carry pollens on their clothes until they change their clothes.

Pollen types range from 6 μm to 60 μm in size and have beautiful artistic shapes and pores as shown here (Table 16.1).

Table 16.1: Sizes and shapes of pollen.

Type of pollen	*Illustration*	*Size range (μm)*
Parthenium		20–28
Eucalyptus		19–31
Casuarina		28–35
Holoptelea		27–33
Acacia		35–45
Cocos		42–52

MOLD-PREVENTIVE MEASURES

Outdoor molds are seasonal and appear in early spring. They grow in moist shady areas, common soil, decaying vegetation and composite piles, rotting wood, and dry fallen leaves.[4] Indoor molds are perennial and prevalent during the winter, found in dark, warm, humid, damp basements, cellars, bathrooms and laundry rooms, refrigerator drip trays, garbage pails, air conditioners, and humidifiers. The mold spore load can be prevented or reduced by removing decaying debris from yard, roof, and gutters. Bathroom should be ventilated and clothes should be dried outdoors. Faucets, pipes, and ductwork should be checked for leaks. Dehumidifier and air conditioner are used to maintain the relative humidity below 50% to reduce the spore counts. Windows should be kept open for several minutes to allow mold spores to disperse when entering the room, which were closed for several weeks or months. Clearing all visible molds from walls and ceilings may help to reduce the mold load. Mold control products should be used to retard the growth of molds such as mildew spray on walls and furniture, tile cleaners to clean the wall tiles, multipurpose spray cleaners to remove

Table 16.2: Sizes and shapes of fungal spores.

Type of fungal spores	*Illustration*	*Size range (μm)*
Aspergillus		3.5–5
Cladosporium		(5–28) × (3–8)
Nigrospora		10–35
Alternaria		(20–60) × (9–18)
Helminthosporium		(50–75) × (2–7)
Fusarium		(25–120) × (2–9)

grease and soils from washable surface disinfectant, and cleaner to effectively remove molds from any surface. Molds also commonly appear in the cupboards with clothes, which were not operated for long time. Mold counts become more in the rooms stored with goods, files or papers, or junk luggage when the room is not operated for a long time.

The spores are smaller than pollens, and their counts depend upon the area and the condition of the area, where molds grow luxuriously and available for inhalation. Molds induce respiratory and sinus infections with long-standing unresolved problems in some population. The shapes of mycelia and spores are illustrated here (Table 16.2).

MITE-PREVENTIVE MEASURES

Mites live and reproduce on mattress, bedding, upholstery, carpets, and curtains. Mites feed on scales of human skin, animal danders, most of the organic debris, and birds. They thrive in warm and humid environments with more than 50% humidity. House dust mites thrive and live in clean homes too. Live, dead, and decaying mite bodies; eggs; and fecal matter that float in the air induce mite allergy on inhalation in sensitive persons.[5] Mite commonly thrives in an environment having humidity more than 52 RH and temperature around 18–24°C. This environment is congenial to make colonies. Mite is a harmless creature, rich in protein and enzymes, mostly found in the GI tract and in fecal particles. They become airborne, when the colony-bound area, such as mattresses, carpets, or upholstery furniture, is disturbed by movements or by sitting, standing, or lying on the respective areas; when they come in contact with nasal and bronchial mucous membrane through inhalation, the sensitized subjects react to the sequence of allergy symptoms. Mite exposure can be reduced by using mite impermeable membrane in the form of pillow covers and mattresses cover. Two micro-gram Der P1 per gram of house dust[6] increases the risk of asthma attack. Acaricides are very effective in controlling mite[4] population by killing mites, thus leading to a reduction in reproduction and excreta and eggs. Vacuuming removes mites tightly adhered to carpets, beddings, and curtains, and also helps in the removal of fecal matter and eggs. A chemical such as tannic acid is effective in decaying mite bodies and fecal particles, and it no longer has a potential to induce allergy. Other chemicals such as benzyl benzoate, pirimiphos-methyl, bioallethrin, and d-phenothrin, and fungicide such as natamycin interfere with the high-protein food supply of mite when spread on the places where mites are suspected.

In tropical countries such as India and Africa, and Gulf countries, the simplest method to kill mites is by their exposure to sunrays and and then beat the article with a sizable stick to remove the dead mites before it is shifted indoors. Sensitive subjects should not be exposed to the beating dust. Ironing with high temperature or dipping in boiling water for a few minutes followed by drying also kills mites (Figs. 16.1 and 16.2).

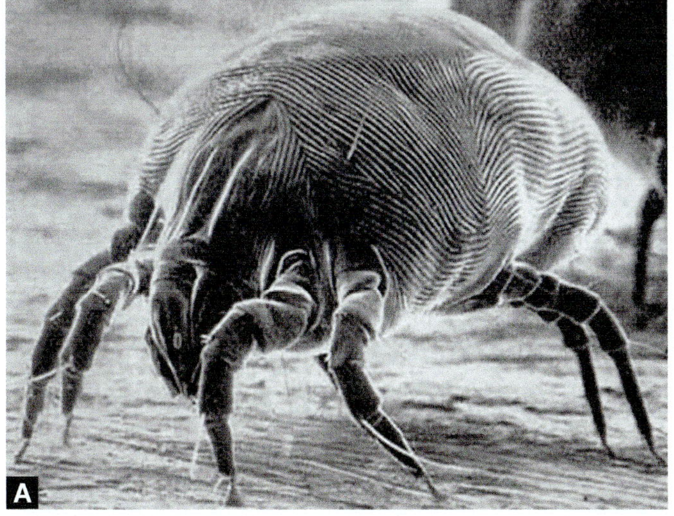

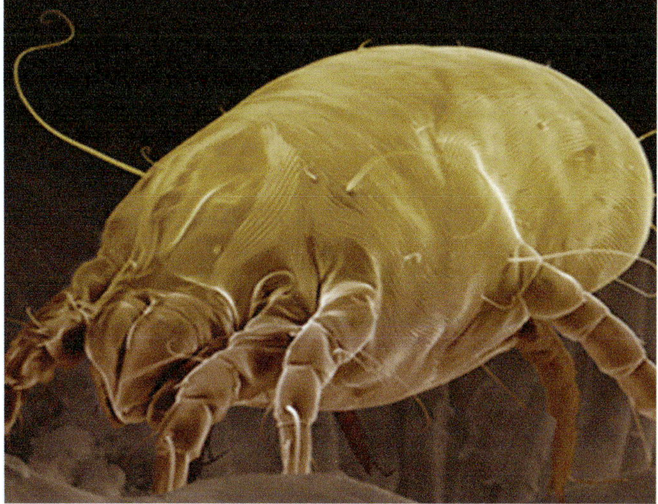

Fig. 16.1A: Mite (mite, mite egg, mite fecal particle, mite impermeable membrane with mite).

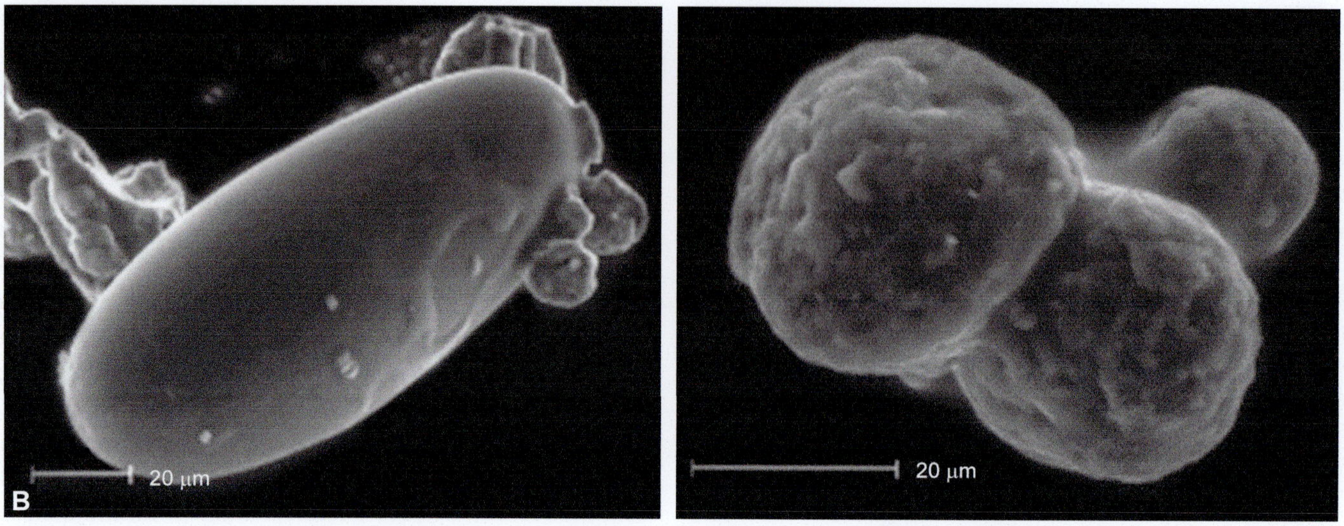

20 μm

B

20 μm

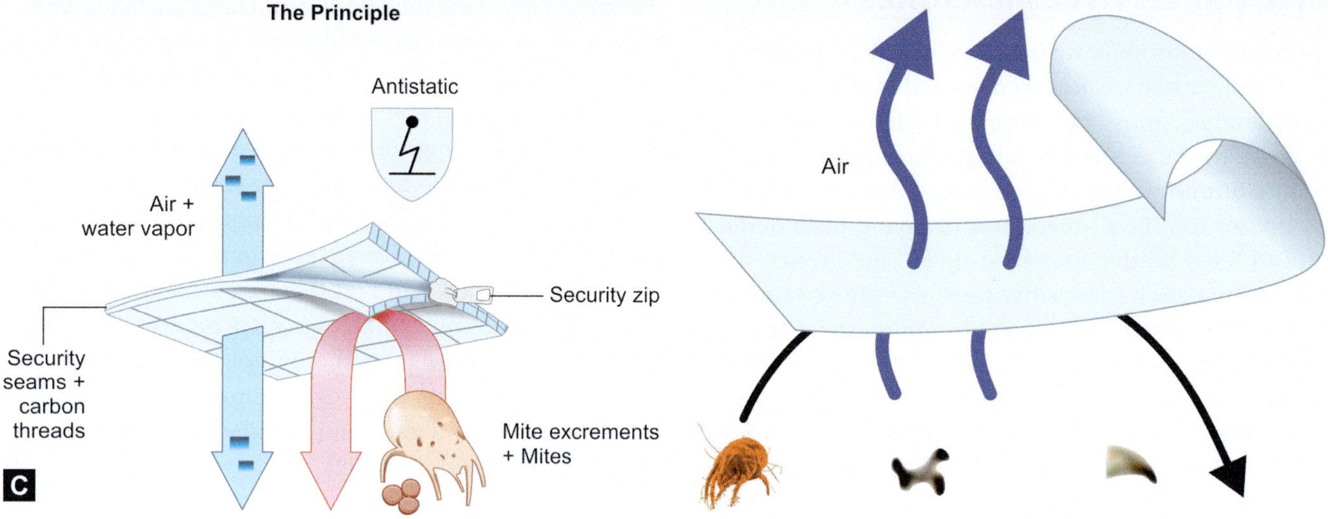

The Principle

Antistatic

Air +
water vapor

Security zip

Security
seams +
carbon
threads

Mite excrements
+ Mites

Air

C

Figs. 16.1B and C: Mite (mite, mite egg, mite fecal particle, mite impermeable membrane with mite).

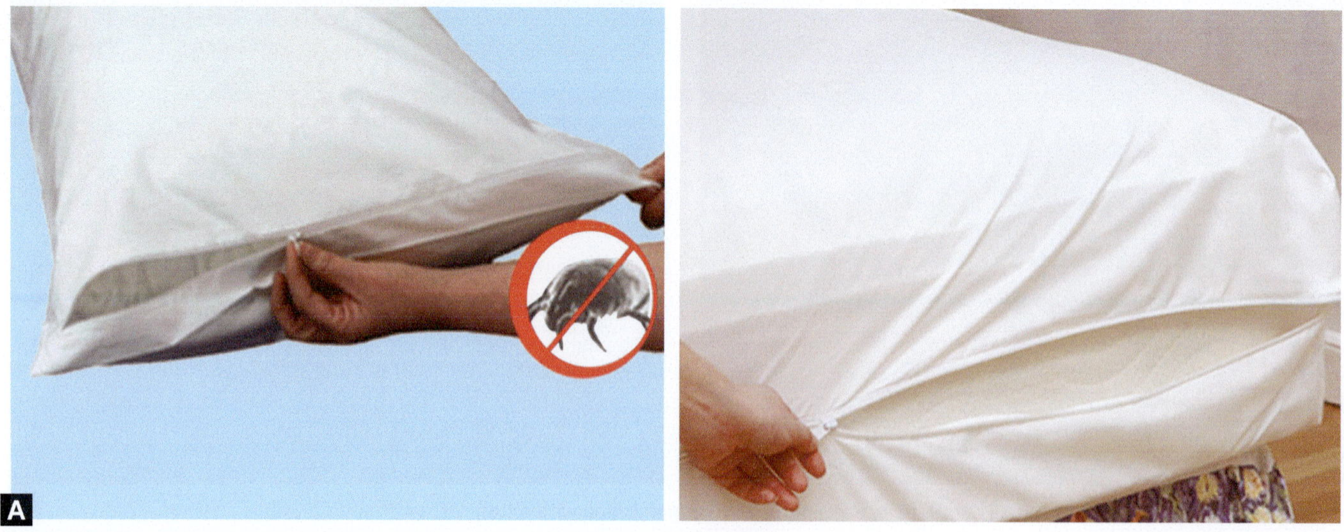

Fig. 16.2A: Mite control (mattresses cover, pillow cover, acaricides to control mite).

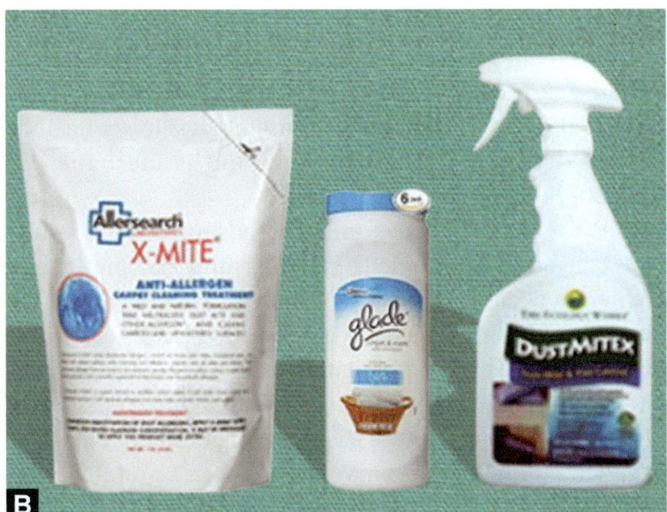

Fig. 16.2B: Mite control (mattresses cover, pillow cover, acaricides to control mite).

INSECT-PREVENTIVE MEASURES

Insects are predominant group in animal kingdom, they thrive everywhere and even adapted to most adverse condition. Insect allergy is mainly due to common indoor insects such as scales, fecal particles, and dead and decaying body particles of cockroaches, rats, moths, houseflies, mosquitoes, and red ants. Today, in most of the urban places of India, people are living in multistory buildings having toilet ducts running in multiple meters, which is a good place for the colonization of cockroach. The illumination with attractive lights in the evening including the street lights attracts moths. Cockroaches, mosquitoes, and moths need not live in the vicinity of the sensitive subjects and become active at dawn and early morning. These insects emit fine scales from their body, which are invisible, lighter, and transport into the air and can be inhaled. Recently, we noticed subjects become sensitized to these insects after house dust mite higher sensitivity. The inhalation to these insect fragments become overloaded in the air and lifestyle of the subjects spending time in indoor than outdoor, which expose to these fragments higher and become sensitized. Controlling insects indoors is slightly difficult in old houses, where insect-hiding places are abundant. Common methods of controlling insects include limiting the spread of food in and around the house and keeping food out of bedroom, keeping food and garbage containers closed, mopping kitchen floor and washing countertops regularly, eliminate water leaks from faucets and pipes, plugging crevices around house to prevent entry of cockroach, use of safe pesticides to prevent insect infestation. Draining stagnant water beneath refrigerator, air conditioners, humidifiers, gardens and pots, and in fountains not functioning in and around house to avoid breeding of the mosquitoes.

PET ALLERGEN-PREVENTIVE MEASURES

Common household pets such as dogs, cats, and birds secrete oil from oil glands, saliva, aerosolized urine, and wither danders, and the secretion contains proteins, which become airborne on drying.[7] Livestock particularly cattle, sheep, goat, and even pig seldom cause allergy disorder. Prevention of pets out of bedrooms, confine them to areas without carpets or upholstered furniture and, if possible, keeping them away from the house will reduce the allergen load indoors. Avoid contact with soiled litter cages, wear mask and gloves near rodents and dust often with damp cloth may reduce floating in the air (Fig. 16.3).

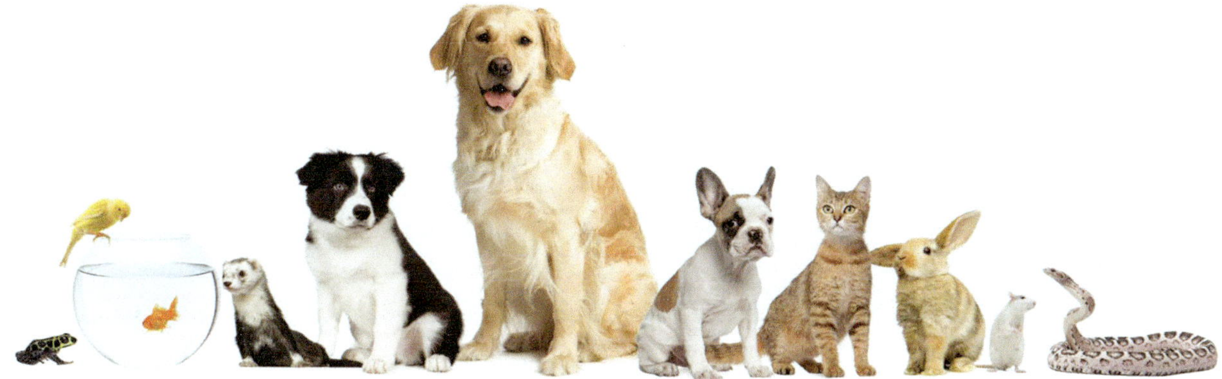

Fig. 16.3: Pets.

FIG PETS

Whatever case may be the source, type, potency, tolerability and nature of allergen in the surrounding. Omnipresence of inhalant in the air and normal human being inhales 15,000–20,000 L of air per day hence every chance for entry of aeroallergen while person inhales air thus poses difficulty in avoidance, since person may differ in tolerance to allergens.

The best way is to avoid inhalant allergens by using personal preventive devices. A novel idea of filtering the air before it enters into the nasal passage was proposed by Albert G Hill in 1955. The concept is very simple, one has to use filters before air enters into the nasal passage. Since the design of first nose filters, there are several advancement, refinement, and improvization and are thoroughly reviewed by the author.[7]

PREVENTIVE DEVICES

They include air filters, which filter particulate matter up to 0.5 μm. Its main function is to filter the particulate matter where the patient is sensitive or irritant to these particles. This filter does not filter the fumes or gases. It is required to be used only when exposure to the air causes irritation.

Filter Mask with Dynamic Activated Carbon Cloth

This is one of the new generation high-tech air filter media with potential protection against inhalation of harmful chemicals in the form of gases, fumes, smoke, vapors, and odors, and to some extent, fine particles. Dynamic activated carbon cloth (DACC) is made out of filament yarn deposited with activated carbon molecules. It is a flexible form of dynamic activated carbon and is mechanically weak but highly porous in nature.

The DACC is effective and has adsorption properties than conventional molded, granular, and palletized and powder activated carbon. It involves fast intra-particle adsorption kinetics, which takes place in gas and liquid phase adsorption. Atoms of pollutants have an affinity toward DACC surface and adsorb like a sponge at room temperature. DACC has ability to capture gas molecules and hold them at room temperature (van der Waals equation), and it warms the cold air and prevents the entry of fog (Fig. 16.4).

The DACC is made of minimum 90% pure form of dynamic activated carbon. Carbon pore size is near to or less than 10 μ. DACC adsorbs 57–85% chemical pollutants. Five grams of activated carbon have surface area of 1,300–2,000 sq. meters. (Football ground area). Filter membrane can be reusable after regeneration. DACC filters pollutants by physical adsorption by weak and bond molecules saturated on the surface of the DACC and are discharged by heating to regenerate DACC. Molecules of pollutants bouncing across the DACC gradually lose energy and finally come to rest on DACC. It adsorbs diesel, kerosene smell, roadside smell and dust, cooking smoke, garbage smell and dust, cigarette smoke, and mold and mildew filtering pollutants. It is good at trapping organic chemicals and chlorine (Fig. 16.5).

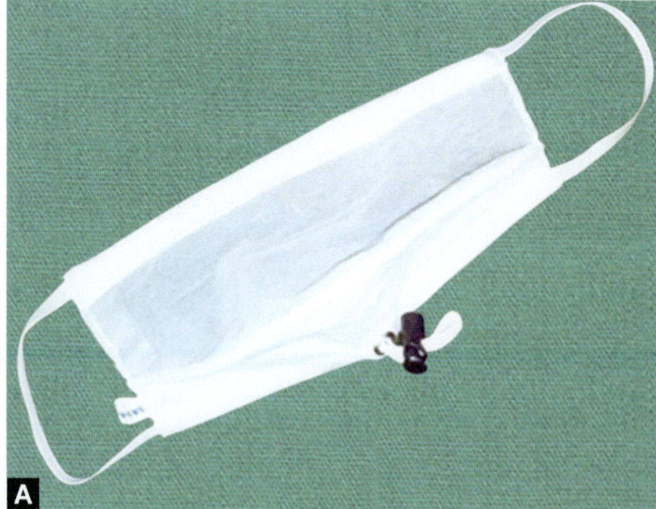

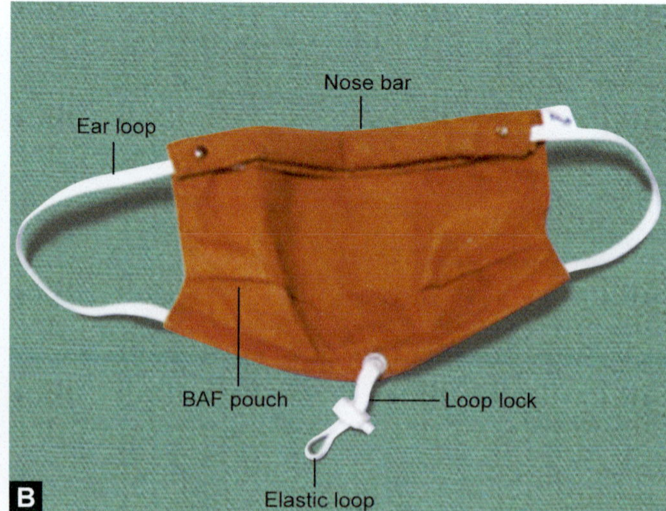

Figs. 16.4A and B: Filter masks (preventive filter mask, chemical filter mask with DACC).

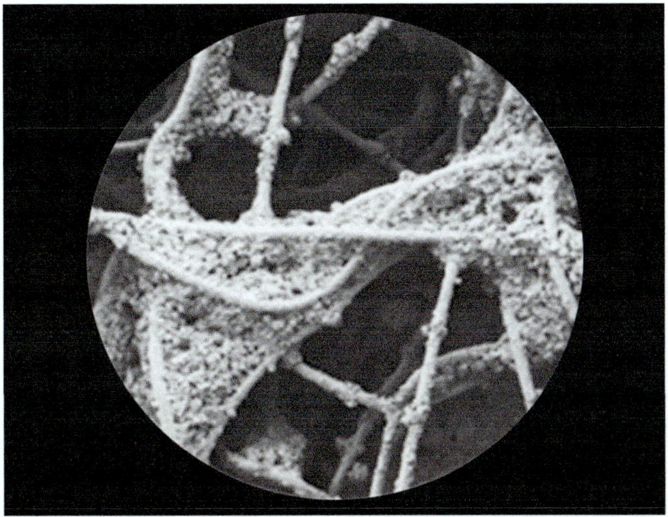

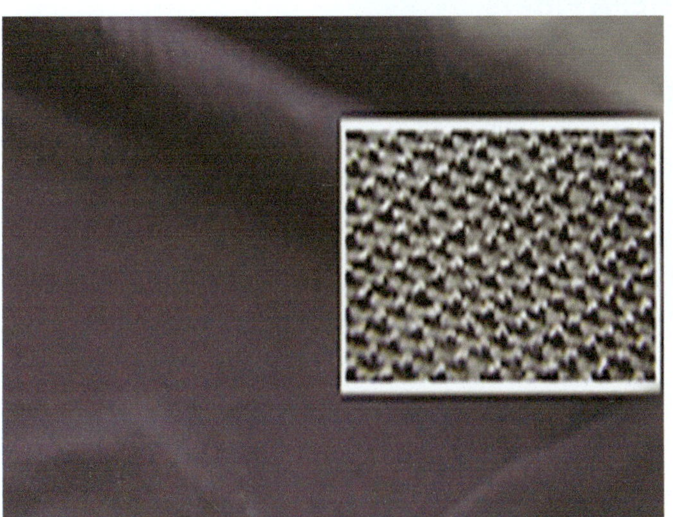

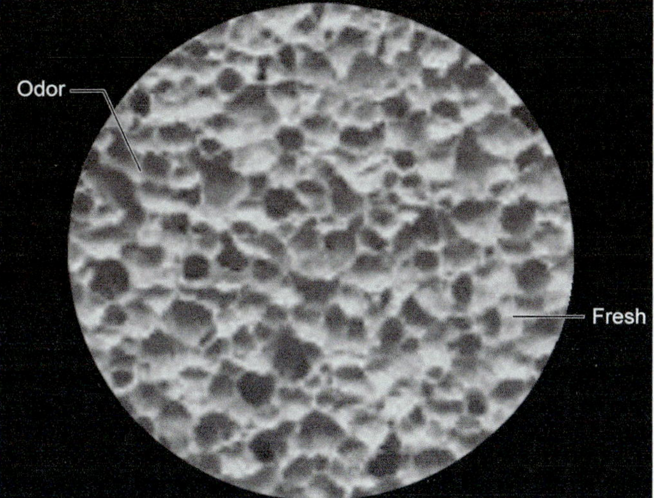

Fig. 16.5: Dynamic activated carbon cloth (DACC) (graph-adsorption).

Nonwoven Nose Filter

The nonwoven nasal filter facilitates easy breathing by providing a larger total surface area of filtration and having more efficient and effective breathing compared to netted (mesh) filters.[8] It was devised and patented by the author.[9] It has a maximum surface filter area with three-dimensional filtration. Attain adaptation of normal breathing with nose filters in a few minutes. Ready-made sizes available to suit everyone. Due to resilient action, nasal secretions and sense of foreign body are very minimum.

The advantage of this filter is its simple procedure for fixing and maintenance. Aesthetic nose appearance is maintained due to flexibility; polymer used to construct the nose filter is clinically acceptable and nonirritant, filters near to 80% of 0.5 μm particulate matter has built in activated carbon, filters fumes, and polluted gases, suitable for indoor and outdoor biological and organic pollutants (Fig. 16.6).

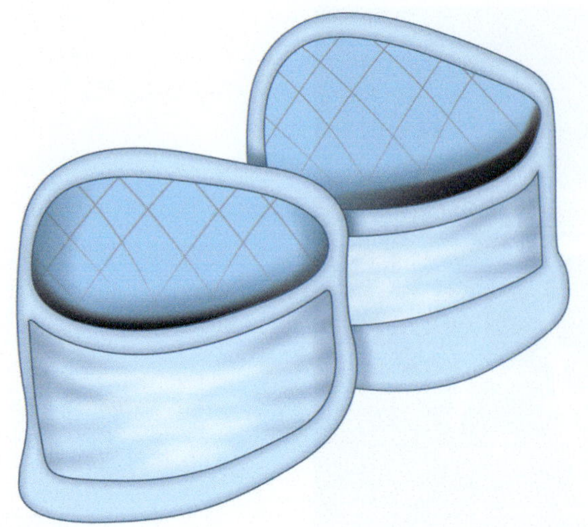

Fig. 16.6: Nonwoven nose filter.

Nasal-Irrigation Solute

Regular irrigation of the nose removes nasal secretions, thus recurrent infections brought down to minimum.[10-12] It also hydrates and decongests the nose to improve airflow and open sinus passage by improving nasal drainage and enhances potential action of nasal medication. Composition of nasal irrigation solute is a blend of sodium chloride, sodium hydrogen carbonate, potassium chloride, and calcium chloride. It is a hypertonic solution, which reduces bacterial growth, rejuvenates nasal cilia, and enhances ciliary's action (Fig. 16.7).

Air purifiers and air cleaners—these devices are effectively used to purify air in living room and bedrooms. There are three phases of air cleaners:

1. Source control of pollutants
2. Air cleaning or filtration
3. Ventilation control to dilute pollutants.

Devices such as air cleaners, air filters, ionizers, and electrostatic precipitators improve air quality by removal of pollutants; however, these are useful as an adjuvant to effective source control and adequate ventilation. Air cleaning alone cannot adequately remove all the pollutants found in indoor air (Figs. 16.8 to 16.10).[13]

HEPA Filters

High-energy particulate accumulator (HEPA) is ultimate in absolute air filtration The media is made of 100% submicronic glass fibers, which is resistance to heat tolerance up to 320°C and resistance to chemicals and moisture. It filters less than 0.3 μm particles up to 99.9% and is operated at a temperature up to 120°C with 100% relative humidity. Ultra-low particulate accumulator filters filter air up to 99.99% of 0.1–0.2 μm particles (Figs. 16.11 and 16.12).

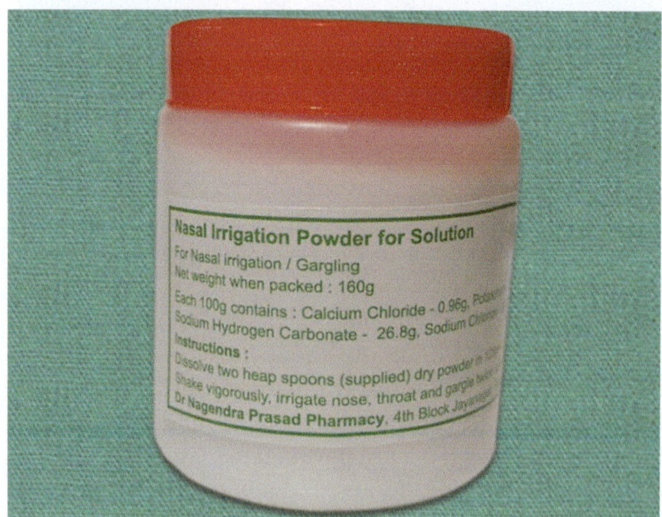

Fig. 16.7: Nasal irrigate solute.

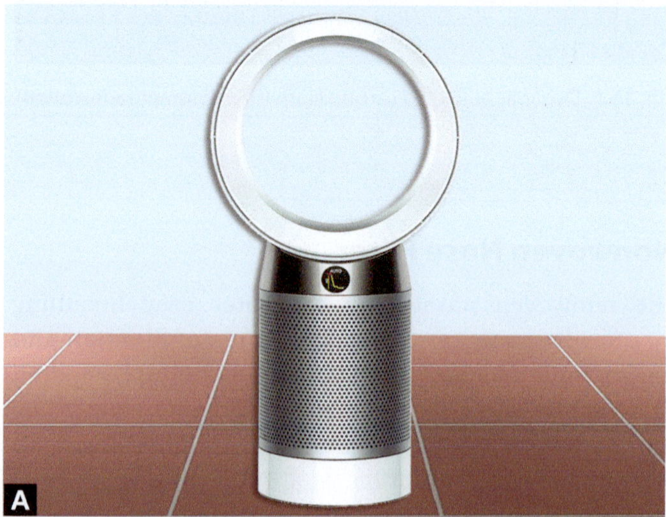

Fig.16.8A: Room air purifiers, vent with high-energy particulate accumulator (HEPA) filters.

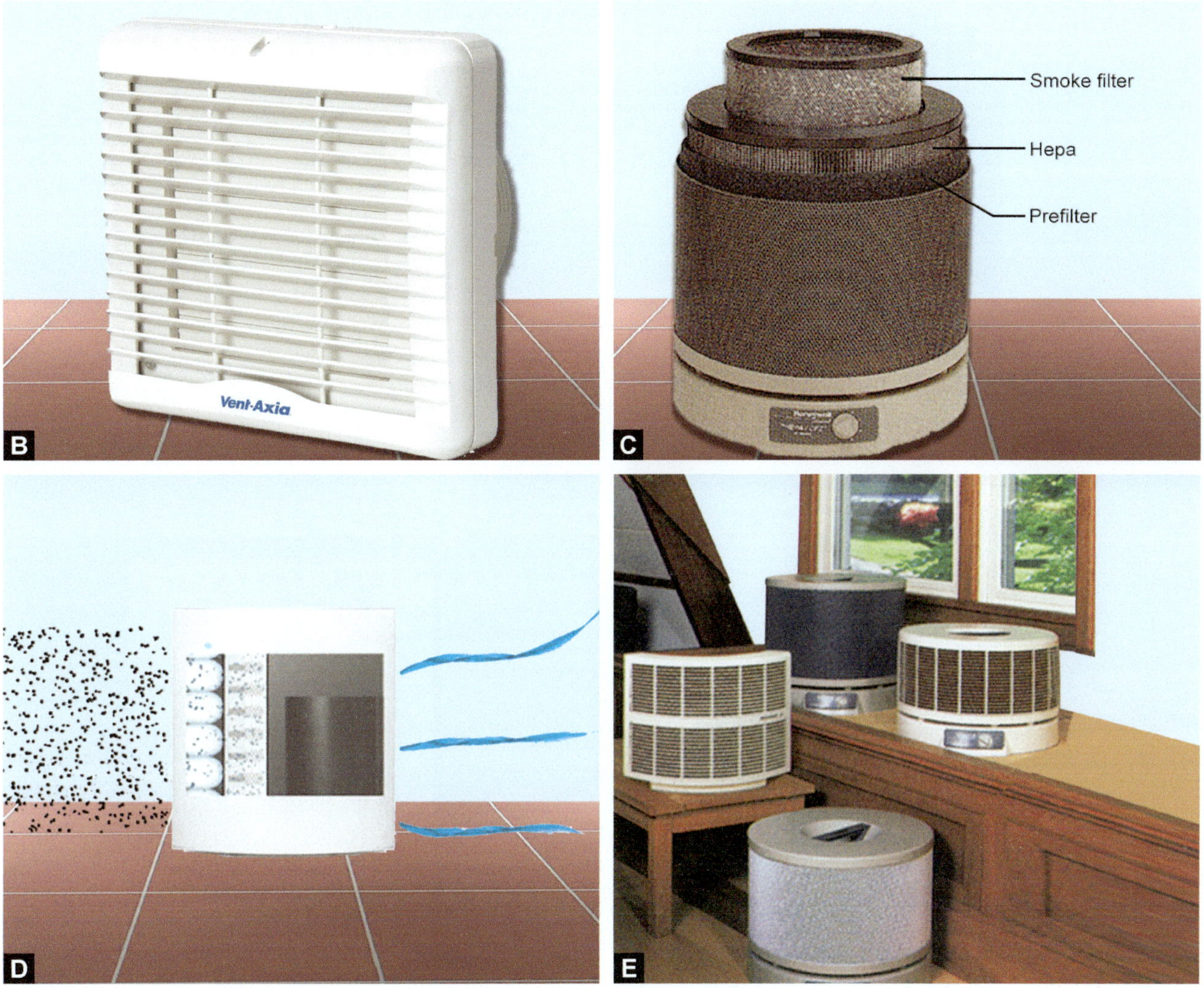

Figs. 16.8B to E: Room air purifiers, vent with high-energy particulate accumulator (HEPA) filters.

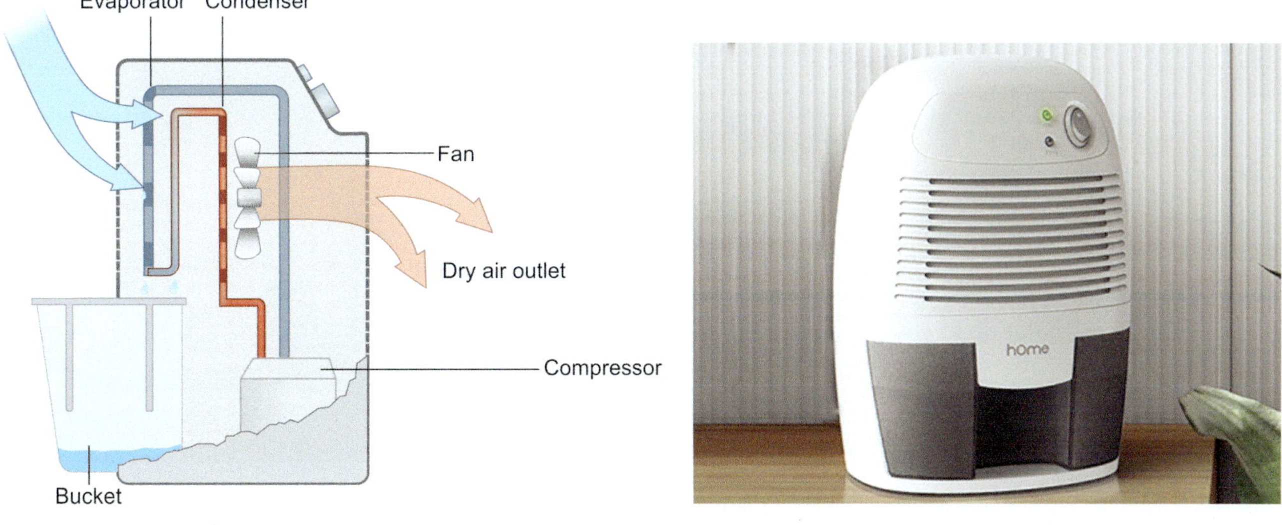

Fig. 16.9: A dehumidifier.

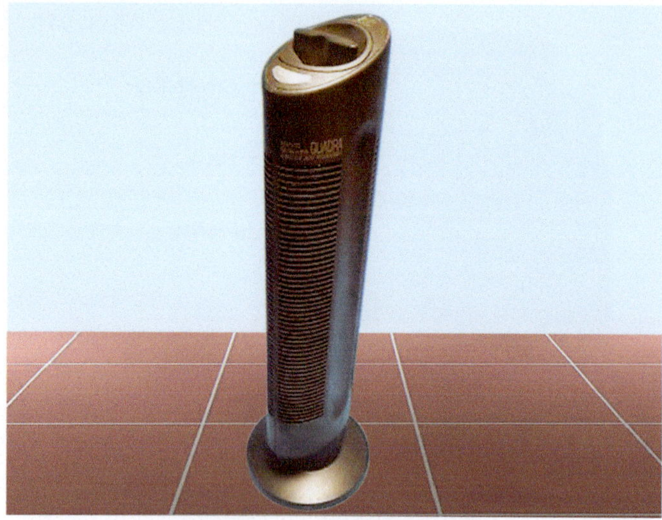

Fig. 16.10: Ionizer.

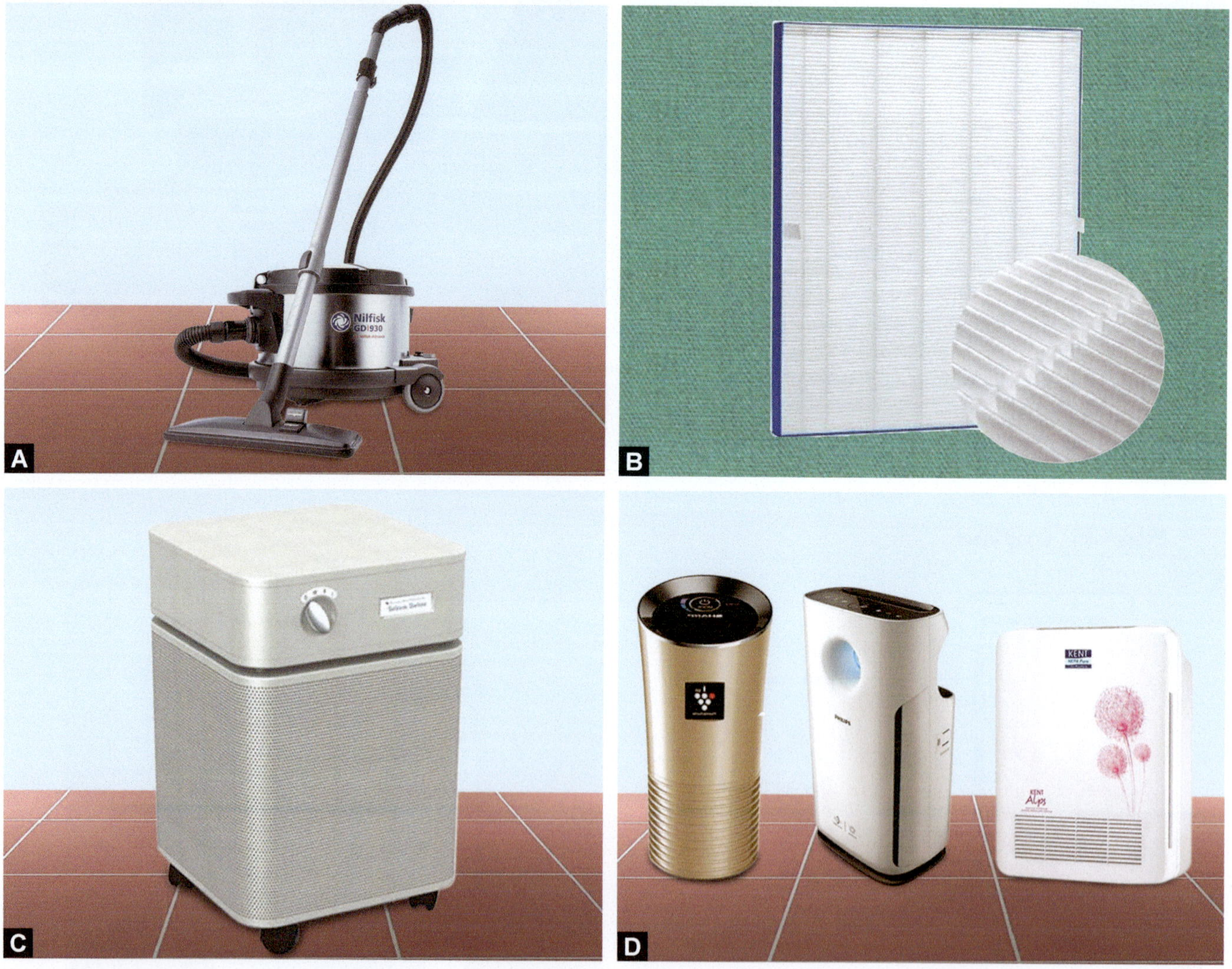

Figs. 16.11A to D: High-energy particulate accumulator (HEPA) filters (models of HEPA filters, HEPA vacuum cleaner).

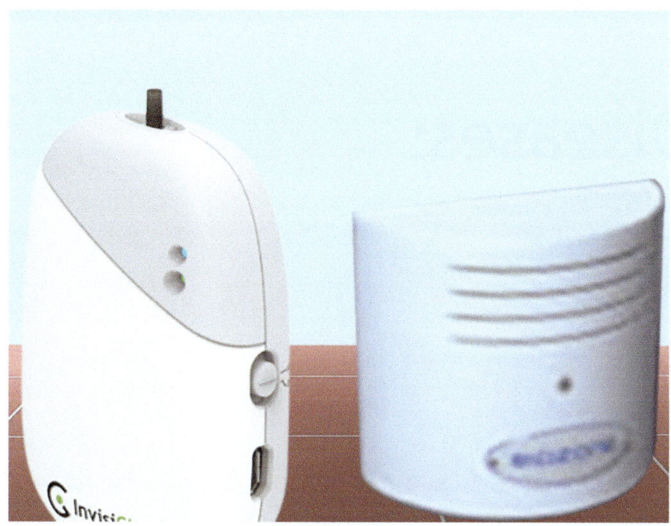

Fig. 16.12: Air purification (table—comparative study).

REFERENCES

1. Lacey J. Agricultural and occupational bioaerosoles: sampling and clinical application. In: Triq, Emberlin J, eds. Clinical Application of Aero-biology. Brussels, Belgium: The UCB Institute of Allergy; 1996:45-55.
2. Stevens WJ. Sensitivity to the Occupational Environment. Brussels, Belgium: The UCB Institute of Allergy Belgium; 1995.
3. Spieksma FTM. Airborne allergen on pauci-micronic particles. In: Triq, Emberlin J, ed. Clinical Application of Aerobiology. Brussels, Belgium: The UCB Institute of Allergy; 1996:15-21.
4. Shripad N. Agashe role of aerobiological monitoring in practice of allergy. In: Prasad R, ed. Advances in Allergy and Asthma. Lucknow, India: Shivam Pub.; 2000:99-100.
5. de Blay F. Domestic animals and their role as trigger of allergy. UCB Inst Aller. 1994:19-29.
6. Ridout S. The efficacy of acaricides in control of house dust mite. Environmental measures in the prevention of allergy. UCB Inst of Aller. 1994;19-29.
7. Albert G. Hill London, Ontario, Canada, United State Patent Office: US patent No. 2715904, August 23, 1995, Patent Information System, Nagpur-6.
8. Nagendra Prasad KV. 'Nose Filter' A device to prevent inhalant allergens. In: Patel RK, ed. Allergy. 30th Annual Convention of Indian College of Allergy and Applied Immunology. Ahmedabad, India: BJ Medical College; 1996:164-88.
9. Nagendra Prasad KV. Allergist, Bangalore Allergy Centre, Richmond Circle, Bangalore-560025. Govt. of India, the Patent Office: Complete Specification No. 173702, 1996.
10. Mabry R. Therapeutic agents in the medical management of sinusitis. Otolaryngol Clin. North Am. 1993;26(4): 561-70.
11. Anglen J, Apostoles S, Christensen G, Ganior B. The efficacy of various irrigation solutions in removing Slime-producing *Staphylococcus*. J. Orthopaed Trauma. 1994;8(5):390-6.
12. Subiza J. Inhibition of the seasonal IgE increase to *Dactylis glomerata* by daily saline nasal—sinus irrigation during the grass pollen season. J Aller Clin Immunol. 1999; 104(3 Pt 1):711-2.
13. Nagendra Prasad KV. Prevention of allergy. In: Prasad R, ed. Advances in Allergy and Asthma. Lucknow, India: Shivam Pub.; 2000:69-74.

CHAPTER 17

Treatment of Allergic Diseases: Antihistaminics

RC Saxena, Mona

INTRODUCTION

Histamine is a diamine, first isolated from ergot mold in 1910 by Sir Henry Dale at Welcome Laboratories,[1] and subsequently, it was found to be present in all tissues (*histos*); hence it is known as histamine. Histamine is widely distributed in nature in both the animal and plant kingdoms. Earlier histamine was considered to play a vital role in pathophysiology of allergic diseases (allergic rhinitis, urticaria) and in asthma.[1] Current studies during the past two to three decades have discovered that this most ancient biomolecule has a broad spectrum of physiological activities in the body,[2] which could have been identified only after the discovery and cloning of various types of subfamilies of histaminergic receptors during the year 1991–2000, namely, H_1, H_2, H_3, and H_4 receptors.[2] Histamine is now known to be involved in:[2]

- Aminergic (monoaminergic as well as diaminergic) neurotransmission;
- Brain functions especially in the sleep–wake cycle;
- Cell differentiation, development, proliferation, and maturation;
- Dilatation of blood vessels, reduction of blood pressure, and cardiac protection;
- Embryonic development and energy of endocrines;
- Fracture, wound healing, and regeneration;
- Gastrointestinal functions and their regulations;
- Hematopoiesis and homeostasis;
- Immunity, inflammatory responses, and allergic manifestations.

Majority of the tissues involved in the above-mentioned functions do express one or the other types of the histaminergic receptors or their subfamilies. These receptors are expressed in such a way that histamine regulates the functions of a specific tissue, e.g., the immune system and its secretions such as interleukins regulate the activity of histaminergic system and vice versa (Fig. 17.1).

HISTAMINERGIC SYNTHESIS, TRANSPORT, AND DISPOSAL: NEWER CONCEPTS

Histamine is synthesized from a semi-essential amino acid called as histidine which is acted upon by histidine decarboxylase (HDC) enzyme. It appears that as the two types of cyclo-oxygenase enzyme[3] involved in cytoprotection and cytodestruction manifested as inflammation, pyrexia, and pain, the two types of HDCs appear to be present in the cells (Fig. 17.2):

1. *Intuitive HDC enzyme*: It is normally present in physiological amounts for performing normal regulatory physiological functions of histamine, which are cytoprotective in nature. Such histamine appears to be produced mostly from non-mast, non-basophil-like cells and has been named as "neo-synthesized histamine."
2. *Inducible HDC enzyme*: It gets activated and induced mostly in pathological states such as infection, antigenic exposure, inflammation, graft rejection, and conditions that are mostly mediated through IL-3. Such histamine is mostly synthesized and liberated from its granular storage sites of mast cells, basophils or eosinophils, and perhaps other alike cells of the body such as dendrites from where they are released.

It is suggested that polymorphic genetic studies must be done to know such types of isoforms of HDC. The above-mentioned histamine is transported from the intracellular site to vesicles by vesicular monoamine transporter (VMAT-2) and from the extracellular site by organic cation transporter (OCT-2) as well as by OCT-3

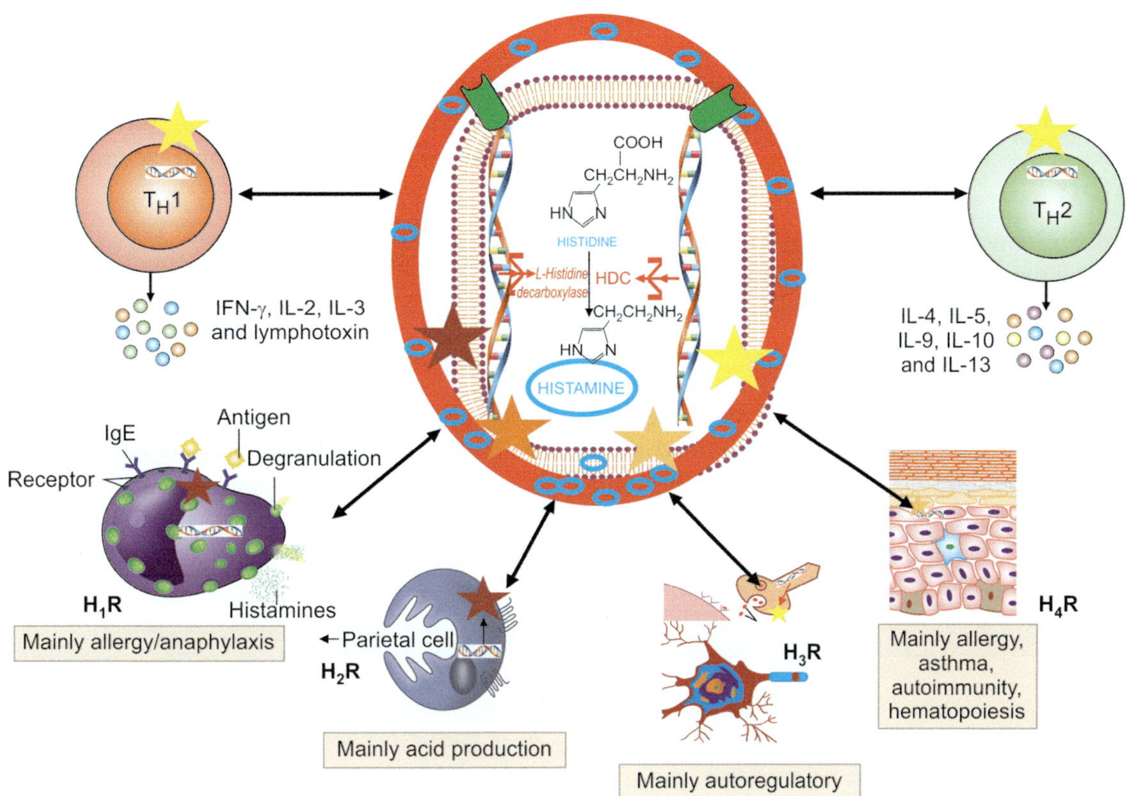

Fig. 17.1: Histamine synthesis: Its regulation of expression of H_1, H_2, H_3, and H_4 receptors, and of TH_1 and TH_2 IL-producing cells and their effects.

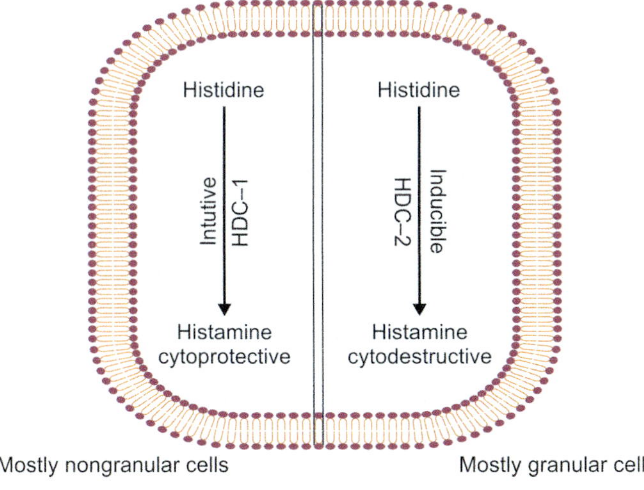

Fig. 17.2: Two types of histidine decarboxylase (HDC).

also called as extraneuronal monoamine transporter.[2] HDC gene-deleted mice were found to be completely devoid of endogenous histamine, whereas VMAT-2 gene-deleted mice did not release histamine.

Histamines from both sources are the same, but their action produced is different depending on the type of the receptor with which this histamine small ligand combines.

Histamine is catabolized by histamine-*N*-methyl transferase enzyme and by diamine oxidase.

PHARMACODYNAMICS

It is a universally known fact that when a female unites with a male, it produces an offspring, which may be good or bad. This is the situation with histaminergic smaller but quick acting ligand, i.e., when it combines with a histaminergic receptor, it produces an effect or a response which may be desirable or undesirable depending on the type of the receptor with which it binds and produces an excessive response, an optimum response, or a lesser response. Further, this response also depends on the type of the tissue (like soil for a seed) and the availability of the type of the receptor and its expression. Thus, it is an interplay between the histaminergic ligand and the specific type of the receptor.

During the past 25 years, due to advancements in recombinant DNA technology, genetics, cloning, and radioligand studies, the four histaminergic receptors have been discovered during 1991–2000 which are listed below.

H_1 Receptors

These are proteins consisting of chains of 487 amino acids embedded in the biomembrane of the granular mast cells, basophils, adrenal medullary cells in addition to endothelial cells of the upper and lower airways, smooth muscle cells of the gut, immune cells, cells of cardiovascular system (CVS), central nervous system (CNS), and similar other cells like skin.[4,5] These receptor biomolecules are transcribed from 3p25 and 3p14–21 chromosomal sites in human beings, and their genes had been cloned in 1993,[2] although H_1 receptors were described long back in the year 1966.

Union of histamine with such receptors at the respective site causes allergies, allergic rhinitis (upper airways), bronchospastic cough and asthma (lower airways), angioneurotic edema, urticaria, anaphylactic shock and other hypersensitivity reactions, and quite often central behavioral changes (Fig. 17.1)

Such allergic disorders are very well treated with classic H_1 receptor-blocking agents,[6] which are listed in Table 17.1.

First-generation Antihistaminics

These are initially discovered classic H_1 antagonists which could cross the blood–brain barrier and could also antagonize their own family receptors H_1 and H_2 causing sedation in the CNS (Fig. 17.3) and being polygamous in nature. Such antihistaminics were also anticholinergics

Table 17.1: Classification of antihistaminic drugs.

Classical H_1 receptor blockers Antiallergic	*H_2 receptor blockers Acid reducers*	*H_3 receptor blockers Alertness producers*	*H_4 receptor blockers Allergy, asthma, autoimmunity reducers*
First-generation (sedatives, anticholinergic, less effective, and less safer) • Chlorpheniramine • Clemastine • Diphenhydramine • Astemizole • Mepyramine maleate *Second-generation (safer, more effective)*[7] • Acrivastine • Cetirizine • Loratadine • Ebastine • Mizolastine *Daytime nonsedatives (don't cross the blood–brain barrier, long half-life, unbind brain cells)* • Fexofenadine (Long $t_{1/2}$, due to enterohepatic circulation) • Levocetirizine (Unbinds brain cells as per PET studies) *Main uses* Antiallergic Anti-anaphylactic (use soluble preparation by intravenous and fast-acting drug in emergency) Some are used for vertigo Others as antiparkinsonian due to anticholinergic effect	• Cimetidine (Crosses blood–brain barrier, hence sedation, rebound, hormonal side effects being polygamous) • Ranitidine • Famotidine • Nizatidine • Tiotidine • Zolantidine *Main uses* Peptic ulcer Hyperacidity Stress ulcers	• Benzonitrile[11] • Clobenpropit • Ciproxifan[1,11] • Conessine[1] • Ergoline[15] • Idophenpropit • JNJ 10181457[11] • JNJ 39220675[25] • Modafinil[11] • Pitolisant[11] • Roxatidine • Tiprolisant[16] (In the third phase clinical trial) • Thioperamide (First one to be discovered) *Main uses* Blockers block autoregulatory inhibitory receptors and bring back accumulation of histamine and alertness. Hence, they are used for sleep–wake disorders and narcolepsy[11] associated with other conditions such as Parkinson's disease, neuropsychiatric disorders,[1] and neuroinflammation	• JNJ 7777120[12,14] • JNJ 28307474[17] • JNJ 10191584 • JNJ 39758979[18,19] (In the second phase clinical trial: selective, safe, and longer acting with more $t_{1/2}$) *Main uses* Asthma even resistant type, chronic arthritis as receptors are also found in chondrocytes and synovial fluid,[17] chronic pruritus of eczema, atopic dermatitis of resistant type (effects like prednisolone if given with H_1 receptor antagonists),[8,17] and in neural pain.

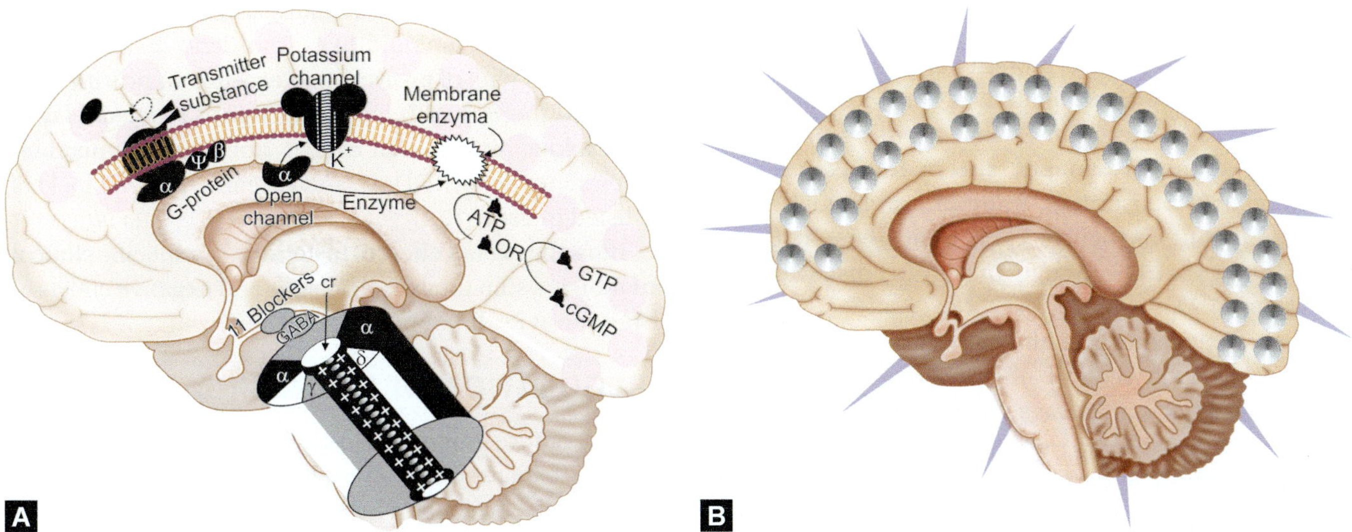

Figs. 17.3A and B: (A) Histamine blockers that cross the blood–brain barrier (BBB) cause sedation; (B) Histamine blockers that do not cross the BBB retain alertness.

producing atropine-like side effects. Thus, despite being effective, these were associated with such undesirable effects such as sedation and dryness, especially in children and daytime working persons. Degree of sedation is dependent on the intensity and the affinity with which these antihistaminics combine with H_1 receptors in the brain and the cholinergic receptors. Due to these undesirable effects, nowadays these are not preferred to second-generation H1 antihistaminics because these are also less effective[7] compared to second-generation antihistaminics. The names of such antihistaminics are given in Table 17.1.

Second-generation Antihistaminics

The names of the second-generation H_1 antihistaminics are given in Table 17.1. These are more effective and safer agents. This group also includes the daytime, nonsedative antihistaminics which do not cross the blood–brain barrier and do not combine with the brain H_1 receptors as observed with positron-emission tomography (PET) imaging such as levocetirizine[8] and fexofenadine having a longer half-life due to enterohepatic circulation.

These agents are important antiallergic agents and are being used in different types of allergies such as insect bites, cough, and anaphylaxis (use soluble antihistaminics with quick onset of action via the intravenous route). In addition, some are used as antivertigo and antiparkinsonian agent due to their anticholinergic properties.

H_2 Receptors

These are also proteins consisting of chains of 359 amino acids embedded in the biomembrane of parietal cells of the stomach (producing acid) and exocrine glands (producing pulmonary secretions), neurons in the CNS, smooth muscles, cardiovascular cells, mast cells, basophils, and allied cells. These receptor biomolecules are transcribed from chromosomal 5 at 5q35.3 in human beings and their genes had been cloned in 1991(Fig. 17.1),[2] although the H_2 receptors were discovered much earlier, and the description of selective H_2 blockers was given in 1970, which was a landmark in the history of pharmacology which set the stage for the modern approach to the treatment of acidic peptic diseases, which is now known to be an infective disorder caused by *Helicobacter pylori*.[9]

When H_2 receptors combine with histamines at the target site mainly in the gastric parietal cells, these produce acid in the exocrine glands to produce secretions; otherwise, H_2 receptor agonists cause suppression of the CVS, smooth muscles, and immune cells. H_2 receptor blockers are mainly used for hyperacidity disorders such as gastroesophageal reflux disease, healing of peptic ulcer, and prophylaxis of stress ulcers[10] such as burns. Among various H_2 blockers listed in Table 17.1, cimetidine crosses the blood–brain barrier and produces sedation and hormonal side effects in addition to rebound phenomenon.[3]

H_3 Receptors

By nature, these are also proteins consisting of chains of 445 amino acids embedded in the biomembranes of the neuron in the brain as well as in the periphery, especially at the presynaptic site in the axon. These receptors are transcribed from chromosomal 20 at 20q13.33 in human beings,[2] and their genes had also been cloned in 1999 though they were discovered in 1983[2] (Fig. 17.1).

When histamines combine with these receptors at the presynaptic sites of all monoaminergic neurons (catecholaminergic, noradrenergic, adrenergic, dopaminergic) of the sympathetic or extrapyramidal system, and serotonergic, diamine histaminergic, or cholinergic nerves of the parasympathetic nervous system, there is inhibition of the release of specific neurotransmitters, i.e., H_3 receptors apply a potent brake.[1,11] Similarly, it happens with peptidergic, gabaminergic, as well as glutamate-releasing neurons. Thus, histamine being an alerting amine, activation of such receptors will cause inhibition of the histamine release and their shortage produces narcolepsy (sleeping disorder) associated with cognitive disorder.[11] Inhibition of glutamate release will also cause CNS depression. Thus, histamine is intimately involved in sleep–wake cycles, and H3 blockers are of value in narcolepsy, Parkinson's disease, neuropsychiatric disorders,[11] as well as neuroinflammatory disorders. H_3 agonists afford cardioprotection by inhibiting the release of norepinephrine similar to α-2 agonist clonidine or α-methyldopa.

For narcolepsy and cognitive disorders, H_3 blockers include modafinil (clinically extensively used),[11] pitolisant, tiprolisant (third phase of clinical trial), ciproxifan, and others,[1,11] which are listed in Table 17.1. Among these, thioperamide was the first one to be discovered.

H_4 Receptors

These are also proteins consisting of 390 amino acids mostly embedded in the biomembrane of immune cells (T and B cells, eosinophils, mast cells),[12] hematopoietic cells, bone marrow cells, spleen, gastrointestinal tract, airways, dermis, epidermis and chondrocytes of articular tissue, and synovial fluid cells.[13] These receptors are expressed in these cells after being transcribed from 18q11.2 chromosomal sites,[2] and their genes had been cloned in 2000. It appears that most of such cells are non-mast, non-granular cells synthesizing "neo-synthesized histamine." Thus, these receptors play a vital role in etiopathogenesis of resistant airway diseases such as bronchial asthma, allergic rhinitis, autoimmune rheumatoid-like disorders, hemopoiesis, and resistant type of pruritus and eczema. In pruritus, the combined therapy with H_1 blockers gives relief similar to prednisolone[14] in cases of cancer, noninsulin-dependent diabetes mellitus (NIDDM), and eczema. Anti-H_4 blockers are listed in Table 17.1.

Thus, the overall effect of histamine in a specific clinical situation is a sum total of all positive and negative effects of histamine at its different receptor sites.

REGULATION OF HISTAMINE

The very nature of the physiology is the same everywhere, i.e., to regulate the physiological functions of the biomolecules available in the body. This, in turn, means that the concentration of the biomolecules must be regulated to keep them in a balanced state. Higher or lower levels cause hyperfunctioning or hypofunctioning, just as with adrenaline, hypertension or hypotension occurs. This holds true for all the ligands in the body including the histamine ligand, which is basically regulated at two levels: *Plasma and interstitial tissue fluid level*: When the concentration of histamine increases beyond the physiological limits in this compartment, histamine itself decreases its cellular synthesis by inhibiting HDC directly or through interleukins secreted by T cells under its influence. This holds true if the concentration of histamine falls below the physiological levels, reverse phenomenon takes place by negative feedback mechanism. By a similar mechanism, there is either a downregulation of receptors in hyperhistaminism and an upregulation of histaminergic receptors in hypohistaminism. However, if this mechanism fails, disease sets in.

Cytoplasmic and synaptic level: All neurotransmitters are released from presynaptic nerve terminals into synapse to act upon postsynaptic receptors. Here also a very powerful negative feedback mechanism exists through H_3 regulatory autoreceptors present. In case there is excess of neurotransmitters causing exaggerated physiological response, autoregulatory receptors immediately apply a potent brake so as to inhibit not only the release and synthesis of histamine but also the release of many of the aminergic, cholinergic, peptidergic, and gabaminergic neurotransmitters,[1] which is a very unique phenomenon with histamine (Fig. 17.2). This is just like presynaptic α-2 inhibitory adrenergic receptors which may perhaps be synergizing with presynaptic inhibitory histaminergic receptors at the adrenergic nerve terminals. In case of histamine, this has been worked out very well with H_3 receptors using radioactive ligands, which proved that overworking of these H_3 inhibitory receptors creates shortage of histaminergic alerting amines so as to create narcolepsy and cognitive disorders. This is being treated with the autoreceptor H_3 receptor blocking antihistaminics such as modafinil and others, which are listed in Table 17.1.

CLINICAL CONDITIONS: ANTIHISTAMINICS AS THERAPEUTIC AGENTS

Today the use of antihistaminics is not only limited in the treatment of different types of allergies and hypersensitivity reactions as it was in the past, but after the discovery of newer types of histaminergic receptors, the use of antihistaminics has extended its spectrum much beyond depending on the type of receptors, its agonist, or the type of a specific antagonist, i.e., the blockers used.

Airway Diseases

Despite the fact that the nasal passage as well as the bronchial passage share common features, but still there is a variable response to classic H_1 antihistaminics. It was earlier thought that intrinsically liberated histamine is different from what we used experimentally to assess the efficacy of bronchodilator effect of antihistaminics in guinea pigs by aerosol method for its usefulness in bronchial asthma. But classic H_1 antihistaminics are not very much effective in bronchial asthma but are the most effective and useful drug in the management of allergic rhinitis and nasal allergies where these H_1 antihistaminics ameliorate itching, sneezing, watery rhinorrhea, and symptoms characteristic of early allergic response to an antigen. However, most antihistaminics are not useful for controlling nasal obstruction, which actually occurs in the late phase of allergic reactions. However, more recent clinical trials with some of the second-generation antihistaminics with antiallergic and anti-inflammatory effects such as desloratadine, fexofenadine, and levocetirizine have been shown to improve nasal symptoms including nasal obstruction in patients with allergic rhinitis.[6]

First-generation antihistaminics are no longer recommended either for the treatment of allergic rhinitis or for asthma. Clinical evidences have shown that long-term use of classic second-generation antihistaminics is more useful and effective even on a "required on-demand basis" both in cases of allergic rhinitis and in bronchial asthma. Some antihistaminics, e.g., azelastine, may also be administered intranasally for short term in the management of seasonal rhinitis.

Current researches, based on the discovery of more of the histaminergic receptors, have shown that H_4 receptor blockers (Table 17.1) are more effective both in allergies and in bronchial asthma (an inflammatory disorder)[3] especially of the resistant type,[17] as H_4 receptors mediate inflammation and Th17 responses and H_4 ligands have great therapeutic potentials.[20]

Allergic Conjunctivitis

Orally given classic H_1 antihistaminics as stated previously are effective not only in allergic rhinitis but also in allergic conjunctivitis to ameliorate the ocular symptoms, which are frequently associated with allergic rhinitis. However, symptoms of allergic conjunctivitis are often best managed with local ophthalmic preparations.

Cold and Cough

Despite the fact that classic first-generation H_1 antihistaminics are most frequently employed for the symptomatic management of common cold, evidence for their effectiveness remains to be clearly established.[6] Although first-generation H_1 antihistaminics with anticholinergic properties having anti-secretomotor effects are considered effective in reducing rhinorrhea and sneezing associated with common cold, these may cause atropine-like side effects such as dryness of nose due to thickening of mucus secretions, making it more difficult to be expectorated and to cough out.

Monotherapy is always safe and dose controllable, and is recommended, but in the market, many of the fixed combinations of antihistaminics along with decongestant, caffeine, analgesics, and anticholinergics are available. However, the use of such combination therapy is often questioned, and no proof exists for their more effectiveness than the use of monotherapy in such cases.[6] Nevertheless some combination products do provide a convenient approach in the management of cold, cough, and flu; the ingredients are provided in therapeutic doses to give symptomatic relief to the patients and do not produce interactions among themselves. It is a well-known fact that dry cough is treated with cough suppressants, and wet cough with sputum is treated with expectorants and often with liquefying mucolytic agents. However, in the market, a large number of cough preparations are available in combination, which are not considered therapeutically sound as two medicines may have opposing therapeutic effects. First-generation H_1 antihistaminics such as diphenhydramine has been extensively and effectively used for dry irritating cough.

Atopic Dermatitis, Eczema, and Urticaria

Atopic dermatitis is a common inflammatory condition seen mostly in children where topical corticosteroid is the first-line management for acute episodes. Classic H_1 antihistaminics are useful to ameliorate allergy as well as insomnia associated in this condition that H_1 antihistaminics give relief in itching and reduce the number, size, and duration of urticarial lesions in chronic urticaria. In all these conditions, even in resistant cases of classical treatment, newer H_4 receptor blockers such as JNJ 39758979, especially along with classic antihistaminics, are found to be most useful, selective, and safe as antipruritic agents, and the effect so produced is comparable to prednisolone in clinical ongoing trials.[17-19] In allergic diseases in children, antihistaminics such as levocetirizine have been found to be well tolerable and satisfactory.[21]

Motion Sickness

Some of the classic H_1 antihistaminics having anticholinergic effects are effective in the conditions such as cyclizine, meclizine, promethazine, and diphenhydramine because in motion sickness, a cholinergic mechanism is involved.

Insomnia

Since histamine is an alerting amine in the brain, classic first-generation H_1 antihistaminics that cross the blood-brain barrier are capable of blocking central histaminergic receptors to produce sleep, and thus, these are useful in insomnia by inducing sleep and drowsiness.

Sleep–Wake Cycle and alike CNS Disorders

Since H_3 autoregulatory receptors apply a potent brake on the release of histamine, it can result in anti-alerting effects such as narcolepsy associated with several neuropsychiatric disorders and Parkinson's disease, where H_3 blockers are found to be useful. Modafinil is widely used in narcolepsy all over the world.[1,11]

Peptic Ulcer

H_2 blockers are well known to be used in this condition.

PRECAUTIONS WHEN OTHER DRUGS COADMINISTERED

Adverse drug reactions can occur with any drug, may it be antihistaminics at either the pharmacokinetic site or the pharmacodynamic site.[22,23]

1. *At metabolic sites:* These antihistaminics are mostly metabolized and hepatically eliminated by proteinous mixed-function oxidases (MFOs) in conjunction with cytochrome P450 (CYP). If antihistaminics as well as the coadministered drugs are metabolized by the same MFO and CYP, one of them can either inhibit the enzyme competitively or enhance the quantity of enzymes by enzyme induction mechanism and thus can affect their hepatorenal elimination, their concentration in systemic circulation, and their effect at the receptor site.[6]
   a. Classic first-generation antihistaminics can combine with greater affinity for CYP2D6 enzyme, which metabolizes other coadministered drugs with weaker affinity to bind with CYP2D6 such as tricylic antidepressants, β-blockers, some antipsychotics, venlafaxine, anti-arrhythmics, and tramadol, and are thus displaced by antihistaminics and are not metabolized. Therefore, the concentration of the coadministered drugs at the site of their action is increased, which produces an exaggerated pharmacological response and toxicity.
   b. In contrast to the above point, adverse effects can occur with commonly CYP3A4 metabolizing pigments for classic second-generation antihistaminics having lesser affinity to bind with the pigment compared to other coadministered drugs having a strong affinity to bind with the pigment. As a result, metabolism of H_1 antihistaminics is inhibited by other firmly bound coadministered drugs that displace the antihistaminics from the enzymic site such as macrolides, antifungals, and calcium channel blockers. Thus, erythromycin, a macrolide, inhibits the metabolism of terfenadine and increases its concentration at the pharmacodynamic site in the heart resulting in fatal *torsades de pointes* and prolonged QT interval.[3] Therefore, terfenadine should never be given together in cold and coryza with secondary infections as I have also witnessed such deaths.

      However, because of high safety margin of these second-generation antihistaminics, generally such serious side effects do not appear especially with fexofenadine (a metabolite of terfenadine), cetirizine, and levocetirizine (a metabolite of hydroxymine), which minimally affect CYP3A4 enzymatic protein, and therefore, these are the safest H_1 antihistaminics.

2. *At receptor sites:* Depending on the physicochemical properties (oil water coefficient, i.e., lipophilicity, molecular weight, etc.), highly lipophilic classic first-generation H_1 antagonists do cross the blood-brain barrier, reach the receptor site, and block widely distributed H_1 receptors in the brain, thus producing sedative effects (Fig. 17.3) associated with coordination problems, dizziness, lack of concentration, and paradoxically agitation and excitability especially in children and elderly subjects.[24] Therefore, in mobile patients (doctors, nurses, machine workers, cyclers, swimmers, drivers, etc.), such drugs must be avoided and daytime antihistaminics should be prescribed. Further, all CNS depressants and alcohol-like substances must be avoided with classic H_1 antihistaminics especially in the alcoholics and the drivers to avoid accidents. However, the sedative property of such first-generation antihistaminics may benefit the patients with insomnia and severe itching at night.

Being polygamous in nature, these antihistaminics also block cholinergic receptors producing atropine-like side effects and which must be taken care of. Initially, H_2 blockers can also cause hormonal side effects. Children, especially under 2 years, and elderly people have developmental and degenerative inabilities, respectively, and are more vulnerable to side effects such as paradoxical CNS stimulation with first-generation antihistaminics, especially promethazine which is frequently prescribed while it must not be used in such cases. It should also be noted that all antihistaminics are chemicals, and they can also produce allergic reactions especially on local application, although a rare phenomenon.

CONCLUSION

There are important differences in the chemical structure, and pharmacokinetic and pharmacodynamic profiles of these antihistaminics. Therefore, these must be prescribed with great caution especially in children below 2 years, elderly population, and hepatorenally diseased patients. It is desirable to keep classic H_1 first-generation antihistaminics in reserve for patients who require sedation at night and prescribe safer, nontoxic, noncardiotoxic second-generation antihistaminics with least chances of drug interactions, namely, fexofenadine and levocetirizine, in routine practice.

H_2 blockers are well known for peptic ulcer, whereas H_3 blockers (modafinil, pitolisant)[3,11] are being widely used in narcolepsy and have potential usability in treating obesity, cognitive dysfunction, attention deficit, and hyperactivity disorders in children. Since H_3 agonists with their three isoforms put a potent brake on the release of various aminergic neurotransmitters, acetylcholine and histamine, these have a potential cardioprotective (heart failure and *myocardial infarction*) and gastroprotective use as well as anti-inflammatory and anticonvulsant use, and also in the management of shock. H_4 inhibitors are being evaluated for their antiallergic effects (in rhinitis, atopic dermatitis) and bronchial asthma (an inflammatory disease), and they act as an antipruritic agent, an eczema ameliorator, and a reliever of autoimmune disorders such as rheumatoid arthritis and for hemopoiesis[12,14,17,20] especially of resistant type.

Thus, histamine, its agonist as well as its antagonist have a great therapeutic future not only in allergy and asthma but also in many other systemic disorders.

REFERENCES

1. Hanuskova E, Plevkova J. Histamine and its effects mediated via H_3 receptor—potential clinical applications of H_3 antagonists. Acta Med Mar. 2013;1:28-36. doi:10.2478/acm-2013-0004.
2. Shahid M, Tripathi T, Sobia F, et al. Histamine, histamine receptors, and their role in immunomodulation: an updated systematic review. Open Immunol J. 2009;2:9-41.
3. Saxena RC, Mona, eds. Compendium of Drugs: A Biochemical Basis, 2nd ed.; Lucknow: NMTC Productions; 2010:138.
4. Saxena RC, Das M, Dixit KS, Bhargawa KP. Involvement of H_1 and H_2 receptors in histamine-induced skin response in human. Ind J Med Res. 1983;78:277-80.
5. Saxena RC, Dixit KS, Bhargawa KP. Nature of histaminergic receptors in human skin. World Conference. London, UK: Clinical Pharmacology & Therapeutics; 1980.
6. Van Schoor J. Antihistaminics: a brief review. Prof Nurs Today. 2012;16:16-21.
7. Diana S, Church MD, Church MK. Pharmacology of antihistaminics. WAO J. 2011;4(3):S22-7.
8. Hiraoka K, Tashiro M, Grobosch T, et al. Brain histamine H_1 receptor occupancy measured by PET after oral administration of levocetirizine, a non-sedating antihistamine. Exp Opin Drug Saf. 2014;14(2):1-8.
9. Chandra M. Helicobacter pylori: concepts and controversies. In: Saxena, RC, Singh R, Mona, eds. International Symposium Chemotherapy: Problems and Perspectives in 21st Century, Lucknow, India; 1999:13-8.

10. Brown NJ, Roberts J. Histamine, Bradykinin and their antagonists. In: Hardman JG, Limbard LE, eds. Goodman & Gilman's the Pharmacological Basis of Therapeutics, 10th ed. New York, NY: McGraw-Hill; 2001:645-58.
11. Lin JS, Sergeeva OA, Haas HL. Histamine H_3 receptors and sleep-wake regulation. JPET. 2011;336:17-23.
12. Hanuskova E, Plevkova J. The role of histamine H_4 receptors as a potential targets in allergic rhinitis and asthma. Open J Mol Integr Physiol. 2013;3:6-14. doi:10.4236/ojmip.2013.31002.
13. Ueno K. Expression and function of the histamine receptors in dermal and articular tissues. Yakugaku Zasshi. 2014;134:1093-108.
14. Matsushita A, Seike M, Okawa H, et al. Advantages of histamine H_4 receptor antagonist usage with H_1 receptor antagonist for the treatment of murine allergic contact dermatitis. Exp Dermatol. 2012;21:714-5. doi:10.1111/j.1600-0625.2012.01559.x.
15. Auberson YP, Troxler T, Zhang X, et al. From ergolines to indoles: improved inhibitors of the human H_3 receptor for the treatment of narcolepsy. Chem Med Chem. 2015;10:266-75. doi:10.1002/cmdc.201402418.
16. Łaż ewska D, Kié-Kononowicz K. New developments around histamine H_3 receptor antagonists/inverse agonists: a patent review (2010-present). Expert Opin Ther Pat. 2014; 24:89-111. doi:10.1517/13543776.2014.848197.
17. Cowden JM, Yu F, Banie H, et al. The histamine H_4 receptor mediates inflammation and Th17 responses in preclinical models of arthritis. Ann Rheum Dis. 2014;73:600-8. doi:10.1136/annrheumdis-2013-203832.
18. Ohsawa Y, Hirasawa N. The role of histamine H_1 and H_4 receptors in atopic dermatitis: from basic research to clinical study. Allergol Int. 2014;63:533-42. doi:10.2332/allergolint.13-RA-0675.
19. Thurmond RL, Chen B, Dunford PJ, et al. Clinical and preclinical characterization of the histamine H_4 receptor antagonist. JNJ-39758979. J Pharmacol Exp Ther. 2014;349:176-84. doi:10.1124/jpet.113.211714.
20. Kiss R, Keseru GM. Novel histamine H_4 receptor ligands and their potential therapeutic applications: an update. Expert Opin Ther Pat. 2014;24:1185-97. doi:10.1517/13543776.2014.959494.
21. Ferrer M, Morais-Almeida M, Guizova M, Khanferyan R. Evaluation of treatment satisfaction in children with allergic disease treated with an antihistamine: an international, non-interventional, retrospective study. Clin Drug Investig. 2010;30:15-34. doi:10.2165/11530910-000000000-00000.
22. Saxena RC, Mukerjee P, Chandra A, Srivastava SN. An extended study of adverse drug reactions in a teaching hospital. Ind J Pharmacol. 1993;1:25-49.
23. Saxena RC. Overview of ADR and its relation with nutrition. In Symposium on Prediction, Detection and Avoidance of Adverse Drug Resections; Proceedings from the World Conference Clinical Pharmacology and Therapeutics, Yokohama, Japan; 1992.
24. White JM, Rumbold GR. Behavioural effects of histamine and its antagonists: a review. Psychopharmacology (Berl). 1988;95:1-14. doi:10.1007/BF00212757.
25. Vanhanen J, Kinnunen M, Nuutinen S, Panula P. Histamine H_3 receptor antagonist JNJ-39220675 modulates locomotor responses but not places conditioning by dopaminergic drugs. Psychopharmacology (Berl). 2014;232:1143-53; Oct 12. [Epub ahead of print].

CHAPTER 18

Allergen Immunotherapy: General Guidelines

VK Jain, Rajendra Prasad, Shubhra Jain

INTRODUCTION

Allergy and its disorders are chronic and systemic in nature, increasing world over, and common in children and adults. Immunity has been stated as protection against some diseases. In the history, initial immunotherapeutic interventions have been used by Jenner, Pasteur, Koch, and von Behring for effective prevention of diseases. These initial immunomodulator models have initiated the later development of allergen immunotherapy (AIT). In the early 1900s, Noon[1] and Freeman[2,3] have used AIT by inoculation of grass pollen for treatment of hay fever for the first time. Numerous well-designed controlled studies have shown the efficacy of AIT in various nasorespiratory and other immunoglobulin (IgE)-mediated allergic disorders.

Allergen immunotherapy is a standard therapeutic approach for the management of patients suffering from allergic diseases. Besides avoidance of exposure of clinically relevant allergens, immunotherapy (IT) provides immunomodulation effects to modify the natural history of atopic allergy leading to immunological shift from T helper type 2 (Th2) to Th1 response. Allergen-specific immunotherapy (ASIT) is a method of treatment for patients suffering from IgE-mediated allergic diseases to control the symptoms and decrease the sensitivity toward allergen (s) by introducing increasing doses of specific relevant therapeutic antigens until a maintenance dose is reached and the treatment continues to achieve clinical efficacy.

Allergen immunotherapy is considered to be a safe method of treatment even though there may be a risk of side effects during the treatment.[4] IT has been known by several names such as allergy vaccine, desensitization, hyposensitization, ASIT, specific IT (SIT), and AIT. Recently, the term "allergy immunotherapy" is proposed universally aiming to induce immune tolerance to allergens. IT can include both allergen-specific and nonspecific approaches.[5] AIT can be administered by different routes, i.e., subcutaneous, sublingual, oral, nasal, and recently lymphatic. However, currently in clinical practice, only subcutaneous IT (SCIT) and sublingual IT (SLIT) are used routinely based on sufficient evidences.[4-12]

Various international and national guidelines are available to practice IT.[4-12] As per international and national regulations, the practice of AIT should only be allowed to those physicians who have undergone specialized training in allergy and IT and also practice only at places where facilities of anaphylaxis management are available.

MECHANISM OF ACTION

The underlying mechanism of IT is complex and related to the route of administration of allergen(s).[5,7,12-14] The basic goal of therapy of immunological diseases, autoimmunity, and organ transplantation is to induce immune tolerance to specific antigens. In the beginning, it was thought that by administration of low doses of antigen, the immune system produces IgG antibodies (blocking antibodies) rather than IgE antibodies resulting in less number of IgE molecules available, not correlated with changes in the levels of IgG and IgE. Now it is well established with evidences that AIT produces a shift from Th2 to Th1 immune response, which leads to a reduction in inflammatory mediators and specific IgE levels and causes clinical improvement by reducing airway hyper-responsiveness to specific allergen(s). After AIT, there is an increase in specific IgG levels. However, an initial increase in IgG4 level indicates poor prognosis, but that of IgG1 means a better prognosis. AIT also reduces IL-4 and

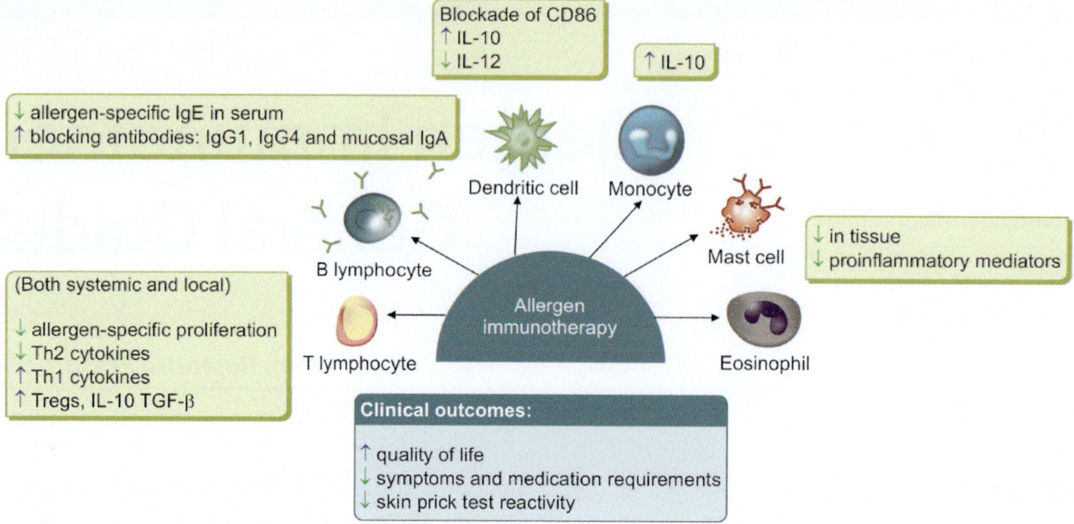

Fig. 18.1: Mechanism of action of allergen immunotherapy.

IL-5 production through CD4+ Th2 cells and shifts toward an increased interferon gamma production by Th1 cells. Th1 subset activation is also associated with increased cell-mediated immunity and is protective for immune response against the development of allergy/allergic disorders. AIT modifies Th4+ T-cell responses by immune deviation, T-cell anergy, or both. Further, a subtype of T cells with immunosuppressive function and cytokine profiles distinct from their Th1 and Th2 cells, termed regulatory/suppressor T cells, has been described. Regulatory T (Treg) cells producing IL-10 and possibly transforming growth factor beta (TGF-β), CD4+ CD25+ T cells, and Th3 cells play a major role in the inhibition of allergic disorders. The expression of FOXP3 on CD4+ CD25+ T cells has also been shown to correlate with the suppressive capacity of Treg cells and clinical efficacy following AIT. Figure 18.1 depicts the mechanism of action of AIT. In the past five decades, a large number of well-controlled trials and immunological studies have provided sufficient scientific explanation to understand the mechanism of IT.

In summary, the following immunological changes have been observed responsible for the relief of allergic symptoms:

- ↑ IgG-blocking antibodies and specific IgG4
- ↑ Secretary IgG and IgA↓ IgE antibodies
- ↓ Specific IgE antibodies with an initial rise
- ↑ INF-γ causes ↓ Th2 response and ↓ IL-4
- Alter in T-cell functions, by ↓ production of both Th1 and Th2 cytokines
- ↓ Production of mediators (histamine, PGD_2, PGF_2, and ECP)
- ↓ in T helper cells or ↑ in T-suppressor cells
- Leads to fall in IgE and release of mononuclear inhibition/mitogen factors
- ↓ Production of cytokines (IL-2) and histamine-releasing factors
- Immune deviation from Th2 to Th1
- ↓ BHR, tissue responsiveness, and target cell reactivity to antigen
- ↑ IL-10 producing T cells within 1 week of SIT and maximum at 4 weeks
- ↑ IL-10 and TGF-β lead to ↑ IgG1, IgG4, and IgA production, and ↓ IgE production
- ↓ Target cell reactivity to antigen challenge as demonstrated, by basophil degranulation/histamine release and provocation/skin tests.

SELECTION OF PATIENTS

Proper selection of patients is important for considering effective IT and should be based on their detailed clinical history and positive skin reactivity preferably to skin prick test (SPT). In clinical practice, routinely positive RAST and/or ELISA tests for specific IgE are not recommended unless skin tests are negative or contraindication to positive clinical history of exposure of allergen(s). The age for AIT is 5 years or more with no upper and lower age limits with an ideal age of 12–45 years in routine clinical practice. Patients symptoms of sufficient duration and severity who failed to avoid exposure to allergens, poor response, and/or adverse drug reactions, and agreed for adherence to long-term therapy are considered for AIT for IgE-mediated specific diseases as per indications. Informed written consent and proper counseling from the patient and/or relatives should be done before skin test, and IT should be initiated based on their risk/benefits.

DIAGNOSTIC TEST FOR IGE-MEDIATED ALLERGEN SENSITIZATION

After proper selection of patients based on their detailed clinical history and examination strongly suspecting disease of allergic etiology, in vivo and in vitro tests should be done in clinical practice for confirmation of diagnosis. In vivo tests, preferably SPT and intradermal test, are performed only in specific conditions. In vitro tests, RAST/ELISA, are done only if skin tests are contraindicated or negative with positive history of exposure to allergens or patient is not willing for skin test with a definite history of exposure to allergens.[11,12,15]

INDICATIONS OF ALLERGEN IMMUNOTHERAPY

A number of various placebo/double-blind trials have confirmed that AIT with SCIT or SLIT is effective in reducing symptoms and medication score, inducing favorable changes in the immune system, and improving the quality of life.[4-12]

- *Allergic rhinitis/conjunctivitis*: Moderate to severe intermittent/mild to moderate-severe persistent rhinitis
- *Allergic bronchial asthma*: (Controlled)
- *Allergic rhinitis and asthma*: As above
- To prevent bronchial asthma in allergic rhinitis
- Insect sting allergy, specially hymenoptera
- Prevention of venom-induced anaphylaxis and local reaction (LR)
- Allergic dermatitis.

CONDITIONS NOT RECOMMENDED FOR IMMUNOTHERAPY

- *Food hypersensitivity*: SCIT is not recommended. However, oral IT/SLIT showing increased tolerance to various foods, i.e., hazelnut/peanut, egg, and milk for children, but no Food and Drug Administration (FDA) approval.
- *Urticaria and angioedema*: Not recommended as clinical trials do not support.

Table 18.1: Contraindications of allergen immunotherapy.[4-12,37]

Diseases/drugs	*Absolute*	*Relative*
Asthma	Poorly/uncontrolled asthma	Partially controlled asthma
Autoimmune disorders	Active forms	Remission
Malignant neoplasms	Malignant disease; but venom immunotherapy is advised highly in high-risk venom allergy patients	–
Cardiovascular diseases	No	Yes
Acquired immunodeficiency	HIV-positive symptomatic patient	HIV-positive asymptomatic patient with CD4 count >200/uL
Pregnancy	Not to initiate but may continue if the patient is already on AIT before pregnancy	–
Lactation	Up to 6 months after delivery but continue if the patient is already on immunotherapy	–
Beta blockers	No	Yes
ACE inhibitors	No	Yes
Monoamine oxidase inhibitors	No	Yes
Children	0–2 years	>2–5 years

ACE, angiotensin-converting enzyme; AIT, allergen immunotherapy; HIV, human immunodeficiency virus; VIT, venom immunotherapy

TYPES OF IMMUNOTHERAPY

There are seven different types of IT, which are as follows:

- SCIT—conventional/rush/cluster
- SLIT
- Oral IT
- Intranasal IT
- Bronchial IT
- Intralymphatic IT
- Epicutaneous IT.

Subcutaneous IT

In SCIT, there are two phases/schedules: The first phase is the buildup schedule, also called updosing or dose-increased phase, where increased doses of allergen vaccine are given during a period of 8–28 weeks. The second phase is the maintenance phase, where vaccine is usually given at an interval of 1–2 months and continued till 3–5 years. In SCIT, there are three types of regimens: conventional, rush IT, and cluster IT.

Conventional Regimen

Commonly Used in Clinical Practice

In India, only aqueous extracts are currently available. AIT is first routinely started with 1:5,000 w/v diluted antigen, and the injections are given twice a week starting from 0.1 mL and increased subsequently subcutaneously to 0.9 mL in graduated syringe or insulin syringe. The second injection containing 1:500 w/v strength is also given twice a week starting from 0.1 mL in the same manner as the first injection. After well tolerance of first and second injection, third injection containing 1:150 w/v is given once a week starting from 0.1 mL to 0.5 mL, and thereafter increasing the dose of vaccine and intervals to achieve the highest maintenance dose, i.e., 1:50-1.0 mL once a month. Usually, the maintenance dose is between 0.5 and 1.0 mL of 1:50 dilution. In cases showing high skin sensitivity with LR after initiation (1:5,000 w/v) of AIT, it is rescheduled/started with higher dilution, i.e., 1:50,000 w/v or even higher, and the first injection is administered in the hospital/clinic having facilities to manage anaphylaxis.

Rush IT Regimen

The advantage of rush IT is to achieve the maintenance dose more quickly within a week with fewer clinic visits. In rush IT, the maintenance dose is achieved very rapidly than conventional and rush therapy regimens. The schedule is using eight injections over 3 days or in a single day.[15] Systemic reaction and LR are reported more. Therefore, these protocols need further studies in terms of risk and benefit ratio to patient.

Cluster IT Regimen

In cluster IT, the maintenance dose is achieved earlier than conventional schedules, and usually two or more injections are given in each visit. The starting dose is similar to that of the perennial AIT regimen. The frequency of LR and systemic reaction are similar or more than that of the conventional regimen. (A) Here, weekly visits are necessary because, at each visit, more than one injection is given at a small interval between injections, varying from 30 minutes to 2 hours. After the maintenance dose is reached in approximately 2 months, the interval between visits is increased. The cluster IT regimen is advantageous to the patients who reside at a significant distance from the physician. There are similar efficacy and immunological changes in the cluster IT regimen as observed with the perennial IT regimen in various studies.[16] However, initial doses are required to be given in a hospital setup able to manage emergencies associated with this form of therapy. Cluster IT schedule with hypoallergenic mite SCIT has also been developed and is found to be safe and well tolerated in routine clinical practice.

Sublingual IT

In recent years, there has been a great interest to advocate IT through a sublingual route. There has been numerous double-blind, placebo-controlled trials which have shown good efficacy. SLIT has been widely practiced in some countries of Europe and in India.[7,17-20] SLIT requires a much higher amount of antigen (50–100 times more than SCIT) to achieve clinical efficacy, whereas SLIT is ineffective when low doses of antigen are administered.[21] In SLIT, vaccine can be given as drops or tablets.[22] SLIT requires only a limited number of allergen for clinical efficacy. Currently, it is not approved in India by the Drug Controller General of India and in the United States by the FDA as well.

Other Uncommon Routes

Oral IT

Various clinical trials[7,4] have been carried out—only few of them showed reasonable efficacy[23,24] and the others showed no efficacy.[25,26]

Adverse reactions in the form of vomiting, diarrhea, and abdominal pain have been reported.[26,27] Therefore, oral IT is currently not recommended.[28]

Bronchial IT

Few clinical trials have been carried out with limited efficacy and high risk of bronchospasm in many patients.[22,29] Thus, this route is not recommended due to the undesirable risk-benefit ratio.

Nasal IT

It is not commonly used in clinical practice and essentially stopped since the introduction of SLIT. Randomized controlled studies with dust mites and pollen extracts have shown the effectiveness in reducing symptoms and medications used. Local adverse reactions are common in this therapy.[7,30-33]

Epicutaneous IT

In this approach, the extracts of allergens in the form of patch applied once a week have been used, and studies have shown higher treatment success in placebo-controlled studies. However, no significant differences in the primary outcome and nasal provocation scores are shown between the groups. The major adverse effect is eczematous reaction at the application sites.[7,34]

Intralymphatic IT

In this approach, intradermal allergen extract is injected into the inguinal lymph nodes. In the uncontrolled study, three injections of grass pollen extract have been used at an interval of 4 weeks[35] and have been significantly effective as the conventional SCIT requiring over 3 years. The total extract dose was more than 1,000-fold less with intralymphatic injections.

SELECTION OF ALLERGENS

Flora and fauna and its airborne pollens are rich in India compared to the Western countries, and they locally vary at every 200 km distance. Environment of the place and soil conditions affect the protein content and antigenicity of the allergens, and vary in urban/rural/hilly/coastal areas. Therefore, it is essential to select the proper allergens for diagnostic skin test and therapeutic vaccine correlating with the symptoms and history of exposure to specific allergens. It is also important to have the knowledge of occupation and residence of the patients and geographical habitat and also the precipitating factors for their allergic symptoms. A document on various aeroallergens (pollens, fungi, insects, and mite allergens) present in different parts of the country has been published. Allergen extracts of nearly 50 pollens, 15–20 fungi, and insects are included in the Indian manufacturer's list, which are most commonly prevalent throughout the country. Two house dust mite species, namely, *Dermatophagoides pteronyssinus* and *D. farinae*, are predominant in regions with high humidity, especially in coastal areas.[12]

STANDARDIZATION AND TYPES OF ALLERGEN EXTRACTS

The allergen extracts used for the purpose of diagnostic skin test and for IT should be standardized in view of biological potency, characterization, stability, and cost-effectiveness. In India, native extracts available as aqueous preparations are used for SCIT and are prepared by extraction of allergenic materials obtained from natural sources with an in-house reference standard. Fifty percent glycerol is used as a good stabilizer of proteins in SPT solutions but cannot be used for therapeutic vaccine. The Drug Controller of India/state units regulated the allergen manufacturer in India. Allergen standardization is regulated by the European Medicines Agency in Europe and the FDA in the United States.[13]

The biologic potency and composition may be affected by the quality and purity of the source materials and also the extraction methods including storage conditions. In addition to aqueous extracts used commonly, depot extracts are used for SCIT in Europe.[7,12] Aqueous allergen extracts are most commonly used worldwide. They are the heterogeneous mixtures of allergens and nonallergic materials, which are rapidly absorbed, less stable, and causing more systemic side effects. Depot and modified vaccines are slowly absorbed, more stable causing less systemic side effects with more LRs, less allergenic, and more immunogenic, and require less injections. These vaccines are modified by physical methods with aluminum, calcium phosphate, tyrosine, and liposome and chemically modified by polymerization (allergoids) with formaldehyde, glutaraldehyde, and alginate and by nonpolymerization with methoxy polyethylene glycol. Sterility test is needed for every new batch of antigen extract. The allergen extracts/vaccines should be stored at 4–8°C, and the antigens are transported using an appropriate cold chain.

SIDE EFFECTS OF IMMUNOTHERAPY

The side effects of allergen vaccines may occur locally and systemically.

Local effects may be early (<30 minutes) or late (>30 minutes, most commonly after 6–24 hours).

The *LRs* (redness, swelling, warmth, pain, and itching) are common and occur with a frequency ranging from 26% to 82% in patients and 0.7–4% of injections. They are usually poor predictors of subsequent systemic reactions at the next injection and do not require dose reduction. However, some patients with greater frequency of large LRs might be at high risk for future systemic reactions. Late LRs may sometimes produce more nodules in depot vaccine preparations.

Systemic reactions may present as intensification of allergic symptoms of rhinitis, bronchial asthma, urticaria, fatigue, shock and anaphylaxis with change in voice, frequent change in posture, hypotension, feeble pulse, mental confusion, sinking feeling, loss of consciousness, and vasovagal attack. The frequency of systemic reaction is low; however, life-threatening and fatal reactions do occur. Systemic reactions are more in rush IT compared to conventional IT.[7] Symptoms of anaphylaxis usually occur within 30 minutes after an injection; therefore, the patient should remain in medical clinic for at least 30 minutes after AIT. Delayed systemic reactions can occur after 30 minutes and are in general not severe. Systemic reactions are less in depot/alum preparation than in aqueous allergen preparation.

Systemic reactions are less in SLIT than in SKIT. LRs in SLIT manifest in the form of oral mucosal redness/pruritus/edema.[7,12,36,37]

DURATION OF IMMUNOTHERAPY

The duration of IT is usually 3–5 years. Some of the patients may require longer treatment to maintain better allergic symptoms and reduction in medicines. The decision of discontinuation of IT should be individualized with proper evaluation of symptoms and medication score.

KEY POINTS FOR PRACTICING ALLERGEN IMMUNOTHERAPY

- Allergy and allergic disorders (IgE mediated) are commonly reported in clinical practice of different specialties.
- Diagnosis is based on a detailed clinical history and a physical examination along with a history of exposure to allergens to be confirmed by skin tests, preferably SPT and in specific cases RAST/ELISA.
- Allergy practice, for both diagnosis and IT, should be practiced only by a trained allergy medical doctor and with facility for managing anaphylaxis.
- A holistic approach of management of allergic disease is based on allergen avoidance, pharmacotherapy, AIT, and patient education.
- The AIT is efficacious and cost-effective, changes the natural course of disease along with immunological changes, and is effective in long-term prevention.
- Only standardized allergen extracts should be used with proper storage conditions for both diagnosis and AIT.
- The specific indications and contraindications should be evaluated properly before starting AIT.
- The duration of AIT is usually 3–5 years with an ideal age for initiation of AIT being 12–45 years.
- Clinical response of AIT is a slow process. Response starts generally after 6 months and should be explained to the patient before initiation.
- Systemic and local side effects should be evaluated properly, explained to patients, and managed accordingly. Patients should be under observation in the clinic for at least 30 minutes.

REFERENCES

1. Noon L. Prophylactic inoculation against hay fever. Lancet. 1911;1:1572-3.
2. Freeman J. Further observations of the treatment of hay fever by hypodermic inoculations of pollen vaccine. Lancet. 1911;2:814-7.
3. Freeman J. "Rush Inoculation," with special reference to hay fever treatment. Lancet. 1930;1:744-7.
4. Bousquet J, Lockey R, Malling HJ. Allergen immunotherapy: therapeutic vaccines for allergic diseases. A WHO Position Paper. J Allergy Clin Immunol. 1998;102:558-62.
5. Burks AW, Calderon MA, Casale T, et al. Update on allergy immunotherapy: American Academy of Allergy, Asthma & Immunology/European Academy of Allergy and Clinical Immunology/PRACTALL consensus report. J Allergy Clin Immunol. 2013;131:1288-96.e3.
6. Zuberbier T, Bachert C, Bousquet PJ, et al. GA^2 LEN/EAACI pocket guide for allergen-specific immunotherapy for allergic rhinitis and asthma. Allergy. 2010;65:1525-30.
7. Cox L, Nelson H, Lockey R, et al. Allergen immunotherapy: a practice parameter third update. J Allergy Clin Immunol. 2011;127:S1-55.
8. Scadding GK, Durham SR, Mirakian R, et al. BSACI guidelines for the management of allergic and non-allergic rhinitis. Clin Exp Allergy. 2008;38:19-42.
9. Pfaar O, Bachert C, Bufe A, et al. Guideline on allergen-specific immunotherapy in IgE-mediated allergic diseases. Allergy J Int. 2014;23:282-319.
10. Jutel M, Agache I, Bonini S, et al. International consensus on allergy immunotherapy. J Allergy Clin Immunol. 2015;136:556-68.

11. Gaur SN, Singh BP, Singh AB, et al. Guidelines for practice of allergen immunotherapy in India. Indian J Allergy Asthma Immunol. 2009;23:1-21.
12. Gaur SN, Kumar R, Singh AB, et al. Guidelines for practice of allergen immunotherapy in India: 2017—An update. Indian J Allergy Asthma Immunol. 2017;31:3-33.
13. Jutel M, Agache I, Bonini S, et al. International consensus on allergy immunotherapy II: mechanisms, standardization and pharmacoeconomics. J Allergy Clin Immunol. 2016;137:358-68.
14. Akdis M, Akdis CA Mechanism of allergen specific immunotherapy: multiple suppressive factor at in immune tolerance to allergens. J Allergy Clin Immunol. 2014;133:621-31.
15. Cox L. Accelerated immunotherapy schedules: review of efficacy and safety. Ann Allergy Asthma Immunol. 2006;97:126-37.
16. Durham SR. Immunotherapy mechanism, plenary immunotherapy: is it a shot in the dark, or just a drop, do we know when to start and when to stop? American College of Allergy, Asthma and Immunology 2006, Annual Meeting; November 6-15, 2006; Philadelphia, PA.
17. Malling HJ. Is sublingual immunotherapy clinically effective? Curr Opin Allergy Clin Immunol. 2002;2: 523-31.
18. Nelson HS. Advances in upper airway diseases and allergen immunotherapy. J Allergy Clin Immunol. 2003;111: S793-8.
19. Khinchi MS, Poulsen LK, Carat F, et al. Clinical efficacy of sublingual and subcutaneous birch pollen allergen-specific immunotherapy: a randomized, placebo-controlled, double-blind, double-dummy study. Allergy. 2004;59:45-53.
20. Demoly P, Passalacqua G, Calderon MA, Yalaoui T. Choosing the optimal dose in sublingual immunotherapy: rationale for the 300 index of reactivity dose. Clin Trans Allergy. 2015;5:44.
21. Passalacqua G, Canonica GW. Allergen immunotherapy: history and future developments. Immunol Allergy Clin North Am. 2016;36:1-12.
22. Crimi E, Voltolini S, Troise C, et al. Local immunotherapy with *Dermatophagoides* extract in asthma. J Allergy Clin Immunol. 1991;87:721-8.
23. Möller C, Dreborg S, Lanner A, Björkstén B. Oral immunotherapy of children with rhinoconjunctivitis due to birch pollen allergy. A double blind study. Allergy. 1986;41:271-9.
24. Giovane AL, Bardare M, Passalacqua G, et al. A three-year double-blind placebo-controlled study with specific oral immunotherapy to *Dermatophagoides*: evidence of safety and efficacy in paediatric patients. Clin Exp Allergy. 1994;24:53-9.
25. Cooper PJ, Darbyshire J, Nunn AJ, Warner JO. A controlled trial of oral hyposensitization in pollen asthma and rhinitis in children. Clin Allergy. 1984;14:541-50.
26. Oppenheimer J, Areson JG, Nelson HS. Safety and efficacy of oral immunotherapy with standardized cat extract. J Allergy Clin Immunol. 1994;93:61-7.
27. Mosbech H, Dreborg S, Madsen F, et al. High-dose grass pollen tablets used for hyposensitization in hay fever patients. A one-year double-blind placebo-controlled study. Allergy. 1987;42:451-5.
28. Nowak-Wegrzyn A, Albin S. Oral immunotherapy for food allergy: mechanisms and role in management. Clin Exp Allergy. 2015;45:368-83.
29. Tari MG, Mancino M, Monti G. Immunotherapy by inhalation of allergen in powder in house dust allergic asthma—a double-blind study. J Investig Allergol Clin Immunol. 1992;2:59-67.
30. Canonica GW, Passalacqua G. Noninjection routes for immunotherapy. J Allergy Clin Immunol. 2003;111: 437-48.
31. Nickelsen JA, Goldstein S, Mueller U, et al. Local intranasal immunotherapy for ragweed allergic rhinitis. I Clinical Response. J Allergy Clin Immunol. 1981;68:33-40.
32. Welsh PW, Butterfield JH, Yunginger JW, et al. Allergen-controlled study of intranasal immunotherapy for ragweed hay fever. J Allergy Clin Immunol. 1983;71: 454-60.
33. Passalacqua G, Albano M, Pronzato C, et al. Long-term follow-up of nasal immunotherapy to *Parietaria*: clinical and local immunological effects. Clin Exp Allergy. 1997;27:904-8.
34. Senti G, Graf N, Haug S, et al. Epicutaneous allergen administration as a novel method of allergen immunotherapy. J Allergic Clin Immunol. 2009;127: 997-1002.
35. Senti G, Prinz Vavarika BM, Erdmann I, et al. Intralymphatic allergen administration renders specific immunotherapy faster and safer: randomized controlled trial. Proc Natl Acad Sci USA. 2008;105:17908-12.
36. Rogala B, Markiewicz-Bendkowska IB, Brzoza Z, et al. Side-effects of injective allergen immunotherapy administered to intermittent or persistent allergic rhinitis patients. Rhinology. 2007:45;134-9.
37. Pitsios C, Demoly P, Bilo MB, et al. Clinical contraindications to allergen immunotherapy: an EAACI position paper. Allergy. 2015;70:897-909.

CHAPTER 19

Cluster Allergen Immunotherapy

PC Kathuria

INTRODUCTION

Allergic disease is a major problem all over the world. Allergen immunotherapy (AIT) has been used to treat allergic diseases since the early 1900s. There is practically no controversy about the use of AIT in the treatment of allergic rhinitis, allergic rhinoconjunctivitis, allergic asthma, and insect hypersensitivity reactions (stinging insect venom). Recent data look promising also for AIT as a diseases-modifying treatment for food allergy and atopic dermatitis. Many medications are available to treat the symptoms of allergic rhinitis and asthma, but AIT is the only potentially immune-modifying and curative (causal) treatment available. Clear evidence has proved for the clinical efficacy, the long-lasting benefit of clinical effects, the (secondary) prevention of bronchial asthma, the reduction of new allergic sensitization, and a good safety profile of subcutaneous immunotherapy (SCIT). The efficacy of this treatment depends on the specific preparation used, the quality and cumulative dose of the allergen extracts administered for immunotherapy (IT), and moreover the dosage schedules—whether conventional schedules or cluster/rush protocols in SCIT.[1]

SUBCUTANEOUS IMMUNOTHERAPY PROTOCOLS

The SCIT is started with the introduction of specific allergen vaccine during which the dose is increased to the maintenance dose. SCIT describes gradually ascending dosages of the allergen extracts and are injected subcutaneously in weekly intervals (up-dose for a period of 6 months) until the individual achieved maximum tolerance dose (MTD). Several dosage protocols have been described, which last from several weeks to months for the initial buildup dose period. The dose is determined by the patient's clinical tolerance to the vaccine as per the degree of sensitivity. Evidence from various studies has shown that a maintenance dose of 5–20 μg can induce clinical benefit.[2,3]

CONVENTIONAL VS. CLUSTER IMMUNOTHERAPY

Why only 9–10% of US patients and 4% of Canadians with allergic rhinitis receive conventional SCIT and many stop it prematurely? Is it because of frequent office visits and the 30-minute waiting time after injections? Is it inconvenience due to time involved? Freeman noted the inconvenience of the weekly buildup schedules and began experimenting with more rapid schedules as "intensive desensitization," in contrast to conventional therapy.[4] In his article, he reported that a 7-year-old girl with horse dander-induced asthma desensitized over 4 days, but developed urticaria, fluttering heat, and felt "funny." The allergen vaccine dose was decreased, but she was able to ride her pony without discomfort. He concluded that the advantages of the "rush" method were time-saving, convenience, and patient compliance.[5] Conventional up-dosing protocols use 12–16 weekly injections during buildup dosing and four to six weekly injections during the maintenance phase, but inconvenience and time are likely the most common reasons for not beginning or discontinuing the conventional form of SCIT. Moreover, this treatment is susceptible for interferences, e.g., in case of viral or bacterial infectious disease during the initial buildup dose period of SCIT, the interval between two injections must be increased to avoid untoward adverse reactions by allergen vaccine. Either the dose has to be reduced or the therapy must be restarted again. The aim of accelerated schedules in SCIT like cluster protocols is to reach the dose maintenance period faster than the conventional method; hence, two to three injections are given per treatment day (with an interval of 30 minutes between the injections) in weekly intervals. So, the individual maximum dose can be reached after 4–5 weeks, depending on the depot allergen or chemically modified allergen preparations (allergoids) or standardized allergen vaccine (*Summary Statement 22*) (Table 19.1). Clinical and physiological improvement can be demonstrated very shortly after the patient reaches a maintenance dose (Table 19.2).[6]

Table 19.2: Conventional vs. cluster protocols.

1	Visits	Thirty visits/ 30 injections	Eight visits/ 18 injections
2	Time waiting	30 minutes wait	2.5–3 hours cluster (30-minute interval)
3	Prophylactic meds	Antihistamine	Prednisone 20 mg × twice a day (BD) Cetirizine 10 mg × BD Zinetac 150 mg × BD Montelukast 10 mg daily
4	Buildup dose	7.5 months	5 weeks

See Cox et al. (2011).

Table 19.1: Cluster allergen immunotherapy (A practice parameter third update).

Visit number	*Volume (mL)*	*Dilution (v/v)*	*Vial color*	*Dose (mg)*	*Cumulative dose (mg)*
1	0.10	1:1000	Green	0.1	0.1
	0.40	1:1000	Green	0.4	0.5
	0.10	1:100	Blue	1.0	1.5
2	0.20	1:100	Blue	2.0	3.5
	0.40	1:100	Blue	4.0	7.5
	0.07	1:10	Yellow	7.0	14.5
3	0.10	1:10	Yellow	10.0	24.5
	0.15	1:10	Yellow	15.0	39.5
	0.25	1:10	Yellow	25.0	64.5
4	0.35	1:10	Yellow	35.0	99.5
	0.50	1:10	yellow	50.0	149.5
5	0.07	1:1	Red	70.0	219.5
	0.10	1:1	Red	100.0	319.5
6	0.15	1:1	Red	150.0	469.5
	0.20	1:1	Red	200.0	669.5
7	0.30	1:1	Red	300.0	969.5
	0.40	1:1	Red	400.0	1,369.5
8	0.50	1:1	Red	500.0	1,869.5

Conventional immunotherapy—7.5 months, 30 injection/30 visits.

January

S	M	T	W	T	F	S
					1	2
3		5	6	7	8	9
10		12	13	14	15	16
17		19	20	21	22	23
24		26	27	28	29	30
31						

February

S	M	T	W	T	F	S
		2	3	4	5	6
7		9	10	11	12	13
14		16	17	18	19	20
21		23	24	25	26	27
28						

March

S	M	T	W	T	F	S
		2	3	4	5	6
7		9	10	11	12	13
14		16	17	18	19	20
21		23	24	25	26	27
28		30	31			

April

S	M	T	W	T	F	S
				1	2	3
4		6	7	8	9	10
11		13	14	15	16	17
18		20	21	22	23	24
25		27	28	29	30	

May

S	M	T	W	T	F	S
						1
2		4	5	6	7	8
9		11	12	13	14	15
16		18	19	20	21	22
23		25	26	27	28	29
30						

June

S	M	T	W	T	F	S
		1	2	3	4	5
6		8	9	10	11	12
13		15	16	17	18	19
20		22	23	24	25	26
27		29	30			

July

S	M	T	W	T	F	S
				1	2	3
4		6	7	8	9	10
11		13	14	15	16	17
18		20	21	22	23	24
25		27	28	29	30	31

(Contd...)

(Contd...)

Cluster immunotherapy—5 weeks, 18 injection/8 visits.

January						
S	M	T	W	T	F	S
					1	2
3		5	6		8	9
10		12	13		15	16
17		19	20		22	23
24		26	27	28	29	30
31						

February						
S	M	T	W	T	F	S
		2	3	4	5	6
7	8	9	10	11	12	13
14	15	16	17	18	19	20
21	22	23	24	25	26	27
28						

See Cox et al. (2011).

CLUSTER CANDIDATES

Any patient, who is considered a candidate for IT, is a candidate for cluster IT, but the following patients/situations may benefit from cluster schedules:

- Poor adherence or systemic reactions with conventional IT.
- Work/life schedule precludes weekly injections for a prolonged time.
- Asthma that can only be controlled long enough to reach a maintenance dose with an accelerated (cluster) schedule.

PREMEDICATION WITH ACCELERATED IMMUNOTHERAPY SCHEDULES

Summary Statement 57: *AIT practice parameter third update*: The occurrence of both local and systemic reactions to cluster IT might be reduced with the administration of antihistamine, while combination with H2 antagonist (ranitidine), leukotriene receptor antagonist (montelukast), and corticosteroid (prednisolone) 2 hours before dosing is effective in reducing the systemic and local reactions during accelerated IT buildup protocols.

Summary Statement 58: Omalizumab pretreatment has been shown to improve the safety and tolerability of cluster IT schedules in patients with moderate persistent asthma and allergic rhinitis, respectively. Additionally, omalizumab used in combination with IT has been shown to be effective in improving symptom scores compared to IT alone.

SAFETY PROFILES OF CLUSTER SCHEDULES OF SPECIFIC AIT

Current controlled studies with both adult and pediatric allergic patients reveal a promising safety profile of cluster schedules comparable with the conventional schedules of dose increase in SCIT allergic children sensitized to dust mites were randomized in two groups. Twenty children were treated with a cluster protocol, whereas 10 children were randomized to a conventional protocol to reach the maintenance dose within 13 weeks only. Children with coexistent allergic asthma were included in this trial. There was no significant difference in the incidence of adverse events. Moreover, the good tolerability of cluster IT in adult patients has been examined in a large retrospective observational multicenter study of Serrano et al. on 1,147 allergic patients who received a total of 6,982 doses. Forty-two systemic reactions (0.6% of all injections) were documented in 39 patients (3.4%) (Table 19.3). There was no systemic reaction in the combined omalizumab with cluster immunotherapy in our observational study done in 65 patients with allergic rhinitis with intermittent bronchial asthma sensitized to dust mites. (*Dermatophagoides farinae* and *D. pteronyssinus*). There was no systemic reaction in the combined omalizumab (anti-IgE) and cluster IT, whereas the systemic reactions in cluster vs. conventional IT (20% vs. 18.7%) were of grade

Table 19.3: Clinical trials with cluster protocols in SCIT.[7,8]

Author	*Year*	*n*	*Study design*	*Allergen*	*Treatment interval for induction phase (weeks)*	*Number of injections in induction phase*	*Systemic adverse events (% of all injections)*	*Clinical and immunological outcome measures*
Tabar et al.	2005	Cluster = 120; conventional = 119	Prospective, randomized, placebo-controlled, double-blind comparative	HDM	12	13	0.15 (no difference between groups)	Rhinitis and asthma symptom scores, skin test reactivity, IgG4 and IGE levels
Serrano et al.	2009	1147	Retrospective, observational	218 HDM, 231 grasses, 640 grasses and olive, 53 olive, 5 others	2–5	4–10	0.6	–
Schubert et al.	2009	Cluster = 20; conventional = 10	Prospective, controlled, randomized, comparative, open label	HDM, children with allergic asthma "head-to-head" comparison	5 13	14 14	3.5 4.6	Blocking CD63 expression, cysteinyl leukotriene level, IgG and IgG4 levels
Pfaar et al.	2009	395	Prospective, controlled, open label	Pollen	5	16	2.05	–
Zhang et al.	2009	Cluster = 48; conventional = 48	Prospective, controlled, randomized, comparative open label	HDM "head-to-head" comparison	6 14	14 (cluster) 15	1 0.9	(Weekly) rhinitis symptom scores, medication scores, Rhinitis Quality of life, global treatment effectiveness (VAS), skin test reactivity, IgE levels
Pfaar et al.	2010	79	Prospective, controlled, open label	HDM	3	12	3.2	–

II and grade III, and well controlled, with epinephrine injection.[9] A recently published study of 395 patients with pollen-induced allergic rhinitis analyzed the safety of a 5-week cluster schedules with another depot allergen preparation. This schedule aims to reduce the time needed for the dose induction phase by 66% compared to conventional schedules. However, after 148 injections (or 2.05% of all injections), systemic reaction occurred with a majority of grade I and grade II reactions (84% and 16%, respectively, in all systemic reactions).[7,8] In a retrospective, observation review in a large multicenter group regarding cluster IT safety was conducted for 441 patients receiving cluster IT. Forty-eight patients (10.9%) experienced systemic reactions (maintenance dose achieved). Immunotherapy Systemic Reaction Grading System, is 38.3% received grade I reaction, 48.9% grade II reaction, and 10.6% grade III reaction (Based on the World Allergy Organization) as compared to systemic reaction (2–7%) in the US study with conventional schedules.[10]

CONCLUSION

Inconvenience is likely the most common reason for not beginning or discontinuing the conventional form of SCIT. Cluster IT is a safe treatment method which is more effective and faster than conventional IT. Clinical effects begin more rapidly due to higher cumulative amount of allergens in the buildup phase in cluster schedules compared with conventional up-dosing protocols. Premedication requires prior administration of each cluster, especially in asthmatic patients. Cluster immunotherapy with both depot allergens (aluminum hydroxide adjuvant) and chemically modified allergen preparations (allergoids), and standardized allergens have convenience, safety profile, efficacious, and better adherence for IT.

REFERENCES

1. Abramson MJ, Puy RM, Weiner JM. Is allergen immunotherapy effective in asthma? A meta-analysis of randomized controlled trials. Am J Respir Crit Care Med. 1995;151:969-74.
2. Cox L. Accelerated immunotherapy schedules: review of efficacy and safety. Ann Allergy Asthma Immunol. 2006;97:126-37.
3. Cox LS. Shooting for a faster approach to the immunotherapy target: will cluster become conventional? Ann Allergy Asthma Immunol. 2009;102:177-8.
4. Freeman J. Rush inoculation with special reference to hay fever treatment. Lancet. 1930;215:744-7.
5. Cox L. Allergen immunotherapy and asthma: efficacy, safety, and other considerations. Allergy Asthma Proc. 2008;29:580-9.
6. Cox L. et al., Allergen immunotherapy a practice parameter third updated. J Allergy Clin Immunal. 2011;Jan 12: 51-5.
7. Schubert R, Eickmeier O, Garn H, et al. Safety and immunogenicity of a cluster specific immunotherapy in children with bronchial asthma and mite allergy. Int Arch Allergy Immunol. 2009;148:251-60.
8. Pfaar O, Mösges R, Hörmann K, Klimek L. Safety aspects of cluster-immunotherapy with semi-depot allergen extracts in seasonal allergic rhinoconjunctivitis. Eur Arch Otorhinolaryngol. 2010;267:245-50.
9. Kathuria PC. Safety of Accelerated Schedules of Cluster Allergen Immunotherapy with house dust mites in sixty five patients with perennial br asthma WISC 2012 World allergy congress. Hyderabad India 6-9 December (Abstract).
10. Cox L, Larenas-Linnemann D, Lockey RF, Passalacqua G. Speaking the same language: the World Allergy Organization subcutaneous immunotherapy systemic reaction grading system. J Allergy Clin Immunol. 2010;125:569-74.

CHAPTER 20

Future of Allergen-specific Immunotherapy

Sagar L Kale, Swati Sharma, Bharti Arora, Naveen Arora

INTRODUCTION

Allergen avoidance, pharmacotherapy, and immunotherapy are the prevalent treatment modalities for allergic diseases. Avoiding the exposure of allergens is the best defense strategy to circumvent allergic symptoms, and it may be best recommended for several food allergens, latex hypersensitivity, etc.; however, it is almost impossible to employ in case of aeroallergens such as pollen, mold, and insect castings.[1] Pharmacological treatments are the mainstay of therapeutic options and offer symptomatic relief; however, the symptoms relapse upon the discontinuation of medicines, and a long-term use is accompanied with side effects.[2] Allergen-specific immunotherapy (AIT) is in practice for over 100 years and currently is the only curative treatment available for allergic diseases.[3] Immunotherapy is the only available treatment that has a potential to modulate the Th2 immune responses underlying allergic diseases. AIT is recommended in the following scenarios: when (a) allergen avoidance is impossible or (b) pharmacotherapy is unable to reduce the symptoms and causes side effects or (c) to avoid the risk of anaphylaxis. Earlier, a natural exposure to high levels of allergens in beekeepers and cat owners was observed to induce tolerance towards the offending allergen.[4] Similarly, tolerance to allergenic antigens can be induced artificially by administering high doses of the respective allergens. AIT involves a gradual administration of increasing dose of specific allergens until the generation of tolerance.[5] Allergen specific immunotherapy (ASIT) is effective for the treatment of allergic asthma, allergic rhinitis and conjunctivitis, and hymenoptera hypersensitivity.[6,7] S-AIT induces a tolerant state in peripheral T cells, characterized mainly by activation-induced death, anergy, or immune response modification by regulatory T cells (Tregs).[8] ASIT involves a repeated administration of sensitizing allergen either by subcutaneous injection or by sublingual application.[9] ASIT involves a buildup phase consisting of weekly injections and a maintenance phase consisting of monthly injections.[5] After natural exposure to allergens, ASIT reduces the recruitment of inflammatory cells such as eosinophils, basophils, and mast cells at the site of exposure. ASIT increases the production of blocking IgG antibodies and subsequently reduces the levels of allergen-specific IgE antibodies.[4] Subcutaneous immunotherapy (SCIT) involves a subcutaneous (usually under the skin) administration of allergen extracts. SCIT is effective in ameliorating allergies caused by insect venom or inhalant allergens [pollens, molds, house dust mites (HDMs)].[10] Studies have reported that SCIT may lead to systemic side effects such as anaphylaxis and is not recommended for food or latex allergies.[11] Sublingual immunotherapy (SLIT) tackles the complexities associated with SCIT, is generally well tolerated, and involves the administration of allergens (prepared as tablets or drops) to the oral mucosa (usually under the tongue) for 1–2 min before swallowing. SLIT is generally taken daily in contrast to SCIT, which is taken 4–6 weekly in the maintenance phase, and is much safer as compared to SCIT as it carries a lesser risk of anaphylaxis.[12] In the past few years, intensive research has been focused to increase the safety and efficacy of ASIT. Current allergen-SIT protocols use whole allergen extracts, and a majority of studies have shown the efficacy of ASIT in treating allergic diseases. For instance, a study evaluated the tolerability and efficacy of ASIT with whole-body mosquito (*Culex quinquefasciatus*) in a randomized controlled trial of 40 patients (sensitized to mosquito and suffering from allergic rhinitis and bronchial asthma) and demonstrated improved symptoms along with a reduced airway hyper-reactivity and an increase in IgG4 antibodies.[13]

Furthermore, a double-blind, placebo-controlled trial using mixture or single allergen for immunotherapy for 1 year in 99 patients demonstrated higher therapeutic efficacy in patients administered with allergen mixture in contrast to those administered with single allergen extract for insect hypersensitivity.[14]

Natural allergen extracts are undefined heterogeneous mixtures of carbohydrates, proteins, and organic compounds. The allergen content in the natural allergen extracts may vary among the batches, which may lead to the inconsistent clinical effects. Administration of these heterogeneous extracts may cause life-threatening anaphylactic reactions and also may induce false-positive reactions during allergy diagnosis and/or additional IgE sensitization in patients during therapy as observed in immunotherapy with birch pollen extract.[14-17] Allergen extracts may contain the contamination of allergens from other sources or with bacterial components such as endotoxins, which may influence the immune response.[18] Allergen immunotherapy is associated with various drawbacks such as adverse IgE-mediated reactions, insufficient efficacy, high costs, and a prolonged duration of treatment (3–5 years), thereby affecting patient adherence to therapy. Novel approaches to ASIT that focused on increasing its efficacy with reduced side effects are under investigation. These include the use of purified allergens,[19-21] recombinant allergens,[22-24] hypoallergenic recombinant allergens, T-cell reactive peptides, allergoids (chemically modified allergens), fragments of major allergens, and chimeric allergens.

CHEMICALLY MODIFIED ALLERGENS

Allergens can be chemically modified to form allergoids. Administration of allergoids for ASIT is associated with a reduced risk of anaphylaxis as evidenced by a number of studies demonstrating greater therapeutic efficacy and safety.[25-27] Oligomerization of allergens by glutaraldehyde or paraformaldehyde distorts or masks IgE epitopes, which subsequently reduces IgE binding, while maintaining its immunogenicity.[28] Carbamylation, a chemical process where the allergens are treated with potassium cyanate at neutral pH, has been exploited for the generation of monomeric allergoids.[29] SLIT with monomeric carbamylated allergoid given as a soluble tablet was effective and safe in mite-induced rhinitis.[30] Maleylation, a process where allergens are treated with maleic acid anhydride that leads to the alteration of ε amino group of lysine residues, has been used in the generation of allergoids. It converts allergens into ligands of scavenger receptor, a pattern recognition receptor expressed by antigen-presenting cells (APCs), and is involved in the recognition of foreign antigens.[31] The composition of allergoids prepared from the whole extracts is undefined and may contain irrelevant proteins. The use of allergoids prepared from the recombinant proteins may solve this issue. Recent studies indicate that low allergenicity of allergoids as compared to their natural extracts may be associated with low immunogenicity due to chemical modification.[32] Despite these drawbacks, allergoid immunotherapy holds a promise for traditional SCIT, and more studies are needed to prove its efficacy.

RECOMBINANT ALLERGENS

Some of the drawbacks of using natural allergen extracts, such as variable composition and contamination by other allergens or by bacterial components, can be overcome by using recombinant allergens individually or in combination.[33,34] Also, some of the allergenic extracts have very few dominant allergens, ranging from 1 (namely, Bet v 1 and Fel d 1, from birch pollen and *Felis domesticus*) to 20 (HDM).[35,36] Administration of the whole extract for immunotherapy in such cases risks additional sensitization. Therapeutic preparations focusing on the part that is majorly involved in IgE responses can prove beneficial in enhancing the safety of the preparation. Recombinant allergens can be chemically defined by determining their physical, chemical, and immunological properties. Activity of a natural allergen extract is determined in terms of concentration and IgE binding of one of the major allergen, whereas the activity of recombinant allergens is determined in terms of concentration and IgE binding of each and every component. Furthermore, as recombinant allergens are produced in a controlled environment, it negates the potential risk of contamination of the extract with foreign and nonallergenic materials, such as pesticides in case of pollen extracts. Collection of the raw materials for natural allergen extracts is difficult and poses a risk of batch-to-batch variation, which is thus circumvented in case of recombinant allergens.[33] However, recombinant allergens have their drawbacks as well. Almost all recombinant proteins are expressed in bacterial systems such as *Escherichia coli*. As seen in the case of an isoform of Bet v 1, a variation in production conditions can strongly influence the characteristics of the recombinant proteins.[37] Furthermore, the bacterial systems lack post-translational modification machinery needed for protein glycosylation. This causes a problem in allergens that are glycoproteins. Also, the use of codon in *E. coli* is different from that in the eukaryotic systems, which may further affect the final protein product. The use of eukaryotic expression systems can overcome these drawbacks and may enhance the quality of expressed protein for immunotherapy.[38]

ALLERGENS MODIFIED GENETICALLY

Site-directed mutagenesis (SDM) has been used to produce hypoallergenic variants of respiratory and food allergens. SDM obliterates IgE binding epitopes retaining intact T-cell epitopes, thus reducing allergenicity while maintaining immunogenicity. A hypoallergenic Bet v 1 generated by SDM displayed a reduced IgE reactivity;[39] similarly, a variant of Par j 1 (*Parietaria judaica* major allergen) generated by mutagenesis of specific cysteine residues showed a reduced skin reactivity and IgE binding.[40] It has been successfully used to reduce allergenicity of Mal d 1 (apple allergen) and Bet v 1.[41] Introduction of point mutations in IgE binding epitopes of Hev b 5, Hev b 6.02 (latex allergens), and Lol p 5 can reduce their allergenicity and maintain T-cell reactivity.[42-44] Recent studies with osmotin, a pathogenesis-related protein used for the development of transgenic crops, showed that mice immunized with mutated B-cell peptides representing linear epitopes of osmotin or with engineered hypoallergenic variants of osmotin containing these epitopes exhibited a reduced production of IgE and IgG1 and a reduced lung infiltration as compared to mice immunized with native osmotin.[22,24] The use of hypoallergenic variants of allergens produced by SDM offers a possibility for safer and efficacious approach for allergen-SIT.

DELETION MUTANTS

Hypoallergens can also be produced by selectively deleting the IgE binding regions in the gene and preserving the regions encoding T-cell epitopes. A hypoallergenic variant of Phl p 5b, a timothy grass pollen allergen, was produced by deleting IgE binding regions of Phl p 5b and showed significantly reduced IgE binding and histamine release from the granulocytes obtained from the patients allergic to grass as compared to wild Phl p 5b.[45] Deletion hypoallergenic mutants have also been made for Per a 1, Lol p 1, and Asp f 3 (*Aspergillus fumigates* major allergen).[46-48]

FUSION PROTEINS

Allergens can be fused with the stimulators of the immune system. The presence of a large number of immune stimulators presents infinite possibilities of combinations to be used in immunotherapy. Der p 1 covalently coupled to Qβ, a bacteriophage-derived protein that forms virus-like particles, administered to volunteers mounted a significant IgG1 and IgG3 antibody response against both the proteins with no induction of IgE in healthy individuals, thereby making it a potential candidate for SIT in allergic patients.[49] Furthermore, SIT with pollen allergoids adjuvanted to monophosphoryl lipid A, a Th1-favoring adjuvant, induced tolerance and a significant production of IgG and IgG4 antibodies after the second course of treatment.[50] Attempts have also been made to fuse allergens with TLR ligands. A study by Creticos et al. demonstrated that immunotherapy in patients allergic to ragweed, with Amb a 1, a major ragweed pollen allergen, conjugated to a TLR-9 ligand, suppressed the induction of ragweed-specific IgE and led to improved allergic rhinitis symptoms during the ragweed season.[51] Ovalbumin fused with flagellin is more prominent in inducing antigen-specific responses as compared to coadministration of ovalbumin and flagellin in mice.[52] Furthermore, ovalbumin fused to flagellin A induces a strong IL-10 response in murine myeloid DCs and has been shown to prevent intestinal allergy in a murine disease model.[53,54] Covalent coupling of rFel d 1 to carbohydrate-based particles prevented the induction of allergic symptoms by inducing a rapid antibody production in mice.[55] Furthermore, mice and rabbits administered with Fel d 1-derived peptides fused with a hepatitis B virus-derived PreS domain showed a reduced IgE-mediated allergenic activity and had a potential in immunotherapy for cat allergy.[56] Mice sensitized with fusion proteins (Cry j 1 and Cry j 2, Japanese cedar pollen allergens) in immunoregulatory liposome demonstrated reduced IgE responses after a challenge with allergen.[57]

ALLERGEN CHIMERA AND DNA SHUFFLING

A chimeric molecule GFD comprising Fel d 1 fused to human IgG1 antibody inhibited Fel d 1 allergen-mediated mediator release from the basophils of cat-allergic donors' blood and cord blood mast cells in a dose-dependent manner. Fel d 1 component of GFD chimera is recognized by FcεRI via IgE and IgG1 components, which in turn is recognized by FcγR that leads to the formation of

FcγR–(GFD)–IgE–FcεRI inhibiting mediator release from the basophils and mast cells.[58] In another study, a chimera comprising B-cell epitope of Der p 1 coupled with antibody against complement-type receptor 1 (CR1, CD35) was able to suppress allergen-specific B lymphocytes. This chimera binds to allergen-specific B cells via the allergen-mimicking peptide and suppresses them via CR1 signaling.[59] A hypoallergenic variant produced by reshuffling of *Dermatophagoides pteronyssinus* group 1 allergen genes decreased IgE and IgG1 in serum and IL-4 and IL-5 in bronchoalveolar lavage fluid in murine model of asthma.[60] Furthermore, a genetically reshuffled engineered Der p 2 produced by reshuffling of two fragments of Der p 2 (aa 1-53 and aa 54-129) in reverse order showed a reduced basophil activation and a reduced allergenicity in skin prick test of mite-allergic patients. The reshuffled Der p 2 molecule when administered to mice or rabbits leads to the production of inhibitory IgG antibodies and a reduction in allergenicity as compared to rDer p 2.[61] Hybrid molecules produced by the reassembly of Der p 1 and Der p 2 fragments without cysteine residues reduced allergic responses without affecting T-cell reactivity. This hybrid molecule leads to the induction of IgG antibodies when administered to rabbits that inhibit IgE reactivity of HDM-allergic patient's sera.[62]

PEPTIDE IMMUNOTHERAPY

Peptide immunotherapy (PIT) comprises immunotherapy with short, synthetic soluble peptides that encompass the immunodominant T-cell epitope from the allergen of interest, holds a therapeutic promise, and is a relatively safe alternative over whole allergen-SIT.[63] T-cell peptides contain T-cell epitopes but lack conformational epitopes required for IgE binding, thereby hampering IgE binding and presenting a definitive advantage over immunotherapy with recombinant or whole native allergens.[63] Several studies have evaluated PIT in patients with cat allergy, bee venom hypersensitivity, and grass pollen allergies.[64] Clinical trials with two synthetic peptides containing the T-cell epitope-rich region of a major cat dander allergen Fel d 1 showed promising results with reduced symptom score reflecting an improvement in lung and nasal symptoms after allergen challenge and reduced IL-4 production by peripheral T cells at a higher dose; however, it was associated with late-phase reactions.[65,66] Another study with 12 short peptides derived from Fel d 1 demonstrated an improvement in quality of life when compared with placebo group with reduced late asthmatic responses.[67,68] Similar approaches have been used for bee venom hypersensitivity using peptides derived from PLA2 and for Japanese cedar pollinosis using peptides derived from Cry j1 and Cry j 2.[69,70] The presentation of peptides by nonprofessional APCs (namely, keratinocytes) or immature DCs, under noninflammatory conditions, induces T-cell anergy or immunosuppressive T cells, thereby leading to tolerance.[71] The advantages of using peptides in immunotherapy are as follows: they (i) show a reduced cross-linking of IgE and a subsequent reduction in mast cell and basophil activation, (ii) can be manufactured and standardized easily, (iii) have negligible side effects, (iv) induce suppressive T cells/ Tregs, and (v) are known to induce IL-10 secretion in human beings.

ALTERNATIVE STRATEGIES FOR SIT: CYTOKINE/ANTICYTOKINE THERAPY

Cytokines play a major role in the manifestation of allergic diseases.[72] Th2 cytokines are known to play a pivotal role in the manifestation of allergy pathogenesis, and molecules capable of antagonizing Th2 cytokines can be beneficial in immunotherapy.[73] Administration of Th1 cytokines may inhibit the induction of Th2 immune responses; conversely, the administration of anti-Th2 cytokines may alleviate allergic responses. Administration of IFNγ, a Th1 cytokine, inhibits IL-4-induced immune response.[74] However, it may lead to adverse side effects. sIL-4Rα binds to IL-4 and blocks its interaction with membrane-bound IL-4R, thus hampering its effects, and has been shown to improve allergic symptoms as compared to placebo group.[75] Reslizumab and mepolizumab, humanized monoclonal anti-IL-5 antibodies, have been evaluated for the safety and efficacy in allergic asthmatic patients. Mepolizumab reduces airway eosinophils but shows no improvement in lung function,[76] whereas reslizumab has shown improvements in lung function and asthma control.[77] Although approaches involving blocking of other inflammatory pathways are under investigation, more studies are needed before these concepts can be taken further in the treatment for allergic diseases.

ANTI-IgE THERAPY

Omalizumab is a humanized anti-IgE antibody that binds to the Fc fragment of IgE and reduces the binding of free IgE to Fcε RI. Administration of omalizumab rapidly reduces free IgE in the serum and expression of high-affinity receptors.[78] Although a number of studies have proved the efficacy of omalizumab, few studies have reported side effects such as pain and bruising.[79] Occurrence of anaphylaxis in 0.1% patients within 24 hours of administration has also been reported.[80]

MODIFYING ALLERGEN ACTIVITY

As proteases (endogenous and exogenous) have been known to play a critical role in pathobiology of allergic diseases,[81-84] the inhibition of protease activity has been used to alleviate allergic symptoms. Recently, a range of protease inhibitors including nafamostat mesilate, gabexate mesilate, and AEBSF have been demonstrated to attenuate allergen-induced airway inflammation in murine model of allergic airway disease.[85-87] APC366, a tryptase inhibitor, reduced histamine release from the mast cells.[88] Another tryptase inhibitor, MOL 6131, reduced Th2 cytokine secretion in mouse model.[89] Many aeroallergens have an intrinsic proteolytic activity that potentiates their allergenicity.[83,90,91] Targeting protease activity has a potential to be used as an adjunct along with conventional therapy for immunomodulation. Immunotherapy with an active or inactive Per a 10, a major cockroach allergen in Per a 10 or cockroach extract-sensitized mice, demonstrated that inactive Per a 10 showed a maximum reduction in systemic and lung inflammation and a maximum induction in IL-10 secretion as compared to immunotherapy with active Per a 10.[92] Inactive proteases can be exploited for immunotherapy, and further studies are warranted to address their safety and long-term clinical efficacy.

CONCLUSION

The quest for developing safe, long-lasting, and efficacious immunotherapy with reduced or negligible side effects has led to a rapid progress with the development of novel methods in immunotherapy for therapeutic intervention of allergic diseases. With knowledge of allergen gene sequences, with three-dimensional structure of allergen, and with the advent of epitope mapping techniques, it is possible to produce hypoallergenic variants of major allergens without affecting their immunogenicity or T-cell reactivity. A lot of studies have focused on increasing safety of SIT and minimizing its IgE binding side effects. Also, newer methods have used Th1 adjuvants coupled with the allergens to shift the immune response away from Th2. These possibilities using modified recombinant allergens or using adjuvants to circumvent Th2 responses hold a promise to treat allergic diseases in the future.

REFERENCES

1. Bousquet, J, Khaltaev N, Cruz AA, et al. Allergic Rhinitis and its Impact on Asthma (ARIA) 2008 update (in collaboration with the World Health Organization, GA(2) LEN and AllerGen). Allergy. 2008;63:8-160.
2. Kale SL. In: Atta-ur-Rahman, ed. Frontiers in Clinical Drug Research–Anti Allergy Agents. Sharjah: Bentham Science Publishers; 2013.
3. Durham SR, Leung, DY. One hundred years of allergen immunotherapy: time to ring the changes. J Allergy Clin Immunol. 2011;127:3-7.
4. van de Veen W, Wirz OF, Globinska A, et al. Novel mechanisms in immune tolerance to allergens during natural allergen exposure and allergen-specific immuno-therapy. Curr Opin Immunol. 2017;48:74-81.
5. Moote W, Kim H. Allergen-specific immunotherapy. Allergy Asthma Clin Immunol. 2011;7:S5.
6. Durham SR, Till SJ. Immunologic changes associated with allergen immunotherapy. J Allergy Clin Immunol. 1998;102:157-64.
7. Lerch E, Muller UR. Long-term protection after stopping venom immunotherapy: results of re-stings in 200 patients. J Allergy Clin Immunol. 1998;101:606-12.
8. Verhagen J, Blaser K, Akdis CA, et al. Mechanisms of allergen-specific immunotherapy: T-regulatory cells and more. Immunol Allergy Clin North Am. 2006;26:207-31.
9. Burks AW, Calderon MA, Casale T, et al. Update on allergy immunotherapy: American Academy of Allergy, Asthma & Immunology/European Academy of Allergy and Clinical Immunology/PRACTALL consensus report. J Allergy Clin Immunol. 2013;131:1288-96.
10. Moingeon P, Mascarell L. Novel routes for allergen immunotherapy: safety, efficacy and mode of action. Immunotherapy. 2012;4:201-12.
11. Incorvaia C, Mauro M, Cappelletti T, et al. New applications for sublingual immunotherapy in allergy. Recent Pat Inflamm Allergy Drug Discov. 2009;3:113-7.
12. Tabatabaian F, Casale TB. Selection of patients for sublingual immunotherapy (SLIT) versus subcutaneous immunotherapy (SCIT). Allergy Asthma Proc. 2015;36: 100-4.
13. Srivastava D, Singh BP, Sudha VT, et al. Immunotherapy with mosquito (Culex quinquefasciatus) extract: a double-blind, placebo-controlled study. Ann Allergy Asthma Immunol. 2007;99:273-80.
14. Srivastava D, Singh BP, Arora N, et al. Clinico-immunologic study on immunotherapy with mixed and single insect allergens. J Clin Immunol. 2009;29:665-73.
15. Moverare R, Elfman L, Vesterinen E, et al. Development of new IgE specificities to allergenic components in birch pollen extract during specific immunotherapy studied

with immunoblotting and Pharmacia CAP System. Allergy. 2002;57:423-30.
16. van der Veen MJ, Mulder M, Witteman AM, et al. False-positive skin prick test responses to commercially available dog dander extracts caused by contamination with house dust mite (Dermatophagoides pteronyssinus) allergens. J Allergy Clin Immunol. 1996;98:1028-34.
17. Osterballe O. Side effects during immunotherapy with purified grass pollen extracts. Allergy. 1982;37:553-62.
18. Trivedi B, Valerio C, Slater JE. Endotoxin content of standardized allergen vaccines. J Allergy Clin Immunol. 2003;111:777-83.
19. Dhyani A, Singh BP, Arora N, et al. A clinically relevant major cross-reactive allergen from mesquite tree pollen. European Journal of Clinical Investigation. 2008;38: 774-81.
20. Kukreja N, Sridhara S, Singh BP, et al. Purification and immunological characterization of a 12-kDa allergen from Epicoccum purpurascens. FEMS Immunol Med Microbiol. 2009;56:32-40.
21. Sudha VT, Arora N, Gaur SN, et al. Identification of a serine protease as a major allergen (Per a 10) of Periplaneta americana. Allergy. 2008;63:768-76.
22. Sharma V, Singh BP, Gaur SN, et al. Molecular and immunological characterization of cytochrome c: a potential cross-reactive allergen in fungi and grasses. Allergy. 2008;63:189-97.
23. Shankar J, Singh BP, Gaur SN, et al. Recombinant glutathione-S-transferase a major allergen from Alternaria alternata for clinical use in allergy patients. Mol Immunol. 2006;43:1927-32.
24. Sharma V, Gupta R, Jhingran A, et al. Cloning, recombinant expression and activity studies of a major allergen "enolase" from the fungus Curvularia lunata. J Clin Immunol. 2006;26:360-9.
25. Rossi RE, Monasterolo G. A pilot study of feasibility of ultra-rush (20-25 minutes) sublingual-swallow immunotherapy in 679 patients (699 sessions) with allergic rhinitis and/or asthma. Int J Immunopathol Pharmacol. 2005;18:277-85.
26. Lombardi C, Gargioni S, Melchiorre A, et al. Safety of sublingual immunotherapy with monomeric allergoid in adults: multicenter post-marketing surveillance study. Allergy. 2001;56:989-92.
27. Passalacqua G, Albano M, Fregonese L, et al. Randomised controlled trial of local allergoid immunotherapy on allergic inflammation in mite-induced rhinoconjunctivitis. Lancet. 1998;351:629-32.
28. Maasch HJ, Marsh DG. Standardized extracts modified allergens–allergoids. Clin Rev Allergy. 1987;5:89-106.
29. Mistrello G, Brenna O, Roncarolo D, et al. Monomeric chemically modified allergens: immunologic and physicochemical characterization. Allergy. 1996;51:8-15.
30. Passalacqua G, Pasquali M, Ariano R, et al. Randomized double-blind controlled study with sublingual carbamylated allergoid immunotherapy in mild rhinitis due to mites. Allergy. 2006;61:849-54.
31. Rajagopal D, Ganesh KA, Subba Rao PV. Modulation of allergen-specific immune responses to the major shrimp allergen, tropomyosin, by specific targeting to scavenger receptors on macrophages. Int Arch Allergy Immunol. 2000;121:308-16.
32. Wurtzen PA, Lund L, Lund G, et al. Chemical modification of birch allergen extract leads to a reduction in allergenicity as well as immunogenicity. Int Arch Allergy Immunol. 2007;144:287-95.
33. Valenta R, Linhart B, Swoboda I, et al. Recombinant allergens for allergen-specific immunotherapy: 10 years anniversary of immunotherapy with recombinant allergens. Allergy. 2011;66:775-83.
34. Wallner M, Pichler U, Ferreira F. Recombinant allergens for pollen immunotherapy. Immunotherapy. 2013;5:1323-38.
35. Andersson K, Lidholm J. Characteristics and immunobiology of grass pollen allergens. Int Arch Allergy Immunol. 2003;130:87-107.
36. Mari A. When does a protein become an allergen? Searching for a dynamic definition based on most advanced technology tools. Clin Exp Allergy. 2008;38: 1089-94.
37. Wallner M, Himly M, Neubauer A, et al. The influence of recombinant production on the immunologic behavior of birch pollen isoallergens. PLoS One. 2009;4:e8457.
38. Schmidt M, Hoffman DR. Expression systems for production of recombinant allergens. Int Arch Allergy Immunol. 2002;128:264-70.
39. Ferreira F, Ebner C, Kramer B, et al. Modulation of IgE reactivity of allergens by site-directed mutagenesis: potential use of hypoallergenic variants for immunotherapy. FASEB J. 1998;12:231-42.
40. Bonura A, Amoroso S, Locorotondo G, et al. Hypoallergenic variants of the Parietaria judaica major allergen Par j 1: a member of the non-specific lipid transfer protein plant family. Int Arch Allergy Immunol. 2001;126:32-40.
41. Son DY, Scheurer S, Hoffmann A, Haustein D, Vieths S. Pollen-related food allergy: cloning and immunological analysis of isoforms and mutants of Mal d 1, the major apple allergen, and Bet v 1, the major birch pollen allergen. Eur J Nutr. 1999;38:201-15.
42. Beezhold DH, Hickey VL, Sussman GL. Mutational analysis of the IgE epitopes in the latex allergen Hev b 5. J Allergy Clin Immunol. 2001;107:1069-76.
43. Karisola P, Mikkola J, Kalkkinen N, et al. Construction of hevein (Hev b 6.02) with reduced allergenicity for immunotherapy of latex allergy by comutation of six amino acid residues on the conformational IgE epitopes. J Immunol. 2004:172:2621-8.
44. Swoboda I, De Weerd N, Bhalla PL, et al. Mutants of the major ryegrass pollen allergen, Lol p 5, with reduced IgE-binding capacity: candidates for grass pollen-specific immunotherapy. Eur J Immunol. 2002;32:270-80.
45. Schramm G, Kahlert H, Suck R, et al. "Allergen engineering": variants of the timothy grass pollen allergen Phl p 5b with reduced IgE-binding capacity but conserved T cell reactivity. J Immunol. 1999:162:2406-14.

46. Wu, CH, Lee MF, Yang JS, Tseng CY. IgE-binding epitopes of the American cockroach Per a 1 allergen. Mol Immunol. 2002;39:459-64.
47. Tamborini E, Faccini S, Lidholm J, et al. Biochemical and immunological characterization of recombinant allergen Lol p 1. Eur J Biochem. 1997;249:886-94.
48. Singh BP, Banerjee B, Naik P, et al. Immune response to n-terminal and c-terminal deletion mutants of Aspergillus fumigatus major allergen ASP F 3. Ind J Clin Biochem. 2006;21:20-7.
49. Kundig TM, Senti G, Schnetzler G, et al. Der p 1 peptide on virus-like particles is safe and highly immunogenic in healthy adults. J Allergy Clin Immunol. 2006;117:1470-6.
50. Rosewich M, Schulze J, Eickmeier O, et al. Tolerance induction after specific immunotherapy with pollen allergoids adjuvanted by monophosphoryl lipid A in children. Clin Exp Immunol. 2010;160:403-10.
51. Creticos PS, Schroeder JT, Hamilton RG, et al. Immunotherapy with a ragweed-toll-like receptor 9 agonist vaccine for allergic rhinitis. N Engl J Med. 2006;355: 1445-55.
52. Huleatt JW, Jacobs AR, Tang J, et al. Vaccination with recombinant fusion proteins incorporating Toll-like receptor ligands induces rapid cellular and humoral immunity. Vaccine. 2007;25:763-75.
53. Schulke S, Waibler Z, Mende MS, et al. Fusion protein of TLR5-ligand and allergen potentiates activation and IL-10 secretion in murine myeloid DC. Mol Immunol. 2010;48:341-50.
54. Schulke S, Burggraf M, Waibler Z, et al. A fusion protein of flagellin and ovalbumin suppresses the TH2 response and prevents murine intestinal allergy. J Allergy Clin Immunol. 2011;128:1340-8.e1312.
55. Thunberg S, Neimert-Andersson T, Cheng Q, et al. Prolonged antigen-exposure with carbohydrate particle based vaccination prevents allergic immune responses in sensitized mice. Allergy. 2009;64:919-26.
56. Niespodziana K, Focke-Tejkl M, Linhart B, et al. A hypoallergenic cat vaccine based on Fel d 1-derived peptides fused to hepatitis B PreS. J Allergy Clin Immunol. 2011;127:1562-70.e1566.
57. Ishii Y. [Allergen-specific immunotherapy utilizing mechanisms for immune regulation]. Nihon Rinsho Men'eki Gakkai kaishi. 2008;31:392-8.
58. Lim HF, Nair P. Efficacy and safety of reslizumab in patients with moderate to severe eosinophilic asthma. Exp Rev Respir Med. 2015;9:135-42.
59. Kerekov N, Michova A, Muhtarova M, et al. Suppression of allergen-specific B lymphocytes by chimeric protein-engineered antibodies. Immunobiology. 2014;219:45-52.
60. Zhao BB, Diao JD, Liu ZM, et al. Generation of a chimeric dust mite hypoallergen using DNA shuffling for application in allergen-specific immunotherapy. Int J Clin Exp Pathol. 2014;7:3608-19.
61. Chen KW, Fuchs G, Sonneck K, et al. Reduction of the in vivo allergenicity of Der p 2, the major house-dust mite allergen, by genetic engineering. Mol Immunol. 2008;45:2486-98.
62. Chen KW, Blatt K, Thomas WR, et al. Hypoallergenic Der p 1/Der p 2 combination vaccines for immunotherapy of house dust mite allergy. J Allergy Clin Immunol. 2012;130:435-43.e434.
63. O'Hehir RE, Prickett SR, Rolland JMT. Cell epitope peptide therapy for allergic diseases. Curr Allergy Asthma Rep. 2016;16:4.
64. Larche M. Peptide immunotherapy for allergic diseases. Allergy. 2007;62:325-31.
65. Marcotte GV, Braun CM, Norman PS, et al. Effects of peptide therapy on ex vivo T-cell responses. J Allergy Clin Immunol. 1998;101:506-13.
66. Pene J, Desroches A, Paradis L, et al. Immunotherapy with Fel d 1 peptides decreases IL-4 release by peripheral blood T cells of patients allergic to cats. J Allergy Clin Immunol. 1998;102:571-8.
67. Oldfield WL, Larche M, Kay AB. Effect of T-cell peptides derived from Fel d 1 on allergic reactions and cytokine production in patients sensitive to cats: a randomised controlled trial. Lancet. 2002;360:47-53.
68. Alexander C, Tarzi M, Larche M, Kay AB. The effect of Fel d 1-derived T-cell peptides on upper and lower airway outcome measurements in cat-allergic subjects. Allergy. 2005;60:1269-74.
69. Kammerer R, Chvatchko Y, Kettner A, Dufour N, Corradin G, Spertini F. Modulation of T-cell response to phospholipase A2 and phospholipase A2-derived peptides by conventional bee venom immunotherapy. J Allergy Clin Immunol. 1997;100:96-103.
70. Kitaoka M, Shin Y, Kamiya N, et al. Transcutaneous peptide immunotherapy of Japanese Cedar Pollinosis Using solid-in-oil nanodispersion technology. AAPS Pharm Sci Tech. 2015;16:1418-24.
71. Moldaver D, Larche M. Immunotherapy with peptides. Allergy. 2011;66:784-91.
72. Bellanti JA. Cytokines and allergic diseases: clinical aspects. Allergy Asthma Proceed. 1998;19:337-41.
73. Smarr CB, Bryce PJ, Miller SD. Antigen-specific tolerance in immunotherapy of Th2-associated allergic diseases. Crit Rev Immunol. 2013;33:389-414.
74. Stirling RG, Chung KF. Future treatments of allergic diseases and asthma. Br Med Bull. 2000;56:1037-53.
75. Borish LC, Nelson HS, Corren J, et al. Efficacy of soluble IL-4 receptor for the treatment of adults with asthma. J Allergy Clin Immunol. 2001;107:963-70.
76. Flood-Page PT, Menzies-Gow AN, Kay AB, Robinson DS. Eosinophil's role remains uncertain as anti-interleukin-5 only partially depletes numbers in asthmatic airway. Am J Resp Crit Care Med. 2003;167:199-204. .
77. Zhu D, Kepley CL, Zhang K, et al. A chimeric human-cat fusion protein blocks cat-induced allergy. Nat Med. 2005;11:446-9.
78. Holgate S, Casale T, Wenzel S, et al. The anti-inflammatory effects of omalizumab confirm the central role of IgE in allergic inflammation. J Allergy Clin Immunol. 2005;115:459-65.
79. Yalcin AD. Advances in anti-IgE therapy. BioMed Res Int. 2015;2015:317465.

80. Cox L, Platts-Mills TA, Finegold I, et al. American Academy of Allergy, Asthma & Immunology/American College of Allergy, Asthma and Immunology Joint Task Force Report on omalizumab-associated anaphylaxis. J Allergy Clini Immunol. 2007;120:1373-7.
81. Kukreja N, Sridhara S, Singh BP, Arora N. Effect of proteolytic activity of Epicoccum purpurascens major allergen, Epi p 1 in allergic inflammation. Clin Exp Immunol. 2008;154: 162-71.
82. Sudha VT, Arora N, Singh BP. Serine protease activity of Per a 10 augments allergen-induced airway inflammation in a mouse model. Eur J Clin Investig. 2009;39:507-16.
83. Kale SL, Arora N. Per a 10 activates human derived epithelial cell line in a protease dependent manner via PAR-2. Immunobiology. 2015;220:525-32.
84. Sagar Laxman Kale NA. Airway epithelial cells: barrier and much more. Ind J Allergy Asthma Immunol. 2013;27:99.
85. Saw S, Kale SL, Arora N. Serine protease inhibitor attenuates ovalbumin induced inflammation in mouse model of allergic airway disease. PLoS One. 2012;7:e41107.
86. Ishizaki M, Tanaka H, Kajiwara D, et al. Nafamostat mesilate, a potent serine protease inhibitor, inhibits airway eosinophilic inflammation and airway epithelial remodeling in a murine model of allergic asthma. J Pharmacol Sci. 2008;108:355-63.
87. Chen CL, Wang SD, Zeng ZY, et al. Serine protease inhibitors nafamostat mesilate and gabexate mesilate attenuate allergen-induced airway inflammation and eosinophilia in a murine model of asthma. J Allergy Clin Immunol. 2006;118:105-12.
88. He S, Gaca MD, Walls AF. A role for tryptase in the activation of human mast cells: modulation of histamine release by tryptase and inhibitors of tryptase. J Pharmacol Exp Ther. 1998;286:289-97.
89. Oh SW, Pae CI, Lee DK, et al. Tryptase inhibition blocks airway inflammation in a mouse asthma model. J Immunol. 2002;168:1992-2000.
90. Kale SL, Agrawal K, Gaur SN, Arora N. Cockroach protease allergen induces allergic airway inflammation via epithelial cell activation. Sci Rep. 2017;7:42341.
91. Agrawal K, Kale SL, Arora N. Protease activity of Per a 10 potentiates Th2 polarization by increasing IL-23 and OX40L. Eur J Immunol. 2015;45:3375-85.
92. Srivastava D, Mehta AK, Arora N, et al. Proteolytically inactive per a 10 allergen of Periplaneta americana modulates Th2 response and enhances IL-10 in mouse model. J Clin Immunol. 2010;30:426-34.

CHAPTER 21

Noninjective Allergen-specific Immunotherapy

Komarla Nagendra Prasad

INTRODUCTION

Rising trends in the incidence of allergy disorders are commonly seen in all walks of life and every corner of the world. The present knowledge of cellular and molecular mechanisms of allergy is a need for effective treatment. Type-I allergies are IgE dependent and are allergy-based inflammation with clinical manifestations of allergy disease such as conjunctivitis, rhinitis, asthma, urticaria, and atopic dermatitis. Allergic asthma is one of the most serious allergy disorders, and it has become an epidemic in many parts of the world with high prevalence in Western countries. Allergic inflammation is driven by exposure to allergens through specific IgE-dependent mechanism, resulting in tissue inflammation by eosinophils and chemical mediators such as vasoactive amines. Allergen-specific IgE plays an important role in eosinophil recruitment during allergic late phase inflammatory response. Eosinophils, in turn, play an important role in pathogenesis of asthma, allergic inflammation by mediating injury to the mucosal surfaces including bronchial mucosa. Eosinophils generate proteins called eosinophilic cationic protein (ECP), increase airway reactions and contribute to bronchoconstriction characteristic of asthma. In addition, B cells producing IgE and infiltrating eosinophils and many other inflammatory cells including the mast cells, basophils, macrophages, dendrite cells, neutrophils, natural killer cells, epithelial cells, and T cells are involved in allergic inflammation. These cells produce more of inflammatory mediators including histamine, cysteine, leukotrienes, chemokine, and cytokines, which are involved in initiating, regulating, and amplifying the allergic inflammatory response.

Recent understanding of T-helper (Th) cells, which produce specific proinflammatory cytokines in response to sensitized allergens by Th2. These Th2 cytokines producing a subset of T-helper cells include interleukin (IL) 4, IL-5, IL-6, IL-9, IL-10, and IL-13. IL-4 cytokine is prominently responsible for stimulating differentiation of Th2 cells from naïve T-helper cells.

In contrast, Th1 cells, another subtype of T helper cells, produce interferon γ (IFN-γ) which tends to oppose the production and reactions of IL-4 and inhibits the allergic response. The Th1 cells from naïve T-helper cell are induced by IL-12, which is produced by macrophages and dendrite cells. IL-12 and IFN-γ inhibit allergen-induced eosinophil recruitment, Th2 cytokine synthesis airway hyper-reactivity, and IgE synthesis. The events that promote Th1 phenotypic bias by promoting the production of IL-12, IFN-γ cytokines, and/or retrieving the production of Th2 cytokines may have a position to limit allergic disease including asthma. The production of IFN-γ antagonizes the effect of IL-4 and IL-5 and leads to IgG2 secretion rather than IgE in allergen-specific immunotherapy and acts rather as a disease-modifying intervention than symptom reducing.[1]

The most efficient mechanisms in allergy management are the avoidance or minimization of the contact with specific sensitized allergens. This is not practicable in most of the cases. Pharmacotherapy provides a well-acting and well-accepted symptomatic treatment, which can be applied locally or systemically over a long period, which reduces active allergy inflammation but without immunomodulation. The allergy inflammation retrieves symptoms on cessation of pharmacotherapy and occasionally induces its own limited adverse events on long-term use. The anti-IgE (omalizumab) is effective in generating passive immunomodulation to reduce allergy inflammation by downregulation of IgE, IgE receptors on mast cells and the sustained efficacy on withdrawal is minimal.

In 1911, Leonard Noon proposed that the inoculation of grass pollen extracts would benefit the patients suffering from hay fever and sensitive to grass pollen.[2] He administered increasing doses of pollen extracts at 7–14 days interval injections over a period of several months and induced 100-fold reduction in conjunctival sensitivity to grass pollen. John Freeman, who followed up 20 subjects during the grass pollen season, reported the clinical condition of Noon's work in the same year.[3] He demonstrated decreased symptoms during pollen season and increased tolerance to conjunctival challenge in 18 subjects. Initially, the inoculation treatment was given a course of weekly injections to few subjects treated during the season. In 1920, perennial treatment showed the advantages of greater efficiency, necessitating fewer injections per year.[4] After a few decades, in 1963 Lowell and Franklin conducted a double-blind study on the effectiveness and specificity of injection therapy in ragweed hay fever.[5] A series of annual studies on ragweed hay fever was conducted by Johns Hopkins in 1963 by comparing the response to preseasonal injections of crude ragweed extract, purified ragweed antigen E (Amb a I), or a placebo-containing histamine.[6] Meta-analysis with 18 prospective, blinded, placebo-controlled studies of immunotherapy for allergic rhinitis (AR) was published in English between 1966 and 1996;[7] among which, seven studies were on grass extracts, six studies on ragweed, two studies on *Dermatophagoides pteronyssinus*, two studies on mountain cedar, and one on Alternaria. Seventeen out of the 18 studies favored the active treatment, symptom improvement with an odds risk of 1.81. Meta-analysis of 20 randomized-controlled trials published between 1977 and 1997 conclude that odds ratio was 3.2 for symptom improvement with all allergens and 4.2 for reduction in medication with house dust mite immunotherapy.[8] The results were confirmed in 67 papers published between 1954 and 1998.[9] Lowell and Franklin established the immune specificity of allergen immunotherapy (AIT).[5] Many studies address the issue of effective doses for AIT and conclude that high doses are more effective than moderate doses or very low doses of allergens.

The World Allergy Organization (WAO) document defines an allergenic extract as follows: "Allergen extract means a preparation of an allergen obtained by extraction of the active constituents from animal or vegetable substances with a suitable menstruum".[10,11] Allergen is a biological product, such as molds, insects, house dust mites, and animal dander, which are capable of inducing allergy symptoms. The allergen extracts are administered to subject for diagnosis, prevention, and treatment of allergy diseases. The WAO adopted the word allergen vaccine to indicate the vaccines that modify or downregulate the immune response for allergic diseases. Evidence based on AIT is the most important published data from the WAO document.[10,11]

The only accepted, curative, and effective immunomodulation in allergy disorder is by allergen specific immunotherapy (ASI) and recently called "allergy vaccine". The subcutaneous immunotherapy (SCIT) undoubtedly has clinical efficacy and proved beyond century but displays several inconveniences such as the need to visit doctor for its administration, invasiveness, which is not tolerated psychologically especially in children. Due to the possible local side effects and rarely systemic effects of SCIT, its recommendation by medical professionals became less popular. In few countries, the use of SCIT by trained professionals was restricted by regulatory agencies with emergency management facility. Noninjection immunotherapy was emerged to avoid these inconveniences and some forms, such as sublingual and intranasal applications, etc., which accomplish the goal successfully. Number of placebo-controlled, double-blind studies demonstrate clinical and immunological efficacy. John Freeman with Leonard Noon described AIT inoculation by subcutaneous routes and later rush desensitization to shorten the time required to reach maintenance dose and to reduce the inconvenience to the subject in which injection was administered every 1½ to 2 hours throughout 14 hours a day for 3–4 days to reach maintenance dose.[12]

NONINJECTIVE ROUTES OF ADMINISTRATION (LOCAL ROUTES)

The problem of subjects with investment of time to visit physician who administer SCIT, money and invasiveness demand the replacement of SCIT. The allergen extracts by local noninjective routes with potential advantage over subcutaneous injection being administered safely at home by the subject, thereby greatly decreasing investment and inconvenience. Four noninjective routes were being studied and two were approved for clinical application.

Oral Immunotherapy

Oral administration of allergen extracts was examined in the beginning of the 1920s but was abandoned by most of the clinicians as it is less effective than the injection therapy and causes gastrointestinal side effects.[13] In the 1980s, the oral immunotherapy was re-examined with birch pollen extract in patients with AR in Scandinavia.[14] Administration of approximately 200 times the conventional SCIT dose over 2 months birch pollen season results in significant reduction in end-organ sensitivity, some reduction in symptoms with increase in allergen-specific IgG, and reduction in the allergen-specific IgE.[15] Many gastrointestinal side effects were reported in several studies and was expensive, and its clinical use was virtually abandoned in the early 1990s.

Bronchial Immunotherapy

In 1950, bronchial immunotherapy (BIT) was proposed, and Double-blind, placebo-controlled (DBPC) was performed in the 1990s.[16] Two DBPC studies were done with dust mites, one group with 22 adult subjects treated for 3 months in which no significant improvement was found. In the other study with 24 adults treated for 2 years, a significant improvement was seen in the majority of the subjects in FEV_1 after BIT. The unfavorable risk/benefit ratio of BIT was completely abandoned.[17,18]

Nasal Immunotherapy

There were 18 DBPC studies on nasal immunotherapy (NIT), 17 studies showed a significant reduction of symptoms and/or drug intake score.[19,20] The clinical efficacy was comparable to SCIT as far as rhinitis is concerned. In some studies, there was a reduction of nasal response to specific challenge. The early initiation of NIT to induce symptoms was overcome with the use of micronized dry powders, which were effective and do not induce rhinitis symptoms. Due to incorrect technique of its application, there were bronchospasms in three cases, which was reported in these studies.[21] The only long-term follow-up study suggested that NIT does not maintain its clinical efficacy once discontinued.[22] Preseasonal course is needed every year. To simplify the mode of administration and to improve the compliance, a schedule with a single and steady dosage was proposed. The dose to be administered is selected by means of the end-point cutaneous technique and then remains fixed for the entire treatment course. NIT requires good training and some precautions in order to avoid inhalation into the deep airways. Premedication with nasal disodium cromoglycate before each dose was suggested. With these setbacks, the NIT was progressively declining in its routine application.

Sublingual Immunotherapy

Sublingual immunotherapy (SLIT) has many advantages over SCIT treatment. It has shown efficacy for AR and asthma sensitive to house dust mites, pollens, and molds. Pollen studies include parietaria, grass, ragweed, and trees pollens. Treatment of children with atopic dermatitis or nasal allergy may even help to prevent the progression of asthma.[23]

Mechanisms of SLIT

The immunological characteristics of the oral mucosa is that it is a immune-privileged organ. Antigens derived from food proteins and different commensal and pathogenic microbes are in regular contact with oral mucosal immune system, immune homeostasis is maintained by local pro-tolerogenic mechanisms counteracting allergic reactions and inflammations.[24] The physical barrier is represented by the squamous epithelium, which lines the masticatory mucosa except at sublingual and vestibular areas are covered by lining mucosa with exocrine glands.[25] The dendritic cells (DCs) which take up antigens in the epithelium of the mucosa migrate to basal lamina to present the antigens to oral lymphoid foci within oral mucosa to T cells to induce effective immune response.[26] It has shown that the antigens stay in the mucosa for up to 20 hours after administration.[27] Tracer studies of radioactive-labeled allergen showed that allergen retained within the oral mucosa for at least 2 hours and up to 18–20 hours following sublingual administration of allergen.[28] Studies using radioactive-labeled parietaria delivered sublingually showed plasma levels peaked in 2 hours.[29] Sublingual antigens act on antigen presenting cells in the mucosa to develop tolerance to the allergens. Local "mucosal immunity" appears to play a significant role.[30]

Oral mucosal DCs are concomitantly stimulated by microbial antigens present under physiological conditions in high numbers in the oral mucosa via toll-like receptor 2 (TLR2) or TLR4, which are highly expressed by oral mucosal DCs in contrast to epidermal DCs.[31] Healthy oral mucosa comprises mainly myeloid DCs, which expressed oral mucosal Langerhans cells (oLCs).[32] Studies on ex vivo isolated human oral mucosal tissue using dye labeled grass allergen phleum pratense (Phl p5) revealed that the capacity of oLCs to take up allergens reaches a threshold after a defined time of allergen contact and at a specific allergen concentration applied.[27] Up to this threshold, a further increase in the applied dose does not enhance the amount of allergen uptake by oLCs any further. This is in line with dose-dependent efficacy seen in clinical studies performed with grass pollen tablets.[33,34] The epithelium of the sublingual region is thinner than that of other oral mucosal sites, resorption of drugs is higher at this site. The ratio of oLCs to mast cells is higher in sublingual region compared to vestibulum.[35] As a consequence, application of the allergens to the vestibular region instead of the sublingual region might be helpful in children below 3 years or in subjects with sublingual swelling and itching in the clinical practice to circumvent or minimize mast cell-related side effects of SLIT.

Lower number of subepithelial mast cells but higher number of T cells was detected in subjects using SLIT.[36] In parallel, the amount of T cells expressing the marker of activated and regulatory T-cell forkhead box protein 3 (FoxP3) was significantly higher in the oral epithelium of SLIT-treated subjects compared to the placebo group. Data obtained with the help of murine model systems revealed that the amount of allergen-specific IgE in the nasal mucosa decreases during SLIT.[37] Enhancement of FoxP3+CD4+CD25+ T-regulatory cells (Treg) and IL-10 in the peripheral blood, and IL-18 and the signaling lymphocytic activation molecule was observed under SLIT.[38-40] An increase in serum IgG4 and peak seasonal IgA1/IgA2 reduced the number of inflammatory cells infiltrating target organs, as well as a reduction in ECP went along with SLIT.[40] Bacterial toxins are useful adjuvants to deliver antigens to major histocompatibility pathways.[41]

Clinically Efficacy of SLIT

The ASI by SLIT is administering allergens by sublingual or vestibular mucosa in the form of drops, sprays, stripes, or tablets. Randomized controlled clinical trials (RCTs) were initiated to evaluate the efficacy of SLIT and were assessed by assessment of symptom severity and rescue medication used during natural exposure to allergens. Double-blind, placebo-controlled (DBPC)-RCT studies are ideal methodological design adopted with results considered the efficacy as per the WAO.[42] In 1986, SLIT was first described in DBPC trial. The subsequent data on efficacy though the studies were heterogenous, expressed significantly improved in 1998 recorded four DBPC studies on SLIT in adults with allergic terms of degree of symptoms and reduction in medication score.[43,44] WAO position paper on rhinitis (AR).[45] AR and its impact on asthma reviewed 10 DBPC studies and indicated the efficacy with high-allergen dose (SLIT at least 100 times the cumulative dose of SCIT) on AR induced by pollens and mites, confirming with safety. Wilson Cochrane meta-analysis on the efficacy and safety of SLIT in AR concludes that SLIT is safe, and it significantly reduces symptoms and medication requirements in AR.[44] In 2006, the WAO recognized the cumulative evidence that SLIT represents a viable alternative to SCIT and encouraged to continue clinical investigation to characterize optimal techniques.[45]

Double-blind, placebo-controlled studies from Europe (Italy and France) began in the 1990s. Tari et al.[46] in 1990 documented dust mite antigens for 12–18 months using SLIT. AR and asthma symptoms improved among children who were treated with SLIT. There was a significant decrease in symptoms as well as medication use. In 1994, after 24 months of treatment, a decrease in specific IgE antibodies to dust mites was found.[47] In India, the author at Bengaluru Allergy Center treated over 100,000 subjects with SLIT for the past 15 years and found a decrease in symptoms and medication scores with enhanced health-related quality of life (HRQL) achieving a sustained effect on cessation after 3–5 years of SLIT.

A review article by Passalacqua and Canonica[48] in 2001 reported on 18 studies using SLIT in double-blind, placebo-controlled trials. Sixteen of these studies involving the most common allergens showed improved symptoms and decrease medication in rhinitis. Studies also showed efficacy for asthma and were reported in adults and children. Safety profiles were good using current dosing regimens.[49-51] No life-threatening reactions have occurred.

The first meta-analysis of SLIT for AR that included 22 trials with 979 subjects concludes that SLIT was significantly more effective than placebo.[52] Meta-analysis in asthma including 25 trials with more than 1000 adults and children demonstrated significant effect of SLIT on symptoms score, medication, and pulmonary function.[53] Subsequently, one meta-analysis focused on children between the age of 4–18 years having AR involving 10 trials enrolling 484 patients showed SLIT to be effective than placebo.[54] A meta-analysis of asthma in children included 9 trials enrolling 441 patients showed a significant reduction in asthma symptoms and medication[55] and all these were heterogeneous trials with varying sample sizes, publication biases and discrepancies in data collection and studies provide suggestive evidence.[56]

There were eight randomized open-label controlled trials, assessing the clinical efficacy of SLIT, compared with controlled group who are on drugs.[57-64] Two demonstrated a significant reduction in nonspecific bronchial hyper-responsiveness.[60-62,64] One study evaluated the safety of non-up-dosing regimen,[59] and another study designed[63] to demonstrate with two non-crossing allergens (birch and grass), which are overall more effective than single allergen in both pollen seasons.

Forty-two trials with a total of 3,958 subjects having allergic conjunctivitis, 2011 had SLIT and 1947 had placebo and showed reduced symptoms of allergic conjunctivitis, redness, itchiness and watery eyes compared to placebo.[65,66]

Comparing SCIT and SLIT

One double-dummy, double-blind study without placebo group conducted grass pollen study showed clinical efficacy of SLIT equivalent to SCIT.[67] Another DBDDPC study with birch pollen compared SLIT and SCIT; symptoms were reduced by about one-third in SLIT group and one-half in SCIT group with no significant difference between treatments. There were three and four adverse reactions with SCIT and none in SLIT group.[68] Four open studies and one by Bernardis P et al., study with Alternaria tenuis with rhinitis were having significant difference in favor of SLIT.[69] A study having 43 subjects with rhinitis, sensitive to mite for immunological observation was significantly in favor of SCIT.[70,71] The open comparison in mite showed that clinical improvement was more with SCIT especially asthma symptoms and SLIT controlled rhinitis symptoms well. Mauro et al.[71] compared SCIT and SLIT in 47 patients with birch allergy and found no difference between the two treatments. In seasonal symptom score although specific IgG4 significantly increased only with SCIT.

A controversial aspect in these published data is variable dose. The dose used with SLIT ranges between 2 and 375 times the amount used with SCIT. Response to low and high dose generated positive and negative results. A clear dose-response relationship has been formally demonstrated for grass extracts, where optimal dose is identified to be 15–25 µg of major allergen per day, which is roughly 50 times the monthly dose of SCIT. There is no consensus on whether the best regimen is preseasonal, co-seasonal, or continuous administration. Majority of trials utilized preseasonal regimen but this cannot be immediately extrapolated to all extracts and to all patients. The maintenance phase without buildup phase with few trials has shown to be safe.

Comparing SLIT with gold standard SCIT, one double-dummy without placebo with grass pollen allergic patients showed clinical efficacy of SLIT equivalent to SCIT.[72] An open trial 12-month study in *Alternaria* allergic patient showed clinical improvement in symptom and medication score in AR.[73] Open trial with mites showed clinical improvement prompt with SCIT in asthma symptoms and SLIT controlled with rhinitis symptoms.[74] In an open-label study with SCIT and SLIT in 47 patients having birch allergy, no difference in seasonal symptom score was found between SLIT and SCIT; allergen-specific IgG4 significantly increased in SCIT.[75]

The cumulative amount of allergen administered in the course of a year is generally 20–200 times greater with SLIT forms of immunotherapy compared with SCIT. In some studies, the daily dose of allergenic protein in micrograms is equivalent to the dose given every 2–4 weeks in SCIT.

A range of allergen doses were evaluated in a dose-exploratory phase I safety study of patients with seasonal allergic rhinoconjunctivitis treated with grass pollen SLIT tablets.[76] Eighty-four subjects were randomized to seven different Timothy grass tablet strengths: 25,000; 75,000; 100,000; 300,000; 500,000; 750,000; and 1 million SQ-T units. In this system, 100,000 SQ-T units was equivalent to ~20 µg phleum p 5, a dose similar to the effective maintenance dose for grass pollen SCIT. No serious or systemic adverse events were observed in the study, providing evidence that daily doses as high as 1 million SQ-T units (~200 µg phleum p 5) were well tolerated by SLIT.

A similar safety study of the 5-grass standardized allergen tablet for SLIT was performed to establish a tolerated dose for subsequent trials.[77] Doses of 100–500 IR were evaluated for safety and tolerability in 30 grass-allergic adults over a 0-day treatment period. Through incorporation of a 5-day up-dosing regimen, high-dose treatment with 500 IR (~42 µg Group 5 major allergens) could be reached without significant untoward adverse events. The majority of adverse events were mild to moderate with the most common being oral pruritus, throat irritation, and tongue swelling. No serious adverse events occurred.

SUMMARY

The present treatment of respiratory allergy is based on allergen avoidance, pharmacological treatment, and immunotherapy. Immunotherapy is an allergen response modifier and the response with sustained effect on withdrawal of therapy. Noninjective immunotherapy—SLIT is gaining popularity over the injective immunotherapy—SCIT due to improved convenience, compliance, and safety. SLIT opens the door for expansion of immunotherapy to a first-line treatment option in allergies. Immunotherapy (SCIT/SLIT) prescribed by a specialist (allergist/allergologist/allergy physician) who were trained well in the field, with clinical history, in vitro (sIgE) and in vivo (SPT) diagnosis established. Remote diagnosis exclusively by sIgE is incomplete and inconclusive and not advisable. SLIT is indicated in type-1 subjects with low compliance with SCIT and subject's choice. ASI by SLIT or SCIT should be the first line of treatment in the early stages of sign and symptoms of Allergy March and never considered as a last choice of treatment when rest of therapy fails. SLIT or SCIT is not an alternative to drugs for controlling the symptoms, but must be used in combination therapy in alleviating allergy symptoms to enhance HRQL.

REFERENCES

1. Haelden BM, Kay AB, Larche M. Peptide-mediated immune responses in specific immunotherapy. Int Arch Allergy Immunol. 2000;122:229-37.
2. Noon L. Prophylactic inoculation against hay fever. Lancet I. 1911;177:1572-3.
3. Freeman J. Further observations on the treatment of hay fever by hypodermic inoculations of pollen vaccine. Lancet II. 1911;178:814-7.
4. Brown A. The Perennial treatment of seasonal hay fever. J Allergy. 1932;3:113-9.
5. Lowell FC, Franklin W. A double-blind study of the effectiveness and specificity of injection therapy in ragweed hay fever. N Engl J Med. 1965;273:675-9.
6. Norman PS, Winkenwerder WL, Lichtenstein LM. Immunotherapy of hay fever with ragweed antigen E: comparisons with whole pollen extract and placebos. J Allergy. 1968;42:93-108.
7. Ross RN, Nelson HS, Finegold I. Effectiveness of specific immunotherapy in the treatment of allergic rhinitis: an analysis of randomized, prospective, single or double blind, placebo-controlled studies. Clin Ther. 2000;22:342-50.
8. Abramson MJ, Puy RM, Weiner JM. Is allergen immunotherapy effective in asthma? A meta-analysis of randomized controlled trials. Am J Respir Crit Care Med. 1995;151: 969-74.
9. Abramson M, Puy R, Weiner JJ. Immunotherapy in asthma an updated systematic review. Allergy. 1999;54:1022-41.
10. Bousquet J, Lockey RF, Malling HJ. eds. WHO position paper-allergen immunotherapy. Therapeutic vaccines for allergic diseases. Allergy. 1998;54:1069-88.
11. Bousquet J, Lockey RF, Malling HJ, eds. Allergen Immunotherapy, therapeutic vaccines for allergic diseases. A WHO Position Paper (edited with the WHO panel members). J Allergy Clin Immunol. 1998;102:558-62.
12. Freeman J. "Rush" inoculation. With special reference to hay fever treatment. Lancet. 1930;215:744-7.
13. Zeller M. Oral ragweed pollen therapy. J. Allergy. 1939;10:579.
14. Taudorf E, Laursen L, Lanner A, et al. Oral Immunotherapy in birch pollen hay fever. J Allergy Clin Immunol. 1987;80:153-61.
15. Taudorf E, Laursen L, Lanner A, et al. Specific IgE, IgG and IgA antibody response to oral immunotherapy in birch pollinosis. J Allergy clin Immunol. 1989;83:589-94.
16. Herexeimer H. Bronchial hypersensitisation and hyposensitisation in man. Int Arch Allergy Appl Immunol. 1951;40:40-57.
17. Crimi E, Voltolini S, Troise C, Gianiorio P, Crimi P. Local immunotherapy with Dermaptophagoides extract in asthma. J Allergy Clin Immunol. 1991;87:721-8.
18. Tari MG, Mancino M, Monti G. Immunotherapy by inhalation of allergen in powder in house dust allergic asthma. A double blind study. J Invest Allergol Clin Immunol. 1992;2:59-67.
19. Canonica GW, Passalacqua G. Non-injection routes of immunotherapy. J Allergy Clin Immunol. 2003;111:437-48.
20. Schumacher MJ, Pain MCF. Intranasal immunotherapy with polymerized grass pollen allergens. Allergy. 1981;37: 241-5.
21. D' Amato G, Lobefalo G, Liccardi G, Cazzola M. A double-blind placebo-controlled trial of local nasal immunotherapy in allergic rhinitis to *Parietaria* pollen. Clin Exp Allergy. 1995;25:141-8.
22. Passalacqua G, Albano M, Pronzato C, et al. Nasal immunotherapy to *Parietaria*: long-term follow-up of a double-blind study. Clin Exp Allergy. 1997;27:904-8.
23. Mastrandrea F, Serio G, Minelli M, et al. Specific sublingual immunotherapy in atopic dermatitis. Results of a 6-year follow-up of 35 consecutive patients. Allergol Immunopathol. 2000;28:54-62.
24. Paster BJ, Boches SK, Galvin JL, et al. Bacterial diversity in human subgingival plaque. J Bacteriol. 2001;183: 3770-83.
25. Lu FX, Jacobson RS. Oral mucosal immunity and HIV/SIV infection. J Dent Res. 2007;86:216-26.
26. Jotwani R, Palucka AK, Al-Quotub M, et al. Mature dendritic cells infiltrate the T-cell-rich region of oral mucosa in chronic periodontitis: in situ, in vivo, and in vitro studies. J Immunol. 2001;167:4693-700.
27. Van Wilsem EJ, Van Hoogstraten IM, Breve J, et al. Dendritic cells of the oral mucosa and the induction of oral tolerance. A local affair. Immunology. 1994;83:128-32.
28. Bagnasco M. Absorption and distribution kinetics of the major *Parietaria* allergen administered by noninjectable routes to healthy human beings. J Allergy Clin Immunol. 1997;100:13-18.
29. Bagnasco M, Mariani G, Passalacqua G, et al. Absorption and distribution kinetics of the major *Parietaria judaica* allergen (Par j 1) administered by noninjectable routes in healthy human beings. J Allergy Cin Immunol. 1997;100:122-9.
30. Scadding GW, Shamji MH, Jacobson MR, et al. Sublingual grass pollen immunotherapy is associated with increases

in sublingual Foxp3 expressing cells and elevated allergen-specific immunoglobulin G4, immunoglobulin A and serum inhibitory activity for immunoglobulin E facilitated allergen binding to B cells. Clin Exp Allergy. 2010;40:598-606.

31. Brown JL, Frew AJ. The efficacy of oromucosal immunotherapy in respiratory allergy. Clin Exp Allergy. 2001;31:8-10.
32. Allam JP, Duan Y, Winter J, et al. Tolerogenic T cells, Th1/Th17 cytokines and TLR2/TLR4 expressing dendritic cells predominate the microenvironment within distinct oral mucosal sites. Allergy. 2010:66:532-9.
33. Allam JP, Novak N, Fuchs C, et al. Characterization of dendritic cells from human oral mucosa: a new Langerhans' cell type with high constitutive Fc epsilon RI expression. J Allergy Clin Immunol. 2003;112:141-8.
34. Allam JP, Wurtzen PA, Reinartz M, et al. Phl p 5 resorption in human oral mucosa leads to dose dependent and time-dependent allergen binding by oral mucosal Langerhans cells, attenuates their maturation, and enhances their migratory and TGF-beta 1 and IL-10-producing properties. J Allergy Clin Immunol. 2010;126:638-45.
35. Didier A, Malling HJ, Worm M, et al. Optimal dose, efficacy and safety of once-daily sublingual immunotherapy with a 5-grass pollen tablet for seasonal allergic rhinitis. J Allergy Cin Immunol. 2007;120:1338-45.
36. Allam JP, Stojanovski G, Friedrichs N, et al. Distribution of Langerhans cells and mast cells within the human oral mucosa: new application sites of allergens in sublingual immunotherapy. Allergy. 2008;63:720-7.
37. Laaksonen K, Junikka M, Lahesmaa R, et al. In vitro allergen-induced mRNA expression of signalling lymphocytic activation molecule by PBMC of patients with allergic rhinitis is increased during specific pollen immunotherapy. J Allergy Clin Immunol. 2003;112:1171-7.
38. Larche M, Akdis CA, Valenta R. Immunological mechanisms of allergen-specific immunotherapy. Nat Rev Immunol. 2006;6:761-71.
39. Akdis CA, Barlan IB, Bahceciler N, Akdis M. Immunological mechanisms of sublingual immunotherapy. Allergy 2006;61:11-4.
40. Moingeon P, Batard T, Fadel R, et al. Immune mechanisms of allergen-specific sublingual immunotherapy. Allergy. 2006;61:151-65.
41. Mascarell L, Van OL, Moingeon P. Novel ways for immune intervention in immune therapy: mucosal allergy vaccines. Immunol Allergy Clin North Am. 2006;26:283-306, viii. Allergy. 2006;61:151-65.
42. Canonica GW, Baena-Cagnani CE, Bousquet J, et al. Recommendations for standardization of clinical trials with allergen-specific immunotherapy for respiratory allergy. A statement of a World Allergy Organisation (WAO) taskforce. Allergy. 2007;62:317-24.
43. Calderon MA, Alves B, Jacobson M, et al. Allergen injection immunotherapy for seasonal allergic rhinitis. Cochrane Database Syst Rev. 2007;CD001936.
44. Wilson DR, Lima MT, Durham SR. Sublingual immunotherapy for allergic rhinitis: systematic review and meta-analysis. Allergy. 2005;60:4-12.
45. Bousquet J. Sublingual immunotherapy: validated. Allergy. 2006;61:5. 2010;125:131-8.
46. Tari MG, Mancino M, Monti G. Efficacy of sublingual immunotherapy in patients with rhinitis and asthma due to house dust mite—A double-blind study. Allergol Immunopathol. 1990;18:277-84.
47. Tari MG, Mancino M, Madonna F, et al. Immunologic evaluation of 24-month course of sublingual immunotherapy. Allergol Immunopathol. 1994;22:209-16.
48. Passalacqua G, Canonica GW. Allergen-specific sublingual immunotherapy for respiratory allergy. Bio Drugs. 2001;15:509-19.
49. Lombardi C. Safety of sublingual immunotherapy with monomeric allergoid in adults: Multi post-marketing surveillance study. Allergy. 2001;56:989-92.
50. Andre C. Safety of sublingual immunotherapy in children and adults. Int Arch Allergy Immunol. 2000;121:229-34.
51. Di Rienzo V. Post-marketing surveillance study on the safety of sublingual immunotherapy in children. Allergy. 1999;54:1110-3.
52. Wilson DR, Torres L, Durham SR. Sublingual immunotherapy for allergic rhinitis. Allergy. 2005;61:3-8.
53. Calamita Z, Saconato H, Bronhara Pela A, Nagib Atallah A. Efficacy of sublingual immunotherapy in asthma. Systematic review of randomized clinical trials. Allergy. 2006;61:1162-72.
54. Penagos M, Compalati E, Tarantini F, et al. Efficacy of Sublingual immunotherapy in the treatment of allergic rhinitis in children. Meta-analysis of randomised controlled trials. Ann Allergy Asthma Immunol. 2006;97:141-8.
55. Penagos M, Passalacqua G, Compalati E, et al. Meta-analysis of the efficacy of sublingual immunotherapy in the treatment of allergic asthma in paediatric patients, 3 to 18 years of age. Chest. 2008;133:599-609.
56. Nieto A, Mazon A, Pamies R, et al. Sublingual immunotherapy for allergic respiratory diseases: an evaluation of meta-analyses. J Allergy Clin Immunol. 2009;124:157-61.
57. D' Ambrosio FP, Ricciardi L, Isola S, et al. Rush sublingual immunotherapy in *Parietaria* allergic patients. Allergol Immunopathol (Madr). 1996;24:146-51.
58. Gozalo F, Martín S, Rico P, et al. Clinical efficacy and tolerance of two-year *Lolium perenne* sublingual immunotherapy. Allergol Immunopathol (Madr). 1997;25:219-27.
59. Guerra L, Compalati E, Rogkakou A, et al. Randomized open comparison of the safety of SLIT in a no-updosing and traditional updosing schedule in patients with *Parietaria* allergy. Allergol Immunopathol (Madr). 2006;34:82-3.
60. Lombardi C, Gargioni S, Venturi S, et al. Controlled study of pre-seasonal immunotherapy with grass pollen extract in tablets: effect on bronchial hyper-reactivity. J Invest Allergol Clin Immunol. 2001;11:41-5.
61. Marogna M, Spadolini I, Massolo A, Canonica GW, Passalacqua G. Randomized controlled open study of sublingual immunotherapy for respiratory allergy in real-life: clinical efficacy and more. Allergy. 2004;59: 1205-10.

62. Marogna M, Spadolini I, Massolo A, et al. Clinical, functional, and immunologic effects of sublingual immunotherapy in birch pollinosis: a 3-year randomized controlled study. J Allergy Clin Immunol. 2005;115:1184-8.
63. Marogna M, Massolo A, Spadolini I, et al. Efficacy of sublingual immunotherapy with single or multiple allergens in polysensitized patients. Ann Allergy Asthma Immunol. 2007;98:274-80.
64. Marcucci F, Sensi L, Di Cara G, et al. Dose dependence of immunological response to sublingual immunotherapy. Allergy. 2005;60:952-6.
65. Calderon MA, Penagos M, Sheikh A, et al. Sublingual immunotherapy for treating allergic conjunctivitis (Review) S Evidence-based Child health. Cochrane Rev J. 2012;7:1041-154.
66. Quirino T, Iemoli E, Siciliani E, et al. Sublingual vs injective immunotherapy in grass pollen allergic patients: a double-blind double-dummy study. Clin Exp Allergy. 1996;26: 1253-61.
67. Khinchi S, Poulsen LK, Carat F, et al. Clinical efficacy of sublingual swallow and subcutaneous immunotherapy in patients with allergic rhinoconjunctivitis due to birch pollen. A double-blind double-dummy placebo-controlled study. Allergy. 2004;59:45-53.
68. Bernardis P, Agnoletto M, Puccinelli P, et al. Injective VS sublingual immunotherapy in *Alternaria tenuis* allergic patients. J Investig Allergol Clin Immunol. 1996:6:55-62.
69. Piazza I, Bizzarro N. Humoral response to subcutaneous, oral and nasal immunotherapy for allergic rhinitis due to *Dermatophagoides pteronyssinus*. Ann Allergy. 1993;71:461-9.
70. Mungan D, Misirligil Z, Gurbuz L. Comparison of the efficacy of subcutaneous and sublingual immunotherapy in mite sensitive patients with rhinitis and asthma: a placebo-controlled study. Ann Allergy Asthma Immunol. 1999;82:485-90.
71. Mauro M, Russello M, Incorvaia C, et al. Comparison of efficacy, safety and immunologic effects of subcutaneous and sublingual immunotherapy in birch pollinosis: a randomized study. Eur Ann Allergy Clin Immunol. 2007;39:112-9.
72. Severino M, Cortellini G, Bonadonna P, et al. Sublingual immunotherapy for large local reactions. Due to honeybee sting. Double-blind placebo controlled trial. J Allergy Clin Immunol. 2008;122:44-8.
73. Sieber J, De Geest S, Shah-Hosseini K, Mösges R. Medication persistence with long-term, specific grass pollen immunotherapy measured by prescription renewal rates. Curr Med Res Opin. 2011;27:855-61.
74. Mun MD, Shin JM, Han DH. Efficacy and safety of a once-daily sublingual immunotherapy without escalation regimen in house dust mite-induced allergic rhinitis International. Forum Allergy Rhinol. 2013;3:177-83.
75. Wilson DR, Torres LI, Durham SR. Sublingual immunotherapy for allergic rhinitis. Cochrane Database Syst Rev. 2003;CD002893. doi:10.1002/14651858.
76. Kleine-Tebbe J, Ribel M, Herold DA. Safety of a SQ-standardized grass allergen tablet for sublingual immunotherapy: a randomized, placebo-controlled trial. Allergy. 2006;61:181-4.
77. Larsen TH, Poulsen LK, Melac M, et al. Safety and tolerability of grass pollen tablets in sublingual immunotherapy—a phase-1 study. Allergy. 2006;61:1173-6.

CHAPTER 22

Sublingual Immunotherapy

BV Balachandra, PK Vedanthan

HISTORY

In the first century BC, Mithridates VI (131–63 BC), king of Pontus in the Asia Minor (presently Turkey), noted that ducks when fed plants known to be poisonous to humans did not manifest any apparent ill effects. While preparing himself for the ever-present possibility of a palace revolt, Mithridates VI sought to gain immunity from poisoning by swallowing small amounts of the poison (toad stool toxins) in gradually increasing doses. So successful was the outcome of his experiments that later he failed to achieve attempted suicide even after ingesting large doses of the same poison.[1] For many centuries, the technique of gaining tolerance or active immunity through incremental dosage schedules continued to be known as "Mithridasation."

INTRODUCTION

Allergen immunotherapy (AIT) was first described by Leonard Noon and John Freeman in 1911. Since that time, there have been several studies demonstrating the efficacy, safety, and dosage of AIT, as well as the development of newer technology in the manufacturing of allergy vaccines. AIT is the only established therapy which is disease-modifying treatment through an immunological mechanism. None of the therapeutic modalities have this distinction for allergic diseases. In spite of this advantage, AIT has not taken a stride; this is mainly due to the delay in clinical relief, time commitments, expenses involved as well as the risk of reactions with the subcutaneous route of administration. Hence, alternate safer methods of administration are being sought, and hence this discussion on sublingual immunotherapy (SLIT).

Depending upon the route of administration, AIT is broadly classified as subcutaneous immunotherapy (SCIT) and SLIT. There are several other forms of AIT, which are mentioned elsewhere.

MECHANISM OF ACTION

The immunological mechanisms of SLIT are similar to SCIT, though the magnitude of the change with SLIT in most parameters is moderately less than that with SCIT.

When SLIT vaccines are placed in the sublingual region and drops are held in this region for about 2 minutes, small amount is absorbed from the mucosa and taken up by dendritic cells (DCs), and the rest of the sublingual vaccines are swallowed or digested.

The precise mechanism by which oral mucosal tolerance is induced is unknown, but the route of allergen processing and presentation seems likely to be an important factor regarding how T cells respond. SLIT skews the immune response from Th2 to Th1. This occurs by the release of proinflammatory cytokines (IL10, TGF Beta) that stimulates Th1 cells and Treg cell activity and suppress Th2 activity.

The development and regulation of T-cell responses are initially controlled by DCs. The interactions between DCs and T cells determine whether the eventual response is active or tolerant. Induction of a tolerogenic phenotype of DCs would therefore seem to be a key immunologic event in SLIT. In humans, the predominant DCs in oral mucosa are conventional Langerhans cells (LCs). Oral LCs differ from skin LCs in their expression of various surface molecules, which indicate that they are immature cells. In vitro studies have shown that immature DCs tend to drive T-cell responses toward tolerance, i.e., toward Th1 response and away from Th2 response. Oral cavity contains mostly immature DCs, and these immature DCs are pro-tolerogenic.

Absorption of grass pollen antigens into human buccal mucosa slows down the maturation of the mucosal LCs and enhances their ability to produce pro-tolerogenic cytokines such as transforming growth factor (TGF)-β1 and interleukin (IL)-10, which again supports the concept of DC-driven tolerance as the main mechanism of SLIT.

When SLIT vaccines are placed in the sublingual region and drops are held in this region for about 2 minutes, small amount is absorbed from the mucosa and taken up by DCs, and the rest of the sublingual vaccines are swallowed or digested. The DCs absorb allergens and later move to regional lymph nodes as confirmed by the radioactively labeled allergen studies.[2] Allergens are taken up by mucosal DCs and then presented to T cells together with IL-12, biasing the response toward a Th1-like profile and away from the Pro-IgE Th2 profile. The increased release of IL-10 drives the immune cells to pro-tolerogenic. Interferon-γ (IFN-γ) and IL-2 secreted from Th1 cells further stimulate specific B-cell production of protective IgG1 and IgG4 antibodies, and decrease the release of the Th2 Pro-IgE cytokines IL-4 (Fig. 22.1). Oral mucosal DCs actively upregulate regulatory T (Treg) cell subtypes, including Forkhead box P3 protein (FOXP3)-expressing T cells, contributing to T-cell anergy mediated by IL-10 and TGF-β. These interconnected pathways lead to a reduction in allergic inflammation and symptoms (Fig. 22.1).

Sequential Effects of AIT

There is a decrease in the Mast cell and Basophil activity for degranulation locally.

- T-cell tolerance, induction of Treg cells, and suppression of Th2 cells.
- Decrease in tissue mast cells and eosinophils and release of their mediators, and decrease in the late-phase response.
- Early increase followed by a decrease in specific IgE.
- Increase in specific IgG4, and in some studies IgA and IgG1.

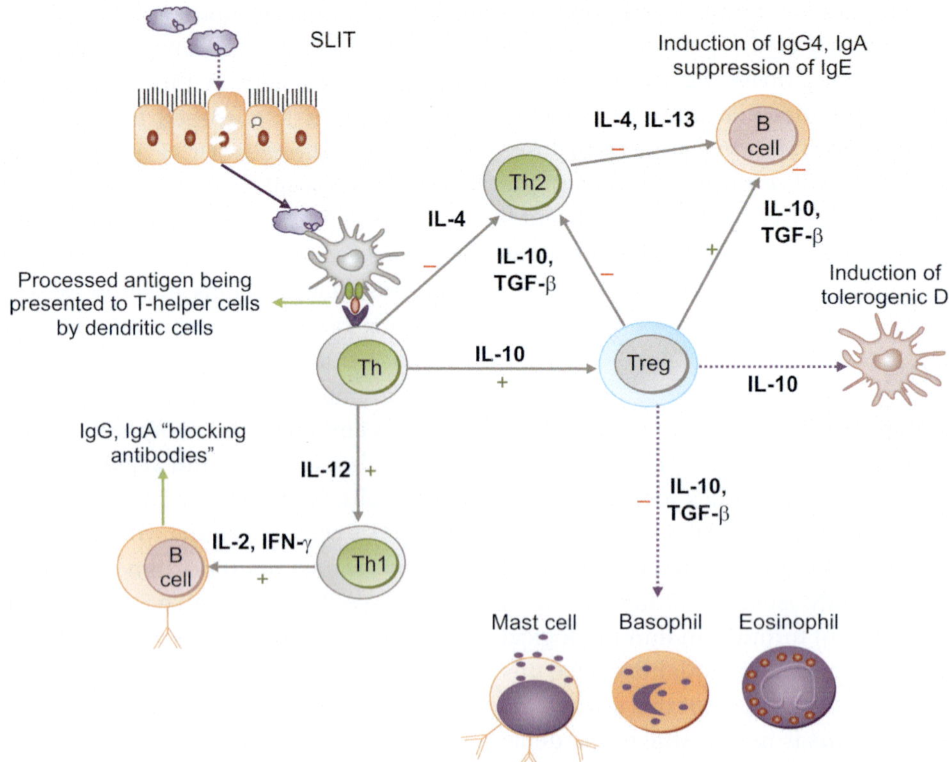

Fig. 22.1: Immune mechanism of sublingual immunotherapy (SLIT): SLIT allergens administered into sublingual region are taken up by mucosal dendritic cells (DCs) and presented to T cells in the cervical lymph nodes. In the presence of interleukin (IL)-12, the response is deviated toward a Th1-like profile. Further, Th1 cells stimulate B cells in the presence of interferon (IFN)-γ and IL-2 to produce immunoglobulin (IgG)- and IgA-blocking antibodies. DCs upregulate regulatory T (Treg) cells, which is an essential step in SLIT. Treg cells suppress proliferation, tissue infiltration, and proinflammatory cytokine production. IL-10 and transforming growth factor (TGF)-β induce IgG4 and IgA from B cells and suppress IgE production. IL-10 and TGF-β suppress the effector cells of allergic inflammation such as mast cells, basophils, and eosinophils. IL-10 induces tolerogenic DCs. (+) = Activation; (–) = Suppression.

Courtesy: M. Prashanth

Summary of Mechanism of Action of SLIT

- SLIT vaccines skew the immune response from Th2 to Th1.
- Treg cells play an important role in inducing T-cell anergy with the help of IL-10 and TGF-β.
- SLIT decreases tissue mast cells and eosinophils, and also reduces mast cell and basophil degranulation.
- Decrease in specific IgE and increase in specific IgG1 and IgG4.

CLINICAL EFFICACY OF SLIT

Overall 77 randomized, double-blind, placebo-controlled (RDBPC) trials of SLIT were conducted till June 2013: 39 with grass, 23 with house dust mite (HDM), 5 with *Parietaria* pollen, and 10 with other allergens (ragweed, cypress, cat, olive, birch, cedar). Of the 77 trials, five trials were found to be totally negative. All the remaining trials consistently reported efficacy to be dose dependent.

At present, eight systematic reviews with meta-analysis assessing the efficacy of SLIT for respiratory allergy have been published. The meta-analysis with the largest number of SLIT studies was conducted by Radulovic et al.[3] In this Cochrane review, the efficacy of SLIT was compared with placebo assessing symptom scores, medication requirements, biomarkers, and safety data. Sixty RDPBC trial met the criteria to be included in the systemic review and 49 trials were suitable for meta-analysis (SLIT n-2,333 and placebo n-2,256). Thirty-four studies were conducted in adults and 15 in children. A significant reduction in symptom scores and medication requirements was found in patients in the SLIT group compared to those who received placebo. SLIT was effective in both adults and children.

Efficacy in Allergic Rhinitis

In a meta-analysis conducted in studies only on children, Penagos et al. evaluated the efficacy of SLIT for the treatment of allergic rhinitis. There was a "significant reduction in both symptoms and medication use in SLIT group compared to placebo."[4] The most comprehensive meta-analysis of SLIT in allergic rhinitis is that of Radulovic et al., which included 22 trials and a total of 979 patients. The overall results favored SLIT over placebo for rhinitis symptoms and medication scores.

Efficacy in Asthma

The meta-analysis by Calmita et al. evaluated the effect of SLIT for asthma in nine studies, including 303 participants (150 SLIT and 153 placebo), and assessed asthmatic symptoms; six studies of 254 participants (132 SLIT and 122 placebo) evaluated asthma medication. There was improvement in asthma symptoms and medication use, but without statistical significance.[5] A meta-analysis on the efficacy of SLIT for allergic asthma in pediatric patients aged 3–18 years was conducted by Penagos et al. Overall, there was a significant reduction in both symptoms and medication use following SLIT compared to placebo.[6]

SLIT Tablets in Moderate Persistent Asthma

HDM (SLIT)-tablet therapy could reduce the use for inhaled glucocorticoids. Six hundred and four subjects 14 years or older with HDM allergic rhinitis and mild to moderate asthma were randomized 1:1:1:1 to double-blind daily treatment with one of three active doses [one, three, or six standardized quality (SQ)-HDM] or placebo who required low to medium doses of inhaled budesonide (100–800 μg per day) were included in the study. The minimal dose of inhaled budesonide required to control asthma symptoms was measured at the onset and after 1 year of HDM SLIT-tablet therapy. There was a modest but statistically significant reduction in the amount of budesonide required (81 μg per day) in the group receiving the highest dose of HDM SLIT (six SQ) compared with placebo, but not in the groups receiving the lower doses (three and one SQ). Thus, based on this limited data, SLIT appears to be well tolerated and possibly helpful in patients with asthma requiring low to moderate doses of inhaled glucocorticoids.[7]

Efficacy of SLIT in Allergic Rhinitis and Allergic Asthma

Compalati et al. conducted a meta-analysis to evaluate the efficacy of SLIT with HDM in allergic rhinitis and allergic asthma. Eight studies met the acceptable criteria for allergic rhinitis, and nine studies met the acceptable criteria for allergic asthma.

Both the studies showed a significant reduction in symptom scores and medication scores.

However, in view of considerable interstudy heterogeneity of studies, no firm conclusion of efficacy can be drawn.[8]

Efficacy of SLIT on Allergic Rhinoconjuctivitis

A Cochrane systematic review and meta-analysis was conducted by Calderon et al. to evaluate the effects of SLIT on ocular symptoms in patients with allergic rhinoconjuctivitis. They showed that SLIT induced a significant reduction in total ocular symptom scores and individual ocular symptom for red eyes compared to placebo. The participants on active treatment showed an increase in the threshold dose for the conjuctival allergen provocation test with no significant reduction in ocular eye drop use.[9]

SLIT in Atopic Dermatitis

A double-blind, placebo-controlled study of 48 children with atopic dermatitis treated with HDM SLIT reported a significant difference from baseline values of analog scores and medication use only in the mild to moderate severity group, whereas the study showed that patients with severe disease had only a marginal benefit.

SLIT in Food Allergy

There are few RDPBC trials conducted with food allergy. Enrique et al. conducted a RDPBC trial for hazelnut allergy. Patients received an escalating dose of 2×10^{-11} to 66.25 mg of hazelnut, yielding a cumulative dose of 119.51 mg or matched placebo. Efficacy was assessed by a DBPC food challenge after 8–12 weeks of treatment. The mean dose of hazelnut required to provoke symptoms increased from 2.29 to 11.56 g in the active group, compared to 3.49–4.14 g in the placebo group.[10]

Kim et al. conducted a RDPBC trial to investigate SLIT in children with peanut allergy. Subjects underwent 6 months of dose escalation of 0.25–2,000 µg and 6 months of maintenance dosing of 2,000 µg followed by DBPC food challenge. During the challenge, the treatment group safely ingested 20 times more peanut protein than the placebo group; there was a decrease in wheal size in skin prick test and decreased basophil responsiveness.[11]

However, few studies have shown promising results. Further studies are needed to evaluate the role of SLIT food allergy in clinical efficacy and safety.

Comparison of SLIT and SCIT

The efficacy of SLIT and SCIT in allergic rhinoconjuctivitis and mild to moderate asthma was compared by several authors; however, due to lack of high-quality, double-blind, randomized control studies, a firm conclusion could not be drawn (Table 22.1).

Table 22.1: Comparison of SLIT and SCIT.

Characteristics	*SCIT*	*SLIT*
Home administration	Never	Always
Route	Subcutaneous injections	Oral
Discomfort	Yes	Rare
Safety	Good safety when used carefully	Better safety profile than SCIT
Death	Reported, less than 40 cases in the past 100 years and millions of patients	Never
Adherence to treatment	Many studies have shown 50% default	Variable—20–80%
Dosage	Lower than SLIT	3–375 times dosage of SCIT
Cost	Direct cost lower, indirect patient monitoring cost higher	Direct cost higher, no indirect cost
Patient acceptance	Lower than SLIT	Higher than SCIT
Efficacy clinical improvement	Good effect	Good effect but may be slightly less than SCIT. More data is needed, and dosage needs to be standardized
Prevention of neo-sensitizations	Proved	Recent data shows that SLIT can prevent new sensitizations
Long-lasting efficacy after discontinuation	Proved	One study has shown the effect lasting after stopping SLIT for 5 years. More studies needed
Efficacy Switching back to Th1 from Th2	Proved	Recent studies have suggested. More studies needed

Yukselen et al. conducted a 1-year, double-blind, double-dummy, RCT to assess the effect of SCIT, SLIT, and placebo on symptoms, medication scores, and biomarkers. SCIT and SLIT group patients received standardized HDM; ten patients were included in each group. SCIT significantly reduced symptoms and medication scores for rhinitis and asthma.

The SLIT also reduced the symptoms associated with rhinitis and asthma, as well as medication usage for rhinitis, but this reduction was not significant compared to placebo, skin reactivity, and serum-specific IgE for HDM in both SCIT and SLIT. Serum IgE was significantly decreased in SCIT group only. SLIT has been shown to hamper the progression of the 'Allergic march' (Figs. 22.2 and 22.3).

Long-term Efficacy of SLIT

Di Rienzo et al. conducted the 10-year, open-label, nonrandomized controlled study in children (mean age 8.5 years) with asthma sensitized to HDM to assess the long-term effect of SLIT. The authors found that the mean peak flow result was significantly higher in the active group compared to the control group. They concluded that SLIT was effective even after discontinuation, and clinical efficacy was maintained for 4–5 years.[12]

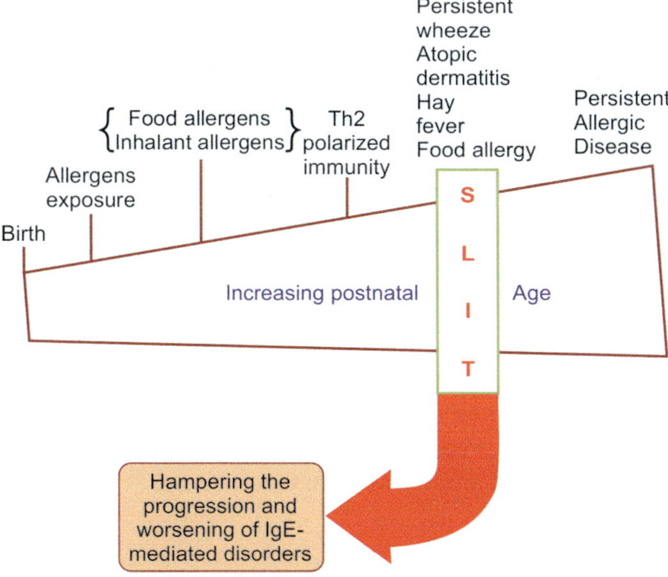

Fig. 22.2: Proposed slowing down of the 'Allergic March' by SLIT administration by immunomodulation.

Courtesy: M. Prashanth

SLIT: Progression of Atopy

There are several studies to demonstrate that SLIT can positively alter the course of atopy. Novembre et al. enrolled 113 children in the age group of 5–14 years with allergic rhinoconjuctivitis monosensitized to grass allergen in an open-label study; patients received SLIT or standardized pharmacotherapy for 3 years. The development of asthma in the third year was 3.8-fold more likely in controls than in patients who received SLIT, strongly suggesting that SLIT can alter the course of the atopic march.[13]

Marogna et al. studied the effects of SLIT in patients with allergic rhinitis with or without asthma in an open-label study where the patients were randomized to medications only, and SLIT and medications for 3 years. There was a significant decline in positive methacholine sensitivity by the third year in the SLIT group, but not in the control group. Additionally, neo-sensitization occurred in 38% of controls versus 5.9% of SLIT patients. This suggests that SLIT can effectively prevent newer sensitizations, as well as the progression toward asthma.[14]

SLIT in Polysensitized Patients

In the present era, it seems that most of them are sensitized to more than one allergenic component. Component-resolved diagnosis could improve the reliability of choosing particular molecular components of allergens for immunotherapy. This method provides specific information on the molecular component of allergens,

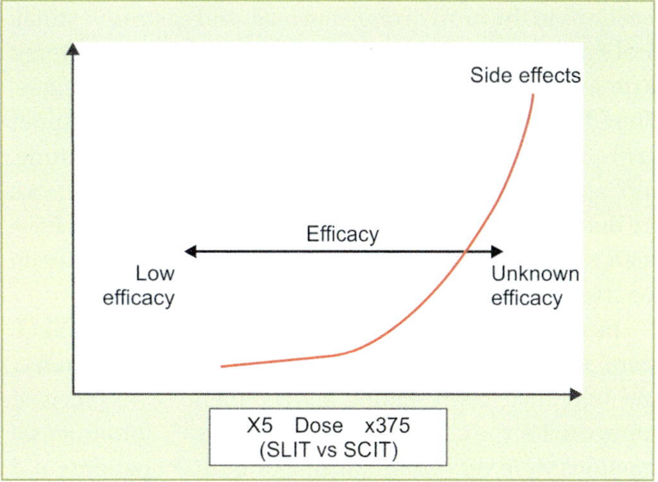

Fig. 22.3: Dose–response curve of SLIT. Efficacy increases with an increase in dose of SLIT, from 5 times the dose of SCIT to 375 times the dose of SCIT. The side effects increase with higher dosage.

Courtesy: M. Prashanth

confirming or excluding true sensitizations. In large-scale clinical studies, polysensitized patients treated with grass pollen tablets are benefitted as much as monosensitized patients.[15] More data are required to validate the efficacy of multi-AIT in polysensitized patients.

Adherence to SLIT

The SLIT is self-administered at home, so there are concerns about compliance. Several studies have quoted compliance of SLIT to be variable from 90% to 15%.

The analyses of sales provided by manufacturers are 15% at 2 years of SLIT and was not affected by the regimen prescribed, allergens utilized, and reimbursement status.[16]

Cost of SLIT

The cumulative dose of allergen given in SLIT is higher than in SCIT, and therefore, the cost of SLIT vaccines is higher than that of SCIT vaccines. However, in SLIT, there is no need for medical and nursing supervision cost, which reduces the overall cost of SLIT in comparison with SCIT.

The treatment with SLIT grass tablets was economically superior to symptomatic treatment alone, after adjusting for the comparable cost differences among national healthcare services.[17] SLIT resulted in significant gain of quality-adjusted life years and in a significant cost saving.

SLIT Safety

The SLIT appears to be safer and better tolerated compared to SCIT. The majority of SLIT adverse effects are local reactions in the form of oral, mucosal, and gastrointestinal. Oral symptoms are in the form of itching of the lips, altered taste sensation, swelling of the lips, swelling of the tongue, altered taste perception, throat irritation, etc. Upper gastrointestinal symptoms are stomach ache, vomiting, and abdominal pain. Lower gastrointestinal symptoms are diarrhea and abdominal pain. Systemic reactions have been reported with SLIT; fortunately, no death has been reported so far.

In a comprehensive review of 104 articles on SLIT, there are 66 studies that provided information on safety and tolerance, representing 4,378 patients who received approximately 1,181,000 SLIT doses,[18] oromucosal reactions were very common affecting 75% of patients and were seen more frequently in the buildup phase.

In the studies that specified the type of reaction, 169 (0.056%) of 314,959 doses administered were classified as producing systemic adverse events (SAEs).

In the SLIT comprehensive review,[18] there were no fatalities, although there were 14 probable SLIT-related SAEs in 3,984 patients treated with a total of 1,019,826 doses. This represents 1.4 SAEs per 100,000 SLIT doses. The most common SLIT-related SAEs were asthmatic reactions (n = 7), one of which required hospitalization; the others were abdominal pain/vomiting (n = 3), uvula edema (n = 1), and urticaria lasting 48 hours. There have been a few case reports of systemic reactions of a severity that should be categorized as anaphylaxis. Two of these four experienced anaphylaxis with the first SLIT tablet.[19]

Since this treatment is administered at home without medical supervision, patients should be provided with specific instructions regarding how to manage adverse reactions, and when and what to report to the physician.

Types of Preparations of SLIT

The SLIT is dispensed as drops, sprays, or tablets (available only for grass/ragweed pollens in the United States, HDM as well as other inhalants in Europe). These products should have a calculated dose of the active ingredients when finally dispensed.

Dosage and Schedule

The monthly dose of SLIT vaccines ranges from 2 to 375 times the usual monthly dose of SCIT; the appropriate dose for efficacy of SLIT has not been completely resolved. One drop of SLIT contains 50 μL of allergen vaccine. SLIT is usually given as daily dose: one drop in the first week, two drops in the second week, three drops in the third week, four drops in the fourth week, five drops in the fifth week. Once a maximum of five drops is attained without adverse effects, then a dose of five drops is maintained for 1–4 weeks; later it will be moved to the next level of concentration.

Another method is to start with the maintenance vial. There is no consensus on the need for the buildup method versus starting with maintenance dose.

Storage

The SLIT vaccines are stored at 2–8°C in a refrigerator. However, SLIT preparations containing glycerol may be stable for several months at room temperature.

Duration of SLIT

The usual course for SLIT is 3–5 years. An open-controlled, 15-year follow-up study of subjects treated with SLIT for 3, 4, and 5 years suggests that a 4-year course appears to be the best option for clinical efficacy and long-term effect.[20]

Patient Selection

Eligibility criteria for SLIT is the same as those for SCIT in which patients refuse to take injections:

- History of symptoms related to allergen exposure documented by positive allergen-specific IgE test.
- The allergen used for immunotherapy must be relevant to the clinical history.
- Patients whose allergy is uncontrolled with pharmacotherapy.
- Patients in whom pharmacotherapy induces undesirable side effects.
- Patients who do not want to be on constant or long-term pharmacotherapy.
- Age does not appear to be a limitation; however, SLIT may not be considered in young infants due to difficulty in identifying systemic reactions.
- Allergens that are difficult to avoid.
- Patient does not want injectable immunotherapy.

Contraindications to SLIT

- When patients' asthma is not well controlled by pharmacotherapy with forced expiratory volume in 1 second <70%.
- Not to initiate immunotherapy during pregnancy; however, if a patient is already on SLIT, then SLIT can be continued without escalating the dose.
- If standardized allergen vaccine extract is not available for SLIT.
- If a patient is on nonselective beta blockers that cannot be changed.

Selection of Relevant Allergens in Polysensitized Patients for Treatment

Generally, it may not be good to mix more than three to four allergen combinations during SLIT.

- The additional extracts will cause dilution of all the extracts so that an effective dose will not be administered.
- There may be deleterious effects of one extract upon another in the mix.
- History before and after skin prick test is required to assess the relevance of skin prick test in a patient.
- Weather symptoms are predominant—indoors or outdoors.
- Weather symptoms are seasonal or perennial or perennial with seasonal exacerbation.
- Do the symptoms correlate with the natural exposure of allergens?
- Is weather seasonal exacerbation of symptoms significant?
- Can the allergens be avoided?

How much quality of life affected? Adverse events explained and advised about immediate management in systemic reaction.

There is a possibility of a limited absorption capacity of the sublingual mucosa, so multiple extracts would compete for absorption for sublingual administration.

Case Scenario

A 10-year-old boy with a history of sneezing, watery nose, nose and throat itching, and redness of eye almost every day from the past 2 years. Symptoms are more severe between July and February. Maternal grandfather is having allergic rhinitis and uncle having allergic rhinitis and asthma.

Child underwent a skin prick test and his tests revealed:

Saline—0 × 0 mm

Histamine—8 × 8 mm

HDM—10 × 8 mm with pseudopods

Cockroach—4 × 5 mm

Child is being treated with intranasal corticosteroids. Symptoms are significantly relieved with intranasal steroid. Mother feels symptoms are better by about 75%.

Parents are interested and want to pursue a specific therapy rather than only pharmacotherapy. Hence, a decision to start specific immunotherapy using the SLIT method was entertained.

Method of Writing a Prescription for SLIT

There are certain basic steps to be taken before writing the actual recipe:

1. *Identification of the culprit antigens*: This can be accomplished by correlating a patient's history and skin reactivity. This may entail a repeat history taking.
2. Determine the concentration of the major antigen and its concentration in the component to be treated (here it is *Dermatophagoides pteronyssinus*: 63 µg/mL of standardized material).[21]
3. Determine the therapeutic dose of the antigen to be treated (*D. pteronyssinus*: 10 µg/maintenance dose).

4. Allergen vaccine is prepared for 10 mL, which could be used for 20 injections as 0.5 mL per dose for 10 months. Hence, initially the dose calculation is done for SCIT and later converted to SLIT dosage for 4 months; actually we are utilizing 10 months dosage of SCIT in 4 months, so we are giving 2.5 times the dose of SCIT.

Note: SCIT preparation and schedule of dosage are not discussed in this chapter.

Selection of the Relevant Antigens for SLIT

Obviously, the culprit antigens are the HDM and cockroach.

Child was advised about the avoidance of cockroach, and SLIT was initiated for only HDM after taking the consent.

Actual Recipe

D. pteronyssinus 10,000AU/mL: 2.00 mL
50% glycerine diluent: 28.00 mL
Total (for 8 weeks supply): 30.00 mL

Dosage—2.5 Times the Monthly Dosage of SCIT

Schedule

1. One drop/day × first week
2. Two drops/day × second week
3. Three drops/day × third week
4. Four drops/day × fourth week
5. Five drops/day onward DAILY
   Five drops/day will be the maintenance dose.
   Advised follow-up: every 2 months

The SLIT dose will always be initiated in the presence of the physician, and the patient is observed for 30 minutes.

The drops need to be placed under the tongue, and the patient is requested to hold the drops for 2 minutes.

At times, practically speaking, 2 minutes is TOO LONG.

Hence, the author is advising his patients to hold the drops for ATLEAST 1 MINUTE and then to swallow.

Patient is also instructed not to eat or drink 1 hour prior and after the SLIT administration.

Proper recording of the dosage, time, date, and any reactions need to be maintained without fail.

SUMMARY

1. Mucosal tolerance and the interactions between DCs and T cells will determine whether the eventual response is active or tolerant.
2. SLIT is beneficial in the treatment of allergic rhinitis, allergic asthma, and allergic rhinoconjuctivitis, and possibly in few cases of atopic dermatitis.
3. SLIT may alter the course of atopic disease toward more tolerant.
4. Effectiveness of SLIT persists even after treatment is discontinued.
5. SLIT is found to be very safe. Local reactions are common. Systemic reactions are rare but can occur.
6. SLIT for food allergy still needs evaluation.
7. SLIT should be prescribed only by a trained allergist.
8. Only standardized allergens should be used for SLIT.
9. Patient selection is the key to success of SLIT.

GLOSSARY

Anergy: A state of immune unresponsiveness.

Allergy: Abnormal immune response by the body to a substance (e.g., pollen, food) resulting in clinical signs and symptoms.

Allergen immunotherapy: Administering increasing doses of allergens to accustom the body to substances that are generally harmless (e.g., grass, pollen, house HDM).

Allergic sensitizations: Presence of IgE antibody to common environmental and food allergens.

Dendritic cells: Antigen-presenting cells.

Langerhans cells: Antigen-presenting cells.

Polysensitizations: Presence of IgE antibody to multiple common environmental and food allergens.

REFERENCES

1. Appian. Chapter 16. Appain's Roman History. Book 12. In: White H, trans. Cambridge, MA: Harvard University Press; 1962:453.
2. Allam JP, Wurtzen PA, Reinartz M, et al. Phl p 5 resorption in human oral mucosa leads to dose dependent and time-dependent allergen dependent allergen binding by oral mucosal Langerhans cells, attenuates their maturation, and enhances their migratory and TGF-β1 and IL 10-producing properties. J Allergy Clin Immunol. 2010;126:638-45.
3. Radulovic S, Calderon MA, Wilson D, Durham S. Sublingual immunotherapy for allergic rhinitis. Cochrane Database Syst Rev. 2010;12:CD002893.
4. Penagos M, Compalati E, Tarantini F, et al. Efficacy of sublingual immunotherapy in the treatment of allergic rhinitis in pediatric patients 3 to 18 years of age: A meta-analysis of randomised, placebo-controlled, double-blind trials. Ann Allergy Asthma Immunol. 2006;97:141-8.
5. Calamita Z, Saconato H, Pela AB, Atallah AN. Efficacy of sublingual immunotherapy in asthma; systemic review of

randomised clinical trials using the Cochrane collaboration method. Allergy. 2006;61:1162-72.

6. Penagos M, Passalacqua G, Compalati E, et al. Meta-analysis of the efficacy of sublingual immunotherapy in the treatment of allergic asthma in the pediatric patients, 3 to 18 years of age. Chest. 2008;133:599-609.
7. Mosbech H, Deckelmann R, de Blay F, et al. Standardized quality (SQ) house dust mite sublingual immunotherapy tablet (ALK) reduced inhaled corticosteroid use while maintaining asthma control: a randomized, double-blind, placebo-controlled trial. J Allergy Clin Immunol. 2014;134:568-75.e7.
8. Compalati E, Passalacqua G, Bonini M, Canonica GW. The efficacy of sublingual immunotherapy for house dust mites in respiratory allergy: results of GA2LEN meta-analysis. Allergy. 2009;64:1570-9.
9. Calderon M A, Penagos M, Sheikh A, et al. Sublingual immunotherapy for treating allergic conjunctivitis. Cochrane Database Syst Rev. 2011;6:CD007685.
10. Enrique E, Pineda F, Malek T, et al. Sublingual immunotherapy for hazelnut food allergy: a randomised double-blind placebo-controlled study with a standardised hazelnut extract. J Allergy Clin Immunol. 2005;116:1073-9.
11. Kim EH, Bird JA Kulis M, et al. Sublingual immunotherapy for pea nut allergy : clinical and immunological evidence of desensitization. J Allergy Clin Immunol. 2011;127: 640-6.
12. Di Rienzo V, Marcucci F, Puccinelli P, et al. Long-lasting effect of sublingual immunotherapy in children with asthma due to house dust mite: a 10-year prospective study. Clin Exp Allergy. 2003;33;206-10.
13. Novembre E, Galli E, Landi F, et al. CO seasonal sublingual immunotherapy reduces the development of asthma in children with rhinoconjuctivitis. J Allergy Clin Immunol. 2004;114:851-7.
14. Marogna M, Spadolini I, Massolo A, et al. Randomised controlled open study of sublingual immunotherapy for respiratory allergy in real-life: clinical efficacy and more. Allergy. 2004;59:1205-10.
15. Calderon MA, Cox L, Casale TB, et al. Multiple-allergen and single-allergen immunotherapy strategies in polysensitized patients: looking at the published evidence. J Allergy Clin Immunol. 2012;129:929-34.
16. Senna G, Lombardi C, Canonica GW, et al. How adherent to sublingual immunotherapy prescriptions are patient? The manufacturer's view point. J Allergy Clin Immunol. 2010;126:668-9.
17. Bachert C, Vestenbaek U, Christensen J, et al. Cost-effectiveness of grass allergen tablet (GRAZAX) for the prevention of seasonal grass pollen induced rhino-conjuctivitis: a northern European perspective. Clin Exp Allergy. 2007;37:772-9.
18. Cox LS, Larenas Linnemann D, Nolte H. Sublingual immunotherapy: a comprehensive review. J Allergy Clin Immunol. 2006;117:1021-35.
19. de Groot H, Bijl A. Anaphylactic reaction after the first dose of sublingual immunotherapy with grass pollen tablet. Allergy. 2009;64:963-4.
20. Marogna M, Spadolini I, Massolo A, et al. Long lasting effects of sublingual immunotherapy according to its duration: A 15-year prospective study. J Allergy Clin Immunol. 2010;126:969-75.
21. Nelson HS. Preparing Subcutaneous Allergen Vaccines, Allergens and Allergen Immunotherapy Subcutaneous, Sublingual, and Oral. 5th ed. Abingdon, Oxfordshire: CRC Press/Taylor & Francis Group; 2014. Florida. USA.

CHAPTER 23

Quality of Life in Allergic Diseases

VK Jain

INTRODUCTION

Allergy is a systemic disease having multiorgan involvement. In the clinical practice over the past three decades, there has been increasing awareness of the importance of health-related quality of life (HRQoL). It is important to evaluate the primary outcome of HRQoL in chronic diseases. HRQoL is a new term but not a new concept to majority of the practicing clinicians. For many generations, clinicians are routinely asking multiple questions related to HRQoL to their patients in clinical practice: Are you feeling well or not? Is there any limitation in your daily activities or sleep? Does this bother you? Are you getting better with medicine? Are your children going to school or not? Have you started going to workplace?

Therefore, the clinician will focus more on specific problems of the patient and will advise better diagnosis and overall management.

Allergy or allergic disease is a public health problem world over. Respiratory allergy is projected to affect 50% of the population. If this problem is continued, it could be the epidemic of the twenty-first century.[1] Restriction of physical activity, absentees from work or school, loss of productivity, and mental attitude due to allergic manifestation will ultimately turn into a poor quality of life (QoL) including the socioeconomic burden.[2,3] Among the respiratory allergies, the most common manifestations include bronchial asthma and rhinitis. In other allergies, skin manifestation and food allergy are also a major concern of HRQoL.

Health is a common theme in most of the cultures but having different concepts of health in various communities world over. The oldest definition of health is "absence of disease". It continues to be a neglected entity. Its value is only understood when it is lost. During the past few decades, there has been a reawakening that health is a fundamental human right having worldwide social goals and is essential to the satisfaction of basic human needs.[4]

DEFINITION OF HEALTH

"Health" is a common term widely used but still most people find difficult to define. Therefore, many definitions of health have been provided from time to time.

WHO Definition

WHO (1948) in its Constitution defined "Health is a state of complete Physical, Mental & Social wellbeing & not merely an absence of disease or infirmity." In 1978, this statement was amplified to include the ability to lead a "Socially & Economically productive life."[5]

NEW PHILOSOPHY OF HEALTH

- Fundamental human right
- Essence of productive life
- Intersectoral and integral part of development
- Concept of QoL
- Involves individual, state, and international responsibilities
- Its maintenance is a major and continuous social investment
- Worldwide social goal.

WHAT IS HEALTH-RELATED QUALITY OF LIFE?

"QoL" is a rather difficult expression, often meaning different things to different persons and makes it very difficult to define. However, most agree that many factors, such as finances, spirituality, and health, contribute to QoL and also affect each other. Considering simply, HRQoL is the component of overall QoL that is determined primarily by a person's health and which can be influenced by clinical interventions. Therefore, Schipper and colleagues simply define it as "The functional effects of an illness and its consequent therapy upon a patient, as perceived by the patient."[6]

METHODS OF SELECTING

QoL Instruments

Many valid instruments for measuring HRQoL are available, yet no best instrument is available. Now we are having multiple valid instruments for measuring HRQoL in patients of asthma and rhinitis but not yet with two conditions together. Each has been developed for different purposes and with different measurement properties. There are two types of HRQoL questionnaires: generic and specific.

Generic Instruments

Generic instruments are designed to be applicable to patients in all health states. The most commonly used and best validated are the Sickness Impact Profile *(SIP)*,[7] the Medical Outcomes Survey Short Form 36 *(SF36)*,[8] the Nottingham Health Profile *(NHP)*,[9] and the McMaster Health Index Questionnaire.[10] Although each profile attempts to measure all important aspects of health-related function, each achieves this in different ways. For instance, the SF-36 contains nine domains that can be combined into two primary functions—mental and physical. In contrast, the SIP has two major domains, physical and psychosocial, that combine to give one overall score.

The great advantage of generic instruments is that burden of illness can be compared across different medical conditions, for example, one can compare the burden of illness experienced by patients with rhinitis and asthma.[11,12] However, generic instruments are needed to be broad in their comprehensiveness, therefore they have very little depth and as a result may not include impairments that are important to a patient with specific condition. So, in many conditions including rhinitis and asthma, generic instruments may be unresponsive to small changes, which are important to patients.[13]

Specific Instruments

Specific instruments have been developed due to lack of depth of focus of generic instruments. These are specific for a group of patients, i.e., elderly, or a particular function, e.g., pain, sneezing, or a specific disease. These are developed by asking the patient and it focuses on the particular impairment and clinically detects important changes in patient problems that requires interventions. The common specific instruments are Standard Gamble, Time Trade Off, and Feeling Thermometer[14] and are useful for measuring the value of patients' place on their own health states.

For the measurement of the value that society places on various health states, we use the quality of wellbeing scale,[15] multi-attribute health utility index,[16] and Euro QoL.[17] Recently, the standard gambling and feeling thermometer have been modified for the use as disease-specific instruments especially in children with asthma.[13]

IMPACT OF ALLERGY AND ALLERGIC DISEASES ON HRQoL

Allergy and allergic diseases not only affect the QoL of the patients but also having impact on the status of family members and community. It may affect persons of all ages irrespective of gender. The impact may be medical in the form of diseases, its complications, and management. It may also have physical, psychological (emotional), social, and economic impacts.[18-21] HRQoL is poor in various allergic disorders especially in rhinitis and asthma.[22-25] The older age and longer duration of symptoms and low BMI[26,27] are considered as risk factors for reduced HRQoL both in allergic rhinitis and asthma.

Medical Impact of Allergic Disorders on HRQoL

Various types of medical impacts have been associated with patients of allergic rhinitis and asthma, and both affect QoL.[11,28-30] Allergic rhinitis causes facial structural changes, i.e., adenoid face, mouth breather, high-arched palate, etc.[31,32] These patients may also have poor oral hygiene, i.e., gingivitis, dental plaques, overcrowding, and malocclusion of teeth.[32-34]

One-fifth of the patients have poor smell and taste,[35,36] and one-third have nasal polyp with faster growth and high rate of relapse after surgery.[37] Acute to chronic sinusitis and otitis media is also common.[38-40]

Obstructive sleep apnea (OSA) is also reported among the patients of allergic rhinitis (AR)[41,42] and depends on the severity of nasal obstruction, which can be corrected by use of regular steroid sprays with the reduction of allergen exposure and immunotherapy. Patients have reported improvements in HRQoL with both sublingual and subcutaneous immunotherapy.[43-47] Fifty percent of the patients of AR may develop bronchial asthma throughout the life.

Asthma patients are also having poor HRQoL with greater impairment in females,[48] obese (more BMI)/underweight,[26,27] and middle to old age groups. HRQoL is markedly reduced in bronchial asthma patients with or without rhinitis and related more with the severity of asthma rather than allergic rhinitis.[24,49] One-third to one-fourth of the patients of allergic bronchial asthma may develop allergic rhinitis. A positive correlation has been observed between pulmonary function test values and HRQoL scores.[50,51] There is no significant difference in HRQoL in atopy versus nonatopic subjects;[49] however, polysensitization is associated with worst HRQoL.[52]

Physical Impact of Allergic Disorders on HRQoL

Patients of allergic disorders may have poor sleep, concentration at work, poor learning and memory, absentees from work in all age groups both in males and females.[13,53-58] Children have poor academic performances with less school activity, limitation in sports, and impaired learning ability in the classroom.[21,28,59] Physical impairment measures are significantly greater in asthma patients and correlate with severity compared with allergic rhinitis.[49,60]

Pyschological Impact of Allergic Disorders on HRQoL

Allergy and allergic disorders may cause various psychosomatic disorders including stress, which is the first reaction followed by anxiety, depression, irritability, mood changes, poor concentration, poor memory, and personality changes with poor decision-making.[61-66]

Mental health score in patients with allergic rhinitis is more compared with asthma.[49,60,67]

Social Impact of Allergic Disorders on HRQoL

One-fourth to one-third of the patients of allergic diseases may have various social problems, i.e., inhibitions to attend various family and community social programs and not actively participating.[16,23,50]

Economic Impact of Allergic Disorders on HRQoL

Allergic diseases may affect the financial status of patients and family, which could be directly related to physician visits, investigations, and procedural, hospitalization, and medication costs. Indirect economic burden may be in the form of lost days of work with decreased productivity and missed school days.[2,3,60]

CONCLUSION

Allergy is a systemic disease having multiorgan involvement. In the past three decades, the awareness regarding QoL has increased among clinicians. Many measuring scales have been developed to evaluate HRQoL in various allergic disorders both in children and adults. Impact of allergy and allergic disorders may be medical, social, physical, and economical. Allergy and allergic diseases are to be recognized as early as possible to reduce complications and their impacts on HRQoL, thereby reducing the overall cost of the management.

REFERENCES

1. Pawankar. Editorial Allergy Clin Immun Int. JWAO. 2005 (Sept. Oct 2005).
2. Bousquet J, Fayol C. Assessment of quality of life in patients with perennial allergic rhinitis. J Allergy Clin Immunol. 1994;74:182-8.
3. World Health Organization Prevention and Control of Chronic Respiratory Diseases at Country Level, Towards a Global Alliance against Chronic Respiratory Diseases (GARD) based on the WHO Meeting on Prevention and Control of Chronic Respiratory Diseases, Geneva, Switzerland. WHO/NMH/ CHP/CPM/CRA/05. 17–19 June, 2004.
4. Park K. Park's Textbook of Preventive and Social Medicine. 23rd Ed. Banarsidas Bhanot Pub. India. Concept of health and diseases; 2015;13-51.
5. WHO. Health for All, Sr. No. 1; 1978.
6. Schipper H, Clinch J, Powell V. Definitions and conceptual issues. In: Spilker B, ed. Quality of Life Assessment in Clinical Trials. New York, NY: Raven Press; 1990:11-24.
7. Bergner M, Bobbitt RA, Carter WB, Gilson BS. The Sickness Impact Profile: development and final revision of a health status measure. Med Care 1981;19:787-805.
8. Stewart AL, Hays R, Ware JE. The MOS short-form general health survey. Reliability and validity in a patient population. Med Care. 1988;26:724-32.
9. Hunt SM, McKenna SP, McEwen J, et al. A quantitative approach to perceived health status: a validation study. J Epidemiol Community Health 1980;34:281-6.

10. Sackett DL, Chambers LW, MacPherson AS, et al. The development and application of indices of health: general methods and summary of results. Am J Public Health. 1977;67:423-8.
11. Bousquet J, Bullinger M, Fayol C, et al. Assessment of quality of life in patients with perennial rhinitis with the French version of the SF-36 health status questionnaire. J Allergy Clin Immunol. 1994;94:182-8.
12. Bousquet J, Knani J, Dhivert H, et al. Quality of life in asthma. 1. Internal consistency and validity of the SF-36 questionnaire. Am J Respir Crit Med. 1994;149:371-5.
13. Juniper EF, Guyatt GH, Feeny DH, et al. Minimum skills required by children to complete health-related quality of life instruments: comparison of instruments for measuring asthmaspecific quality of life. Eur Respir J. 1997;10:2285-94.
14. Torrance GW. Measurement of health state utilities for economic appraisal. J Health Econ. 1986;5:1-30.
15. Kaplan RM, Anderson JP, Wu AW, et al. The quality of well-being scale: application in AIDS, cystic fibrosis and arthritis. Med Care 1989;27:S27-43.
16. Feeny D, Furlong W, Barr RD, et al. A comprehensive multi-attribute system for classifying the health status of survivors of childhood cancer. J Clin Oncol. 1992;10:923-8.
17. The EuroQol Group. A new facility for the measurement of health-related quality of life. Health Policy 1990;16:199-208.
18. Baiardini I, Braido F, Brandi S, et al. Allergic diseases and their impact on quality of life. Ann Allergy Asthma Immunol. 2006;97:419-29.
19. Juniper EF. Impact of upper respiratory allergic diseases on quality of life. J Allergy Clin Immunol. 1998;101 Suppl 2:386-91.
20. Guyatt GH, Feeny DH, Patrick DL. Measuring health-related quality of life. Ann Intern Med. 1993;118: 622-9.
21. Silva CH, Silva TE, Morales NM, et al. Quality of life in children and adolescent with allergic rhinitis. Braz J Otorhinolaryngol. 2009;75:642-9.
22. Chen H, Katz PP, Eisner MD, et al. Health related quality of life in adult rhinitis:The role of perceived control of disease. J Allergy Clin Immunol. 2004;114:845-50.
23. Blaiss MS. Outcome analysis in asthma. JAMA. 1997;278;1874-80.
24. Elkholy MM, Khedr MH, Halawa A, Elbaramawy A. Quality of allergic rhinitis on quality of life in patients with bronchial asthma. Int J Health Sci (Qassim). 2012;6:194-202.
25. Leynaert B, Neukirch C, Liard R, et al. Quality of life in allergic rhinitis and asthma. A population-based study of young adults. Am J Respir Crit Care Med. 2000;162:1391-6.
26. Kalpaklioğlu AF, Kara T, Kurtipek E, Saygun M. Effect of body mass index on quality of life in allergic/asthmatic patients. Allergy Asthma Proc. 2006;27:499-503.
27. Ford ES, Mannino DM, Redd SC, et al. Determinant of quality of life among people with asthma: findings from behaviroal risk factors survelliance system. J Asthma. 2004;41:327-36.
28. Meltzer EO. Quality of life in adults and children with allergic rhinitis. J Allergy Clin Immunol. 2001;108:45-53.
29. Juniper EF. Measuring health-related quality of life in rhinitis. J Allergy Clin Immunol. 1997;99:742-9.
30. Bousquet J, Khaltaev N, Cruz AA, et al. Allergic rhinitis and its impact on asthma (ARIA) 2008 update (in collaboration with World Health Organization, GA2LEN and AllerGen). Allergy 2008;63:8-160.
31. Bresolin, D, Shapiro PA, Shapiro GG, et al. Mouth breathing in allergic children: its relationship to dentofacial development. Am J Orthod. 1983;334-40.
32. Bresolin, D, Shapiro GG, Shapiro PA, et al. Facial characteristics of children who breathe through the mouth. Pediatrics 1984;73:622-5.
33. Gulati, MS, Grewal N, Kaur A. A comparative study of effects of mouth breathing and normal breathing on gingival health in children. J Indian Soc Pedod Prev Dent. 1998;16:72-83.
34. Wagaiyu EG, Ashley FP. Mouthbreathing, lip seal and upper lip coverage and their relationship with gingival inflammation in 11-14 year-old schoolchildren. J Clin Pedod. 1991;18;698-702.
35. Apter, AJ, Mott AE, Frank ME, Clive JM. Allergic rhinitis and olfactory loss. Ann Allergy Asthma Immunol. 1995;75:311-6.
36. Cowart, BJ, Flynn-Rodden K, McGready SI, Lowry LD. Hyposrnia in allergic rhinitis. J Allergy Clin Immunol. 1993;91:747-51.
37. Ferrell BP. Endoscopic sinus surgery: sinonasal polyposis and allergy. Ent J. 1993;72:389-99.
38. Ruggeri, et al. Relations between allergic rhinitis and otitis media with effusion. The role of the Eustachian tube. Minerva Pediatr. 1990;42:481-3.
39. Tomonaga, K, Kurono Y, Mogi G. The role of nasal allergy in otitis media with effusion: a clinical study. Acta Otolaryngol. 1988;458:s41-7.
40. Lombardi, E, Stein RT, Wright AL, et al. The relation between physician-diagnosed sinusitis, asthma, and skin test reactivity to allergens in 8-year-old children. Pediatr Pulmonol. 1996;22:141-6.
41. Kushida CA, Guilleminault C, Clerk AA, et al. Nasal obstruction and obstructive sleep apnea: a review. Allergy Asthma Proc. 1997;18:69-71.
42. McNicholas WT, Tarlo S, Cole P, et al. Obstructive apneas during sleep in patients with seasonal allergic rhinitis. Am Rev Respir Dis. 1982;126:625-8.
43. Dahl R, Kapp A, Colombo G, et al. Efficacy and safety of sublingual immunotherapy with grass allergen tablets for seasonal rhinoconjunctivitis. J Allergy Clin Immunol. 2006;118:434-40.
44. Srivastava D, Singh BP, Sudha VT, et al. Immunotherapy with mosquito (*Culex quinquefasciatus*) extract: a double-blind, placebo-controlled study. Ann Allergy Asthma Immunol. 2007;99:273-80.
45. Srivastava D, Singh BP, Arora N, Gaur SN. Clinicoimmunologic study on immunotherapy with mixed and single insect allergens. J Clin Immunol. 2009;29:665-73.
46. Srivastava D, Singh BP, Arora N. Current immunological approaches for management of allergic rhinitis and bronchial asthma. Inflamm Res. 2009;58:523-36.
47. Parasuramalu BG, Gangaboraiah, Balaji R, Someswara GM. Assessment of quality of life among patients with

respiratory allergy, receiving sublingual and subcutaneous immunotherapy. Ind J Allergy Asthma Immunol. 2011; 25:21-7.

48. Ford ES, Mannino DM, Redd SC, et al. Determinants of quality of life among people with asthma: findings from the behavioral risk factor surveillance system. J Asthma 2004;41:327-36.
49. Kalpaklioglu AF, Baccioglu A. Evaluation of quality of life: impact of allergic rhinitis on asthma. J Investig Allergol Clin Immunol. 2008;18;168-73.
50. Nalina N, Satish Chandra MR, Umashanker. Assessment of quality of life in bronchial asthma patients. Int J Med Pub Health. 2015;5:93-7.
51. Katz PP, Eisner MD, Henke J, et al. The Marks asthma quality of life questionnaire: further validation and examination of responsiveness to change. J Clin Epidemol. 1999;52:667-75.
52. Cirillo I, Vizzaccaro A, Klersy C. Quality of life and polysensitization in young men with intermittent asthma. Ann Allergy Asthma Immunol. 2005;94:640-3.
53. Gerth Van Wijk R. Allergy: a global problem. Quality of life. Allergy 2002;57:1097-10.
54. Jenney MEM, Campbell S. Measuring quality of life. Arch Dis Child. 1997;77:347-54.
55. Derebery MJ, Berliner KI. Allergy and health-related quality of life. Otolaryngol Head Neck Surg. 2000;123:393-9.
56. Ferreira LN, Brito U, Ferreira PL. Quality of life in asthma patients. Rev Port Pneumol. 2010;16:23-55.
57. Hazell M, Frank T, Frank P. Health-related quality of life in individuals with asthma related symptoms. Respir Med. 2003;97:1211-8.
58. Merikallio VJ, Mustalahti K, Remes ST, et al. Comparison of quality of life between asthmatic and healthy school children. Pediatr Allergy Immunol. 2005;16:332-40.
59. Klymenko VA, Karpushenko JV. The quality of life of children with allergic diseases. J Asthma Allergy. 2014;3.
60. European Academay of Allergology and Clinical Immunology. The impact of allergic rhinitis on quality of life and other airway diseases: summary of a European conference. Allergy 1998;53:S1-31.
61. Oğuztürk Ö, Ekici A, Kara M, et al. Psychological status and quality of life in elderly patients with asthma. Psychosomatics 2005;46:41-6.
62. Amore M, Antonucci C, Bettini E, et al. Disease control in patients with asthma is associated with alexithymia but not with depression or anxiety. Behav Med. 2013;39:138-45.
63. Trzcińska H, Przybylski G, Kozłowski B, Derdowski S. Analysis of the relation between level of asthma control and depression and anxiety. Med Sci Monit. 2012;18:CR190-4.
64. Di Marco F, Santus P, Centanni S. Anxiety and depression in asthma. Curr Opin Pulm Med. 2011;17:39-44.
65. Urrutia I, Aguirre U, Pascual S, et al. Impact of anxiety and depression on disease control and quality of life in asthma patients. J Asthma. 2012;49:201-8.
66. Noriega NH. Association between anxiety and depression in allergic diseases. Ann Depress Anxiety. 2015;2:1047.
67. Juniper EF. Quality of life in adults and children with asthma and rhinitis. Allergy. 1997;52:971-7.

CHAPTER 24

Allergic Rhinitis

Ashok Shah

INTRODUCTION

Rhinitis is defined as inflammation of the membranes lining the nose and is characterized by nasal congestion, rhinorrhea, sneezing, itching of the nose, and/or postnasal drip.[1] Atopy is an important risk factor for rhinitis, and allergic rhinitis (AR) is the most common form.[2] AR, although a cause of significant and widespread morbidity, is often viewed, rather erroneously, as a trivial disease.[3] It may significantly affect the quality of life of the patient by causing fatigue, headache, cognitive impairment, and other associated symptoms.[4]

Atopic diseases often occur with associated conditions, and AR is no exception. Of all the atopic disorders, AR is most commonly associated with asthma. Estimates show that up to 38% of patients with AR have concomitant asthma, and 60–78% of asthmatics suffer from AR.[3] The clinical association of the allergic form of rhinitis with asthma is well recognized, and inadequate treatment of AR is known to result in suboptimal control, thus making it an important risk factor for the disease.[5] The increasing awareness of the importance of AR in patients of bronchial asthma resulted in a Joint World Health Organization and the World Allergy Organization initiative entitled "Allergic Rhinitis and Its Impact on Asthma (ARIA)."[6] The ARIA workshop report emphasized the importance of early diagnosis and management of AR for the effective management of asthma.

EPIDEMIOLOGY IN INDIA

In a multicenter study by the Asthma Epidemiology Study Group of the Indian Council of Medical Research, the prevalence of bronchial asthma in Indian adults was observed to be 2.38%. In the same study, the authors also observed that "recurrent coryza" occurred in 3.45%, "recurrent skin rashes" in 2.1%, and "recurrent eye itching" in 2.78% of Indian adults. Considering a population of 1.2 billion, these numbers suggest that the burden of rhinitis as well as asthma in India is immense.[7]

On the basis of temporal variation of symptoms during the year, AR was traditionally divided into seasonal allergic rhinitis (SAR) and perennial allergic rhinitis (PAR).[1,6] Based on the earlier classification, the prevalence of SAR varied from 1% to 40%, whereas the prevalence of PAR ranged from 1% to 18% in different populations around the world.[8] SAR is believed to be more common in children and adolescents, whereas PAR is more common in adults. Children of patients with AR carry double the risk of developing AR as compared to others.[9]

The International Study on Asthma and Allergy in Childhood Conducted in India

The International Study on Asthma and Allergy in Childhood (ISAAC) research program, established in 1991, is a worldwide collaborative research project involving more than 100 countries and 2 million children.[10-12] This is a unique international initiative to monitor time trends and determinants of the prevalence of asthma and allergies in children. ISAAC developed simple methods for measuring the prevalence of childhood asthma, AR, and atopic eczema for international comparisons, suitable for different geographical locations and languages. Data on nasal symptoms, hay fever, and allergic rhinoconjunctivitis were obtained through a standardized questionnaire. Nasal symptoms were said to be present if the child ever had sneezing, or a runny nose, or a blocked nose in the absence of a cold or the flu. Since there were no widely agreed criteria for the diagnosis or classification of rhinitis, then the term "hay fever" was applied for symptoms pertaining to SAR. If nasal complaints were accompanied by itchy, watery eyes, it was classified as allergic rhinoconjunctivitis. The study comprised children in two age groups: 6–7 years age group and 13–14 years age group. For the 6–7 years age group, there were 91 collaborating centers in 38 countries; whereas in the 13–14 years age group, 155 centers from 56 countries participated.

Phase I (1994–1995)

The ISAAC[11] described the prevalence and severity of asthma, AR, and eczema in children using a standard methodology across the world. The prevalence of rhinitis in patients with itchy, watery eyes ("rhinoconjunctivitis") ranged from 0.8% to 14.9% in the 6–7 years age group and from 1.4% to 39.7% in the 13–14 years age group.

The first phase of ISAAC (1994–1995)[11] in India was conducted in 14 centers. The prevalence of "nasal symptoms ever," "hay fever ever," and "allergic rhinoconjunctivitis" was recorded in two age groups: 6–7 years (*n* = 37,171) and 13–14 years (*n* = 30,879). The prevalence of "nasal symptoms ever" was 12.5% in the 6–7 years age group and 18.6% in the 13–14 years age group; the prevalence of "hay fever ever" was 5.5% in the 6–7 years age group and 8.0% in the 13–14 years age group; and the prevalence of "allergic rhinoconjunctivitis" was 3.3% in the 6–7 years age group and 6.3% in the 13–14 years age group (Table 24.1). These figures were much lower compared with those in the West. In the multicenter study[7] on epidemiology of bronchial asthma in Indian adults, the prevalence of "recurrent coryza" ranged from 1.4% to 7.6%.

Phase II

Not conducted in India.

Phase III (1999–2004)

In the third phase of ISAAC,[12] conducted in 19 centers in the country, the prevalence of current nose symptoms increased from 12.5% to 12.9% in the 6–7 years age group, whereas in the 13–14 years age group, it increased from 18.6% to 23.6%. The prevalence of allergic rhinoconjunctivitis increased to 3.9% and 10.4% in the 6–7 years and 13–14 years age groups, respectively (Table 24.1).

Table 24.1: ISAAC studies in India.[11,12]

Disease symptoms	*Phase I 1994–1995: 14 centers*	*Phase III 1999–2004: 19 centers*
13–14 years	*n* = 37,171	*n* = 30,879
Nasal symptoms ever	18.6	29
Hay fever ever	8.0	17.9
Allergic rhinoconjunctivitis	5.6	10
6–7 years	*n* = 52,098	*n* = 46,761
Nose symptom ever	12.5	15.6
Hay fever ever	5.5	7.6
Allergic rhinoconjunctivitis	3.3	3.9

When compared with countries in the Asia Pacific and the Oceanic regions, it was seen that the prevalence in India was lower (Table 24.2).[13]

CLASSIFICATION

The ARIA workshop report[6] proposed to replace the traditional classification of AR, namely, SAR and PAR with "intermittent" and "persistent" categories. This was based on number of days per week during which the symptoms occur (Box 24.1). The report emphasized the need for epidemiological evidence to link AR with other atopic diseases like asthma, allergic conjunctivitis, and eczema, and stressed upon the need for use of new categorization for epidemiological studies. The new classification, however, lacked validation in daily practice.[14]

Since all symptoms may not be present in every patient with AR, Mygind,[15] in 1979, proposed for the first time that patients with perennial rhinitis could be categorized into two groups as per their most troublesome symptoms. Those who predominantly had sneezing and watery discharge as their most troublesome symptoms were classified as "sneezers," whereas those with nasal blockage and mucous secretions as their main symptoms were described as "blockers." In 1994, the International Consensus Report[1] acknowledged the division of patients into "sneezers and runners" and "blockers," and provided clinical features to distinguish between the two entities. In the ARIA workshop report,[6] this subdivision was included in the diagnosis and assessment of severity of rhinitis and was advocated as an important part of clinical history. The report observed that patients with AR could be more commonly found

Table 24.2: ISAAC: Prevalence of allergic rhinoconjunctivitis in the Indian subcontinent, Asia Pacific, and the Oceanic countries.[11,12]

	Phase I (1994–1995)		*Phase III (1999–2004)*	
Age group	13–14 years	6–7 years	13–14 years	6–7 years
India	6.3	3.2	10.0	3.9
Hong Kong	24.0	13.7	22.6	17.7
Indonesia	5.3	3.8	4.8	3.6
Japan	14.9	7.8	17.6	10.6
Malaysia	13.9	4.1	16.2	4.8
Singapore	15.1	8.5	16.5	8.7
South Korea	10.2	9.8	11.6	8.7
Taiwan	11.7	14.6	17.8	24.2
Thailand	15.5	7.3	21.0	10.4
New Zealand	19.1	9.5	18.0	11.4

BOX 24.1: Classification of allergic rhinitis based on "Allergic Rhinitis and Its Impact on Asthma."[6]

Intermittent: symptoms <4 days/week, and <4 weeks duration

Persistent: symptoms >4 days/week, and >4 weeks duration

Mild disease

Normal sleep

Normal daily activities

Sport, leisure

Normal work and school

No troublesome symptoms

Moderate–severe disease

(One or more items should be present)

Abnormal sleep

Impairment of daily activities, sport, leisure

Problems caused at work and school

Troublesome symptoms

in the "sneezers and runners" category. However, the epidemiological evidence for such a subdivision was previously lacking in the literature.

We compared the clinical and epidemiological profiles of "sneezers and runners" and "blockers."[16] In addition, the earlier classification, namely, SAR and PAR, was compared with the newly proposed categories, i.e., "intermittent" and "persistent." In our study,[16] based on clinical history, almost two-thirds of the 114 patients studied were classified as "sneezers and runners." A significant number of patients in this group were categorized as SAR, but as per the ARIA workshop report,[6] more of these patients were classified as "moderate-severe intermittent." However, a quarter of "sneezers and runners" who were traditionally classified as PAR were now classified as "intermittent." Most of the "blockers" were classified as PAR, and as per the ARIA workshop report classification,[6] more than half were classified as "mild persistent." Thus, patients in our study were better represented when they were classified according to duration and severity of symptoms as per the ARIA categorization.

Patients who are predominantly "sneezers and runners" often report sneezing and anterior rhinorrhea along with itchy nose and itchy eyes as their main symptoms. More patients with SAR are categorized as "sneezers and runners." A significant number of "sneezers and runners" described by us had an atopic family background.[16] In contrast, "blockers" are troubled by severe nasal blockage and thick nasal mucus, which often leads to postnasal drip and breathlessness. The symptoms are constant during the day but may worsen during the night. Further, because of associated breathlessness, these patients could be mistakenly diagnosed as having asthma only, with the possibility of rhinitis being overlooked. Early identification of such patients assumes importance, since morbidity that results from misdiagnosis can be avoided. "Blockers" had significantly more sensitization to perennial allergens, such as fungi and house dust mite. More patients with PAR were categorized as "blockers."

"Sneezers and runners" are often accompanied by ocular symptoms, skin allergy, and throat and palatal itching, whereas patients categorized as "blockers" complain more of mouth breathing, loss of smell, postnasal drip, and breathlessness.[17]

ALLERGENS AND TRIGGER FACTORS

Allergens are antigens that induce and react with specific IgE antibodies. Common aeroallergens arise from a variety of sources, namely, pollens, animals, insects, and fungi, and are often implicated in the pathogenesis of AR.[18] It has been postulated that, worldwide, the increase in domestic aeroallergens like the house dust mite, is responsible for an increase in the prevalence of respiratory allergies.[19]

Tobacco smoke exposure, both active and passive, can lead to increase in risk of allergic diseases in which age is an important factor. In a recent systematic review and meta-analysis, it was observed that both active and passive smoking were associated with a modest increase in the risk of AR in children and adolescents. It has been postulated that the immaturity of the respiratory, nervous, and immune systems in children may make them vulnerable to the health hazards of smoking. In addition, unlike adults, children have limited options to avoid passive smoking, and they are also unable to reduce the quantity of products inhaled.[20]

Skin Test Reactivity in AR in India

The SAR, also known as hay fever, is caused by an IgE-mediated reaction to seasonal aeroallergens like pollens and molds. Length of seasonal exposure to these allergens is dependent on geographical location. In India,[21] there are mainly two pollen seasons: February–April and September–December. In the former season, trees are the dominant aeroallergens, whereas in the latter season, weeds and grasses are the dominant aeroallergens. Molds do not show any definite seasonal trend and are present throughout the year, but definitely show seasonal exacerbation in summer and winter months. Indoor fungi are, however, mainly perennial in nature depending on the source of availability. PAR is caused by aeroallergens, which are present all the year round in the environment. These aeroallergens are commonly found indoors. They include dust mites, molds, animal allergens, or certain pollens and occupational allergens in areas where they may be predominantly present throughout the year. Skin test reactivity in our 114 patients with allergic rhinitis[16] revealed that all patients were sensitive to at least three aeroallergens. Among these, 25 (22%) were positive against three aeroallergens, whereas 39 (34%), 26 (23%), and 24 (21%) were positive against four, five, and six aeroallergens, respectively. Seventy-nine patients (69%) were sensitive to pollens, which were significantly more in sneezers–runners (61, 85%) ($p = 0.02$). In this group, among the pollens, weeds were positive in 49 patients (68%) ($p = 0.03$), grasses in 51 patients (71%) ($p = 0.03$), and trees in 39 patients (54%) ($p = 0.04$). "Blockers" had significantly more sensitization to fungi (26, 62%) and house dust mite (17, 40%) ($p = 0.04$). Sensitization to insects (75, 66%) ($p = 0.08$), kapok cotton (6, 5%) ($p = 0.13$), and wool (4, 3%) ($p = 0.16$) was more in "sneezers and runners," but the difference was not statistically significant.

Skin testing against locally prevalent common aeroallergens in our patients with AR showed that sensitivity was highest with pollens, fungi, and house dust mite.[16,22,23] Among *Aspergilli*, sensitization to *Aspergillus flavus* was more common than other species.[23] All patients were sensitive to at least three aeroallergens. In our study comparing "sneezers and runners" with "blockers," we found that "blockers" had significantly more sensitization to fungi (62%) and house dust mite (40%) ($p = 0.04$).[16] Sensitivity to insects (66%), kapok cotton (5%), and wool (3%) was more in "sneezers and runners," but the difference was not statistically significant (Table 24.3). In 207 patients with AR, we found that sensitization to pollens was significantly positive among patients with intermittent disease; whereas sensitization to insects, fungi, and house dust mite was significantly more among those with persistent disease.[23] Overall, house dust mite was demonstrated to be the most common allergen.[16,23]

We also studied the relation between skin test reactivity to *Aspergillus* antigens and sinusitis in patients with AR.[24] Skin testing in 131 subjects demonstrated that *Aspergillus* sensitization was significantly higher in the "blockers" group as compared to "sneezers and runners," and also significantly higher in those with associated sinusitis. Furthermore, the CT Scan of the Paranasal Sinuses (CT-PNS) scores were significantly higher in *Aspergillus*-positive "blockers" with sinusitis as compared to the *Aspergillus*-negative. This comparison was not statistically significant in "sneezers and runners." The fact that sensitization to *Aspergillus* antigens increases the severity of sinusitis associated with AR could have important clinical implications as these patients may possibly be at an increased risk for developing allergic *Aspergillus* sinusitis.

Table 24.3: Skin testing with common aeroallergens among "sneezers and runners" and "blockers."[16]

Aeroallergen	*Sneezers and runners*	*Blockers*	*Statistical significance*
Pollens*	61 (85%)	18 (43%)	$p < 0.05$
Insects	48 (67%)	27 (64%)	NS
Fungi	21 (29%)	26 (62%)	$p < 0.05$
Dusts	13 (18%)	18 (43%)	$p < 0.05$
House dust mite	11 (15%)	17 (40%)	$p < 0.05$
Kapok cotton	4 (6%)	2 (5%)	NS
Wool	3 (4%)	1 (2%)	NS

*includes grass, weed, and tree pollens.
NS, not significant.

The menace of indoor pollution has assumed great importance in recent years as most of the time is spent indoors by humans.[25] Tobacco smoke, fuel- or wood-burning stoves, and cooking gas also contribute to indoor pollution, and have been associated with worsening of symptoms.[26] Outdoor pollution by noxious fumes and gases like ozone, sulfur dioxide, and nitrogen dioxide was also documented to affect symptoms in AR.[27,28] Automobile pollution due to fossil fuel combustion may enhance allergic inflammation of airways,[29] and thus could be an important contributor to the increased morbidity in asthma and AR. Use of certain drugs, especially the nonsteroidal anti-inflammatory drugs, was reported to cause worsening of symptoms in patients with asthma and AR alike.[30]

CLINICAL FEATURES

An individual having AR suffers from a symptom complex, of which sneezing is the most characteristic symptom.[2] It may arise without warning and may have paroxysms of 10–20 sneezes. Rhinorrhea is typically continuous, profuse, thin discharge, which may irritate the skin covering the upper lip and nose. However, nasal congestion, which may be the only symptom in perennial disease, is the most troublesome symptom. It may be intermittent, becoming more disturbing in the evening and night. Severe nasal congestion leads to interference with aeration of sinuses and eustachian tube, and is responsible for most of the complications such as sinusitis, mouth breathing, and otitis media. Itching of the nose, especially in children, is characterized by frequent rubbing of the nose in upward and outward direction, and is known as the "allergic salute."[2] This often leads to the development of "nasal crease," a horizontal crease across the lower half of the bridge of the nose. Eye symptoms such as sore or tired eyes and lacrimation are often associated with AR. Other features such as hacking, nonproductive cough due to postnasal drip, fatigue, headache, loss of sleep, poor concentration, anorexia, and abdominal discomfort may also be observed. Periodicity is a characteristic feature of this symptom complex, coinciding temporally with the allergen. Allergen rhinitis tends to increase in severity for 2–3 years and then stabilizes, but may occasionally disappear spontaneously. The history should also include questions on loss of smell, snoring, and sleep problems. Significant nocturnal sleep disturbances, excessive daytime sleepiness, and impairment of sleep-specific Quality of Life have been documented in patients with AR.[31] These features were significantly greater in those with associated sinusitis, persistent disease, and urticaria/eczema. Occurrence of chronic cough, sinusitis, and conjunctivitis must also be looked into. The possibility of associated asthma should always be excluded, and an occupational history should be recorded.

Patients who are predominantly "sneezers and runners" often report sneezing and anterior rhinorrhea along with itchy nose and itchy eyes as their main symptoms. The symptoms are worse during the day and improve during the night. More patients with SAR are categorized as "sneezers and runners." A significant number of "sneezers and runners" described by us had an atopic family background, and in most of them symptoms commenced before the age of 20 years.[16] Significantly, more were born between June and September and were sensitized to pollens, and in a significant number of these patients, the symptoms were aggravated on exposure to dust. A significant history of associated allergic manifestations, such as eye, ear, throat, palate, and skin itching, was a key feature of this group. In contrast, "blockers" are troubled by severe nasal blockage and thick nasal mucous, which often leads to postnasal drip. The symptoms are constant during day and night but may worsen during the night. In our study,[16] "blockers" had a significant history of breathlessness and mouth breathing, were troubled by loss of smell, and also had a history of prior nasal surgical procedures without relief. Early identification of such patients assumes importance, since morbidity that results from unnecessary surgical procedures can be avoided. Further, because of associated breathlessness, these patients could be mistakenly diagnosed as having asthma only, with the possibility of rhinitis being overlooked. It has also been postulated that chronic nasal obstruction and continuous postnasal drip that lead to mouth breathing may play an important role in the development of asthma. These patients could perhaps be at a greater risk of developing asthma. "Blockers" had significantly more sensitization to perennial allergens, such as fungi and house dust mite. This could lead to chronic persistent inflammation in these patients throughout the year even during symptom-free periods. More patients with PAR are categorized as "blockers."

Physical findings are mostly present during acute stage of illness. Nasal endoscopy reveals pale to purple nasal mucosa with increased vascularity, enlarged and boggy inferior turbinates, micropolyps, and edema of middle meatus or watery secretions along the posterior pharyngeal wall. Occasionally, conjunctival congestion may also be seen. Perennial rhinitis may lead to formation of transverse nasal crease and dark crease under the eyes, which are caused by venous stasis secondary to constant nasal congestion ("allergic shiners"), or gaping appearance due to constant mouth breathing. Prominent creases below the inferior eyelids, known as Dennie-Morgan lines, are also associated with AR. Polyps and posterior pharyngeal wall lymphoid follicles may also be found.[1,6] Findings due to associated conditions like nasal polyposis, sinusitis, otitis media, upper respiratory infection apart from asthma, and conjunctivitis may also be present.[2]

COMORBIDITIES

Asthma

Of all the atopic disorders, AR is most commonly associated with asthma.[6,32,33] An editorial[3] entitled "Rarely does one hear a wheeze without a sneeze" succinctly described the close link between the two entities. Nasal symptoms have been reported to occur in 28–78% asthmatics, whereas 17–38% of patients with AR have coexistent asthma.[34] The presence of AR significantly increases the likelihood of having asthma currently or in future by up to 40%.[9]

A questionnaire-based study[35] determined the co-occurrence of AR in 646 outpatient asthmatics (405 children and 241 adults) reporting to our institute. Symptoms of rhinitis were present in 75% of the children and 80% of the adults. Three-fourths of children and 55% of adults with asthma and associated AR had simultaneous onset of both diseases. It was thus observed that AR occurred commonly with asthma and could be an independent risk factor for the development of asthma. In another study[36] in 111 children with AR and/or asthma, both diseases co-occurred in 83 (74%) patients, whereas 9 (8%) had asthma only and 19 (17%) had AR alone. We also found that exposure to environmental tobacco smoke led to significant feeling of suffocation in 7/9 (78%) patients with asthma, 73/83 (88%) patients with asthma and AR, and 15/19 (79%) patients with AR alone.

Sinusitis

The presence of sinusitis further aggravates the morbidity caused by rhinitis and/or asthma. We studied 216 patients with AR and/or asthma for the occurrence of sinusitis.[22] All patients underwent spirometry with reversibility and CT-PNS. As a part of the workup, both investigations were performed in all enrolled patients, prior to commencement of standard therapy. A computed tomography (CT) staging system[37] for noting the extent of rhinosinusitis, with the total score ranging from 0 to 24 depending on the number of sinuses involved, was adopted. Twenty-seven patients had asthma only (group 1), 131 had AR (group 2), and 58 had asthma with AR (group 3). On CT-PNS, sinusitis was present in 20 (74%), 88 (67%), and 48 (82%) of patients, respectively. Sinusitis on CT-PNS was present in more than two-thirds of the 189 patients with AR in groups 2 and 3 (136/189). Postnasal drip (62/88 vs. 15/43, $p < 0.05$) and sneezing (52/88 vs. 7/43, $p < 0.05$) were significantly higher in these patients as compared to those without sinusitis. Coexistent sinusitis increased the severity and morbidity caused by AR, especially in those who were predominantly "blockers."[38]

Nasal Polyposis

Sinusitis is often complicated by the presence of nasal polyps.[39] Nasal polyps are growths developing from the membranes lining the nose and sinuses and extend into the nasal cavity causing symptoms of nasal obstruction.[40]

Study conducted at our institute recruited 220 patients with the diagnosis of bronchial asthma and/or allergic rhinitis. Allergic rhinitis was diagnosed in 43 patients out of the recruited 220 patients and nasal polyps occurred in 30 of these patients.[41]

ALLERGIC RHINITIS AND QUALITY OF LIFE

Allergic rhinitis often results in restrictions on the physical, psychological, and social aspects of the patients' life and can also impact their functions at work. These "quality of life" issues provide information that is not usually obtained by conventional clinical and functional measures. They provide insight into the socioeconomic burden of rhinitis on the individual and also focus on patients' own perception of disease. Several disease-specific questionnaires that objectively measure the impact of rhinitis on health-related quality of life have been developed.[42-45] It was observed that adult patients were bothered by missed or unproductive time at work, sleep disturbances, daytime exhaustion, thirst, poor concentration, and headache. These patients experienced annoying practical problems like having to blow their noses and carrying tissues were limited in their daily activities and felt frustrated and irritable. Adolescents had more problems with concentration, particularly with schoolwork. Although younger children were less disturbed by emotional dysfunction and disturbances in daily routine, they were more troubled by taking medications and carrying tissues. These children have decreased involvement in outdoor activities. Moreover, their parents appeared to be more bothered than the children themselves.[9,44]

For the first time in India, we assessed the quality of life in 34 patients with AR and found that AR caused significant practical problems, emotional distress, and limitation in activities.[45] The disease adversely affected behavior, work performance, and lifestyle of these patients. Appropriate treatment along with patient education resulted in significant improvement in the quality of life at 4 weeks, which continued at 8 weeks. We observed that Indian adults were bothered by problems at work and by the fact that it affected their feeling of general well-being. This was in contrast to the study by Juniper et al.,[43] where the authors reported that adults did not consider these problems as important. Our patients were troubled by their disease, which caused hindrance at work, repeated blowing of the nose, and the need to rub their eyes and nose. They were, however, less troubled by the lack of a good night's sleep and the need to carry handkerchief. This could possibly be due to cultural variations. Allergic rhinitis when occurring concurrently with asthma is likely to further affect the quality of life in such patients.[45] Treatment of AR may have a positive impact on asthma-specific quality of life. A diagnosis of AR thus should always be considered in all patients with asthma.

Recent studies suggest that AR adversely affects sleep-related QoL of patients.[46-48] We assessed the sleep-related quality of life impairment in patients with AR by means of questionnaires.[49] Nocturnal sleep, excessive daytime sleepiness, and sleep-specific QoL disturbances were assessed using the Pittsburgh Sleep Quality Index (PSQI), Epsworth Sleepiness Score (ESS), and Nocturnal Rhinoconjunctivitis Quality of Life Questionnaires (NRQLQ), respectively. The PSQI, ESS, and NRQLQ scores significantly correlated with the presence of nasal obstruction, thick nasal discharge as compared to watery rhinorrhea, and postnasal drip. In addition, the NRQLQ score positively correlated with the number of sneezing episodes per day as well as number of sneezes during each episode. All patients were subjected to CT-PNS for the presence of sinusitis. In 207 patients with AR, we found coexistent sinusitis in 132 (63.7%) patients. Patients with concomitant sinusitis had significant impairment in their nocturnal sleep disturbances and had excessive daytime sleepiness as compared to those without sinusitis.[49]

In addition, the presence of nasal polyposis in patients with AR and sinusitis deteriorates the QoL and sleep further. A marked deterioration in the mean Lund Mackay score, Global Visual Analog Scale score, Sino-Nasal Outcome Test 22 score, and QoL scores has been observed in these patients. Sleep disturbances are also more distressing in this subset of patients.[50]

Effect of Allergic Rhinitis on School-going Children

In 112 school-going children with asthma, AR was documented in 100 (89%) children, 65/100 (65%) of them had confirmed sinusitis on CT-PNS. Of the 12 patients with bronchial asthma only, 7 (58%) had sinusitis. The presence of sinusitis was associated with greater impairment in the quality of life due to increased severity of asthma symptoms and emotional dysfunction.[51]

Allergenic rhinitis also hampers the process of learning and school performance. In children, AR affects the quality of sleep and often can lead to daytime fatigue and sleepiness. It leads to increased school absenteeism and distraction during class hours. Associated conditions like sinusitis, asthma, conjunctivitis, eczema, eustachian tube dysfunction, and otitis media add to the morbidity associated with AR.[52]

DIAGNOSIS AND LABORATORY FINDINGS

Although there is no specific test that is diagnostic of AR, laboratory findings can aid in reaching a definite diagnosis.

Allergy Testing

Determination of immediate hypersensitivity to clinically important local aeroallergens, with proper quality control measures, is a simple, rapid, and cheap method of establishing an allergic cause of the disease.[53] It also aids in determining specific allergic triggers in susceptible individuals. Several methods of skin testing are available, but skin prick–puncture tests (SPTs) are now recommended for routine testing for diagnosis of IgE-mediated diseases.[53] In some cases (e.g., in weak allergen solutions), intradermal skin tests may be used instead of SPT. Although they are more sensitive than SPT, they are less safe, correlate less well with clinical symptoms, and may induce false-positive reactions.[54]

Serum IgE

Raised serum IgE levels are found in patients with AR, but this test is neither sensitive nor specific for AR.[2] Around 35–50% of patients with AR may have normal total IgE levels, whereas 20% of asymptomatic individuals can have elevated total IgE levels.[55] It has also been suggested that levels greater than 50 IU/mL in infants or 200 IU/mL in older children and adults may correlate better with the presence of atopy.[56] This test is generally not used alone to establish the diagnosis of AR, but the results can be helpful in some cases when combined with other factors. Serum IgE can be measured using radioimmunoassay such as radioallergosorbent test, which indirectly measures the quantity of specific IgE antibodies against a particular antigen, or by enzyme-linked immunosorbent assay.[57] Serum allergen-specific IgE is of more importance and correlates closely with skin tests and nasal challenges. The specificity and sensitivity of these tests may reach up to 85%.[58]

It has been observed that more than half of patients with AR may have negative serum IgE or skin testing. This is explained by the existence of "local allergic rhinitis" associated with the production of allergen-specific IgE antibodies limited to the nasal mucosa. This requires the measurement of specific IgE in nasal fluid, restricted to research now and may be available in future.[59]

Total Eosinophil Counts

Eosinophils are the predominant cells in nasal cytology smears. Peripheral blood eosinophilia of 4–12% may be seen in patients with AR. Although an elevated eosinophil count supports the diagnosis of AR, it is neither sensitive nor specific for diagnosis.

Nasal Provocation Tests

These may help in confirming sensitivity to allergens but are of limited clinical utility. They are, however, important in diagnosing occupational rhinitis.

Radiological Imaging

Radiographic studies are not usually needed to establish the diagnosis of AR, but can be helpful for evaluating possible structural abnormalities or to help detect complications or comorbid conditions, such as sinusitis or adenoid hypertrophy. Plain radiographs can be helpful for diagnosing acute sinusitis, but CT of the sinuses is more sensitive and specific for the diagnosis of major sinonasal disorders.[60] Magnetic resonance imaging, generally less helpful than CT, is useful in fungal sinusitis.[61]

Other tests include upper airway endoscopy and acoustic rhinometry that objectively measure functional obstruction to airflow in the upper airway but are not used for routine evaluation of patients.

DIFFERENTIAL DIAGNOSIS

There are many conditions that mimic the presentation of AR. The differential diagnosis of AR is summarized in Box 24.2.[62]

MANAGEMENT

Goals of management for AR include restoration of nasal patency, control of nasal secretions, treatment of nasal complications related to obstruction, and prevention of recurrent symptoms. Principles of management are allergen avoidance, control and rescue medications (pharmacotherapy), and immunotherapy in selected patients.

BOX 24.2: Differential diagnosis of allergic rhinitis.[62]

- Vasomotor rhinitis or nonallergic rhinitis
- Gustatory rhinitis (vagally mediated)
- Rhinitis medicamentosa (e.g., due to topical decongestants, antihypertensives, cocaine abuse)
- Hormonal rhinitis (e.g., related to pregnancy, hypothyroidism, oral contraceptive use)
- Anatomic rhinitis (eg., deviated septum, choanal atresia, adenoid hypertrophy, foreign body, nasal tumor)
- NARES
- Immotile cilia syndrome (ciliary dyskinesis)
- Cerebrospinal fluid leak
- Nasal polyps
- Granulomatous rhinitis (e.g., Wegener granulomatosis, sarcoidosis).

BOX 24.3: Stepwise management of allergic rhinitis (with increasing severity).[6]

1. Allergen avoidance
2. Antihistamines: oral/topical
3. Topical decongestants: short course
4. Topical sodium cromoglycate
5. Topical steroids
6. Anti-inflammatory drugs
   Oral steroids: short course
   Antileukotriene agents
   Anti-IgE: omalizumab
7. Immunotherapy.

Based on the classification of symptoms, the ARIA document[6] proposed an evidence-based and stepwise approach of pharmacological treatment of allergic rhinitis (Box 24.3).

Allergen Avoidance

A wide range of allergens have been associated with AR; of which, house dust mites are the most important allergen.[19] Avoiding allergens reduces the symptoms and the need for drug treatment, but benefits may take several weeks to be perceived. Allergen avoidance should be an integral part in the management strategy for AR. House dust mite reduction can be achieved by washing blankets, curtains and bed linen, removal of carpets, control of humidity, and improving ventilation.

Pharmacotherapy

Topical and oral antihistamines, nasal decongestants, and topical as well as oral corticosteroids, along with anticholinergic drugs, comprise the armamentarium available against AR.[63] The efficacy of various drugs available for allergic rhinitis is highlighted in Table 24.4.[6]

Nasal Decongestants

These are α_1-agonist drugs, which reduce the thickness of nasal mucosa by decreasing blood flow and producing vasoconstriction. These may be used systemically or topically. Topical nasal decongestants, besides relieving nasal blockage, allow other topical preparations to penetrate effectively into the nasal cavity. They should not be used for more than a week to 10 days for the fear of rebound phenomenon and rhinitis medicamentosa. Systemic nasal decongestants should be used with caution as they may cause elevated blood pressure, palpitations, loss of appetite, tremors, and sleep disturbances.

Oral Antihistamines

Antihistamines are common initial treatment for patients with AR. The newer oral antihistamines improve patients' quality of life by their effectiveness against most symptoms, namely, rhinorrhea, sneezing, nasal itching, and eye symptoms that are chiefly mediated by histamine.[63] They are, however, less effective for nasal congestion. The first-generation antihistamines usually cause sedation and anticholinergic symptoms like dry mucous membranes, urinary retention, or blurred vision. Narrow-angle glaucoma or prostatic hypertrophy can also be exacerbated. Newer antihistamines are more effective with superior safety.

Cetirizine

A piperazine derivative is a longer acting antihistamine with no cardiac or anticholinergic activities. It provides a positive impact on work/school-related productivity and activity impairment in patients with pollen-induced rhinitis.[64] In the multicenter, double-blind, randomized, placebo-controlled Early Treatment of the Atopic Child (ETAC) trial,[65] cetirizine, after 18 months of treatment, was shown to halve the number of atopic children developing asthma in those sensitized to grass pollens or house dust mite. Cetirizine has also been reported to be of benefit in concomitant eczema and allergic conjunctivitis.

Table 24.4: Efficacy of various agents in allergic rhinitis.[6]

Symptoms	*Nasal decongestants*	*Antihistamines*	*Topical steroids*
Rhinorrhea	–	++	+++
Itching	–	++	+++
Sneezing	–	++	+++
Blockage	++++	+	+++
Impaired smell	–	–	+
Eye symptoms	–	++	++

Levocetirizine

In the treatment of SAR, by comparison with other dosages, levocetirizine, 5 mg once daily, has an optimal benefit/risk ratio and is effective in relieving nasal congestion in patients with PAR.[66] The effect of levocetirizine administered for over 6 months to 551 patients with moderate-to-severe persistent allergic rhinitis (XPERT study)[67] showed that compared to placebo, levocetirizine improved nasal symptoms including nasal obstruction and quality of life (RQLQ and SF-36) and reduced medical costs involved in the long-term management. It was seen that levocetirizine had no effect on cognitive and psychomotor functions in healthy volunteers[68] and on driving performance.[69]

Fexofenadine

Adverse effects of terfenadine on the cardiac rhythm led to introduction of fexofenadine, a metabolite of terfenadine that generally does not cause QTc interval prolongation or any interactions with macrolides and ketoconazole. Fexofenadine, 120 mg once a day, is effective in relieving eye symptoms and nasal congestion, and also improves the quality of life.[70] It improves itchy, watery, red eyes, and nasal congestion symptoms more effectively than loratadine.[71] It has an excellent safety profile and lacks sedating effects. Inability to cross the blood-brain barrier might explain the fact that, at even very high doses, it does not cause sedation and does not impair driving performance. The high selectivity of fexofenadine for peripheral H_1 receptors and the lack of interaction with muscarinic receptors might offer a potential advantage compared with other newer antihistamines.[71]

Desloratadine

A dosage of 5 mg daily provides significant 24-hour relief in SAR. It reduces nasal congestion and bronchial symptoms during the pollen season in patients with seasonal asthma and rhinitis.[72] It is free of adverse effects on psychomotor performance and subjective sleepiness, and is also suitable for those involved in skilled activity, driving, and transportation.[73] Pharmacodynamic interactions have not been documented with ketoconazole, erythromycin, or azithromycin.[74]

Ebastine

In pollen-induced rhinitis, ebastine, 20 mg once daily, is considered significantly superior to loratadine. It improves the total rhinitis symptom score throughout the day and does not alter objective measures of psychomotor and cognitive function.[75] There is no effect on food intake or clinically relevant changes in the QTc interval with ebastine.

Rupatadine

This newer antihistamine may have the potential to provide better control of symptoms than other oral H_1 antihistamines due to its proposed dual pharmacologic profile, which includes antagonism of the H_1 receptor and platelet-activating factor.[76] In a dosage of 10 mg per day, it was effective in alleviating the symptoms of SAR over a 2-week period.

Olopatadine

It is a second-generation antihistamine, having a potential role in the treatment of allergic rhinitis. It antagonizes histamine at the end organ, and also inhibits the release of histamine and other proinflammatory mediators from human mast cells.[77] It significantly suppresses sneezing, rhinorrhea, and nasal congestion.[78]

Topical Antihistamines

Topical antihistaminic sprays have a rapid onset of action (less than 15 minutes), and the action lasts for 12 hours.

Thus, twice daily therapy is required to maintain a satisfactory clinical response. As their action is limited to the target organ, systemic side effects are minimal. However, adverse effects like nasal irritation and bitter after taste are not uncommon. These sprays are now mainly recommended for mild organ-limited disease, as an "on-demand" medication, in conjunction with continuous medications.[79]

Azelastine, a second-generation antihistamine, is available in the form of an intranasal spray. It improves nasal symptoms of rhinitis, including congestion and postnasal drip. When used in combination with fluticasone nasal spray, azelastine provided greater benefit for patients with moderate-to-severe symptoms than either drug alone.[80]

Olopatadine Spray

It is another second-generation antihistamine, available in the form of 0.6% nasal spray. The duration of action is 12 hours and is administered in a dosage of two sprays in each nostril twice a day. It is well tolerated, and safety profile is similar to azelastine. Olopatadine may be more acceptable than azelastine in some patients.[81]

Corticosteroids

Corticosteroids can be used either topically or as systemic agents.[63] Systemic corticosteroids are not indicated for routine treatment of AR. However, a short course of oral steroids (30 mg of oral prednisolone every morning for 3–7 days) may be used to treat moderate–severe disease.[6]

Topical Corticosteroids

Intranasal corticosteroid sprays (INCSs) are the mainstay of treatment of AR.[63] The rationale for using INCS in the treatment of AR is that high drug concentrations can be achieved at receptor sites in the nasal mucosa, with minimal risk of systemic adverse effects. They inhibit both early and late phases of inflammatory response, and are more effective than H_1 antihistamines in reducing all the symptoms of rhinitis, including nasal congestion. Because of their mechanism of action, efficacy appears after 7–8 hours of dosing, but maximum efficacy may require up to 2 weeks. Evidence shows that the long-term use of INCS is free of the concerns associated with the long-term use of oral glucocorticosteroids.[63] Topical preparations do not interfere with skin testing while they continue to suppress the nasal symptoms. Topical preparations of beclomethasone dipropionate (BDP), budesonide (BUD), fluticasone (FP), mometasone (MF), and ciclesonide are currently available as nasal sprays in India. In patients with AR, allergen exposure varies throughout the year, and there are periods in which there is little exposure. Even though symptom free, these patients present with minimal persistent inflammation of the nose and thus should receive INCS on a regular basis.[82] However, compliance to long-term usage of steroid-based preparations has been an area of concern as undue fear, anxiety, and misconception about steroid usage exist among both patients and treating physicians.[83] Studies have shown that patients' perception of their treatment is an important factor for gaining compliance and achieving success in the management of AR.[84-86] This perception is determined not only by the effectiveness and safety of the nasal spray but also by patients' preference for a particular drug. The INCSs that are currently available differ little by way of efficacy and safety profiles, and no consistent studies are available that show superiority of one drug over another.[6,63] However, they vary in their sensory perceptions and studies carried out in this regard highlighted the patients' preference and liking for the drug which appealed most to sensory and physical attributes such as taste, aftertaste, irritation, and odor.[84-86] It is presumed that patients are likely to persist with the drug that is acceptable to them, and this may be an essential factor in successful treatment outcome.[87] Although drug efficacy remains the most important guiding force, many physicians now acknowledge the role of sensory attributes in distinguishing INCS, which may determine the product choice for an individual patient.[88] The preference and acceptability of the four INCSs (BDP, BUD, FP, and MF) based on their sensory perceptions was recently evaluated[86] for the first time in Indian patients with AR. The study found that a significant number of patients preferred MF to the other INCS due to less irritation, odor, and aftertaste, along with superior moistness. This led to a greater overall acceptance of MF as compared to other INCS.[86] In patients with AR, assessment of sensory perceptions could thus play a crucial role in promoting compliance with therapy.

Adverse effects of INCS include transient symptoms of nasal stinging, throat irritation, dry nose, nasal bleeding, and nasal septal perforation.[89] There is no evidence of atrophy of nasal mucosa or nasopharyngeal infection including candidiasis after regular use of BDP or BUD even for 5 years. In children, a reduction in rate of growth was reported earlier[90] in those regularly treated twice a day with intranasal BDP over 1 year. However, no growth slowing has been observed in those treated with FP or MF.[91-92]

In the elderly, the risk of steroid-induced osteoporosis is low and, at the recommended dosages, is not associated with an increased risk of fractures.[93]

Topical Anticholinergic Agents

Anitcholinergics can reduce watery rhinorrhea especially in gustatory and vasomotor rhinitis but have no effect on nasal blockage, itching, or sneezing.[94,95] Ipratropium bromide is the commonly used topical anticholinergic as an isotonic nasal spray. Systemic effects of ipratropium are uncommon due to its low lipid solubility and poor absorption in the systemic circulation. It has been used in combination with terfenadine and beclomethasone with better results.[95] Nasal dryness, irritation, and burning are the most common side effects, followed by dry mouth and headache. Ipratropium bromide is now primarily recommended for patients with rhinorrhea as their primary symptom and in particular gustatory rhinitis. The daily dose ranges from 120 to 320 μg in 3–6 administrations.[96]

Sodium Cromoglycate

Topical instillation of 4% solution of sodium cromoglycate is used as prophylactic agent as it inhibits degranulation of sensitized mast cells, thereby preventing the release of inflammatory mediators.[97] It is more effective in adults with concomitant conjunctivitis, children, and pregnant females. The therapy should begin at least 1 week before the expected exposure time in SAR as it normally takes 4–7 days for relief to be perceived. Regular and round-the-clock administration of the drug is important because it does not relieve symptoms once the allergic reaction has begun.[97]

Leukotriene Antagonists

Leukotrienes, especially LTC4 and LTD4, are more potent than histamine in causing nasal obstruction. Antileukotrienes like zafirlukast and montelukast, as well as the 5-lipoxygenase inhibitor, zileuton, may be useful in relieving nasal symptoms, especially nasal obstruction, in patients with AR. These agents have the advantage of oral route of administration. Montelukast when used concomitantly with loratadine has been shown to significantly improve eye symptoms, nighttime symptoms, individual daytime nasal symptoms, global evaluation, and quality of life in patients with SAR.[98] Combined treatment of montelukast with cetirizine is effective in preventing nasal symptoms when used prophylactically in SAR and reduces allergic inflammation in the nasal mucosa during natural allergen exposure.[99] Currently, these agents are recommended for patients with aspirin-sensitive rhinitis, those with asthma, and those who remain symptomatic despite treatment with antihistamines and INCS.[100] These agents are less effective than INCS in AR, and have an efficacy similar to oral H_1 antihistamines. Adverse effects include vasculitis and allergic reactions in few patients.[6] Montelukast does not modify skin prick test results and therefore does not need to be discontinued before skin testing.[101]

A word of caution about antileukotrienes is their potential to cause Churg–Strauss syndrome (CSS). So far, more than 100 cases of CSS possibly related to antileukotrienes have been recorded by the US Food and Drug Administration (FDA).[102] The onset of CSS ranged from 2 days to 15 months of antileukotriene therapy. It has been postulated that these cases of CSS may result from the unmasking of an underlying incipient "forme fruste" of the vasculitis, during the steroid withdrawal or tapering made possible by antileukotrienes, or from a direct causal role of antileukotrienes.

Humanized Monoclonal Antibodies against IgE

The recombinant humanized monoclonal anti-IgE antibody, omalizumab, is a novel therapy used in patients with SAR.[103] It acts by forming complexes with free IgE, blocking its interaction with mast cells and basophils, and lowering free IgE levels in the circulation. Omalizumab decreases all nasal symptoms and has been proposed to improve the quality of life in patients with rhinitis induced by birch and ragweed pollens as well as those with sensitization to outdoor allergens. However, the relative efficacy compared to H_1 antihistamines and INCS needs to be established. Specific immunotherapy and treatment with monoclonal anti-IgE antibodies have complementary modes of action and may prove useful in sensitized patients.[104] The US FDA, in a postmarketing adverse events survey, documented anaphylactic reactions associated with omalizumab in a total of 124 patients with asthma.[105] Most of the cases had a delayed reaction (after 2 hours), and many were characterized by a protracted regression.

Immunotherapy

Allergen-specific immunotherapy is the practice of administering gradually increasing quantities of an allergen to an allergic subject in order to ameliorate symptoms subsequent to exposure.[6] Immunotherapy using inhalant allergens has been found to be effective in patients with AR. It is indicated as a supplement to allergen avoidance when patients do not respond completely to conventional pharmacologic therapy. It should be started early in the course of rhinitis to reduce the risk of side effects and progression of disease. Injectable subcutaneous-specific immunotherapy may be indicated in severe or prolonged AR, especially those associated with asthma.[6] Individuals with good correlation between history and the presence of specific IgE antibodies are potential candidates for immunotherapy.

A recent Cochrane review,[106] a meta-analysis of 51 randomized double-blind, placebo-controlled trials involving 2,871 subjects with SAR or controls, showed that immunotherapy resulted in a significant improvement in overall symptoms, medication use, and quality of life, more so in patients with SAR. In part, this could possibly reflect the difficulty in determining the extent to which allergy is responsible for perennial symptoms. Nevertheless, clinical trials have shown a definite benefit in appropriately selected subjects.

When more than one allergen is combined into a single mixture for administration, it should be ensured that the components are compatible, and the potency of each individual allergen is not diminished by the presence of other components or due to excessive dilution. Though there is individual variability, a 3- to 5-year treatment is appropriate for most patients, and if a patient does not improve after 1 year of immunotherapy, it should be discontinued.[6] This modality should be avoided in serious immunodeficiency diseases, malignancy, cardiovascular diseases, and those who are on β-blockers. It is not indicated in children and should not be started during pregnancy.

Combination Therapies

Combination therapy with different drugs, with different effects and mechanisms of action may lead to additive or synergistic benefit to the patient.[107] It is indicated in patients with AR who have inadequate response to monotherapy.[108] Recently, FDA approved the use of azelastine hydrochloride and fluticasone propionate nasal spray in a single device. In randomized trials, it has been observed that the combination of an intranasal antihistamine plus an intranasal glucocorticoid is superior to either agent alone.[9] Also, a study of combination therapy with decongestant oxymetazoline and the corticosteroid mometasone furoate nasal spray revealed decreased nasal congestion, improved quality of life without significant risk for rhinitis medicamentosa. The risks involved with combination therapies include increased costs, ineffective combinations, drug interactions, and increased side effects.[108]

Inferior Turbinate Reduction

Inferior turbinate reduction is a surgical alternative for those patients with AR with nasal airway obstruction and enlarged inferior turbinates who have failed medical management.[108]

Non-pharmacological Therapy

Acupuncture has found its role as a non-pharmacological therapy for patients with AR.[108] It helps in reduction of symptoms, improvement in QoL, avoidance of medication use, and its potential medication side effects. It is indicated in patients who are not willing for pharmacological treatment.

FUTURE PERSPECTIVES

New Routes for Administration of Specific Immunotherapy

Intralymphatic Route

In a randomized controlled trial[107,109] of 165 patients with AR due to grass pollen allergy, intralymphatic allergen injections were compared to conventional subcutaneous immunotherapy. Intralymphatic immunotherapy produced long-lasting and comparable effects after only three intralymphatic injections as compared to 3 years of subcutaneous immunotherapy. This also leads to fewer allergic reactions and better patients' adherence and compliance to treatment.

Sublingual Route

In this route, allergen is kept under the tongue for 1–2 minutes and then swallowed. It is easier and safer to administer than given subcutaneously (SCIT), and it can also be given without medical supervision. Though it was recently approved route for grass or ragweed allergy in the United States, it is still not approved for use in India.[9]

Epicutaneous Administration

In a placebo-controlled, double-blind trial in patients with AR, epicutaneous administration in the form of patches filled with grass pollen extract applied on the skin with a self-adhesive tape was found to be safe, better tolerated, and induced significant amelioration of symptoms as compared to placebo.

Cytokine Inhibition

Cytokines have a role in allergic inflammation, and interleukin 33 (IL-33) can induce Th2 cytokine production in Th2 cells, mast cells, basophils, and eosinophils. Considering the role of IL-33, anti-IL-33 treatment is an option for future as evidenced by benefits in an experimental animal model.

Histamine H_3 and H_4 Receptor Antagonists

Histamine H_3 receptors are involved in modulating vascular contractile responses in human nasal mucosa. Therefore, H_3 receptor antagonism may provide clinical benefit to the patient. In animal models, combinations of H_1/H_3 receptor antagonism inhibit nasal congestion. PF-03654746, an H_3 receptor antagonist, along with fexofenadine, was able to reduce nasal symptoms after allergen challenge in humans.

H_4 receptors are found mainly in hematopoietic cells particularly mast cells, basophils, and eosinophils. Pharmacological studies have suggested the role of H_4 receptor antagonists in the treatment of inflammatory diseases. Clinical trials are going on, for UR-63325, an H_4 receptor antagonist. Currently, none of H_3 or H_4 receptor antagonists is approved for treatment of AR.

Phosphodiesterase 4 Inhibitors

Phosphodiesterase 4 (PDE4) is an intracellular enzyme and is expressed in most of the inflammatory cells. It is involved in degradation and inactivation of cyclic adenosine monophosphate (cAMP). PDE4 inhibitor inhibits the inflammatory processes by elevating cAMP levels. In a randomized, double-blind, placebo-controlled study in 25 patients[110] with AR, exposed to allergen challenge, roflumilast, a PDE4 inhibitor has been found to be effective.

Toll-like Receptors Targeted Treatment

Toll-like receptors (TLRs) are a family of pattern recognition receptors expressed by various cells. TLR8 activator molecule, VTX1463, is currently under development for the treatment of AR as nasal spray.

CONCLUSION

Allergic rhinitis is not an insignificant disease. An independent diagnosis of AR in our country is yet to be commonly accepted. In spite of causing a major impact on the quality of life in Indian patients, AR is rarely given the importance it warrants. It causes significant practical problems, limits patients' activities, and has adverse effects on emotions. Troublesome systemic symptoms are also frequently encountered. Patients fail to attribute the ill-health to symptoms of AR, and this disease continues to remain neglected. In India, it is often treated as an "orphan" disease as AR falls in the gray area between the otorhinolaryngologist and the pulmonologist resulting in lack of focus on research in AR by both the specialties.[111] The current approach to classification is likely to play an important role in formulating management strategies in AR. Topical corticosteroids, which reduce all the symptoms and have no significant adverse effects, are now recognized as the cornerstone of the treatment for AR. Appropriate treatment improves patients' well-being not only when AR is the primary condition but also when it occurs concomitantly with other allergic disorders, especially with asthma.[112] However, in India, AR, a not-so-trivial disease constellation, is often neglected and still does not receive the attention it deserves by both patients and clinicians.[113]

REFERENCES

1. International consensus report on diagnosis and management of rhinitis. International rhinitis management working group. Allergy. 1994;49:1-34.
2. Dykewicz MS, Fineman S. Diagnosis and management of rhinitis: parameter documents of the joint task force on practice parameters in allergy, asthma and immunology. American Academy of Allergy and Immunology. Ann Allergy Asthma Immunol. 1998;8:463-518.
3. Shah A. Editorial—Rarely does one hear a wheeze without a sneeze. Indian J Chest Dis Allied Sci. 2000;42:143-5.
4. Juniper EF. Quality of life in adults and children with asthma rhinitis. Allergy. 1997;52:971-7.
5. Grossman J. One airway, one disease. Chest. 1997;111: 11S-6S.

6. Bousquet J, van Cauwenberge P, Khaltaev N, et al. ARIA workshop group; World Health Organization. Allergic rhinitis and its impact on asthma. J Allergy Clin Immunol. 2001;108:S147-334.
7. Aggarwal AN, Chaudhary K, Chhabra SK, et al. Prevalence and risk factors for bronchial asthma in Indian adults: a multicentre study. Indian J Chest Dis Allied Sci. 2006;48:13-22.
8. Sibbald B. Epidemiology of allergic rhinitis. In: Burr ML, ed. Epidemiology of Clinical Allergy. Monographs in Allergy. Basel: Karger; 1993:61-9.
9. Wheatley LM, Togias A. Allergic rhinitis. N Engl J Med. 2015;372:456-63.
10. Asher MI, Keiln U, Anderson HR, et al. International Study of Asthma and Allergies in Childhood (ISAAC): rationale and methods. Eur Respir J. 1995;8:483-91.
11. Strachan D, Sibbald B, Weiland S, et al. Worldwide variations in prevalence of symptoms of allergic rhinoconjunctivitis in children: the International Study of Asthma and Allergies in Childhood (ISAAC). Pediatr Allergy Immunol. 1997;8:161-76.
12. Ait-Khaled N, Pearce N, Anderson HR, et al. Global map of the prevalence of symptoms of rhinoconjunctivitis in children: the International Study of Asthma and Allergies in Childhood (ISAAC) Phase Three. Allergy. 2009;64:123-48.
13. Asher MI, Montefort S, Björkstén B, et al. Worldwide time trends in the prevalence of symptoms of asthma, allergic rhinoconjunctivitis, and eczema in childhood: ISAAC Phases One and Three repeat multicountry cross-sectional surveys. Lancet. 2006;368:733-43.
14. Demoly P, Allaert FA, Leasble M, et al. Validation of the classification of ARIA (allergic rhinitis and its impact on asthma). Allergy. 2003;58:672-5.
15. Mygind N. Perennial rhinitis. In: Mygind N, ed. Nasal Allergy. 2nd ed. Oxford: Blackwell scientific publications; 1979:224-32.
16. Khanna P, Shah A. Categorization of patients with allergic rhinitis: a comparative profile of "sneezers and runners" and "blockers". Ann Allergy Asthma Immunol. 2005;94: 60-4.
17. Modi N, Shah A. Assessment of disease severity in patients with allergic rhinitis when categorized as "sneezers and runners" and "blockers". Respirology. 2009;14:A160.
18. Horwitz RJ, Bush RK. Allergens and other factors important in atopic disease. In: Patterson R, Grammer LC, Greenberger PA, eds. Allergic Diseases: Diagnosis and Management, 5th ed. Philadelphia, PA: Lippincott – Raven; 1997:75-129.
19. Colloff MJ, Ayres J, Carswell F, et al. The control of allergens of dust mites and domestic pets: a position paper. Clin Exp Allergy. 1992;2:1-28.
20. Saulyte J, Regueira C, Montes-Martínez A, et al. Active or passive exposure to tobacco smoking and allergic rhinitis, allergic dermatitis, and food allergy in adults and children: a systematic review and meta-analysis. PLoS Med. 2014;11:e1001611.
21. Singh AB, Kumar P. Aeroallergens in clinical practice of allergy in India. An overview. Ann Agric Environ Med. 2003;10:131-6.
22. Sahay S, Bhargava SK, Shah A. Co-occurrence of sinusitis in patients with asthma and/or allergic rhinitis in Delhi, India. Proceedings of the Korean Academy of Asthma, Allergy and Clinical Immunology (KAAACI) and World Allergy Organisation (WAO) Joint Congress 2006 and the 9th West Pacific Allergy Organisation; Seoul, South Korea; November 3–5, 2006:263 [Abstract].
23. Jamal D, Shah A. A description of skin tests to common aeroallergens among patients with allergic rhinitis from Delhi, India. Indian J Allergy Asthma Immunol. 2007;21:105-6 [Abstract].
24. Sahay S, Shah A. Allergic rhinitis: *Aspergillus* sensitisation increases the severity of sinusitis in "blockers" as compared to "sneezers and runners". Allergy. 2008;63: S73 [Abstract].
25. Ostro BD, Lipsett MJ, Mann JK, et al. Indoor air pollution and asthma. Results from panel study. Am J Respir Crit Care Med. 1994;149:1400-06.
26. Wardlaw AJ. Air pollution and allergic disease. Report of a Working Party of the British society for Allergy and Clinical Immunology. Clin Exp Allergy. 1995;25:6-8.
27. McBride DE, Koenig JQ, Luchtel DL, et al. Inflammatory effects of ozone in the upper airways of subjects with asthma. Am J Respir Crit Care Med. 1994;149:1192-7.
28. Hajat S, Haines A, Atkinson RW, et al. Association between air pollution and daily consultations with general practitioners for allergic rhinitis in London, United Kingdom. Am J Epidemiol. 2001;153:704-14.
29. Seaton A, MacNee W, Donaldson K, et al. Particulate air pollution and acute health effects. Lancet. 1995;345:176-8.
30. Spector SL, Wangaard CH, Farr RS. Aspirin and concomitant idiosyncrasies in adult asthmatic patients. J Allergy Clin Immunol. 1979;64:500-6.
31. Jamal D, Shah A. Nocturnal sleep disturbances, excessive daytime sleepiness and impairment in sleep specific quality of life in patients with allergic rhinitis [Abstract]. Allergy. 2007;62:488.
32. Passalacqua G, Ciprandi G, Canonica GW. The nose-lung interaction in allergic rhinitis and asthma: united airways disease. Curr Opin Allergy Clin Immunol. 2001;1:7-13.
33. Kariyawasam HH, Rotiroti G. Allergic rhinitis, chronic rhinosinusitis and asthma: unravelling a complex relationship. Curr Opin Otolaryngol Head Neck Surg. 2013;21:79-86.
34. Wallace DV, Dykewicz MS, Bernstein DI, et al. The diagnosis and management of rhinitis: an updated practice parameter. J Allergy Clin Immunol. 2008;122:S1-84.
35. Shah A, Panjabi C, Maurya V. Asthma and rhinitis: the co-occurrence in Delhi. Proceedings of the Third Malaysian Congress of Allergy and Immunology; Kuala Lumpur, Malaysia; January 25–27; 2002:54 [Abstract].
36. Sharma A, Shah A. The co-occurrence of bronchial asthma and allergic rhinitis and the effect of environmental tobacco smoke in these patients. Abstract presented at the 9th Asian Research Symposium in Rhinology and 10th Biennial Congress of the Trans-Pacific Allergy and Immunology Society, Mumbai, India; November 19–23, 2004.

37. Lund V, Kennedy D. Quantification for staging sinusitis. Ann Otol Rhinol Laryngol. 1995;167:17-22.
38. Sahay S, Gera K, Bhargava SK, Shah A. Occurrence and impact of sinusitis in patients with asthma and/or allergic rhinitis. J Asthma. 2016;53:635-43.[Epub ahead of print].
39. Slavin RG. Nasal polyps and sinusitis. JAMA. 1997;278: 1849-54.
40. Bachert C, Hormann K, Mosges R, et al. An update on the diagnosis and treatment of sinusitis and nasal polyposis. Allergy. 2003;58:176-91.
41. Behera S. Occurrence and effects of nasal polyps in patients with bronchial asthma and/or allergic rhinitis. World Allergy Organization Journal. 2013;6:213.
42. Juniper EF. Development and testing of a new measure of health status for clinical trials in rhinoconjunctivitis. Clin Exp Allergy. 1991;21:77-83.
43. Juniper EF, Guyatt GH, Dolovich J. Assessment of quality of life in adolescents with allergic rhinoconjunctivitis: development and testing of a questionnaire for clinical trials. J Allergy Clin Immunol. 1994;93:413-23.
44. Juniper EF, Thompson AK, Ferrie PJ, et al. Development and validation of the mini rhinoconjunctivitis quality of life questionnaire. Clin Exp Allergy. 2000;30:132-40.
45. Deepak D, Shah A. Allergic rhinitis: a neglected disease. Indian J Allergy Appl Immunol. 2000;14:1-6.
46. Craig TJ, Hanks CD, Fisher LH. How do topical nasal corticosteroids improve sleep and daytime somnolence in allergic rhinitis? J Allergy Clin Immunol. 2005;116:1264-6.
47. Valovirta E, Pawankar R. Survey on the impact of comorbid allergic rhinitis in patients with asthma. BMC Pulm Med. 2006;30:S1-3.
48. Storms W. Allergic rhinitis-induced nasal congestion: its impact on sleep quality. Prim Care Respir J. 2008;17:7-18.
49. Jamal D, Shah A. Disturbances in nocturnal sleep, excessive daytime sleepiness and sleep-specific quality of life impairment in patients with allergic rhinitis. World Allergy Organization Journal. 2007;1:S73 [Abstract].
50. Ashok Shah. [Editorial] Allergic rhinitis, chronic rhinosinusitis and nasal polyposis in Asia Pacific: impact on quality of life and sleep. Asia Pac Allergy. 2014;4:131-3.
51. Mir E, Shah A. Effect of sinusitis on quality of life in school-going children with asthma. Allergy. 2013;68:25.
52. Mir E, Panjabi C, Shah A. Impact of allergic rhinitis in school-going children. Asia Pac Allergy. 2012;2:93-100.
53. Position paper: allergen standardization and skin tests. The European Academy of Allergology and Clinical Immunology. Allergy. 1993;48:48-82.
54. Dreborg S, Backman A, Basomba A, et al. Skin tests used in type 1 allergy testing. Position paper of the European Academy of Allergy and Clinical Immunology. Allergy. 1989;44:1-69.
55. Johansson SG, Berglund A, Kjellman NI. Comparison of IgE values as determined by different solid phase radioimmunoassay methods. Clin Allergy. 1976;6:91-8.
56. Bousquet J, Coulomb Y, Arrendal H, et al. Total serum IgE concentrations in adolescents and adults using the phadeb as IgE PRIST technique. Allergy. 1982;37:397-406.
57. Zetterstrom O, Johansson SG. IgE concentrations measured by PRIST in serum of healthy adults and in patients with respiratory allergy. A diagnostic approach. Allergy. 1981;36:537-47.
58. Eriksson NE. Allergy screening with Phadiatop and CAP Phadiatop in combination with a questionnaire in adults with asthma and rhinitis. Allergy. 1990;45:285-92.
59. Rondón C, Campo P, Togias A, et al. Local allergic rhinitis: concept, pathophysiology, and management. J Allergy Clin Immunol. 2012;129:1460-67.
60. Naclerio RM, deTineo ML, Baroody FM. Ragweed allergic rhinitis and the paranasal sinuses. A computed tomographic study. Arch Otolaryngol Head Neck Surg. 1997;123:193-6.
61. Shapiro MD, Som PM. MRI of the paranasal sinuses and the nasal cavity. Radiol Clin North Am. 1989;27:447-75.
62. Bellanti JA, Wallerstedt DB. Allergic rhinitis update: epidemiology and natural history. Allergy Asthma Proc. 2000;21:367-70.
63. van Cauwenberge P, Bachert C, Passalacqua G, et al. Consensus statement on the treatment of allergic rhinitis. European Academy of Allergology and Clinical Immunology. Allergy. 2000;55:116-34.
64. Passalacqua G, Canonica GW, Bousquet J. Structure and classification of H_1-antihistaminics and overview of their activities. Clin Allergy Immunol. 2002;17:65-100.
65. Allergic factors associated with the development of asthma and the influence of cetirizine in a double-blind, randomised, placebo-controlled trial: first results of ETAC. Early Treatment of the Atopic Child. Pediatr Allergy Immunol. 1998;9:116-24.
66. Potter PC, Study group. Levocetirizine is effective for symptom relief including nasal congestion in adolescent and adult (PAR) sensitized to house dust mites. Allergy. 2003;58:893-9.
67. Bachert C, Bousquet J, Canonica GW, et al. Levocetirizine improves quality of life and reduces costs in long-term management of persistent allergic rhinitis. J Allergy Clin Immunol. 2004;114:838-44.
68. Gandon JM, Allain H. Lack of effect of single and repeated doses of Levocetirizine, a new antihistamine drug, on cognitive and psychomotor functions in healthy volunteers. Br J Clin Pharmacol. 2002;54:51-8.
69. Verster JC, Volkerts ER, Van Oosterwijck AW, et al. Acute and subchronic effects of Levocetirizine and diphenhydramine on memory functioning, psychomotor performance, and mood. J Allergy Clin Immunol. 2003;111:891-9.
70. van Cauwenberge P, Juniper EF. Comparison of the efficacy, safety and quality of life provided by fexofenadine hydrochloride 120 mg, loratadine 10 mg and placebo administered once daily for the treatment of seasonal allergic rhinitis. Clin Exp Allergy. 2000;30:891-9.
71. Meeves SG, Appajosyula S. Efficacy and safety profile of fexofenadine HCl: a unique therapeutic option in H_1 receptor antagonist treatment. J Allergy Clin Immunol. 2003;112:S69-77.
72. Salmun LM, Lorber R. 24-hour efficacy of once daily desloratadine therapy in patients with seasonal allergic rhinitis. BMC Fam Pract. 2002;3:14.

73. Nayak AS, Schenkel E. desloratadine reduces nasal congestion in patients with intermittent allergic rhinitis. Allergy. 2001;56:1077-80.
74. Simons FE, Prenner BM, Finn A Jr. Efficacy and safety of desloratadine in the treatment of perennial allergic rhinitis. J Allergy Clin Immunol. 2003;111:617-22.
75. Hindmarch I, Shamsi Z. The effects of single and repeated administration of ebastine on cognition and psychomotor performance in comparison to triprolidine and placebo in healthy volunteers. Curr Med Res Opin. 2001;17: 273-81.
76. Guadano EM, Serra-Batlles J, Meseguer J, et al. Rupatadine 10 mg and ebastine 10 mg in seasonal allergic rhinitis: a comparison study. Allergy. 2004;59:766-71.
77. LaForce CF, Carr W, Tilles SA, et al. Evaluation of olopatadine hydrochloride nasal spray, 0.6%, used in combination with an intranasal corticosteroid in seasonal allergic rhinitis. Allergy Asthma Proc. 2010;31:132-40.
78. Yamamoto H, Yamada T, Kubo S, et al. Efficacy of oral olopatadine hydrochloride for the treatment of seasonal allergic rhinitis: a randomized, double-blind, placebo-controlled study. Allergy Asthma Proc. 2010;31:296-303.
79. Weiler JM, Meltzer EO. Azelastine nasal spray as adjunctive therapy to azelastine tablets in the management of seasonal allergic rhinitis. Ann Allergy Asthma Immunol. 1997;79:327-32.
80. Bernstein JA. Azelastine hydrochloride: a review of pharmacology, pharmacokinetics, clinical efficacy and tolerability. Curr Med Res Opin. 2007;23:2441-52.
81. Meltzer EO, Garadi R, Laforce C, et al. Comparative study of sensory attributes of two antihistamine nasal sprays: olopatadine 0.6% and azelastine 0.1%. Allergy Asthma Proc. 2008;29:659-68.
82. Ciprandi G, Buscaglia S, Pesce G, et al. Minimal persistent inflammation is present at mucosal level in patient with symptomatic rhinitis and mite allergy. J Allergy Clin Immunol. 1995;96:971-79.
83. Boulet P. Perception of role and potential side effect of inhaled corticosteroid among asthmatic patients. Chest. 1998;113:587-92.
84. Gerson I, Green L, Fishken D. Patient preference and sensory comparisons of nasal spray allergy medications. J Sensory Stud. 1999;14:491-6.
85. Blaiss MS. Efficacy, safety, and patient preference of inhaled nasal corticosteroids: a review of pertinent published data. Allergy Asthma Proc. 2001;22:S5-10.
86. Khanna P, Shah A. Assessment of sensory perceptions and patient preference for intranasal corticosteroid sprays in allergic rhinitis. Am J Rhinol. 2005;19:316-21.
87. Kaliner MA. Patient preferences and satisfaction with prescribed nasal steroids for allergic rhinitis. Allergy Asthma Proc. 2001;22:S11-15.
88. Kaliner MA. Physician prescribing practices: the role of patient preference in the selection of nasal steroids. Allergy Asthma Proc. 2001;22:S17-22.
89. Deepak D, Panjabi C, Gudwani S, et al. Nasal septal perforation in a patient with allergic bronchopulmonary aspergillosis and rhinitis on long-term corticosteroids. Asian Pac J Allergy Immunol. 2001;19:287-90.
90. Skoner D, Rachelefsky G, Meltzer E, et al. Detection of growth suppression in children during treatment with intranasal beclomethasone dipropionate. Pediatrics. 2000;105:e23.
91. Schenkel EJ, Skoner DP, Bronsky EA, et al. Absence of growth retardation in children with perennial allergic rhinitis after one year treatment with mometasone furoate aqueous nasal spray. Pediatrics. 2000;105:e22.
92. Allen DB, Meltzer EO, Lemanske RF Jr, et al. No growth suppression in children treated with the maximum recommended dose of fluticasone propionate aqueous nasal spray for one year. Allergy Asthma Proc. 2002;23:407-13.
93. Suissa S, Baltzan M, Kremer R, et al. Inhaled and nasal corticosteroid use and the risk of fracture. Am J Respir Crit Care Med. 2004;169:83-8.
94. Mygind N, Borum P. Intranasal ipratropium: literature abstracts and comments. Rhinol. 1989;9:37-44.
95. Bronsky EA, Druce H, Findlay SR, et al. A clinical trial of ipratropium bromide nasal spray in patients with perennial nonallergic rhinitis. J Allergy Clin Immunol. 1995;95:1117-22.
96. Kirkegaard J, Mygind N, Molgaard F, et al. Ordinary and high-dose ipratropium in perennial nonallergic rhinitis. J Allergy Clin Immunol. 1987;79:585-90.
97. Moqbel R, Cromwell O, Walsh GM, et al. Effects of nedocromil sodium on the activation of human eosinophils and neutrophils and the release of histamine from mast cells. Allergy. 1988;43:268-6.
98. Meltzer EO, Malmstrom K, Lu S, et al. Concomitant montelukast and loratadine as treatment for seasonal allergic rhinitis: a randomized, placebo-controlled clinical trial. J Allergy Clin Immunol. 2000;105:917-22.
99. Kurowski M, Kuna P, Gorski P. Montelukast plus cetirizine in the prophylactic treatment of seasonal allergic rhinitis: influence on clinical symptoms and nasal allergic inflammation. Allergy. 2004;59:280-8.
100. Wilson AM, O' Byrne PM, Parameswaran K. Leukotriene receptor antagonists for allergic rhinitis: a systemic review and meta-analysis. Am J Med. 2004;116:338-44.
101. Hill SL III, Krouse JH. The effects of montelukast on intradermal wheal and flare. Otolaryngol Head Neck Surg. 2003;129:199-203.
102. Pagnoux C, Guilpain P, Hauser T, et al. Churg–Strauss syndrome and leukotriene-modifying agents. Clin Pulm Med. 2004;11:349-54.
103. Casale TB, Condemi J, Laforce C, et al. Effect of omalizumab on symptoms of seasonal allergic rhinitis: a randomized controlled trial. JAMA. 2001;286:2956-67.
104. Bousquet J, Khaltaev N, Cruz AA, et al. Allergic Rhinitis and its Impact on Asthma (ARIA) 2008 update. Allergy. 2008;63:8-160.
105. Limb SL, Starke PR, Lee CE, et al. Delayed onset and protracted progression of anaphylaxis after omalizumab administration in patients with asthma. J Allergy Clin Immunol. 2007;120:1378-81.

106. Calderon MA, Alves B, Jacobson M, et al. Allergen injection immunotherapy for seasonal allergic rhinitis. Cochrane Database Syst Rev. 2007:CD001936.
107. Ridolo E, Montagni M, Melli V, et al. Pharmacotherapy of allergic rhinitis: current options and future perspectives. Expert Opin. Pharmacother. 2014;15:73-83.
108. Seidman MD, Gurgel RK, Lin SY, et al. Guideline Otolaryngology Development Group. AAO-HNSF. Clinical practice guideline: allergic rhinitis. Otolaryngol Head Neck Surg. 2015;152:S1-43.
109. Senti G, Prinz Vavricka BM, Erdmann I, et al. Intralymphatic allergen administration renders specific immunotherapy faster and safer: a randomized controlled trial. Proc Natl Acad Sci USA. 2008;105:17908-12.
110. Schmidt BM, Kusma M, Feuring M, et al. The phosphodiesterase 4 inhibitor roflumilast is effective in the treatment of allergic rhinitis. J Allergy Clin Immunol. 2001;108:530-6.
111. Shah A, Pawankar R. Allergic rhinitis and comorbid asthma: perspective from India – ARIA Asia-Pacific workshop report. Asian Pac J Allergy Immunol. 2009;27:71-7.
112. Panjabi C, Shah A. Assessment of health-related quality of life in Indian patients with bronchial asthma and allergic rhinitis. Chest India. 2001;Suppl 2:S41.
113. Shah A. Editorial. Current trends in upper airways and ocular allergic inflammation. Asia Pac Allergy. 2011;1: 105-7.

CHAPTER 25

Ocular Surface Immune Response and Allergies

Manila Khatri, Swati Priyadarshini, Ankita, Sandeep Saxena

INTRODUCTION

The components mediated in the immune system include the tear film, the lacrimal functional unit, a complex comprising the lacrimal glands, ocular surface (cornea, conjunctiva, and Meibomian glands), and eyelids connecting these structures.[1]

TEAR FILM IMMUNOLOGY

The normal tear film contains a variety of elements, complement cascade, proteins, growth factors, and cytokines. The expression of growth factors, prostaglandins, neuropeptides, and proteases is increased in various immune disorders of the cornea and ocular surface. Trafficking signals to immune cells are mediated through critical mediators like chemokines, which are classified functionally based on the recruitment of various cells mediated in the immune response[1] such as neutrophil recruitment (e.g., IL-8); T helper-1 (Th-1) lymphocyte recruitment and activation [macrophage inflammatory protein-1 (MIP-1)]; monocyte–macrophage recruitment [monocyte chemotactic protein-1 (MCP-1)]; and eosinophil recruitment (eotaxin).

OCULAR SURFACE IMMUNOLOGY

The ocular surface immunoregulation is mediated by the responses of the innate and adaptive arms of the ocular immune response.

Conjunctiva

The conjunctiva is a part of the mucosa-associated lymphoid tissue like the lacrimal gland. Humoral immunity involves IgA produced by the lacrimal gland, and cellular immunity is dominated by CD4+ T cells.[2]

The conjunctiva contains polymorphonuclear leukocytes, lymphocytes [regulatory T cells (T_{reg} cells)], macrophages, plasma cells, and mast cells. The conjunctival stroma contains dendritic antigen-presenting cells (APCs), also found in the epithelium known as Langerhans cells, which are specialized of both antigen uptake and priming of naive T lymphocytes.[1] So, the dendritic cells are the sentinel cells of the immune system of the ocular surface. The trafficking of immune cells and antigens to the draining lymph nodes is aided by the rich vascular and lymphatic supply of conjunctiva. The adaptive immune response is generated at lymph nodes through the recruitment of T_{reg} cells, which modulate and suppress the local immune response.[1,3]

Cornea

The cornea also contains dendritic cells, like the conjunctiva, and the corneal epithelium contains Langerhans cells, concentrated in the corneal periphery and limbus. Besides dendritic cells, lymphocytes are also present in the peripheral epithelium and anterior stroma of the cornea. The chemokines and vascular endothelial adhesion molecules regulate the recruitment of the leukocytes from the intravascular compartment into the limbal matrix.[2]

Unlike the conjunctiva, the normal cornea is considered an immunologically privileged site, called so because the generation of innate and adaptive immune response to foreign antigens is relatively suppressed. Immune privilege at the ocular surface and in the anterior chamber of the eye is due to the multiple anatomical, physiological, and immunoregulatory factors.

- Absence of MHC class II^+ APCs in the graft.
- Absence of blood and lymphatic channels in graft and its bed.

- Expression of the CD95 ligand (FasL or Fas ligand) on endothelium that can induce apoptosis of activated lymphocytes and neutrophils, other apoptosis-inducing ligands include tumor necrosis factor-related, apoptosis-inducing ligand and programmed death ligand-1.
- Expression of immunosuppressive agents TGF-β2, α-MSH, vasoactive intestinal peptide, and calcitonin gene-related peptide.
- Anterior chamber-associated immune deviation involving the downregulation of delayed-type cellular immunity stimulates suppressor T cells. APCs upon recognition of antigens enter the venous circulation and induce regulatory T cells in the spleen, bypassing the lymphatic system.[1,3]

Thus, the immunological "blind spots" created by immune privilege lead to immune unresponsiveness or immunologic tolerance and to put the eye at risk for infections.

The cornea can neither produce an acute allergic reaction as it does not contain mast cells nor a typical Arthus reaction as devoid of blood vessels. However, the corneal response through humoral and cellular immune responses occur that enter the periphery from the limbus. So, immune-mediated disorders of the cornea occur primarily in the corneal periphery and limbus. Leukocytes can pass through the ciliary body and the iris root and the plasma proteins through the breakdown of the blood-ocular barrier to gain access to the cornea.[1,2] The cornea acts as an immunologic blotter, soaking up antigens from the ocular surface, first described by Wessely in 1911. Upon injection of a foreign antigen into the cornea of a previously sensitized animal, a ring-shaped infiltrate formed in the corneal stroma, concentric to the injection site called a Wessely immune ring; the infiltrate contains complement factors and neutrophil.[1]

Sclera

Scleral involvement is associated with immune-complex deposition, granulomatous inflammation, and occlusive vasculitis.[1]

TISSUE-SPECIFIC MANIFESTATIONS OF OCULAR ALLERGY

Ocular allergy is one of the most common ocular surface diseases seen in a primary eye care practice.

Numerous factors attributed include genetics, air pollution, pets, and early childhood exposure. Studies have estimated the prevalence of allergic conjunctivitis to range between 15% and 40% of the population.[4] Mild cases of ocular allergy can produce irritating symptoms, and severe forms, such as atopic keratoconjunctivitis (AKC), could lead to vision loss.[5] However, this common condition is often underdiagnosed[4] and undertreated until it reaches severe levels.

The allergen is typically airborne. It enters the tear film and comes into contact with conjunctival mast cells. Degranulation of mast cells releases histamine and other inflammatory mediators that promote vasodilation, edema, and recruitment of inflammatory cells, such as eosinophils.[3] In a presensitized individual, the activation and degranulation of mast cells can be triggered within minutes of allergen exposure and histamine release, thus dilating conjunctival microvasculature leads to conjunctival hyperemia and chemosis. Various immune-related disorders of eye are summarized in Table 25.1.

Contact Dermatoblepharitis

Pathogenesis

Local allergic reactions may occur following the exposure to topical medication, cosmetics, and environmental substances. This may occur as an anaphylactic reaction, as type I (IgE)-mediated hypersensitivity. It may also begin 24–72 hours after exposure to the sensitizing agent, due to a type IV T-cell-mediated hypersensitivity reaction.[3]

Clinical Presentation

Type I immediate hypersensitivity reactions typically occur within minutes after exposure to an allergen.

Symptoms and Signs

Itching, eyelid erythema and swelling, and conjunctival hyperemia and chemosis can occur. In rare cases, systemic anaphylaxis may occur with topical anesthetics and antibiotics such as bacitracin, cephalosporins, and sulfacetamide but often resolve spontaneously.

A delayed type IV hypersensitivity reaction to a medication usually begins 24–72 hours following sensitization by previous exposure. An acute eczematous reaction develops with erythema, cutaneous thickening, and eyelid scaling.

Table 25.1: Various immune-related diseases of the eye.

Part	*Disease*	*Mechanism*
Eyelids	Contact dermatoblepharitis	Type I/IV hypersensitivity
	Atopic dermatitis	Type IV HS
Conjunctiva	Hay fever conjunctivitis and perennial allergic conjunctivitis	Type I/IV hypersensitivity
	Vernal keratoconjunctivitis	Type I/IV hypersensitivity
	Atopic conjunctivitis	Type IV hypersensitivity
	Ligneous conjunctivitis	Immune mediated
	SJS/TEN	Immune mediated/Type IV HS
Sclera	Scleritis and episcleritis	Immune complex mediated
Cornea	Peripheral ulcerative keratitis	Autoimmune
	Mooren ulcer	Autoimmune
Uvea	Infective uveitis Noninfective uveitis	Type I hypersensitivity Immune complex mediated
Retina	Retinitis, retinal vasculitis Eales disease	Immune complex mediated
	Sympathetic ophthalmitis	Type IV hypersensitivity

Sequelae: Hyperpigmentation, dermal scarring, lower-eyelid ectropion, papillary conjunctivitis, and mucoid or mucopurulent discharge, punctate epithelial erosions on the inferior cornea may develop.

Medications causing allergy include the following: *Cycloplegics*: Atropine, homatropine; aminoglycosides—neomycin, gentamicin, and tobramycin; antiviral agents such as idoxuridine; preservatives such as thimerosal and ethylenediaminetetraacetic acid (EDTA).[1]

Management

Identification and discontinuation of the offending agent/allergen is mandatory. Adjunctive therapy includes cold compresses, artificial lubricants, and topical antihistamines. Mast-cell stabilizers and/or nonsteroidal anti-inflammatory drugs (NSAIDs) can be given.[1] In severe cases, a brief course of mild topical corticosteroids is given or tacrolimus ointment is applied over the eyelids and periocular skin to speed up recovery.[1]

Atopic Dermatitis

Pathogenesis

It is a chronic condition in genetically susceptible individuals that usually begins in infancy or childhood. It involves a type IV hypersensitivity reaction, increased IgE hypersensitivity, increased histamine, and impaired cell-mediated immunity.[3]

Clinical Presentation

Findings include pruritus, lesions on the eyelid and other sites (e.g., joint flexures in adolescents and adults, face and extensor surfaces in infants and young children), and a personal or a family history of other atopic disorders, such as asthma, allergic rhinitis, nasal polyps, and aspirin hypersensitivity. It also includes periorbital darkening, exaggerated eyelid folds, meibomianitis, ectropion, and chronic papillary conjunctivitis.[3]

Skin manifestation varies in different age groups: Infants have erythematous rash, children present with eczematous dermatitis and secondary lichenification have scratching, and adults have scaly patches, as well as thickened and wrinkled dry skin.[1]

Management

Allergen avoidance, moisturizing lotions for skin hydration is used. Acute lesions may require topical corticosteroid cream or ointment; long-term use may cause skin thinning. Topical tacrolimus ointment is also effective.

Oral antipruritic agents (antihistamines and mast-cell stabilizers) relieve itching. An allergist's opinion is required in these cases.

SEASONAL AND PERENNIAL ALLERGIC CONJUNCTIVITIS

Allergic Conjunctivitis

Seasonal allergic conjunctivitis (SAC) is the most common form of all ocular allergic diseases, triggered by the environmental allergen exposure.[6] It usually occurs in spring. SAC is induced by exposure to indoor antigens like dust mites, fungi, animal epithelial, and/or occupational allergens.[6] The affected person has symptoms throughout the year with acute seasonal exacerbation.[3]

Clinical Presentation

It presents with itching, redness, and swelling of the conjunctiva (Fig. 25.1). Intense itching is the hallmark. Other criteria include a family or a personal history of atopy (with allergic rhinitis or asthma), a skin allergen challenge test, response to antiallergic treatment, and serum IgE elevation.[1]

Atopic Keratoconjunctivitis

The atopic dermatitis may have associated keratoconjunctivitis. The most characteristic sign in AKC is swelling in the periorbital region, with lower lid swelling called as Dennie–Morgan folds and is associated with redness, itching swelling, and eczema.[3] Loss of lashes due to scratching leads to the Hertoghe sign.[1]

Vernal Keratoconjunctivitis

Vernal keratoconjunctivitis (VKC) is a chronic, seasonally exacerbated, bilateral, at times, asymmetrical, and allergic inflammation of the ocular surface.[7] It is often self-limiting and may leave sequelae or visual impairment in about 5–6% of the patients. It is more frequent in young males, usually starts before the age of 10 years.[7] VKC is rare in adults. Pathophysiology is not precisely known, though two hypersensitivity mechanisms seem to be involved (type I and type IV hypersensitivity).[3] Recent data suggest T-helper type 2 cells and their cytokines, corneal fibroblasts, and epithelium along with various growth factors play an important role in the pathogenesis of VKC.[7]

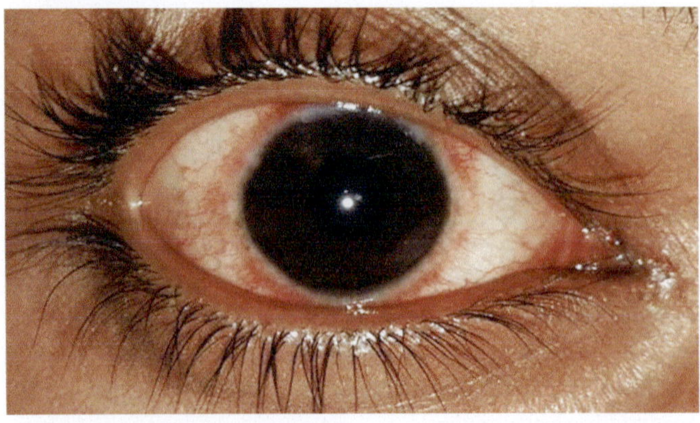

Fig. 25.1: Conjunctival congestion.

Clinical Features

The hallmark in VKC is giant cobblestone papillae that appear in upper palpebral conjunctiva.[7] Thick mucus hypersecretion leading to "ropy discharge" is characteristic of VKC.[7] Trantas dots appear as small gelatinous nodules at limbus and consist of necrotic eosinophils, neutrophils, and epithelial cells. Corneal involvement may lead to punctate epithelial erosions, pannus formation, or noninfectious epithelial ulcer oval shield shaped so called shield ulcer.[3]

Giant Papillary Conjunctivitis

Giant papillary conjunctivitis (GPC) is a noninfectious inflammatory disorder of the ocular surface, related to the presence of foreign body such as contact lens, ocular prosthesis, and sutures.[6] Papillae occur on the upper palpebral conjunctiva. Papillae larger than 0.3 mm in diameter are considered abnormal, and more than 1 mm diameter papillae are giant papillae. GPC can manifest at any age and shows no race or gender predilection. It can affect both atopic and nonatopic individuals, though atopic individuals have severe manifestation.[1]

Management

Approach to treatment involves supportive treatment with cold compresses and artificial tears and avoidance of allergen, and appropriate drugs.[7] The first line of defense and antihistamine and mast cell stabilizers are fast and effective. When symptoms continue to persist or are particularly severe, adding an anti-inflammatory can help enhance the effects of the antihistamine/mast cell stabilizers until the patient's condition improves.

Dual-action drugs: In recent years, combination drugs are increasingly effective for ocular allergy like dual-action topical antihistamines and mast-cell stabilizers.[7,8] This group includes olopatadine, ketotifen, azelastine, epinastine, and bepotastine.[7] Combination dual-action eye drop therapy is more convenient so increases compliance, with a rapid action to block the histamine receptor and help reduce symptom severity.[1]

Fast-acting drugs: Drugs with very fast onset of action (about 3 to 5 minutes) can improve immediate patient comfort and compliance and help prevent the symptoms of itching and redness. Oral and topical antihistamines can be given.

Preventive options: Patients known to have a history of seasonal ocular allergy may be given prophylactic medications beforehand, which provides some protection and reduces the intensity of the allergic response, and avoids/terminates exposure to the allergen.

Therapeutic Options

Anti-allergic therapy: Anti-allergic drugs include olopatadine 0.2%, which is a dual-action drug. Bepotastine is a potent dual-action antiallergic drug. Alcaftadine is a broad-spectrum antihistamine. Other agents include epinastine eye drops and azelastine.[1]

Corticosteroids strategy: In cases with frequent and severe exacerbations, newer and safer topical corticosteroids can help suppress some of the acute-phase (as well as the late-phase) reactions. Steroids block most mediators of inflammation and work effectively in the acute phase of AC. By inhibiting phospholipase A, they block the arachidonic acid pathway, preventing the synthesis of prostaglandins and leukotrienes. They impede the migration of leukocytes to inflammatory sites, minimizing the release of inflammatory mediators from macrophages.[1] Because of the complications associated with their prolonged use, like steroid-induced cataract, glaucoma, and increased susceptibility to viral and fungal infections, they are not given as first-line drugs. The "soft steroids" are loteprednol etabonate and fluorometholone, which can be given topical in a lower concentration with a decreased likelihood of causing side effects.[7] More potent corticosteroids can be reserved for intractable cases.

Nonpharmacologic measures: Simple cool compresses can be very relieving. Preservative-free chilled artificial tears provide some symptomatic relief and flush out the allergen.[7] Environment modification with air conditioning or coolers can be helpful.

Ligneous Conjunctivitis

Pathogenesis

A rare chronic disorder, characterized by the formation of firm, yellowish fibrinous pseudomembranes with wood-like consistency on the conjunctiva. The membrane is an admixture of fibrin, fibrin-bound tissue plasminogen activator (tPA), epithelial cells, and mixed inflammatory cells that adhere to the conjunctiva.[1] It has been linked to severe deficiency in type I plasminogen and deficiency in plasmin-mediated fibrinolysis as primary defect. It is associated with plasminogen gene defect (PLG)6q26.[1]

Clinical Presentation

Patients present with ocular irritation and foreign-body sensation can affect all age groups. There are yellowish, platelike masses over palpebral surfaces on eversion of the eyelid. It is generally bilateral and can recur after surgical excision.[1]

Management

Culture of material is done to exclude a bacterial pseudomembranous or membranous conjunctivitis.

In surgical excision with or without adjunctive cryotherapy, many cases resolve spontaneously over years. Use of purified plasminogen, fresh frozen plasma, heparin, corticosteroids, azathioprine, and amniotic membrane has been reported.[1]

Stevens–Johnson Syndrome and Toxic Epidermal Necrolysis

Pathogenesis

Stevens–Johnson syndrome (SJS) and toxic epidermal necrolysis (TEN) are hypersensitivity reactions to drugs or infections leading to severe mucocutaneous reaction. Both are two ends of a clinical spectrum, differing only by the extent of skin involvement.[9] It results from MHC class I-restricted antigen presentation, leading to infiltration of the skin with cytotoxic T lymphocytes and natural killer cells, which lead to keratinocyte apoptosis via Fas signaling cascade and granulysin release.[10] SJS/TEN is mostly caused by drugs, but *Mycoplasma pneumoniae* and herpes simplex virus infections are well-documented causes and few rare cases in which the etiology remains

Table 25.2: Agents known to elucidate Stevens–Johnson syndrome (SJS) and toxic epidermal necrolysis (TEN).

Pharmacologic	*Infectious*
• Anticonvulsants • Carbamazepine • Phenytoin • Lamotrigine • Barbiturates • Sulfonamides • Nonsteroidal anti-inflammatory drugs	• Bacterial • Mycoplasma pneumoniae • Group A β-hemolytic strep • Viral • Cytomegalovirus • Herpes simplex virus • HIV

unknown.[9, 11] Various agents commonly implicated are elucidated in Table 25.2.

Clinical Presentation

It usually occurs in the children and adult and with female preponderance. The history of exposure to the offending agent can be elicited. Patient presents with rapid-onset pain, redness, photophobia, itching, and foreign-body sensation.[3] On ocular examination, mucopurulent conjunctivitis and episcleritis are commonly noted. Severe inflammation may lead to conjunctival and corneal epithelial sloughing, thus predisposed to infections. Long-term sequelae lead to ocular surface cicatrization, symblepharon, trichiasis, and poor tear film dynamics leading to dry eye.[1]

Treatment

Immediate discontinuation of the offending agent, general measures for systemic stabilization, systemic therapy to combat dehydration and superinfection. The primary therapy for ocular manifestation includes lubrication with preservative-free artificial tears and ointments, topical steroids for inflammation and angiogenesis, topical antibiotics for prophylaxis, and amniotic membrane transplantation for moderate to severe cases is considered.

Diagnostic Approach

Immune-mediated ocular disorders may be associated with a systemic disease. The workup includes proper history taking and examination. The atopic individuals may need an allergen challenge test. In a patient presenting with ocular inflammation, systemic vasculitis needs to be worked up, though antineutrophil cytoplasmic autoantibody tests (Table 25.3) are recommended for early detection and therapy.[2]

Table 25.3: Common laboratory tests for suspected systemic immune-mediated disease.

Common laboratory tests	*Systemic immune-mediated disease*
Erythrocyte sedimentation rate or C-reactive protein	Raised in systemic inflammation
Rheumatoid factor (RF)	Autoantibodies (IgG, IgA, or IgM) against epitopes of the Fc portion of IgG
Antinuclear antibody (ANA)	Antibodies against cell nuclear antigens (inflammatory bowel disease, SLE, etc.)
Antineutrophil cytoplasmic autoantibody (ANCA)	c-ANCA (Wegener granulomatosis) p-ANCA (generally indicative of small-vessel vasculitis [microscopic angiitis])
Urinalysis	Check for casts, red blood cells, etc. (active nephritis)
Complete blood count	Abnormally high or low values in systemic disease

The corneal and ocular surface morbidities may result from underlying autoimmune disease. In cases with suspicion of systemic disease, a multidisciplinary approach with the opinion of an allergist, an ophthalmologist, a dermatologist, a rheumatologist, or an internist must be taken.

REFERENCES

1. Basic and Clinical Science Course. External Disease and Cornea. San Francisco, CA: American Academy of Ophthalmology; 2014–2015.
2. Rahi AHS, Garner A. Textbook of Immunopathology of the Eye. North Balwyn, VIC: Blackwell Scientific Publications; 1976.
3. Silverstein, AM. Allergic reactions of the eye. In: Gell PG, Coombs RRA, eds. Clinical Aspects of Immunology. 2nd ed. Oxford: Blackwell; 1968:1160-75.
4. Rosario N, Bielory L. Epidemiology of allergic conjunctivitis. Curr Opin Allergy Clin Immunol. 2011;11:471-6.
5. Leonardi A, Bonini S. Is visual function affected in severe ocular allergies? Curr Opin Allergy Clin Immunol. 2013;13:558-62.
6. Mishra GP, Tamboli V, Jwala J, Mitra AK. Recent patents and emerging therapeutics in the treatment of allergic conjunctivitis. Recent Pat Inflamm Allergy Drug Discov. 2011;5:26-36.
7. Kumar S. Vernal keratoconjunctivitis: a major review. Acta Ophthalmol. 2009;87:133-47.

8. Barney NP, Graziano FM. Allergic and immunologic diseases of the eye. In: Adkinson NFJ, Yunginger JW, Busse WW, Bochner BS, Holgate ST, Simons FE, eds. Middleton's Allergy: Principles & Practice. Vol. 2. St. Louis, MO: Mosby; 2003:1599-617.
9. Harr T, French LE. Toxic epidermal necrolysis and Stevens-Johnson syndrome. Orphanet J Rare Dis. 2010;5: 39. doi:10.1186/1750-1172-5-39.
10. Chung WH, Hung SI, Yang JY, et al. Granulysin is a key mediator for disseminated keratinocyte death in Stevens-Johnson syndrome and toxic epidermal necrolysis. Nat Med. 2008;14:1343-50.
11. Hazin R, Ibrahimi OA, Hazin MI, Kimyai-Asadi A. Stevens-Johnson syndrome: pathogenesis, diagnosis, and management. Ann Med. 2008;40:129-38.

CHAPTER 26

Urticaria

Ramji Gupta

INTRODUCTION

Urticaria is an erythematous eruption, which is usually sudden, itchy, and varies in size and shape from very small circular lesions to very large irregular areas (Fig. 26.1). These lesions are transient and disappear within 24 hours even without any treatment, though fresh ones may continue to appear. Severe attacks may be associated with abdominal pain, nausea, vomiting, headache, and in children high fever. In adults, fever is infrequent. These are all mediated by histamine. Most cases of urticaria are type I hypersensitivity reaction, which are mediated by IgE antibodies fixed on the surface of tissue mast cells and basophils. As a result of the antigen–antibody reaction on the mast cells, degranulation of mast cells occurs, leading to the release of histamine that causes itching, vasodilatation, and increased permeability of blood vessels resulting in the formation of wheals. Sometimes urticaria is due to type III hypersensitivity reaction and is mediated by IgG antibodies, which form immune complexes with antigens leading to the release of vasoactive substances from complement components, which release histamine with the formation of wheals. Such type of urticaria is usually associated with arthritis, arthralgias, albuminuria, and fever even in adults.

Angioedema is a variant of urticaria where the edema occurs deep in the subcutaneous tissues. The lesions are larger, do not itch, and take 1–7 days to disappear. Commonly it occurs on the face (Fig. 26.2) and hand or forearm as one or two areas of swelling; however, it may be seen anywhere on the body. If lesions involve lips and tongue, there is a risk of edema extending to the larynx, leading to the obstruction of air passages that may result in death. Such cases must be immediately treated.

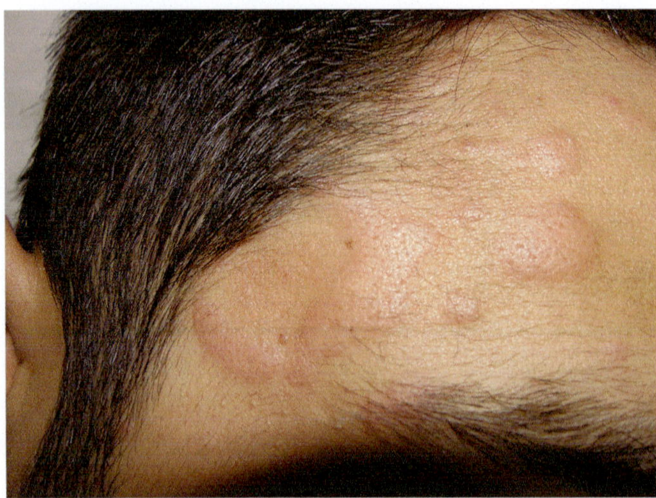

Fig. 26.1: Urticaria.

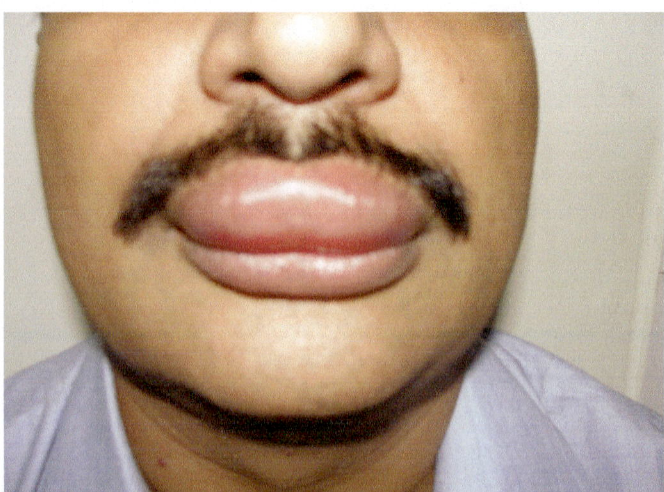

Fig. 26.2: Angioedema.

ETIOLOGY

Various causes of urticaria/angioedema include the following:

Drugs

A large number of drugs like salicylates, penicillin, sulfonamides, tetracycline, and a few others are known to produce urticaria. Most of the time, this type of urticaria is produced by the antigen-antibody reaction, i.e., by the allergic mechanism, but sometimes it may be due to nonallergic mechanisms due to direct degranulation of mast cells by drugs like salicylate, polymyxin B, morphine, curare, and codeine. Urticaria due to drugs most often is of short duration and disappears soon once the drug is withdrawn. However, urticaria due to salicylate and penicillin usually persists for several weeks.

Foods

As with the drug, the mechanism may be allergic or nonallergic as with fish, which can produce direct histamine release as well as allergic reaction. Food items like meat, fish, shellfish, eggs, milk, wheat, rice, pulses, nuts, potato, chocolate, pork, strawberries, and cheese, which contain sufficient amounts of protein, can cause urticaria. Food additives like tartrazine and azodyes and preservatives like benzoates, hydroxybenzoates, and sulfites can also cause urticaria. The frequency of urticarial attacks varies from several attacks in a day to one attack for several days depending upon the frequency with which the food is ingested.[1] The interval between the intake of food and the manifestation of urticaria depends upon the time taken for the digestion and absorption of food from the gastrointestinal (GI) tract. It varies from a few minutes to even 16–18 hours. The urticaria usually disappears within 24–48 hours after further ingestion of the causative food is stopped.

Inhalants

A large number of substances like pollen, fungal spores, fragment of insects, and human and animal dander present in the dust can enter into the body through the respiratory tract and can cause urticaria. The urticaria due to insects and dander usually occurs throughout the year, while it is seasonal due to pollen or fungal spores. However, the pollen content in the atmosphere also varies from place to place, thus a patient may get attack only at a particular place and recover completely at other places.[2]

Infection

The presence of bacterial infection in any part of the body especially the urinary tract, bones, teeth, paranasal sinuses, tonsils, and gallbladder can produce urticaria by releasing bacterial antigen in the circulation from time to time. These attacks can occur any time in a day, and the frequency varies from several attacks in a day to one attack for several days. There may be no clinical evidence of the infection. The proof lies in the disappearance of urticaria with antibiotic[3,4] or on the surgical removal of the focus of infection.

GI Parasite

There is no conclusive evidence that the parasite in the GI tract causes the urticaria. However, when they pass through lungs or skin during their larval stage, may cause the urticaria.

Emotional Upset

Sometimes, urticaria may be precipitated by emotional upset like waiting for an interview or an examination or during a bout of anger.

Pressure

Prolonged and sustained pressure as from a tight belt, brassiere strap, elastic band of socks, watch straps, and other similar objects may produce urticarial wheals. In these situations, the urticaria occurs only after the release of the pressure. Pressure urticaria responds very poorly to treatment, however, spontaneous remission is very frequent.

Cholinergic Urticaria

It is supposed to be due to the release of acetylcholine at the sympathetic nerve ending. The wheals are as a rule very small, 1–3 mm in size (Fig. 26.3), and occur due to sweating induced by heat of sunlight or other sources, physical exertion, emotional tension, or gustatory stimuli. The urticaria persists for a few minutes to an hour. After a severe attack, further exertion may not be able to precipitate the urticaria during the next 24 hours or more.

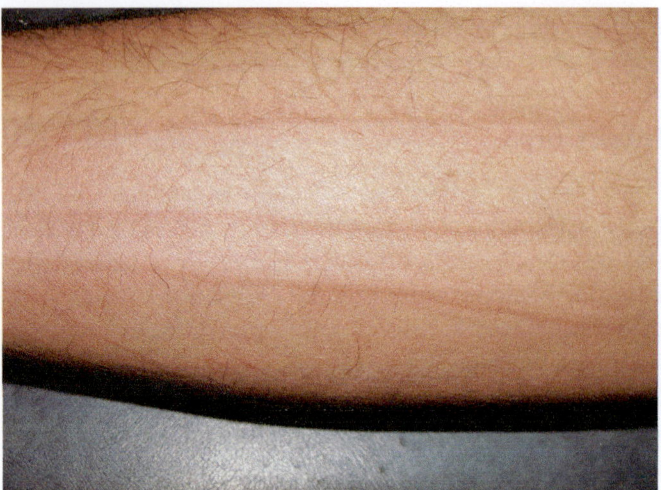

Fig. 26.3: Cholinergic urticaria.

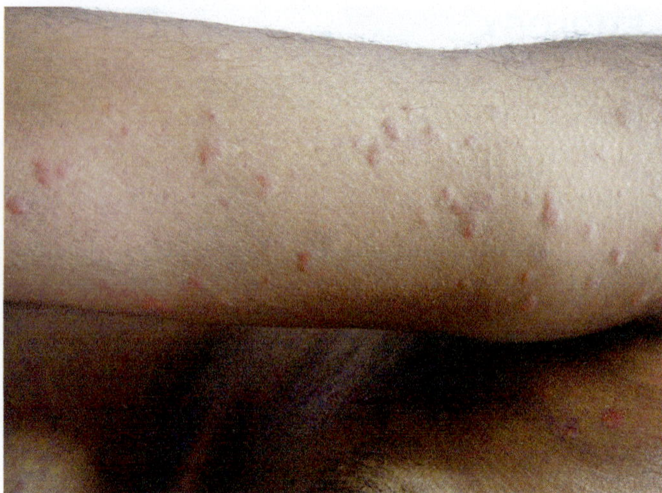

Fig. 26.4: Dermographism.

The urticaria keeps on coming for some months or years and then tends to disappear spontaneously.

Solar Urticaria

It is rare and precipitated by heat from sunlight and not by the heat from any other sources. The lesions are usually limited to sun-exposed areas only.

Heat

Some patients develop urticaria on being exposed to heat from room heater, oven, stove, or even from sun.

Aquagenic Urticaria

It is very rare and is precipitated by contact due to water irrespective of its temperature.

Cold Urticaria

It occurs in two forms (1) familial and (2) acquired. Familial cold urticaria is extremely rare and manifests any time after the birth as huge urticarial swelling along with fever, headache, arthralgia, and leukocytosis on exposure to cold. It occurs in families and transmitted as an autosomal dominant character. Some cases of acquired cold urticaria are due to the presence of cryoglobulins and occur in association with lymphomas, secondary syphilis, or other diseases, but majority of cold urticaria patients are perfectly normal. The urticarial attack in these patients is precipitated by taking cold water bath, washing hand in cold water, exposure to cold wind in early morning or late evening, visit to hill station, entering to an air-conditioned room, exposure to wind after getting drenched in rain or sitting under fan while sweating, intake of ice-cold food or drink, or even touching or holding cold objects. In most of these cases, urticaria occurs during the winter months.

Dermographism

It literally means writing on the skin. In almost every normal individual, firm stroking of the skin with a blunt object gives rise to "triple response of Lewis" with a wheal and flare. However, some patients develop wheal even with light stroking of the skin. Urticarial wheals in these cases correspond to the area of stroking and are thus linear (Fig. 26.4). The patients usually complain of wheal and itching at the site of trauma, friction with clothing, after scratching, or after repeated rubbing. Dermographism may last for months or even indefinitely.

MANAGEMENT

In each and every case of urticaria, a detailed history is very important in an attempt to trace the cause. Urticaria due to food may occur regularly after one or each meal, and the frequency may vary from one or two attacks in a week to several attacks in a day. When the urticaria is suspected to be due to specific food item, it can be confirmed by the disappearance of urticaria within 48 hours after stoppage of the causative food (*diet elimination test*) or by giving a particular food and recurrence of urticaria. This is known as *provocation test*. The easiest way to treat food urticaria is to stop eating the particular offending item of food in all its forms. If it is not possible to avoid that food, specific desensitization with the antigen prepared from the food can be tried. Urticaria due to inhalants may be seasonal or throughout the year. However, it improves spontaneously when the patient goes to other places where the particular antigen is absent or its amount is less. It can be confirmed by breathing through an ordinary cloth mask for 48 hours[5] to see if the urticaria disappears or by intradermal tests with the respective antigen. The simplest way to treat these patients is either to avoid the place where the antigens are plenty or to use the nasal filter[6] or cloth to filter the antigen from inhaled air or desensitize the patient with the respective antigen(s). Stool examination for the presence of parasites or the cysts confirms their presence in the GI tract, which should be treated with appropriate medicine. Urticaria due to cold can be confirmed by the appearance of urticaria on the skin of these patients by the cryostimulation test[7] or by an ice-filled test tube. In cholinergic urticaria, there is an exaggerated response to intradermal carbachol or to exercise.[8] When urticaria is due to the physical agents like cold, heat, sunlight, pressure, or friction, it is better to avoid the causative agent as far as possible or antihistamine may be used if needed. Urticaria due to drug is usually of short duration. It disappears soon after the drug is withdrawn.[8] It occurs at regular intervals depending upon the frequency of drug intake. It can be confirmed by oral provocation tests done with due precautions. Avoidance of the causative and related drugs is best for stopping recurrences. In the case of urticaria due to septic foci, it usually disappears either by surgical removal of the foci or by giving a course of antibiotic for 1–2 weeks. An acute attack of urticaria is controlled by administration of adequate doses of antihistamine orally or intramuscularly, and the same is continued till urticaria disappears completely. The antihistamines control almost all varieties of urticaria.

REFERENCES

1. Gupta R, Urticaria due to tomato. J Pakistan Assoc Dermatol. 2014;24:99-100.
2. Gupta R, Gupta S. Urticaria due to inhalant antigens. Indian J Dermatol, Venereol, Leprol. 2003;69:429.
3. Pasricha JS, Gupta R. Urticaria and urinary tract infection. Indian J Dermatol Venereol Leprol. 1981;47:329.
4. Gupta R, Gupta S, Khera V. Urticaria/Angio-edema due to urinary tract infection. Indian J Dermatol. 2006;50:S53-4.
5. Gupta R. Allergic Disorders in Textbook of Dermatology, 3rd ed. New Delhi, India: Ane Books Pvt. Ltd.; 2011:149-64.
6. Pasricha JS, Gupta R. Allergic Dermatoses in IIlustrated Textbook of Dermatology, 4th ed. New Delhi, India: Jaypee Brothers; 2013:73-96.
7. Gupta R, Manchanda RK. Allergic Disorders in Textbook of Dermatology for Homeopaths, 4th ed. New Delhi, India: B Jain Publishers (P) Ltd; 2011:146-62.
8. Gupta R. Allergic Disorders in Comprehensive Dermatology and Sexually Transmitted Diseases, 1st ed. New Delhi, India: Ane Books Pvt. Ltd.; 2010:122-37.

CHAPTER 27

Angioedema

PC Kathuria

DEFINITION

- Angioedema (AE) is an acute, localized swelling of skin, mucosa, and submucosa caused by extravasations of fluid into the affected tissues (upper respiratory or gastrointestinal tract) and has predilection for the area of more loosely attached skin. It is not pitting but erythematous or skin colored with ill-defined margins due to an increase in vascular permeability secondary to IgE-mediated, mast cell-stimulated histamine release or from activation of the complement system and an elevation in bradykinin [hereditary angioedema (HAE)] it often resolves in hours to days, but can be life-threatening if the upper airway is involved.[1]

CLASSIFICATION, CLINICAL FEATURES AND DIFFERENTIAL DIAGNOSIS

Classification of angioedema (AE)	*Important clinical features in evaluation of AE*	*Differential diagnosis*
1. Allergic AE 2. Drug-related [angiotensin-converting enzyme (ACE)-I, nonsteroidal anti-inflammatory drugs (NSAIDs), salicylates] 3. CI inhibitor deficiency [hereditary angioedema (HAE), acquired angioedema (AAE)] 4. Autoimmune [thyroid disease, connective tissue disease (SLE, vasculitis)] 5. Gleich's syndrome 6. Clarkson syndrome 7. Idiopathic	• Speed of onset • Association with urticaria/without urticaria • Site of AE facial/peripheral/abdominal pain • Precipitating factors • Natural history of attack • Age of first onset • Response to treatment (antihistamines/ steroids/epinephrine) • Drug history—ACE inhibitors/ Angiotensin receptor blocker antagonist/ salicylates and NSAIDs • Family history	• Anaphylaxis • Urticaria (with AE in 40–50% of patients) • Allergic contact dermatitis • Facial cellulitis • Cellulitis • Superior vena cava syndrome • Hypoproteinemia-related edema • Dermatomyositis • Systemic amyloidosis • Eosinophilic fasciitis • Crohn's disease

CAUSES OF ANGIOEDEMA WITH CLINICAL AND LABORATORY FINDINGS[2-5]

Type	*Description (Figs. 27.1 A and B)*	*Laboratory results*
Hereditary angioedema (HAE) type 1	Represents an estimated 80–58% of HAE cases; family history in 75% of patients does not response to antihistamine, corticosteroid, or epinephrine. Most often affects arms, legs, hands, feet, abdomen, and genitourinary systems; attacks typically last 2–5 days; not associated with urticaria; bradykinin mediated.	C4 level—decrease Antigenic C1 INH—decrease Functional C1 INH—decreased Complement component 1q (C1q)—normal

(Contd...)

(Contd...)

Type	*Description (Figs. 27.1 A and B)*	*Laboratory results*
HAE type 2	Represents an estimated 15–20% of HAE; family history in 75% of patients; does not respond to antihistamine, corticosteroids, or epinephrine; most often affects arms, legs, hands, feet, abdomen, genitourinary system; attacks typically last 2–45 days; not associated with urticaria; bradykinin-mediated.	C4 level—decreased Antigenic C1 INH—normal or elevated Functional C1 INH—decreased C1q—normal
HAE with normal C1 INH	Formerly known as HAE type III, variant HAE estrogen-dependent or estrogen-associated angioedema, or inherited AE with normal C1 INH levels. Family history of AE Few reported cases; found mostly in women; does not respond to antihistamines, corticosteroids, or epinephrine; Not associated with urticaria; bradykinin mediated.	C4 level—normal Antigenic C1 INH—normal Functional C1 INH—normal C1q—normal
Acquired C1 inhibitory deficiency	Also known as acquired angioedema (AAE) types 1 and 2; type 1 usually linked to an underlying lymphoproliferative disorder; AAE type 2 occurs when autoantibodies destroy C1 INH function; attacks similar to HAE onset middle age or later; absence of family history does not respond to antihistamines or corticosteroids; not associated with urticaria; bradykinin mediated.	C4 level—decreased Antigenic C1 INH—decreased or normal Functional C1 INH—decreased C1q—decreased
Allergic AE	Associated with food, venom, latex, drugs, or environmental allergens; usually, accompanied by urticaria and sometimes anaphylaxis; may be pruritic attacks typically last 24–48 hours. Responds antihistamine/corticosteroids.	C4 level—normal Antigenic C1 INH—normal Functional C1 INH—normal C1q—normal
Idiopathic AE	Accompanied sometimes with urticaria; swelling lasts up to 48 hours; attack may occur daily; may respond to histamines and corticosteroids.	C4 level—normal Antigenic C1 INH—normal Functional C1 INH—normal C1q—normal
AE with urticarial vasculitis	Accompanied usually with urticaria; skin may show petechiae or purpura after swelling resolves; often there are other symptoms consistent with underlying vasculitis.	C4 level—decreased Antigenic C1 INH—normal Functional C1 INH—normal C1q—decreased
Drug-induced AE	Angiotensin-converting enzyme (ACE)-1 inhibitor; history of ACE use; tend to affect face and tongue. Nonsteroidal anti-inflammatory drug (NSAID). Typically accompanied by urticaria.	C4 level—normal Antigenic C1 INH—normal Functional C1 INH—normal C1q—normal

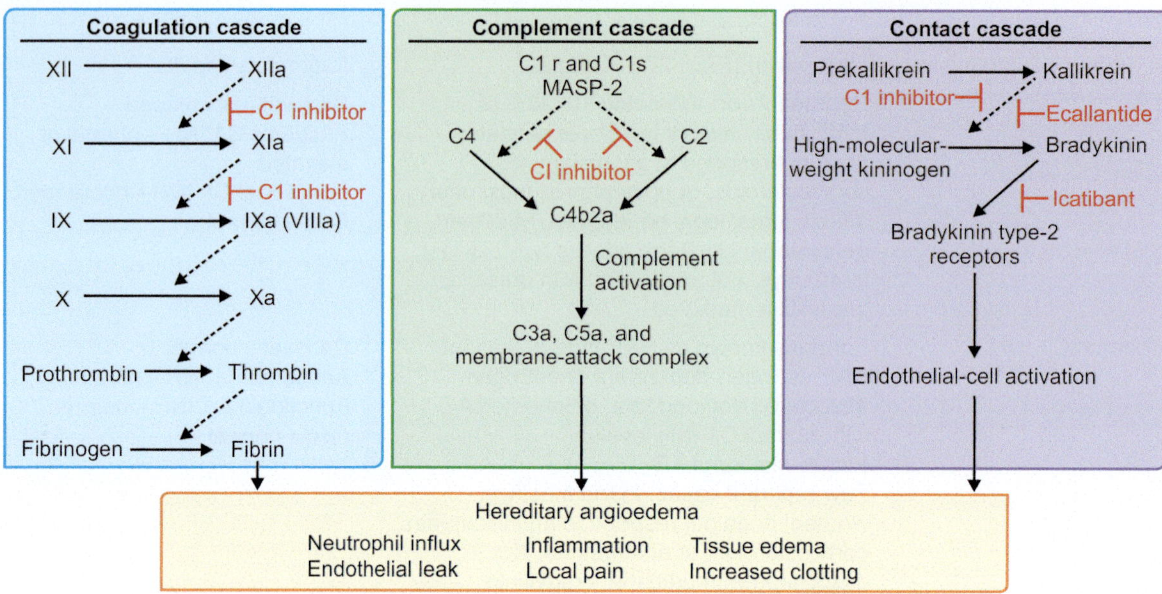

Fig. 27.1A: Dysregulation of coagulation, complement, and contact cascades in hereditary angioedema.

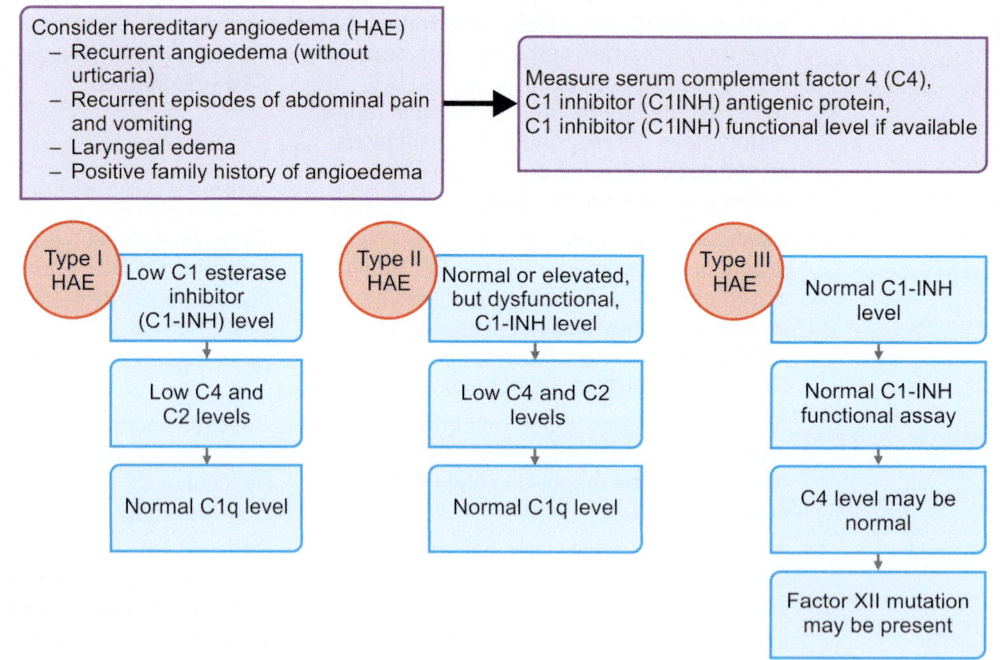

Fig. 27.1B: Diagnostic algorithm for hereditary angioedema.

DIAGNOSIS OF ANGIOEDEMA[6,7]

One of the most important procedures to diagnose AE is to separate allergic from nonallergic AE and to exclude other pathologies such as infection, tumors, and diseases of large salivary glands. These procedures usually follow the initial emergency care, e.g., monitoring of vital function, determination of the status of AE, intubation, oxygen supply, and pharmacotherapy with antihistamines, nebulized adrenaline, and corticosteroids. Besides a detailed physical examination preferably including laryngoscopy, several blood measurements, some imaging procedures, and an extensive anamnesis focusing on the patient's family history and current medications should be performed. A detailed physical examination should reveal whether the swelling is itchy or painful, which indicates allergic AE or inflammatory conditions, respectively. Signs of urticaria usually exclude the determination of C1-INH (C1-inhibitor) activity, and eventually, C1-INH concentration and markers of inflammation (e.g., C-reactive protein, leukocyte count). A reduced activity of plasma C1-INH is indicative of either HAE or AAE and should be examined further, e.g., by genotyping or determination of accompanying diseases such as lymphoma. In some assumed drug-induced cases [angiotensin-converting enzyme (ACE-1)], it might also be helpful to determine serum ACE activity. As for diagnostic imaging procedures, ultrasound visualization of the edema region is usually sufficient, but uncertain cases and/or abdominal pain should undergo magnetic resonance tomography. A first suspicion of HAE is given by mucosal swelling and/or unclear abdominal pain in patients at a young age and those with a family history, a lack of concomitant drug therapy, and the absence of urticaria as well. Following eventually necessary emergency treatment, the diagnostic procedure for HAE (types 1 and 2) requires the measurement of both C1-INH serum concentration and function. Furthermore, plasma levels of the complementary factor C4 in the serum are reduced in a vast majority of the cases. This factor is frequently reduced to approximately 25% of the normal value during the acute episode of AE. Furthermore, other rare conditions, such as Crohn's disease of the mouth and lips, facial cellulitis, and the superior vena cava syndrome should be excluded. An illustration of different manifestations of bradykinin-induced AE is depicted in Flowcharts 27.1 to 27.3.

Flowchart 27.1: Different algorithm of bradykinin-induced AE is depicted.

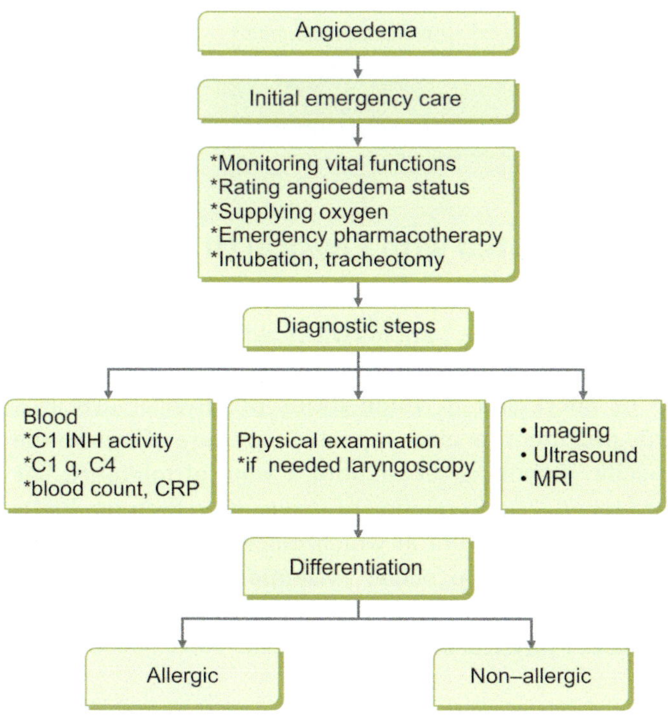

Flowchart 27.2: Different algorithm of bradykinin-induced AE is depicted.

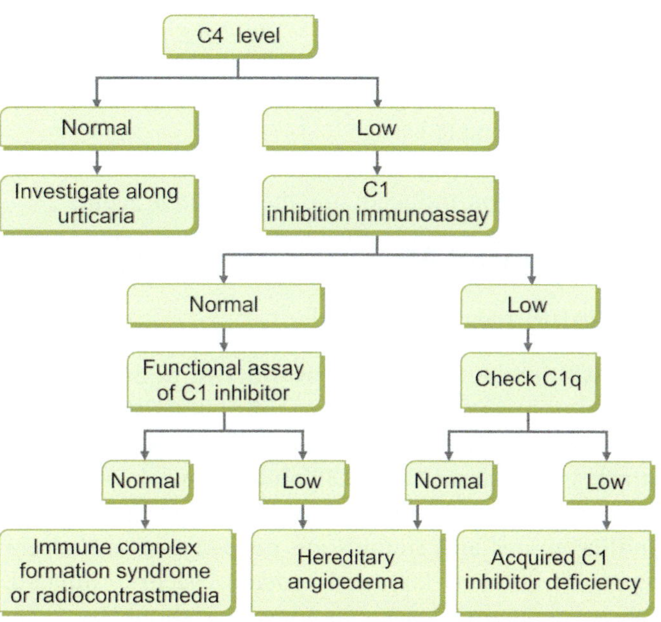

Flowchart 27.3: Different algorithm of bradykinin-induced AE is depicted.

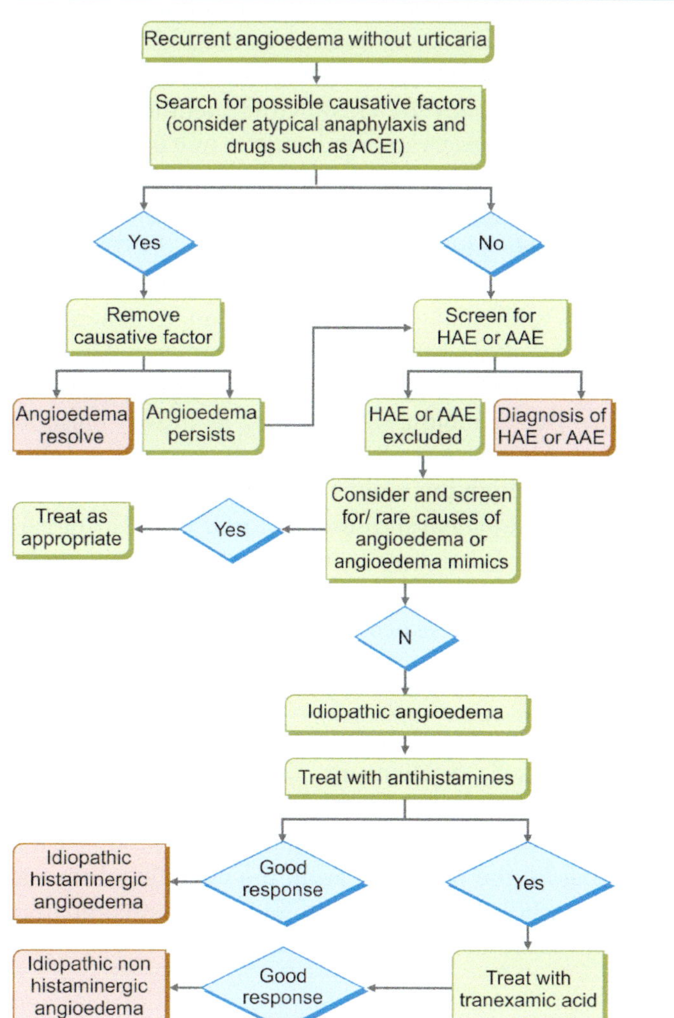

MANAGEMENT OF ANGIOEDEMA[7-9]

Acute allergic AE *(with airway compromise)*

- Epinephrine 1:1,000, 0.3 mL IV or solu-medrol 40 mg IV.
- Glucocorticoids (hydrocortisone 200 mg IV or solu-medrol 40 mg IV).
- Diphenhydramine 50 mg IV.
- If medication-induced, stop the causative agent.

Drug-induced AE

ACE Inhibitor-induced AE

The ACE inhibitor should be withdrawn in any patients who present with AE, however mild and however long after the introduction of the ACE inhibitor. In a very mild attack, withdrawal of the ACE inhibitor may be sufficient to control the problem, however very often intravenous antihistamines and steroids are needed and sometimes repeatedly when laryngeal edema occurs, inhaled, subcutaneous, or intravenous adrenaline should be given. The dose of subcutaneous adrenaline is 0.01 mL per kg body weight of 1:1,000 aqueous adrenaline, and it may be repeated every 15–20 minutes as needed oral or nasal intubation tracheotomy or retrograde intubation over a guide-wire through the cricothyroid membrane may be needed. Close observation in intensive unit is advisable in extremely severe cases. Intravenous saline infusion should be started if hypotension is present. The course can be unpredictable and the AE may worsen rapidly. There may be a poor response to the initial treatment, especially if the AE is well established at presentation. In general, the AE resolves after 1 or 2 days and does not recur if the ACE inhibitor is withdrawn. It is not advisable to replace the original ACE inhibitor with another, as further episodes are likely to occur. A medic alert bracelet is useful and clear instruction about the avoidance of ACE inhibitors should be given to the patient and other doctors involved in the care of the patient. When the situation is stable, the patient may be discharged with a short course of oral antihistamines and a tapering course of oral corticosteroids.

NSAID-Induced AE

Angiodema caused by aspire in is occasionally seen. The proposed mechanisms include cyclo-oxygenase inhibition leading to amplified mast-cell degranulation and enhanced biosynthesis of lipoxygenase products. It is essential for the patient to avoid the offending drug and also the whole group of nonsteroidal anti-inflammatory drugs in the future.

AE with Lupus Erythematosus

The management is basically directed to treat the underlying cause. The treatment of the AE per se may involve the use of antihistamines, systemic steroid, and adrenaline.

AE with Hypereosinophilia

Patients with AE and urticaria associated with markedly elevated peripheral blood eosinophil counts have been reported. Skin biopsies showed infiltration of dermis with eosinophils deposition of proinflammatory major basic protein in the dermis appeared to be responsible for the AE in these cases. The body weight of the patient may increase during attacks, which are associated with fever. The condition responds to systemic prednisolone.

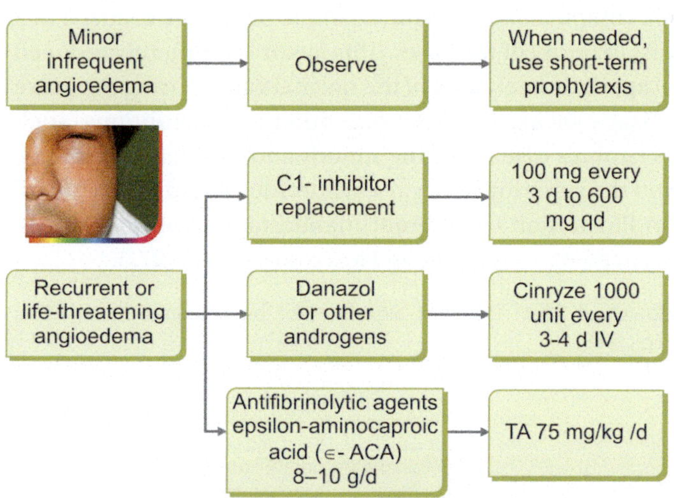

Fig. 27.2: Management of AE.[11,12]

AE Associated with Physical Urticarias

Severe AE can often be prevented by avoidance of the cause, for example, patients with cold urticaria should not swim in cold water. Tolerance treatment has been reported to be successful in some forms of physical urticaria. This treatment involves repeated exposure of skin to the specific provoking factor until a state of tolerance has developed. The frequency of exposure is then gradually reduced to the point at which reactivity to the physical stimulus begins to occur. Systemic antihistamine may be effective in reducing the itching associated with AE caused by physical stimuli.

Idiopathic Recurrent AE

It is important to ensure a patent airway first. Adrenaline should be administered; it may be given as self-injection by the patient. Adrenaline may abort the acute attack. If adrenaline does not work, intravenous antihistamines and hydrocortisone should be given.

- First-generation antihistamines for acute AE (cause drowsiness): oral doxepin (sinequan) may be effective for AE (10–25 mg at bedtime).
- Older children and adults: hydroxyzine (atarax 5 mg/mL, 25 mg tablets) 10–25 mg t.i.d., or diphenhydramine (benadryl) 25–50 mg q6h.
- Second-generation H_1 blockers: fexofenadine (allerga) 180 mg/d b.i.d., loratadine (claritin) 10 mg/d, cetirizine (zyrtec) 10 mg/d, desloratadine (clarinex) 5 mg/d (3) [C]; use with caution in pregnancy and in the elderly.

MANAGEMENT OF HEREDITARY ANGIOEDEMA[10-13]

- If mild to moderate attack, give only demand therapy but if moderate to severe and life-threatening, give long-term prophylaxis. With the advent of serological and modern drugs, if early diagnosis and early treatment is given to a patient of HAE, the duration of each attack is reduced to 1–3 hours from duration of 3–5 days, and the patient can have a normal healthy life.

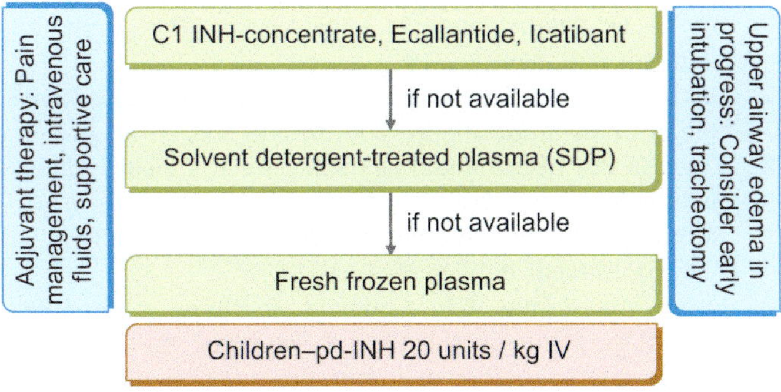

Fig. 27.3: Hospitalization is recommended due to risk of laryngeal edema (Treatment algorithm for HAE).[12]

HAE Chronic Prophylaxis

Long-term prophylaxis is considered only in selected cases if the disease is progressive (moderate to severe), attack of laryngeal edema, or impairment in daily normal activities. Androgens (danazol/stanozolol) are started in higher dose (400–600 mg/day) and taper to minimum effective doses (50–200 mg, twice a week), with regular monitoring of LFT and lipid profile (Fig. 27.2). If there is absolute contraindication to the use of androgens, then only therapy is C1-inhibitor concentrate as a long-term prophylaxis (not available in India). Even the patients are on along-term prophylaxis, they may get acute attack of life-threatening laryngeal edema, where either a nanofiltered plasma-derived C1 INH (pd C1 INH) concentrate or an antikallikrein inhibitor (Ecallantide) and bradykinin Beta2 receptor antagonist (lcatibant) are given on demand therapy (not available in India). We still manage our patients with fresh frozen plasma (FFP) at the time of acute attacks though it is not an ideal therapeutic agent.

Oral danazol 50–200 mg/day or oral stanozolol 2 mg/day is used as lowest effective dose. Side effects include headache, weight gain, liver dysfunction, hirsutism, and menstrual disturbances. For dose of danazol >200 mg/day, monitor CBC, liver function test, creatinine kinase, lactic dehydrogenase, fasting lipid profile, and urinalysis at baseline and q6mo. Abdominal ultrasound should be performed annually or q6mo. Danazol is not to be used in children, during first two trimesters of pregnancy, during lactation, and in patients with hepatitis or cancer. If patients cannot tolerate attenuated androgens, antifibrinolytic agents (plasmin inhibitors), such as tranexamic acid (not approved by the FAD in the USA) 25–50 mg/kg/day divided b.i.d. or t.i.d. (3–6 g/day maximum) or e-aminocaproic acid could be used. They are less effective than attenuated androgens and have many side effects. On rare occasions, they have been linked to (but not proven to cause) thrombophlebitis.

HAE Short-term Prophylaxis

- In cases of any surgical intervention (elective/emergency like gallbladder, head and neck surgery), the drug of choice is pd C1 inhibitor concentrate (not available in India). We give solvent/detergent-treated plasma (SDP) or FFP 1–6 hours before the procedure at the rate of 10 mL/kg (400–800 mL in adults).
- Minor procedures (dental work): If C1 INH is available, no prophylaxis; otherwise: danazol 2.5–10 mg/kg/day (maximum 600 mg/day), stanozolol 4–6 mg/day, for 5 days prior to and 2–5 days after the event (Fig. 27.4).
- Major procedures (including intubation): C1 INH1 concentrate is given 6 hours prior with additional dose on hand during procedure. If it is unavailable, use

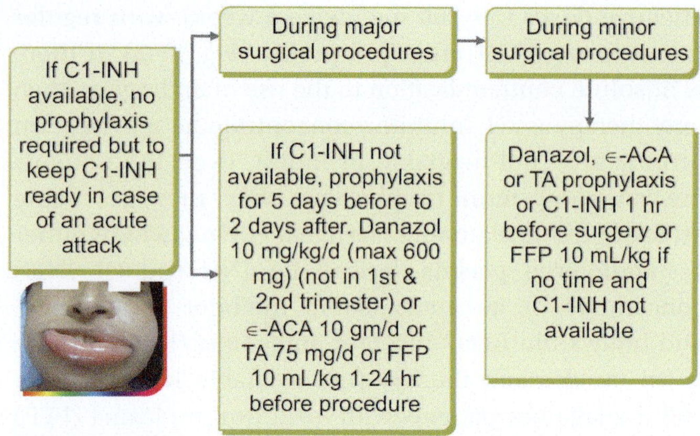

Fig. 27.4: Management and treatment of hereditary angioedema.

danazol 2.5–10 mg/kg/day (max. 600 mg/day), and if SDP is unavailable, use FFP 10 mL/kg; 2–4 units (400–800 mL) for an adult 1–6 hours before.

Acute HAE Treatment

- C1 inhibitor concentrate IV (inter venous), dosed at 1,000 units if <50 kg; 1,500 units if 50–100 kg; 2,000 (units if >100 kg)[2] [C]; a pasteurized human pd C1 INH (berinert), dosed at 20 units/kg (available in 500 units/10 mL, max infusion rate of 4 mL/min IV via peripheral vein (Fig. 27.3). Do not shake (will denature the protein). Worsening of HAE pain was reported as the most severe adverse event[4,6] [B].
- Kalbitor (ecallantide), a kallikrein inhibitor, is dosed in patients >16 years old at 30 mg SC with three separate 10 mg/mL injections in the abdomen, thigh, or upper arm and rotation; second 30-mg dose may be repeated within 24 hours if needed.
- Antihistamines and glucocorticoids typically do not benefit HAE patients.
- Epinephrine can offer transient stabilization/improvement in laryngeal AE, but is not sufficient for full treatment.
- A bradykinin receptor-2 antagonist (icatibant), dosed SC and supplied in a prefilled 3-mL syringe for home administration has received favorable response from the Food and Drug Administration (FDA) advisory.

Acute AAE Treatment

- C1 INH concentrate and FFP.
- Treatment of underlying lymphoproliferative disease is often curative in AAE type I.
- Immunosuppressive therapy to suppress antibody production.
- Clinical trials underway with recombinant human C1-INH (rhucin) concentrate.

SUMMARY

The management of AE is becoming more specific as more is learned about the biology of the development and progression of AE. The future of AE management is likely genotypic characterization in certain cases to determine appropriate therapy to be safer and effective. It is hoped to bring us closer to a cure for AE with all potential improvement in research.

REFERENCES

1. Zingale LC, Beltrami L, Zanichelli A, et al. Angioedema without urticaria: a large clinical survey. CMAJ. 2006;175:1065-107.
2. Bork K, Meng G, Staubach P, Hardt J. Hereditary angioedema: new findings concerning symptoms, affected organs, and course. Am J Med. 2006;119:267-74.
3. Craig T, et al. World Allergy Organ J. 2012;5:185-199; Lang DM, et al. Allergy Asthma Immunol. 2012; 109:395-402; Cicardi M, et al. Allergy. 2012;67:147-57.
4. Cicardi M, et al. Allergy. 2012;67:147-157; Craig T. et al. J Allergy Clin Immunol. 2009; 124:801-808; Lumry WR, et al. Ann Allergy Asthma Immunol. 2011;107:529-37.
5. Frigas E, Park M. Idiopathic recurrent angioedema. Immunol Allergy Cin North Am. 2006;26:739-51. [PMID: 17085288].
6. Au TS. Dr. Management of Angio-edema. H K Dermatol Venereol Bull. 1998;6:4-10.
7. Bas M, Adams V, Suvorava T, et al. Nonallergic angioedema: role of bradykinin. Allergy. 2007:62:842-56.
8. Kathuria PC. Urticaria and its management. Indian J Allergy Asthma Immunol. 2011;25:33-7.
9. Kathuria PC. Food Allergy, Raipur: Advance in Allergy & Asthma, Shivam Publications:134-51.
10. Lunn ML, Santos CB, Craig TJ. Is there a need for clinical guideline in the United States for the diagnosis of hereditary angioedema and the screening of family members of affected patients? Ann Allergy Asthma Immunol. 2010;104(3):211-4.
11. Dardana N, Craig TJ. Recent advances in management and treatment of hereditary angioedema. Pediatrics. 2011;128(6);1173.
12. Zuraw BL. Clinical practice. Hereditary angioedema. N Engl J Med. 2008;359:1027-36.
13. Bowen T, Cicardi M, Farkas H, et al. 2010 International consensus algorithm for the diagnosis, therapy and management of hereditary angioedema. Allergy Asthma Clin Immunol. 2010;6(1):24.

CHAPTER 28

Atopic Dermatitis

Mahesh Goyal, Aditya Goyal, Srishti Sareen

INTRODUCTION

Atopic dermatitis (AD) is a chronic inflammatory skin disorder that manifests as a relapsing eczematous rash. The inherited tendency to respond to small amounts of common environmental proteins including pollen, house dust mites, and food allergens by production of immunoglobulin E (IgE) antibodies is called *atopy*. The latter of the two words, *dermatitis*, can be broken down to the Greek word "derma", which means *skin*, and "itis," which means *inflammation*. Only about 50% of the patients with the disease have allergic sensitization and elevated IgE, hence *atopic dermatitis* is not a definitive term.[1] It occurs more frequently in children than in adults.

The International Study of Asthma and Allergies in Childhood (ISAAC) estimated the prevalence of AD worldwide in children between 6 and 7 years. It was found to be <2% in Iran and China compared to 20% in Australia, England, and Scandinavia. More than 37,000 children from India were studied at 14 different centers as part of phase 1 of the ISAAC study. All centers reported a 12-month period prevalence between 2.4% and 6%, whereas Kottayam reported a prevalence of >9%.[2] Approximately, 70% cases of AD begin in children <5 years of age, although 10% of cases seen in hospital settings start in adults.[3] Moreover, approximately 30% children with AD develop asthma and about 35% develop allergic rhinitis while reaching adulthood.[4]

RISK FACTORS

Genetic and environmental factors play a role in the susceptibility to AD. The concordance in dizygotic twins is 30%, while in monozygotic twins it is increased to 75%, emphasizing the role of genetic factors in increasing susceptibility to AD.[5] A number of genes have been shown to be associated with AD, but the strongest association has been reported with the *filaggrin (FLG)* gene located on chromosome 1.[6] Furthermore, two FLG mutations, R501X and 2282del4, have been reported to be carried by 16.7–56% of all individuals with AD.[7] Around 10% of general population carries at least one null mutation in the *FLG* gene, which leads to disruption of its normal function that is to form intracellular FLG proteins aggregate keratin filaments, which lead to keratinocyte compaction and in turn formation of the stratum corneum, which is a crucial skin barrier.[8] The *FLG* gene mutations are associated with asthma, early onset, and persistent AD along with certain phenotypic characteristics like hyperlinearity of hands.

Environmental factors also play a crucial role in the etiology of AD. The rapid rise in AD prevalence has been thought to be due to a proposed hygiene hypothesis, which attributes the increased susceptibility to AD in early childhood to decreased exposure to proteolytic infections. This hypothesis is further supported by evidence showing that children growing up in an environment with wide exposure to a variety of microflora like unpasteurized cow's milk, livestock, etc., seem protected, at least to some extent against developing the disease and other allergic diseases in general.[9,10] Some studies also showed a higher risk of AD in children with high socioeconomic status.[11]

PATHOGENESIS

Among several proposed hypotheses, two have been postulated to explain the disease development of AD.

Defective skin barrier hypothesis states that AD occurs as a result of disruption of the epidermal barrier function where the disease evolves from the outside in. Reported primary defect is the impaired structural barrier.

An intact epidermis is required to prevent the environmental allergens from entering the body. Proteins like filaggrin and serine protease inhibitors like SPINK5, optimal epidermal hydration, and optimal pH are required to maintain an intact skin. A disruption of any of these components through factors like decreased humidity, trauma, inherited defects, alteration of pH, or infection can interfere with the ability of the epidermis to function as an effective barrier. Any interference that occurs allows the environmental allergens to come in contact with the cells of the immune system triggering the pathophysiological mechanisms leading to AD. In patients with AD, decreased epidermal hydration leads to dry skin, causing pruritus and scratching, which then causes cutaneous trauma leading to the release of inflammatory mediators and worsening of the pruritus. This sets up a vicious cycle and leads to the persistence of the disease.[12-16]

Another hypothesis of AD, primarily immunological, caused by imbalance of T cells, particularly T helper cell types 1, 2, 17, and 22 and regulatory T cells, has been suggested.[17] It has been found that a predominant Th2 differentiation of naive CD4+ T cells occurs in the acute state of AD, which causes an increased downstream production of interleukins, primarily IL-4, IL-5, and IL-13. This interleukin surge leads to an increased level of IgE corresponding to inhibition of Th1 differentiation.

CLINICAL FEATURES

Although this description fits many with the disease, the clinical presentation of AD is often more elaborate with a large variation in the morphology and distribution of the eczema combined with various other features. However, many patients with AD have a general tendency to present with the dry skin (xerosis) due to the low water content and an excessive water loss through the epidermis. The skin is pale because of increased tension in the dermal capillaries

AD clinically presents with varied morphology and distribution of eczema along with the presence of other features. The most common presentation of AD is xerosis or dry skin. As discussed earlier, this occurs due to excessive water loss, resulting in low water content throughout the epidermis. Furthermore, the increased tension in dermal capillaries causes the skin to appear pale, and the ability to sweat is decreased. Patients usually have dry fragile hair and may also have hyperlinearity of palms and feet. Dermographism or *skin-writing,* an increased cholinergic response to scratch resulting in hives at the affected site, can usually be elicited. Along with this, under-eye circles may be present and are attributed to postinflammatory hyperpigmentation. A double skinfold underneath the inferior eyelid called the Dennie–Morgan fold can often be appreciated especially during increased disease activity.

Patients with AD come with a wide spectrum of presentations like *pityriasis alba,* which manifests as dry, pale patches on the face and upper arms, and *keratosis pilaris,* which is characterized by small, rough keratotic papules particularly on the upper arms and thighs. Patients also present with *Dermatitis plantaris sicca,* also known as atopic winter feet. It is characterized by symmetric eczema on the weight-bearing areas of the soles of the feet and is usually seen in school-going children. Eczema of the earlobe, the nipple, and around the margins of the mouth (cheilitis) are other commonly seen presentations and often involve staphylococcal infection that can be bothersome to the patient given the distribution. Eye conditions like keratoconus and cataracts sometimes complicate AD.[1]

AD can essentially be divided into three stages based on the presenting age groups:

1. *Infantile stage*: From infancy to 2 years
2. *Childhood stage*: This stage is from 2 to 12 years
3. *Adult stage*: This stage is for people older than 12 years[18]

In all the stages of AD, there are xerosis, pruritus, and lichenification, and the area of involvement remains the main differentiating feature in all stages.

In the *infantile stage,* the disease is highly pruritic, scaly, crusted, and usually involves patches on the extensor surfaces of the extremities and the cheeks. The diaper area is usually spared.

In the *childhood stage,* there are lichenified plaques involving flexural areas (popliteal and antecubital fossa, volar surface of ankles, wrist and neck). Plaques that are thickened show excoriation.[18]

In the *adult stage,* patients can present with the history of two types: the history of two types either few or no previous skin problems since childhood, or they may have had a chronic relapsing-remitting course. Lichenification is present in the flexural areas and is usually associated with involvement of the face. Involvement of ankles, feet, hands, fingers, and toes may also be seen.[18]

DIAGNOSIS

While there exists no gold standard test, the diagnosis of AD is essentially based on some of the criteria. Different criteria are available for diagnosis. First criterion was introduced by Hanifin and Razka in 1980, which is based on the diagnosis of AD in the presence of 3 or 4 major and at least 3 of 23 minor criteria (Box 28.1).[19] Even though, the Hanifin and Rajka criteria are often used in clinical trials, some of the minor criteria have been poorly specified. Therefore, the American Academy of Dermatology suggested a revised version of these criteria in 2003, which since has been more widely accepted.[20]

BOX 28.1: Hanifin and Razka criteria for diagnosis of AD.

Major criteria (must have three)

1. Pruritus
2. Dermatitis with typical morphology and distribution
   - Flexural lichenification or linearity in adults
   - Facial and extensor involvement in infants and children
3. Chronic or chronically relapsing dermatitis
4. Personal or family history of atopy (asthma, allergic rhinitis, atopic dermatitis)

Minor criteria (must have three)

1. Xerosis
2. Ichthyosis, palmar hyperlinearity, or keratosis pilaris
3. Immediate (type I) skin-test reactivity
4. Raised serum IgE
5. Early age of onset
6. Tendency toward cutaneous infections (especially *S. aureus* and herpes simplex) or impaired cell-mediated immunity
7. Tendency toward nonspecific hand or foot dermatitis
8. Nipple eczema
9. Cheilitis
10. Recurrent conjunctivitis
11. Dennie–Morgan infraorbital fold
12. Keratoconus
13. Anterior subcapsular cataracts
14. Orbital darkening
15. Facial pallor or facial erythema
16. Pityriasis alba
17. Anterior neck folds
18. Itch when sweating
19. Intolerance to wool and lipid solvents
20. Perifollicular accentuation
21. Food intolerance
22. Course influenced by environmental or emotional factors
23. White dermographism or delayed blanch

Diagnosis of AD required the presence of 3 of the 4 major and at least 3 of the 23 minor criteria.

Patients with presumptive diagnosis of AD should be confirmed based on the criteria summarized in Box 28.2. On certain occasions, use of skin biopsy specimens or tests such as serum IgE, potassium hydroxide preparation, patch testing, and/or genetic testing may be helpful to rule out associated skin conditions.[20]

Currently, the diagnosis of AD largely remains clinical as there is no reliable biomarker to distinguish it from other similar diseases. Among laboratory tests, elevated total

BOX 28.2: American Academy of Dermatology criteria for diagnosis of AD.

Essential features (must be present)

- Pruritus
- Eczema (acute, subacute, chronic)
- Typical morphology and age-specific patterns*
- Chronic or relapsing history

Important features (seen in most cases, add support to the diagnosis)

- Early age of onset
- Atopy
- Personal and/or family history
- Immunoglobulin E reactivity
- Xerosis

Associated features (help to suggest the diagnosis of atopic dermatitis (AD) but are too nonspecific to be used for defining or detecting AD for research and epidemiologic studies)

- Atypical vascular responses (facial pallor, white dermographism, delayed blanch response)
- Keratosis pilaris/pityriasis alba/hyperlinear palms/ichthyosis
- Ocular/periorbital changes
- Other regional findings (perioral changes/periauricular lesions)

Exclusionary conditions (a diagnosis of AD depends on excluding these conditions)

- Scabies
- Seborrheic dermatitis
- Contact dermatitis
- Ichthyoses
- Cutaneous T-cell lymphoma
- Psoriasis
- Photosensitivity dermatosis
- Immune deficiency diseases
- Erythroderma of other causes

*Patterns include the following:

1. Facial, neck, and extensor involvement in infants and children.
2. Current or previous flexural lesions in any age group.
3. Sparing of groin and axillary regions.

or allergen-specific serum IgE level is the most common finding; however, it is only seen in 80% of the patients. IgE blood levels, although correlate with disease severity, do not serve as a robust indicator as many patients maintain a normal value even during severe disease. Moreover, serum IgE may also be elevated in several nonatopic conditions including parasitic infections, certain cancers, and autoimmune diseases.[21]

Continued research on novel biomarkers for AD has yielded certain cytokines and chemokines, some of which have shown positive correlation with AD disease severity. Those reported include serum levels of CD30, macrophage-derived chemoattractant, activation-regulated chemokine, and interleukins (IL)-12, -16, -18, and -31. However, none of these have shown reliable sensitivity or specificity for AD to support their general clinical use for diagnosis or monitoring.[22]

DIFFERENTIAL DIAGNOSIS

Atopic dermatitis must be differentiated from the following skin conditions:[23]

1. *Seborrheic dermatitis of infancy*: In this condition, the diaper area is typically involved. It manifests as velvety red patches in infants younger than 4 months, which later clear off in a few months.
2. *Adult-type seborrheic dermatitis*: The causative agent is Malassezia yeast and lesions are found in areas like eyebrows, ear canals, etc., where there is a predominance of seborrheic glands.
3. *Allergic contact dermatitis*: It is a type IV hypersensitivity reaction. The history of contact and localization of contact help in formulating the diagnosis.
4. Scabies.
5. Insect bites.

TREATMENT

Current treatment focuses on providing symptomatic relief, prevents any exacerbations, reduces/prevents any recurrences, and provides a long-term management.[24] The standard treatment involves hydration and moisturization of the skin and use of topical anti-inflammatory preparations. However, certain patients with very severe form of the disease require systemic treatment/phototherapy.[25,26]

Therapeutic Options

- AD can be triggered by a variety of factors like house dust mites, stress, certain foods, and seasonal factors.[27] Avoidance of these factors can help to prevent any acute flares.
- Keeping the skin well hydrated with regular application of moisturizers is very important in treating AD. Emollients must be applied regularly and each time after activities like bathing and swimming. They help in reducing itching and alleviating symptoms.[24]
- Topical steroids are used intermittently with emollients as part of the standard regimen in treating AD. They are usually prescribed for short-term intermittent use because of their safety concern with continuous application.[24] Their side-effect profile includes cutaneous manifestations like skin atrophy/thinning, increased hair growth, telangiectasia, hypopigmentation, etc. The systemic side effects include Cushing's syndrome, cataracts, glaucoma, avascular femoral necrosis, and growth retardation.[28-32]
- For severe cases that do not respond to topical therapy, systemic corticosteroids or cyclosporine/azathioprine can also be used. Phototherapy can also be used in severe cases. Antihistamines can also prove beneficial in providing relief from pruritus. Oral treatment with antibiotics can be given in those with *Staphylococcus aureus* colonization.[24]
- Topical calcineurin inhibitors like tacrolimus and pimecrolimus are not known to cause skin atrophy or other side effects of topical steroids. Hence, they are useful in long-term prescriptions to prevent disease progression.[24]
- Psychological support throughout the disease course must be provided to patients with AD.

REFERENCES

1. Thomsen SF. Atopic dermatitis: natural history, diagnosis, and treatment. ISRN Allergy. 2014;2014:354250.
2. The International Study of Asthma and Allergies in Childhood (ISAAC) Steering Committee. Worldwide variation in prevalence of symptoms of asthma, allergic rhinoconjunctivitis, and atopic eczema: ISAAC. Lancet. 1998;351:1225-32.
3. Bannister MJ, Freeman S. Adult-onset atopic dermatitis. Australas J Dermatol. 2000;41:225-8.

4. Luoma R, Koivikko A, Viander M. Development of asthma, allergic rhinitis and atopic dermatitis by the age of five years. A prospective study of 543 newborns. Allergy 1983;38:339-46.
5. Thomsen SF, Ulrik CS, Kyvik KO, et al. Importance of genetic factors in the etiology of atopic dermatitis: a twin study. Allergy Asthma Proc. 2007;28:535-9.
6. Palmer CN, Irvine AD, Terron-Kwiatkowski A, et al. Common loss-of-function variants of the epidermal barrier protein filaggrin are a major predisposing factor for atopic dermatitis. Nat Genet. 2006;38:441-6.
7. Irvine AD. Fleshing out filaggrin phenotypes. J Invest Dermatol. 2007;127:504-7.
8. Candi E, Schmidt R, Melino G. The cornified envelope: a model of cell death in the skin. Nat Rev Mol Cell Biol. 2005;6:328-40.
9. Strachan DP. Hay fever, hygiene, and household size. BMJ. 1989;299:1259-60.
10. Bach JF. The effect of infections on susceptibility to autoimmune and allergic diseases. N Engl J Med. 2002;347:911-20.
11. Hammer-Helmich L, Linneberg A, Thomsen SF, Glümer C. Association between parental socioeconomic position and prevalence of asthma, atopic eczema and hay fever in children. Scand J Public Health. 2014;42:120-7.
12. Cork MJ, Robinson DA, Vasilopoulos Y. New perspectives on epidermal barrier dysfunction in atopic dermatitis: gene-environment interactions. J Allergy Clin Immunol. 2006;118:3-21; quiz 22-3.
13. Flohr C, England K, Radulovic S, et al. Filaggrin loss-of-function mutations are associated with early-onset eczema, eczema severity and transepidermal water loss at 3 months of age. Br J Dermatol. 2010;163:1333-6.
14. Loden M. The skin barrier and use of moisturizers in atopic dermatitis. Clin Dermatol. 2003;21:145-57.
15. Rawlings AV, Harding CR. Moisturization and skin barrier function. Dermatol Ther. 2004;17:43-8.
16. Verdier-Sevrain S, Bonte F. Skin hydration: a review on its molecular mechanisms. J Cosmet Dermatol. 2007;6: 75-82.
17. Eyerich K, Novak N. Immunology of atopic eczema: overcoming the Th1/Th2 paradigm. Allergy. 2013;68:974-82.
18. Rudikoff D, Lebwohl M. Atopic dermatitis. Lancet. 1998;35:1715-21.
19. Rudzki E, Samochocki Z, Rebandel P, et al. Frequency and significance of the major and minor features of Hanifin and Rajka among patients with atopic dermatitis. Dermatology. 1994;189:41-6.
20. Eichenfield LF, Hanifin JM, Luger TA, et al. Consensus conference on pediatric atopic dermatitis. J Am Acad Dermatol. 2003;49:1088-95.
21. Kabashima K. New concept of the pathogenesis of atopic dermatitis: interplay among the barrier, allergy, and pruritus as a trinity. J Dermatol Sci. 2013;70:3-11.
22. Eichenfield LF, Tom WL, Chamlin SL, et al. Guidelines of care for the management of atopic dermatitis: section 1. Diagnosis and assessment of atopic dermatitis. J Am Acad Dermatol. 2014;70:338-51.
23. Williams HC. Clinical practice. Atopic dermatitis. N Engl J Med. 2005;352:2314-24.
24. Ellis C, Luger T, Abeck D, et al. International Consensus Conference on Atopic Dermatitis II (ICCAD II): clinical update and current treatment strategies. Br J Dermatol. 2003;148:3-10.
25. Charman C. Clinical evidence: atopic eczema. BMJ. 1999;318:1600-4.
26. Sudilovsky A, Muir JG, Bocobo FC. A comparison of single and multiple applications of halcinonide cream. Int J Dermatol. 1981;20:609-13.
27. Langan SM, Williams HC. What causes worsening of eczema? A systematic review. Br J Dermatol. 2006;155:504-14.
28. Bode HH. Dwarfism following long-term topical corticosteroid therapy. JAMA. 1980;244:813-14.
29. Hill CJ, Rostenberg A Jr. Adverse effects from topical steroids. Cutis. 1978;21:624-8.
30. McLean CJ, Lobo RF, Brazier DJ. Cataracts, glaucoma, and femoral avascular necrosis caused by topical corticosteroid ointment. Lancet. 1995;345:330.
31. Queille C, Pommarede R, Saurat J-H. Efficacy versus systemic effects of six topical steroids in the treatment of atopic dermatitis of childhood. Pediatr Dermatol. 1984;1:246-53.
32. Ruiz-Maldonado R, Zapata G, Lourdes T, Robles C. Cushing's syndrome after topical application of corticosteroids. Am J Dis Child. 1982;136:274-5.

CHAPTER 29

Drug Allergy

Sitesh Roy

INTRODUCTION

A drug allergy, or an allergic drug reaction, is an adverse drug reaction that results from a specific immunologic response to a medication.

"Drug hypersensitivity" is a general term that includes both allergic and pseudoallergic drug reactions, which are a subset of idiosyncratic drug reactions.

"Drug pseudoallergy": A pseudoallergic drug reaction is a reaction that is similar or identical in presentation to an immunologic reaction, but is *not* mediated by the immune system. The term "nonimmune-mediated hypersensitivity" is also used. Pseudoallergic reactions, such as those to nonsteroidal anti-inflammatory drugs (NSAIDs), can be as severe as IgE-mediated anaphylaxis and are managed acutely in the same manner (i.e., with epinephrine, steroids). However, the evaluation and future prevention of these reactions is different from that of immunologic reactions.

CATEGORIES OF ADVERSE DRUG REACTIONS

An adverse drug reaction is a general term referring to any untoward reaction to a medication. Adverse drug reactions may be broadly divided into two types: type A and type B (Table 29.1)

Type A Reactions

Type A reactions make up 85–90% of all adverse drug reactions. These can affect any individual, given sufficient dose and exposure, and are predictable from the known pharmacologic properties of a drug. Examples of type A reactions include diarrhea in response to antibiotics, gastritis in association with long-term use of NSAIDs, or aminoglycoside nephrotoxicity.

Type B Reactions

Type B reactions make up 10–15% of adverse drug reactions. These are hypersensitivity reactions, mediated by immunologic or other types of mechanisms, which occur in a susceptible subgroup of patients, have signs and symptoms that are different from the pharmacologic actions of the drug, and usually cannot be predicted.

Most type B reactions are unpredictable, although notable exceptions are the predictable hypersensitivity reactions with allopurinol, carbamazepine, dapsone, abacavir, and flucloxacillin in patients with certain human leukocyte antigen (HLA) types. Hence, HLA testing of patients is recommended before administering abacavir and carbamazepine in populations in which there is appreciable prevalence of the genotype.

Type B (hypersensitivity) reactions may be further subdivided as follows:

Exaggerated Sensitivity to Known Drug Toxicities/Intolerance

Some patients experience the pharmacologically predictable toxicity of a drug (or several drugs) at low and sometimes subtherapeutic doses. An example would be the individual who develops tinnitus in response to a single dose of aspirin. This putatively reflects altered drug metabolism or increased end-organ sensitivity.[1]

Idiosyncratic Drug Reactions

Idiosyncratic drug reactions are qualitatively distinct from the known pharmacologic toxicities of the drug. These reactions can arise from genetic differences in the patient, such as primaquine causing nonimmune hemolytic anemia in patients with glucose-6-phosphate dehydrogenase deficiency or azathioprine toxicity

Table 29.1: Classification of adverse drug reactions.

Drug reaction	*Examples*
Type A: Reactions occurring in most normal patients, given sufficient dose and duration of therapy: Common and predictable	
Overdose	Hepatic failure (acetaminophen)
	Metabolic acidosis (aspirin)
Side effects	Nausea, headache (with methylxanthines)
	Oral thrush or vaginal candidiasis (with glucocorticoids)
	Nephrotoxicity (with aminoglycosides)
Secondary or indirect effects	Diarrhea due to alteration in GI bacteria after antibiotics
	Phototoxicity (with doxycycline or thiazide diuretics)
Drug interactions	Macrolide antibiotics increasing theophylline, digoxin, or statin blood levels
Type B: Drug hypersensitivity reactions restricted to a small subset of the general population: Rare and mostly unpredictable	
Intolerance*	Tinnitus after a single aspirin tablet
Idiosyncrasy† (pharmacogenetics)	G6PD deficiency: Hemolytic anemia after antioxidant drugs (e.g., dapsone)‡
	TMPT deficiency: Toxicity during azathioprine therapy‡
	Pseudoallergic reaction (with NSAIDs)
Immunologic drug reactions (allergy)	Anaphylaxis from beta-lactam antibiotics
	Photoallergy with quinidine
	Immune-mediated thrombocytopenia (with heparin)
	Serum sickness (with antivenom preparations)
	Vasculitis (with phenytoin)
	Stevens–Johnson syndrome (with trimethoprim–sulfamethoxazole)
	Drug-induced hypersensitivity syndrome (with allopurinol in HLA-B*58:01 individuals)‡

GI, gastrointestinal; G6PD, glucose-6-phosphate dehydrogenase; TPMT, thiopurine methyltransferase; NSAIDs, nonsteroidal anti-inflammatory drugs.
*Side effects at sub-therapeutic doses.
†Drug effect not attributable to known pharmacologic properties of drug and not immune medicated.
‡This is an example of a type B reaction that is predictable.

developing in patients with thiopurine methyltransferase deficiency.[2-4]

Aside from a few well-described examples, the mechanisms of most idiosyncratic drug reactions remain obscure and probably reflect complex interactions of metabolic and constitutional factors. NSAIDs causing pseudoallergic reactions is an example of the same.

Immunologic Drug Reactions (Drug Allergy)

Drug allergies result from specific immunologic responses to medications. Allergic drug reactions account for about 6–10% of all adverse drug reactions but up to 10% of fatal reactions.[5] Allergic drug reactions are the focus of the remainder of this review.

DEFINITION AND CLASSIFICATION OF DRUG ALLERGY

A drug allergy, or an allergic drug reaction, is a type B adverse drug reaction that results from a specific immunologic response to a medication. The term "immunologic drug reaction" is also used to describe these reactions. Immunologic drug reactions can be mediated by IgE, IgG, or lymphocytes. There are different systems of classifying immunologic drug reactions.

Based on Immunologic Mechanism

Historically, immunologic reactions, whether caused by drugs, infections, or autoimmune processes, have been divided into four categories (I–IV) according to the Gell and Coombs system (Table 29.2).

Type I: Immediate in onset and mediated by IgE and mast cells and/or basophils.

Type II: Delayed in onset and caused by antibody (usually IgG)-mediated cell destruction.

Type III: Delayed in onset and caused by IgG:drug immune complex deposition and complement activation.

Type IV: Delayed in onset and mediated by T cells. Of note, this classification was established before a detailed analysis of T-cell subsets and functions was technically possible. As new immunologic tools were developed, type IV reactions were further subdivided into types IVa, IVb, IVc, and IVd.[6]

Medications cause types I and IV reactions far more commonly than types II and III, which usually follow prolonged, higher dose therapy. Most medications cause just one type, although certain drugs, such as penicillin, can induce all four types.

Based on Timing of Symptom Onset

The World Allergy Organization (WAO) has recommended dividing immunologic drug reactions into immediate reactions (i.e., onset within 1 hour of exposure) and delayed reactions (onset after 1 hour), based on the timing of the appearance of the symptoms.[7]

Immediate

The WAO distinction between immediate and delayed drug reactions is intended to distinguish IgE-mediated type I reactions from other types. Type I reactions classically

Table 29.2: Gell and Coombs classification of immunologic drug reactions.

Type	*Description*	*Mechanism*	*Clinical features*
I Immediate reaction (within 1 hour)	IgE-mediated, immediate-type hypersensitivity	Antigen exposure causes IgE-mediated activation of mast cells and basophils, with release of vasoactive substances, such as histamine, prostaglandins, and leukotrienes.	Anaphylaxis Angioedema Bronchospasm Urticaria (hives) Hypotension
II	Antibody-dependent cytotoxicity	An antigen or hapten that is intimately associated with a cell binds to antibody, leading to cell or tissue injury.	Hemolytic anemia Thrombocytopenia Neutropenia
III	Immune complex disease	Damage is caused by formation or deposition of antigen–antibody complexes in vessels or tissues. Deposition of immune complexes causes complement activation and/or recruitment of neutrophils by interaction of immune complexes with Fc IgG receptors.	Serum sickness Arthus reaction
IV	Cell-mediated or delayed hypersensitivity	Antigen exposure activates T cells, which then mediate tissue injury. Depending upon the type of T-cell activation and the other effector cells recruited, different subtypes can be differentiated (i.e., types IVa–d).	Contact dermatitis, some morbilliform reactions, severe exfoliative dermatoses (e.g., SJS/TEN), AGEP, DRESS/DiHS, interstitial nephritis, drug-induced hepatitis, other presentations

IgE, immunoglobulin E; Fc IgG, Fc portion of immunoglobulin G; SJS/TEN, Stevens–Johnson syndrome/toxic epidermal necrolysis; AGEP, acute generalized exanthematous pustulosis; DRESS/DiHS, drug rash with eosinophilia and systemic symptoms/drug-induced hypersensitivity syndrome.

Source: Weiss ME, Adkinson NF. Immediate hypersensitivity reactions to penicillin and related antibiotics. Clin Allergy. 1988;18:515.

begin within 1 hour of the first administered dose. However, some IgE-mediated reactions appear after 1 hour up to 4 hours after ingestion of a drug, particularly after oral administration of a drug. In addition, taking the medication with food further slows absorption. Nevertheless, this period of 1 hour identifies the majority of IgE-mediated reactions, which carry the risk of anaphylaxis if the patient is re-exposed.

Delayed

Reactions appearing after 1 hour are classified as delayed, although most delayed reactions begin after 6 hours and typically after days of treatment. As an example, delayed reactions to amoxicillin classically start on day 7 to day 10 of treatment and may even begin 1–3 days after cessation of treatment. These reactions may be caused by several different mechanisms, but they are not IgE mediated. Types II, III, and IV immunologic reactions are all considered as delayed reactions.

Some delayed reactions begin after weeks of continuous treatment. One such disorder is "drug rash with eosinophilia and systemic symptoms" (DRESS), which is a systemic drug reaction that begins after 1–12 weeks in continuous treatment.[8] This reaction, which is also called "drug-induced hypersensitivity syndrome" (DiHS), is characterized by fever, rash, and multiorgan involvement, and may or may not be associated with eosinophilia and lymphocytosis. The liver (hepatitis) and heart (hypersensitivity myocarditis) may be affected. These reactions can persist for weeks to months, even after the medication is stopped. Some of these delayed reactions can also be life-threatening, and as a group, delayed reactions probably account for more deaths than anaphylaxis.

TYPE I REACTIONS

Type I reactions require the presence of drug-specific IgE. A minority of patients form drug-specific IgE upon exposure to a medication, while most do not even with prolonged treatment.

Once formed, drug-specific IgE occupies surface receptors on mast cells and basophils throughout the body. If the drug is encountered again, it (or its metabolite) may bind to these IgE molecules, causing cross-linking of the receptors and activation of the cells, resulting in symptoms. IgE-mediated reactions are dose dependent, although this may not be clinically apparent because even very low doses can cause severe systemic symptoms.

Clinical Features

The signs and symptoms of type I reactions are directly attributable to the immunochemical mediators released by mast cells and basophils. The most common signs and symptoms are urticarial rash; pruritus; flushing; angioedema of the face, extremities, or laryngeal tissues (leading to throat tightness with stridor, or rarely asphyxiation); wheezing; gastrointestinal symptoms; and/or hypotension.

Anaphylaxis is the most severe presentation of an IgE-mediated drug reaction. Mast cell tryptase and histamine can be elevated in the circulation in the first several hours after anaphylaxis, and the detection of these mediators implicates mast cells and basophils in the reaction, supporting the diagnosis of anaphylaxis.

The presence of urticaria is useful in identifying IgE-mediated reactions, because the classical wheal and flare are hallmark signs of mast cell degranulation. However, other skin findings in drug reactions can mimic urticaria, and it can be difficult to discern if a rash was truly urticarial based on history alone. Many delayed reactions involve a pruritic exanthem or rash that causes diffuse swelling of the skin, and affected patients will report raised, itchy areas of skin. However, these delayed-onset edematous exanthems are not urticarial rashes. In addition, they are generally not dangerous, provided the skin does not blister or slough, and there are no signs of organ inflammation. Conversely, urticarial rashes may be altered in appearance or suppressed by ongoing antihistamine therapies, such that in such patients the absence of urticaria should not be taken as evidence against anaphylaxis.

Neither fever nor elevations in serum C-reactive protein are seen with IgE-mediated reactions. The absence of these features can help distinguish IgE-mediated reactions from some other adverse drug reactions.

Timing

The timing of onset of type I reactions is rapid but varies with the clinical setting and presentation. IgE-mediated reactions occur rapidly after the last administered dose, which underlies the designation of immediate by the WAO. The time to onset is influenced by the route of administration; intravenously administered medications may cause symptoms in seconds to minutes, while the same drug administered orally may cause symptoms in 3–30 minutes if taken on an empty stomach; and in 10–60 minutes if taken with food.

- IgE-mediated anaphylactic reactions should not begin several days into a course of therapy, if the patient's exposure to the drug has been continuous. However, if several doses are skipped, symptoms can appear when the drug is resumed.
- Urticaria appearing within minutes to hours after drug intake can also be seen in "pseudoallergic" reactions.
- Isolated urticarial skin eruptions can occur late during continuous therapy.
- The delayed appearance of urticarial rashes with known allergenic drugs such as beta-lactam antibiotics may reflect time required for significant IgE responses (similar to late-occurring serum sickness reactions).
- Urticaria appearing 1–2 weeks after therapy, and accompanied by arthralgias, and fever suggest serum sickness.
- Urticarial eruptions, often appearing days after the start of therapy, sometimes also have maculopapular features. These urticarial rashes typically occur with drugs that rarely cause acute allergy (e.g., macrolide antibiotics) and are unlikely to be IgE mediated. T cells may also be involved, although the pathogenesis is not known.

Commonly Implicated Drugs

The drugs most commonly implicated in type I reactions include the following:

- Beta-lactam drugs (penicillins and cephalosporins)
- Neuromuscular blocking agents
- *Quinolones*—Quinolone antibiotics have been implicated as a common cause of hypersensitivity reactions in Europe, but less commonly in the United States, so there may be important geographical variations that will become more apparent over time.[9] Only some of these reactions are IgE mediated.[10-11]
- Carboplatin and oxaliplatin and other platinum-containing chemotherapeutic agents.
- Foreign proteins, including chimeric antibodies, such as cetuximab and rituximab.

Previous Exposure to the Suspect Drug

IgE-mediated reactions generally require previous exposure to the drug in question. However, the absence of a known prior exposure does not exclude an IgE-mediated reaction, because sensitization may have occurred from exposure to a cross-reactive compound, even though the patient showed no signs of allergy to the sensitizing product.

The following examples illustrate this phenomenon:

- A significant percentage of patients experiencing anaphylaxis upon first exposure to neuromuscular blocking agents are believed to have been previously sensitized through the use of various cosmetics, personal products, and nonprescription cough remedies (e.g., pholcodine in Norway) that contain tertiary and quaternary ammonium groups.[12-14] The ammonium groups shared by all of these agents are highly immunoreactive and can induce cross-reactive IgE antibodies.
- Some patients develop anaphylaxis to cetuximab and appear to have been previously sensitized to oligosaccharides present in the drug.[15] The same oligosaccharides (e.g., alpha-d Gal) are found on several non-primate mammalian proteins, such as beef, pork, and lamb. The source of the original sensitization is still uncertain, although bites of certain tick species (e.g., the lone star tick) have been implicated.

TYPE II REACTIONS

Type II reactions are uncommon and involve antibody-mediated cell destruction. Type II reactions may arise when drugs bind to surfaces of certain cell types and act as antigens. Subsequent binding of antibodies to the cell surface results in the cells being targeted for clearance by macrophages. Type II reactions may involve complement activation, but this is variable.

Clinical manifestations require the presence of high titers of preformed drug-specific IgG (or rarely IgM) antibodies, which are only made by a small percentage of individuals and usually in the setting of high-dose, long-term, or recurrent drug exposure. The factors predisposing individuals to form these antibodies are not fully understood.

Clinical Features and Timing

Type II drug reactions usually present as hemolytic anemia, thrombocytopenia, or neutropenia, since these are the cell types that are most often affected.

The clinical presentation can vary widely in severity; patients may be asymptomatic or present with fulminant illness. Symptoms usually appear at least 5–8 days after exposure but may begin after much longer periods of treatment. Symptoms can start within hours if the causative drug is stopped and then restarted.

Specific Presentations

Specific manifestations depend upon the cell type involved:

- *Drug-induced hemolytic anemia*: Hemolytic anemia may present with dyspnea, varying degrees of fatigue, pallor, jaundice, dark urine, splenomegaly, or signs and symptoms of the hyperdynamic state, such as bounding pulses, palpitations, and "roaring in the ears."

  The drugs most commonly implicated in hemolytic anemia are cephalosporins, penicillins, NSAIDs, and quinine–quinidine.
- *Drug-induced thrombocytopenia*: Thrombocytopenia typically presents with petechial bleeding in the skin and buccal mucosa and isolated thrombocytopenia, often severe (i.e., <20,000/μL) in a patient taking one or several medications. There may be splenomegaly and hepatomegaly due to platelet sequestration in these organs.

  Drugs implicated in thrombocytopenia include heparin, abciximab, quinine and quinidine, sulfonamides, vancomycin, gold compounds, beta-lactam antibiotics, carbamazepine, NSAIDs, and others.
- *Drug-induced neutropenia or agranulocytosis*: Severe neutropenia or agranulocytosis due to type II drug reactions is present days to weeks after beginning the medication, often with acute and clinically apparent symptoms of infection, such as fever, stomatitis, pharyngitis, pneumonia, or sepsis. Rechallenge or inadvertent subsequent administration is associated with a prompt recurrence, even with low doses.

  Culprit drugs include propylthiouracil, the antimalarial drug amodiaquine and one of its major metabolites, mono-desethyl amodiaquine, and flecainide.

TYPE III REACTIONS

Type III reactions are mediated by antigen–antibody complexes and usually present as serum sickness, vasculitis, or drug fever. These reactions are uncommon and usually seen in the context of high-dose, prolonged drug administration, similar to type II reactions.

In a type III reaction, the drug (including biologicals) is believed to act as a soluble antigen. In this capacity, the drug binds drug-specific IgG, forming small immune complexes that can activate complement and precipitate in various tissues, including blood vessels, joints, and renal glomeruli. These immune complexes bind to Fc-IgG receptors of inflammatory cells and/or activate complement, and an inflammatory response ensues. Re-exposure to similar or higher doses of the same drug can cause a more rapid and severe recurrence.

Timing

Signs and symptoms take one or more weeks to develop after drug exposure, since significant quantities of antibody are needed to generate symptoms related to antigen–antibody complexes.

Clinical Presentation

Type III reactions can take several forms:

Serum Sickness

Classic serum sickness involves fever, urticarial or purpuric rash, arthralgias, and/or acute glomerulonephritis. Alternatively, just one or two of these features may be apparent. Other findings include lymphadenopathy, low serum complement levels, and an elevated erythrocyte sedimentation rate. Serum sickness is a complication of several antitoxins, including those for rabies, botulism, and venoms.

Vasculitis

Drug-induced hypersensitivity vasculitis typically presents as palpable purpura and/or petechiae, fever, urticaria, arthralgias, lymphadenopathy, elevated erythrocyte sedimentation rate, and low complement levels. Purpuric lesions often affect the lower extremities. Uncommonly, other organs are involved, such as the gastrointestinal tract or kidneys. The most common culprits are penicillins, cephalosporins, sulfonamides (including most loop and thiazide-type diuretics), phenytoin, and allopurinol.

Arthus Reaction

An Arthus reaction is a localized type III hypersensitivity reaction in which antibody-antigen complexes that fix complement are deposited in the walls of small blood vessels, causing acute inflammation, infiltration of neutrophils, and localized skin necrosis. Arthus reactions were initially described in hyperimmunized laboratory animals. Whether significant local reactions to booster doses of modern vaccines are true, Arthus reactions have not been demonstrated conclusively. Typically, such reactions present as painful local swelling and erythema beginning within a few hours and usually peaking by 24 hours at sites of booster injections of a vaccine. This type of reaction has been reported with tetanus, diphtheria, and hepatitis B vaccines.[16-18]

TYPE IV REACTIONS

Type IV reactions are not mediated by antibodies, in contrast to the other three types above. Type IV drug reactions involve the activation and expansion of T cells, which requires time (normally many hours or days after antigen exposure), hence the name delayed-type hypersensitivity. In some cases, other cell types (e.g., macrophages, eosinophils, or neutrophils) are also involved. Type IV reactions can take many different forms, which vary in significance from inconvenient to life-threatening.

Timing

Type IV reactions are typically delayed in onset by at least 48–72 hours and sometimes by days to weeks following exposure to the culprit drug. Upon rechallenge, symptoms may appear within 24 hours. The time to symptom onset for reactions depends in part upon the number of T cells activated by the drug. These responses are polyclonal, and symptoms appear rapidly if the drug stimulates a large number of different T-cell clones. In contrast, a drug that activates just a few clones may not cause clinical symptoms until these T cells have proliferated for several weeks.

Stevens–Johnson syndrome/toxic epidermal necrolysis (SJS/TEN) and DRESS/DiHS, the most dangerous of the delayed drug hypersensitivity reactions, often appear after weeks of uncomplicated treatment, at which point patients suddenly develop signs and symptoms of a fulminant immune reaction. This presentation results from uncontrolled expansion of oligoclonal T cells that have been massively stimulated by the drug, reminiscent of superantigen-like stimulation.[19]

Subcategories of Type IV

T cells can orchestrate different forms of inflammation depending upon the cytokines produced and the other types of cells that become involved, leading to the subcategories of types IVa–d (Fig. 29.1).[6]

Clinical Presentations

Reactions involving T cells have prominent skin findings, because the skin is a repository for an enormous number of T cells.[20] Many cutaneous T cells are primed memory-effector cells, which react rapidly if immunogenic agents penetrate the skin barrier or diffuse into the skin from the circulation.[21]

Recognized patterns of cutaneous involvement include the following:

Contact Dermatitis

Contact dermatitis is a reaction to topically applied drugs, which is characterized by erythema and edema with vesicles or bullae that often rupture, leaving a crust.[22] Subacute and chronic contact dermatitis are characterized by lichenification, erythema, and scaling.

Maculopapular (Including Morbilliform) Eruptions

Maculopapular eruptions are one of the most common forms of delayed drug reactions and may arise from type IV immunologic reactions, as well as from other mechanisms. They are often called "rashes", a term which includes exanthems with varying degrees of cell infiltrations and thus papular component (maculopapular).

SDRIFE

Symmetrical drug-related intertriginous and flexural exanthem (SDRIFE), formerly called baboon syndrome, is a distinctive drug eruption that typically develops within a few hours to days of drug exposure and presents with demarcated, V-shaped erythema in the gluteal/perianal or inguinal/perigenital areas, often with the involvement of at least one other flexural area, such as the axillae, elbows, or knees.

Some forms of SDRIFE may be related to neutrophilic inflammations, such as acute generalized exanthematous pustulosis (AGEP).

Acute Generalized Exanthematous Pustulosis

The AGEP is a rare type of reaction characterized by superficial pustules, usually appearing within 24 hours after the administration of the culprit drug. Antimicrobial drugs amoxicillin, antimalarials, and calcium channel blockers are the most frequently reported triggers of AGEP.

Drug Fever

Fever can be the sole symptom or the most prominent symptom of drug hypersensitivity, accompanied in a minority of cases by nonurticarial rash or other organ involvement. Medications implicated in causing drug fever include azathioprine, sulfasalazine, minocycline, trimethoprim-sulfamethoxazole, sirolimus, and tacrolimus. Patients with active HIV infection or cystic fibrosis appear to be at particular risk, with higher rates of drug fever to antiretroviral drugs and piperacillin-tazobactam, respectively.[23]

Stevens–Johnson Syndrome and Toxic Epidermal Necrolysis

Severe blistering dermatitides, such as SJS and TEN, are potentially life-threatening reactions characterized by fever and mucocutaneous lesions leading to necrosis and sloughing of the epidermis.

Drug-induced Hypersensitivity Syndrome

The DiHS, also called DRESS, is a severe drug hypersensitivity reaction involving rash, fever (38–40°C), and multiorgan failure. The liver, kidneys, heart, and/or lungs are most often affected in DiHS/DRESS. It is discussed briefly here and reviewed in more detail elsewhere.

Debate is ongoing about the most accurate name for this syndrome, as only about 70% of cases show peripheral eosinophilia (e.g., those caused by abacavir or lamotrigine typically do not). The presence of atypical lymphocytes (activated CD8+) is a more consistent finding, which may persist for months after drug withdrawal.

Drugs that have been implicated in causing DRESS/DiHS include several antiepileptics (including carbamazepine, phenytoin, lamotrigine, and phenobarbital), minocycline, allopurinol, dapsone, abacavir, and nevirapine.

HLA associations: Some DiHS/DRESS reactions occur more frequently in patients with certain HLA types, since the drugs have been shown to bind to the certain HLA allele itself predominantly (e.g., allopurinol/oxypurinol to the HLA-B*58:01) or exclusively (abacavir and HLA-B*57:01),[24] a phenomenon that is also seen in SJS and TEN. Specific examples include:

- DiHS/DRESS and SJS/TEN to allopurinol is associated with HLA-B*58:01.[25] This B*58:01 association is less stringent in Caucasians (approximately 60%), in whom other alleles are also involved in SJS/TEN due to allopurinol.[26]
- DiHS/DRESS, and in some cases SJS/TEN, to carbamazepine disproportionately affects several groups.
  - Han Chinese patients with HLA-B15:02,[27] as well as Thai, Malaysian, and Indian patients with this same allele.[28-30]
  - Japanese and European patients with HLA-A*31:01.[31-32]
- DiHS/DRESS to abacavir occurs exclusively in patients with HLA-B*57:01; milder reactions to this drug are not associated with a certain HLA allele.
- Dapsone hypersensitivity syndrome disproportionately affects Chinese patients with HLA-B*13:01.[33]

  Once a patient has been identified as having a high-risk HLA profile, family members of that patient should also be advised to avoid the relevant drug, as familial occurrence of such hypersensitivity reactions has been noted. Recommendations have been made for screening patients for specific alleles prior to administration of carbamazepine, oxcarbazepine, abacavir, and allopurinol.[34]

Single Organ Involvement

Occasionally with T-cell mediated hypersensitivity, organ involvement occurs in the absence of skin findings, or skin findings are minor and overlooked. Presentations include isolated, drug-induced hepatitis, isolated interstitial nephritis, and isolated pneumonitis. As examples, flucloxacillin, as well as the combination drug amoxicillin-clavulanate potassium, may elicit cholestatic hepatitis, while allopurinol can cause nephritis,[35] and abacavir and nitrofurantoin can cause pneumonitis. Identification of this presentation as drug allergy can be challenging.

Association with Viral Infections

There is a higher risk of several type IV drug allergic reactions (ranging from simple exanthema to SJS/TEN) during generalized viral infections and exacerbations of autoimmune diseases, disorders in which T-cell reactivity is enhanced by widespread immune activation of T cells, high cytokine levels, and an increased expression of major histocompatibility complex and co-stimulatory molecules.

Viral infections that predispose patients to reactions to certain drugs include the following:

- Epstein–Barr virus (EBV) (with amoxicillin);
- Cytomegalovirus (with antibiotics);[36]

- Human herpes virus 6 (with anticonvulsants and other agents);
- HIV infection (with trimethoprim-sulfamethoxazole and other agents);
- In young children, treatment with amoxicillin (and to a lesser extent with other antibiotics) often elicits exanthematous reactions. Most of these children tolerate the same drug if given again later on.[37] It is likely that systemic viral infections are facilitating these reactions as well, although this has not been conclusively demonstrated. Rhinoviruses, which cause only local infections of the nasopharynx and respiratory tract, are unlikely to have this effect because they do not stimulate the immune system to the same degree.

Impact of Dose and Duration of Treatment

Dose seems to play an important role in developing delayed hypersensitivity reactions. Most delayed drug hypersensitivity reactions occur to drugs which are given in daily doses of 100–1000 mg. Allopurinol and lamotrigine are two examples.[38-40] In contrast, drugs that are dosed lower than 10 mg daily are rarely involved in delayed hypersensitivity reactions.

In allopurinol hypersensitivity, there are clinical and in vitro data to suggest that starting dose may also be relevant for developing hypersensitivity.[38,39] Thus, for drugs such as allopurinol or lamotrigine, lower initial doses may lower the incidence of hypersensitivity.

Length of treatment also appears to be a factor, as more than 10 days of administration of gemifloxacin caused maculopapular exanthema in nearly one-third of females in one study, while this was rare with 3 days of treatment.[11]

OTHER TYPES OF IMMUNOLOGIC REACTIONS

Two additional types of immunologic drug reactions that cannot be readily classified within the Gell and Coombs system are drug-induced autoimmunity and fixed drug eruption.

Drug-induced Autoimmunity

Drugs can induce autoimmune diseases.[41] Despite intensive scrutiny, the pathogenesis of these reactions has not been elucidated, although the finding that drug binding to HLA molecules can induce changes of the presented peptides has opened new pathways of research.[24,42] However, a definitive link between these findings and drug-induced autoimmune diseases has not yet been established.

- The best known example is a lupus-like disease, which can develop after exposure to procainamide, phenytoin, isoniazid, sulfasalazine, amiodarone, minocycline, and penicillamine.[41,43-45]
- Penicillamine can also cause a pemphigus-like disorder.
- IgA bullous dermatosis has been associated with vancomycin and various other drugs, including ceftriaxone, ciprofloxacin, and metronidazole.

Fixed Drug Eruption

Fixed drug eruption is a relative common reaction, which is characterized by erythematous and edematous plaques with a grayish center or frank bullae. Lesions recur at exactly the same sites (typically lips and tongue, genitalia, face, and acral areas) with drug re-exposure. These site(s) develop post-inflammatory pigmentation. Fixed drug eruption can occur in response to sulfonamides, anticoagulants, and many other drugs.[46] The mechanism is unknown, although T cells residing in the skin produce interferon gamma.[47-48]

PSEUDOALLERGIC REACTIONS

Pseudoallergic drug reactions are adverse drug reactions with signs and symptoms that mimic immunologic drug allergies, but in which immunologic mechanisms have not been demonstrated. They are a subset of type B, idiosyncratic reactions and are also called "nonimmune hypersensitivity reactions."[7]

Pseudoallergic reactions are difficult to distinguish clinically because they are similar or identical in presentation to true allergic reactions. Some pseudoallergic reactions arise from direct (rather than immunologic) activation of immune and inflammatory cells, so the final steps in pathogenesis and the resultant clinical features are indistinguishable from those of allergic reactions (*see* Table 29.2). The complete mechanisms underlying most of them are not known and may differ from one another. However, the diagnosis, prognosis, and prevention may be different from true allergic reactions. In particular, pseudoallergic reactions cannot be diagnosed with skin or in vitro allergy testing and do not worsen with repeated exposure.

Reactions that Resemble Anaphylaxis

Idiosyncratic reactions that mimic IgE-mediated, type I allergic reactions are the most important for clinicians to understand. Like IgE-mediated reactions, nonimmunologic activation of mast cells and basophils results in the release of vasoactive mediators. These pseudoallergic reactions range in severity from mild to fatal. Accordingly, acute nonimmunologic anaphylaxis should be treated in the same manner as immunologic anaphylaxis.

Nonimmunologic reactions resembling anaphylaxis are often referred to as "anaphylactoid." Unfortunately, the term anaphylactoid has been widely misinterpreted to mean a reaction that was similar to anaphylaxis but less severe, and has led to the undertreatment of patients with nonimmunologic anaphylaxis. *Therefore, the term anaphylactoid is now discouraged, and the concept of nonimmunologic anaphylaxis is preferred.* Clinicians should understand that all forms of anaphylaxis are potentially life-threatening.

It is unclear how certain drugs elicit these reactions. Some affected patients have underlying dermographism and seem to have an "instability" of their mast cells, which degranulate already upon pressure or by exposure to various small molecules.

Common Culprit Drugs

Drugs that can cause nonimmunologic anaphylaxis are radiocontrast agents, opiates, NSAIDs, vancomycin, local anesthetic agents, chemotherapeutic agents, monoclonal antibodies, and other biologic therapies used in cancer therapy.

MANAGING DRUG ALLERGIES

The onset of hives within a few hours of taking a new medication is easily recognized as possible drug hypersensitivity. However, many clinical presentations of drug hypersensitivity are more complex or take place in the setting of illness and/or polypharmacotherapy. The patient in intensive care who develops a rash while receiving multiple medications, or the ambulatory patient with complex chronic diseases, who develops a new and unexplained symptom while taking many medications, illustrates two common presentations of drug allergy.

The main questions that arise in such situations include the following:

- Is the adverse event related to a drug?
- If so, which drug is responsible?
- Is the reaction due to an immune response to the drug (i.e., true drug allergy) or due to another mechanism, such as pseudoallergy?
- If the reaction is a drug allergy, what is the likely mechanism?
- How can necessary therapy for the underlying medical problem be continued?

The classification of a drug allergic reaction is important in determining appropriate diagnostic procedures, options for further treatment, and possible cross-reactivity with similar medications.

RISK FACTORS FOR DRUG ALLERGY

Risk factors for the development of drug allergy include the female sex, prior history of drug allergic reactions, recurrent drug exposure, genetic factors, and certain disease states.

Female Sex

Women are at greater risk than men for allergic reactions to some drugs, for reasons that are not well defined. Women can experience higher rates of both immediate and delayed reactions. As an example of the latter, women of childbearing age developed delayed-onset rashes to gemifloxacin (a quinolone) in 30% of administrations, compared with 3% in men.[49] Intraoperative reactions to neuromuscular blocking agents are also much more frequent in women. In contrast, neither immediate nor delayed allergic reactions to penicillins differ by gender.

Prior History of Allergic Drug Reactions

A prior history of allergic reactions to one or more drugs increases the risk of developing additional drug allergies. This is obviously true in patients with past drug reactions who are subsequently given the same or a related medication. It is also true with pseudoallergic reactions due to NSAIDs, since structurally different NSAIDs may cause similar reactions.

Multiple Drug Allergy Syndrome

The term "multiple drug allergy syndrome" has been used to describe different conditions:

- It was initially used to describe patients with past drug allergic reactions, especially immunoglobulin E (IgE)-dependent reactions, who were at increased risk for reactions to unrelated drugs.[50] One prospective study showed that patients with antibiotic sensitivity by history had a tenfold increased risk for allergic reactions to unrelated antibiotics.[51] A wide variety of clinical reactions were observed in these patients.

- Other researchers applied the term "multiple drug allergy syndrome" to patients who reacted to antibiotics and often various NSAIDs.[52] These reactions were typically urticaria or mild, transient rashes. Some of these patients had underlying chronic urticaria, which is a main differential diagnosis in patients with recurrent "rashes" after various, chemically unrelated medications. The majority of such patients are classified as having pseudoallergic reactions to NSAIDs or NSAID intolerance, but some appear to react to other drugs as well.
- Subsequently, the term "multiple drug allergy syndrome" has been used more narrowly to describe persons who had experienced well-documented immunologic drug reactions (of any Gell and Coombs type) to two or more chemically unrelated medications.[53,54] This appears to arise because of an enhanced responsiveness of the patient's T cells to pharmaceutical substances.[55,56] The implicated drugs are often antibiotics, although hypnotics, antidepressants, local anesthetics, glucocorticoids, and other drug classes were also reported. In a typical clinical scenario, a patient might initially develop drug-induced hypersensitivity syndrome/drug reaction with eosinophilia and systemic symptoms (e.g., DiHS/DRESS, a type IV reaction) to an antiepileptic drug. After this event, the patient develops additional drug allergies. The nature of subsequent reactions depends upon the structure/type of allergy normally associated with the drug in question. For example, if the same patient is later given amoxicillin, the reaction is typically an exanthema. If given phenytoin, another DiHS/DRESS reaction may ensue.

Multiple drug allergy syndrome should *not* be applied to the numerous patients who report adverse reactions to many drugs, in whom symptoms are often not typical of immunologic reactions. Rather, "multiple drug intolerance" may be a more appropriate description.

When multiple unrelated drugs elicit very similar symptoms, with immediate or slightly delayed onset, a role for conditioned responses needs to be considered. It is not immunologically plausible that structurally unrelated drugs should produce exactly the same syndrome, so when this is the history given by the patients (often with more than two drugs), classical Pavlovian conditioning is the most likely diagnosis, especially if the original reaction was frightening or traumatic in any way. Another clue to this diagnosis is a history of allergic-like symptoms to many drugs, including some that uncommonly cause true immunologic drug reactions (e.g., macrolide antibiotics, glucocorticoids, and local anesthetics).

In conclusion, multiple drug allergy syndrome should only be used to describe patients with immunologic reactions to at least two (usually more) unrelated drugs, because such patients often need special attention and management.

Recurrent Drug Exposure

Repeated courses of therapy with the same drugs or related drugs are associated with higher rates of drug allergy.[57,58] As an example, patients with cystic fibrosis who require recurrent courses of the same or related antibiotics are at increased risk for developing allergies to those drugs.

HLA Type

There is evidence for a familial propensity to develop immunologic drug reactions.[59] Data on a variety of drugs and severe drug allergies demonstrated that certain HLA-B alleles represent highly significant risk factors for severe side effects to a particular drug, and are also involved in presenting the drug to the immune system.[27,60]

- SJS/TEN caused by carbamazepine in Han Chinese patients shows a strong association with HLA-B*15:02.[61] However, HLA-B*15:02 is not increased among Han Chinese patients with milder, maculopapular drug eruptions, nor is it associated with SJS/TEN in European Caucasians.[62] Instead, European carriers of the HLA-A*31:01 allele have an increased risk of developing DiHS/DRESS.[32,63]
- SJS/TEN and possibly DiHS/DRESS caused by allopurinol also show a strong association with HLA-B*5801.[25,64]
- A severe hypersensitivity syndrome is caused by the reverse-transcriptase inhibitor abacavir and is highly associated with HLA-B*57:01 in Caucasians.[65,66] Typing of HLA-B*57:01 reduced the incidence of side effects dramatically.[67] The same allele is also implicated in flucloxacillin-induced hepatitis, but with a very low penetrance of the disease. Thus, typing is not recommended.[68]

There are now multiple instances of associations between HLA alleles (mostly class I) and hypersensitivity reactions to specific medications.[69] Some associations have a high specificity (e.g., dapsone hypersensitivity, HLA-B*13:01, and the dapsone hypersensitivity syndrome),[33] although for the majority, the odds ratio is rather low

(<10), implying that besides HLA alleles, other still unknown factors play a crucial role. The pathophysiologic mechanisms that may underlie these associations are discussed separately.

Certain Disease States

Some allergic drug reactions are much more likely to occur if the drug is administered to patients with particular underlying conditions.

- Reactions to aminopenicillins occur more commonly in patients with atypical or abnormal lymphocytes (e.g., in massive immune stimulations, such as EBV infection or leukemia).[33,70]
- Patients with acquired immunodeficiency syndrome (AIDS) have very high rates of dermatologic reactions to sulfonamides and other drugs.[21,71-74] Human immunodeficiency virus (HIV) infection may create an inflammatory milieu that enhances drug allergy.[51,75] A similar phenomenon is seen in generalized herpes virus infections. Indeed, activated, atypical lymphocytes are frequently found in circulation in persons infected with either of these viruses. Other contributing factors may include reduced hepatic glutathione levels due to polypharmacy and immunologic dysfunction associated with AIDS.[74,76,77]

  A common problem is exanthematous skin reactions in small children treated with antibiotics, in particular, penicillins. These mostly mild and transient skin reactions appear to be due to a combined effect of the drug use and various viral infections causing immune stimulation.[78] The vast majority of children will tolerate penicillins if given them again later.

Drug Metabolism

It is unclear if genetic differences in drug metabolism are a risk factor for drug allergy. Although some initial studies suggested that slow acetylation or low glutathione levels might influence the frequency of drug hypersensitivity to sulfonamides and other drugs, later studies did not confirm these theories. Therefore, typing for pharmacogenetic predisposition (e.g., cytochrome p450 polymorphism) has not yet entered clinical practice for the purposes of assessing the risk of drug allergy.

Atopy

Atopy may be defined as an inherited phenotype that includes the predisposition to develop allergen-specific IgE to inhaled or ingested allergens. Patients with atopic/allergic disorders, such as allergic asthma or food allergy, are not at increased risk for the development of drug allergy. However, atopic conditions may aggravate the clinical manifestations of IgE-mediated drug allergies. As an example, positive penicillin skin tests do not occur more frequently in atopic individuals,[79] but an atopic background is a substantial risk factor for severe and fatal penicillin anaphylaxis.[80]

Age

Age is *not* known to be an independent risk factor for drug allergy, but data are confounded by very different patterns of drug use in various age groups. Pediatric drug reactions (in particular mild exanthems) appear to be transient (i.e., not recurrent upon repeated exposure) more often than reactions that occur in adulthood.

SYSTEMATIC APPROACH TO THE PATIENTS

A systematic approach to the evaluation of putative drug allergy in patients receiving multiple medications begins with the following questions:

1. Is the presentation consistent with drug hypersensitivity? If so, what type? Are the signs and symptoms suggestive of an immunologic response (i.e., drug allergy)? Is the drug to which the patient was recently exposed known to cause such symptoms, or does it usually cause pseudoallergic reactions (e.g., NSAIDs)? The different presentations of drug allergy and pseudoallergic reactions are summarized in the table and presented separately (Table 29.3).
2. How severe is the reaction and what organ systems are involved? This can be assessed with a meticulous skin examination, followed by further evaluation of any other organ system that appears to be affected. A complete blood count and tests for liver and renal function should be obtained. This evaluation is indicated if the exanthema is substantial, bullous or pustular, confluent, involves a substantial portion of the body surface area, or if general symptoms (malaise, skin pain, lymphadenopathy) are present.
3. Which drug is responsible? This assessment can be approached in a stepwise manner:
   - Gather detailed medical history and review detailed medical records.

Table 29.3: Common examples of pseudoallergic drug reactions.

Drug	*Clinical reaction(s)*	*Presumed mechanism*
Aspirin and other NSAIDs	Exacerbations of rhinitis and asthma (in patients with aspirin-exacerbated respiratory disease) Urticaria/angioedema (Note: urticaria may also result from a Type I, IgE-mediated allergic reaction)	Inhibited prostaglandin production and enhanced leukotriene production
Opiates	Pruritus, urticaria	Direct stimulation of mast cells and/or basophils causing release of mediators
Vancomycin	Flushing during infusion	Direct stimulation of mast cells and/or basophils causing release of mediators
Radiocontrast media	Anaphylaxis, shock (Note: some may be Type I, IgE-mediated allergic reactions)	Unknown mechanism
Ciprofloxacin	Urticaria (most reactions)	Direct stimulation of mast cells and/or basophils causing release of mediators
Local anesthetics	Syncope	Vasovagal reflex
Protamine	Hypotension, pulmonary hypertension	Unknown mechanism
Choline	Pruritus, urticaria	Unknown mechanism
Isoniazid	Hepatitis	Unknown mechanism

Source: Celik G, Pichler WJ, Adkinson NF Jr. Drug Allergy. In. Adkinson NF, et al. ed. Middleton's Allergy Principles & Practice, 7th ed. Philadelphia: Mosby Elsevier, 2009:1205-26. Illustration used with permission of Elsevier Inc.

- Examine the medical record to see if temporal relationships between symptoms and the administration of specific drugs are apparent.
- For each suspect drug, consider the likelihood of its causing the type of allergic reaction in question, based on the published literature.
- Stop or substitute any/all suspect drugs with known allergic potential that demonstrate a temporal relationship with the symptoms. Observe the consequences of stopping these medications.

Assess if the Testing Possible

For reactions that are suspected to be IgE mediated, consider skin testing. Both skin and in vitro tests (if available) to identify the eliciting drug are normally done after the reaction has resolved completely.[81] In vitro tests are available for some type II, III, and IV reactions.

If there is ambiguity surrounding which drug induced an immunologic reaction and multiple drugs were stopped, plans should be made to continue the evaluation after the patient's convalescence, particularly for drugs that the individual may need in the future. Entering multiple "possible" drug allergies in the medical record will lead to confusion and is not in the patient's best interest.

Identification of the Suspect Drug

The suspect drug is identified using the patient's clinical history of present and past drug reactions and review of the medical record for temporal associations between administration and symptoms, combined with an understanding of what types of drugs cause various reactions. If available, objective tests (e.g., skin testing, in vitro testing) may also support the diagnosis.

Clinical History

The initial step involves determining all the medications to which the patient has had adverse reactions in the past. Additional history can sometimes be obtained from relatives or primary care providers. This information should be documented in the patient's permanent medical record.

The following specific questions should then be answered for each of the reported drugs in question:

- What were the symptoms and signs? What is known about the reaction?
- How long ago did the reaction take place?
- Did the patient require medical treatment or hospitalization because of the reaction?
- Why was the medication taken (indication for use)?

- The dose and route of medication taken (if known).
- Had the patient taken the medication on a previous occasion?
- Was the patient taking other concurrent medications when the reaction occurred? Were any of these newly started?
- The timing of onset of the reaction (from both the precipitating dose and the initiation of that course of therapy).
- Any treatment given and response to that treatment (including the duration of reaction)?
- Has the patient received that medication or a related medication again since the reaction? If so, were there recurrent symptoms?
- Any prior or subsequent history of exposure to other agents in that class, and presence or absence of any associated reaction(s)?

Review the Medical Record

The medical record should be reviewed if possible. In critically ill patients who cannot communicate, it may be the only available source of information.

One approach is the creation of a timeline of medication start and stop, on which the appearance and resolution of symptoms are also charted. It is important to note the onset of fever or the appearance of relevant laboratory abnormalities, such as blood eosinophilia or urine eosinophilia or hematuria.

Limitations of the Clinical History

History alone is often not sufficient for establishing current drug sensitivity. Studies performed on large series of patients with histories of drug allergy have shown that less than 20% actually react to the offending drug(s) upon direct challenge.[82,83] There are multiple reasons why a previously reactive patient may tolerate a drug upon subsequent administration:

1. The suspect drug may never have caused symptoms, but was implicated based on a temporal association. This is probably the most common reason.
2. The patient could have had a true IgE-mediated reaction in the past, but has lost sensitivity to the drug over time. Approximately 80% of patients with IgE-mediated penicillin allergy have lost the sensitivity after 10 years.
3. Biologic states required for reactivity may wane over time and render the patient less vulnerable. For example, aspirin and NSAIDs often aggravate chronic idiopathic urticaria, but are well tolerated once the urticaria remits.
4. IgE-mediated, immediate-type allergic reactions can appear with the first known encounter with a drug, even though these types of reactions require pre-existing sensitization (i.e., formation of IgE antibodies) to the drug. This most often occurs with drugs that are administered intravenously. The explanation for this phenomenon is that sensitization has occurred as a result of exposure to a different but cross-reacting compound, typically a different medication or a cosmetic. The best studied example is that of muscle relaxants (i.e., neuromuscular blocking agents), which can trigger anaphylaxis upon first exposure because patients can become sensitized to over-the-counter cough remedies (pholcodine in Europe) or cosmetics (in the United States).[14]

Another example of individuals with preformed IgE molecules reacting upon first exposure to a drug was identified in patients with anaphylaxis to cetuximab.[15] Some of these patients had antibodies against the oligosaccharide galactose alpha-1,3-galactose found in the drug and developed anaphylaxis upon intravenous administration of cetuximab. This oligosaccharide is also found in beef, pork, and lamb, and a subset of patients had experienced allergic reactions when eating these meats. Because most of the affected patients lived in the southeastern United States, it has been postulated that patients become sensitized to the oligosaccharide as a result of bites from ticks or other ectoparasites.[84]

Drugs with High Allergenic Potential

The different types of immunologic drug reactions and the categories of drugs that are most commonly implicated in each are summarized in Table 29.2.

Objective Testing

Objective testing may be appropriate for some types of allergic drug reactions. Skin testing for type I reactions is supported by extensive clinical experience, but is not standardized or validated for most drugs. The majority of in vitro tests for drug allergy are investigational. In addition, immunodiagnostic tests for drug allergy can require experience to interpret properly.

Testing for Immediate Reactions

Type I, IgE-mediated reactions typically begin within 1 hour of the first administered dose, as discussed previously.

Markers of Anaphylaxis

Elevations in tryptase (serum or plasma) may be detectable in blood samples collected within several hours of an acute allergic event, because this mediator is released by mast cells and basophils. Histamine may also be detectable, but assays are less reliable, and elevations are seen only during a very short time interval after the reaction.

Any elevation of tryptase is consistent with anaphylaxis, although normal levels do not exclude the diagnosis. Tryptase levels should be tested again after the reaction has resolved, to detect a relative increase as well as to exclude indolent mastocytosis, an important risk factor for severe anaphylaxis. Elevations are most likely to be detectable following anaphylaxis with hemodynamic changes, and if blood is collected 1–3 hours from the onset of symptoms.[85] The interpretation of tryptase in the diagnosis of anaphylaxis is not always straightforward. As an example, a tryptase level of 9 ng/mL during anaphylaxis and 3 ng/mL the following day is suggestive of anaphylaxis, even though both levels are below the upper limit of normal (i.e., 11.4 ng/mL). In this example, the serum level tripled, which may be meaningful, since personal tryptase levels are usually quite constant.

Skin Testing for Drug-specific IgE

A variety of medications can be used to perform prick and/or intradermal skin testing for the purpose of determining if the drug interacts with drug-specific IgE bound to cutaneous mast cells. This type of testing is only used to evaluate suspected type I allergic reactions. A positive wheal-and-flare response appearing within 15–20 minutes indicates the presence of drug-specific IgE on the patient's mast cells and supports the diagnosis of a type I reaction.

The clinician must first ascertain that the medication does not cause direct mast cell degranulation, as described with opioids, quinolones, and vancomycin. Medications that activate mast cells directly cannot be studied with this type of skin testing. In addition, the drug solution used for testing should not be nonspecifically irritating to the skin. Nonirritating concentrations of several antibiotics have been determined.[86]

For most drugs, the full range of metabolites and intermediate forms of the drug to which patients may become allergic have not been defined, and testing reagents are not available. Thus, just the native (unmetabolized) form of the drug is used in testing, and this may only detect a fraction of allergic patients. Penicillin is the one exception to this, and the important metabolites and metabolite/protein complexes that are required to detect allergic patients have been characterized. Penicillin skin testing is discussed in detail separately.

Despite this limitation, medications for which skin testing for immediate reactions with the native (unmetabolized) form have proven useful in identifying a subset of allergic patients, include the following:

1. Other beta-lactam antibiotics (cephalosporins and imipenem);
2. Neuromuscular blockers and dyes used to localize lymph nodes intraoperatively (i.e., patent blue, isosulfan blue, and methylene blue);
3. Carboplatin and other platin drugs;
4. Pyrazolones, such as metamizole;[87]
5. Local anesthetics;
6. Thiobarbiturates;
7. Therapeutic monoclonal antibodies, even if fully humanized, can still elicit immune reactions. The majority of reactions involve immunoglobulin G (IgG) antibodies, some neutralizing the efficacy of the therapeutic antibody. IgE-mediated reactions do occur, but are rather rare.

The results of skin testing with one of the above agents should be interpreted as follows:

- A positive result is indicative of allergy, provided nonirritating concentrations of the drug were used.
- A negative result does *not* exclude allergy, because the patient may be allergic to metabolites of the medication or metabolite/protein complexes, as explained previously.

Skin testing may be falsely negative if performed too soon after an anaphylactic reaction. For this reason, a period of 2–4 weeks should be allowed between a severe reaction and skin testing to the suspect drug. However, if skin testing is performed in this period, positive results are still valid. False-negative results can also occur in patients taking medications that blunt immediate skin responses, such as H_1 and H_2 antihistamines and tricyclic antidepressants.

In Vitro Tests

In vitro tests for immediate drug reactions are available, but these are largely considered investigational, as mentioned previously.

- Solid-phase immunoassays, such as the radioallergosorbent test (RAST) and enzyme-linked immunosorbent assay (ELISA), have been developed for a wide variety of drug-specific IgE, using sera from skin test-positive patients for standardization. These tests have been useful in research settings.[11,88,89] However, only for beta-lactam antibiotics and pyrazolone (analgesics not available in the United States), in vitro test results have been systematically compared with skin tests, with in vitro tests consistently proving less sensitive.[88,90] Many immunoassays for drug-specific IgE have been commercialized without published validation, and some of these are highly suspect since IgE-mediated reactions have never been documented.
- Flow cytometry assessing drug-induced basophil activation by means of increase in surface markers, such as CD63, has been studied in the diagnosis of immediate drug allergy.[91-98] Determination of cysteinyl leukotrienes released from blood leukocytes after drug incubation has been suggested to increase the diagnostic value of flow cytometry alone.[99] However, these tests are not yet standardized.

Testing for Delayed Reactions

A maculopapular rash appearing several days into a course of a systemic medication is the most common form of delayed-onset drug allergy.[100,101] Most of these reactions are mediated by T cells (type IV). In contrast to IgE-mediated reactions, delayed drug reactions can recur after decades, even in the absence of interim reexposure.[102]

- Type II reactions (antibody [usually IgG]-mediated cell destruction)
- Type III (immune complex deposition and complement activation)

Type IV reactions—The majority of drug reactions involve dermatitis and/or hepatitis, occasionally with systemic involvement (e.g., DiHS/DRESS). They are principally mediated by T cells and are classified as type IV reactions (*see* Table 29.2). Type IV reactions may be evaluated with various diagnostic tests, including patch testing, intradermal testing with delayed cutaneous readouts, or lymphocyte activation assays.

Patch Testing

Drugs to be used in patch testing are mixed with petrolatum or 0.9% saline, applied to a small area of skin under occlusion for 48 hours, and then removed. The site is examined 48–96 hours after placement. Concentrations of various drugs for use in patch testing have been established.[103]

Patch testing with drug preparations may be useful in evaluating patients with maculopapular exanthema, AGEP, DiHS/DRESS, and flexural exanthema. Mild systemic reactions (e.g., transiently appearing generalized exanthema) can occur even after patch (or intradermal) tests in patients with very high sensitivity (e.g., patients with DiHS/DRESS). It is only occasionally positive if the delayed-appearing skin reaction was mainly macular (no or only moderate cutaneous cell infiltration) or urticarial, or isolated hepatitis or nephritis. Patch testing to evaluate DiHS/DRESS is reviewed separately.

Patch testing to the culprit drug is less likely to be positive (9–23%) in patients with past blistering reactions, such as SJS and TEN. It is not dangerous to perform such testing, contrary to previous belief.[104,105]

Intradermal Testing with Delayed Readout

This type of testing should only be performed if a commercially available injectable form of the drug is available. The concentration used should be known to be nonirritating, and a prick test should be performed initially to assure there is no immediate response.[106] A positive result consists of erythema and induration at the site, and the site is examined at 24–48 hours after placement.[103]

Intradermal testing with delayed readout is slightly more sensitive than patch testing, but somewhat less specific.[101] It has the same indications as patch testing and may be used in evaluating exanthems, acute generalized exanthematous pustulosis, DRESS/DiHS, fixed drug eruption, and symmetrical drug-related intertriginous and flexural exanthema. It has low sensitivity for blistering skin reactions as well as for isolated macular or urticarial skin eruptions. Some patients with DRESS/DiHS may show a slight reappearance of symptoms, even if the dose was minimal.

Only a few preparations of drugs for skin testing are commercially available, so preparations are often made by individual clinicians or centers. This makes it difficult to standardize the procedure or compare results. Overall, patch and intradermal testing with delayed readout appear to have good drug-related specificity, although they can be positive even when recent drug treatment did not cause a reaction. In addition, more work is needed to increase their sensitivity.[101,107-113]

In Vitro Tests for Delayed Reactions

In vitro tests for delayed reactions include lymphocyte transformation/activation tests, upregulation of activation markers on T cells (e.g., CD69), cytokine production, and drug-induced cytotoxicity assays.[114] These tests are done in certain centers only, need to be done with a preparation of pure drug, and are still considered research tools. If available, such tests may help in diagnosis, as they can be positive when skin tests are negative. Their specificity for most drug classes seems to be very good (mostly >95%), but the sensitivity needs to be improved.[111]

Where available, in vitro testing may be useful in evaluating patients with maculopapular exanthema, acute-generalized exanthematous pustulosis, DiHS/DRESS, and flexural exanthema. The sensitivity of tests based on cell expansion, cell activation, or cytokine release is high in DiHS/DRESS, but low in blistering reactions. The role of tests evaluating drug-induced cytotoxic reactions needs to be further evaluated, and may be particularly interesting for bullous skin reactions,[115] as well as for isolated drug-induced hepatitis or nephritis, where skin tests are often negative.

GRADED CHALLENGE

Graded challenge (also called drug provocation testing) involves administering a medication to a patient in a graduated manner under close observation. It is based on the principle that a certain amount of the medication is needed to elicit symptoms.

Indications

Graded challenge is used to exclude allergy to the medication in question and is most appropriate for a patient who is *unlikely to be allergic* to that drug. Graded challenge should *not* be performed in a patient with a positive response in a prior drug allergy test (skin or in vitro).

Graded challenge does *not* modify the allergic response to the drug or prevent recurrent reactions. Therefore,

1. Patients who tolerate a drug upon graded challenge prove that they are not allergic to the drug given at the dose used.
2. A challenge procedure in a patient with a suspected IgE-mediated drug allergy could potentially induce anaphylaxis and should be performed by an allergy expert in a setting equipped to manage possible reactions.

Contraindications

Graded challenge to the suspect drug is contraindicated in patients with the following types of reactions:

- Blistering dermatitis (e.g., SJS, TEN);
- Sloughing of the skin;
- Severe generalized hypersensitivity reactions involving internal organs (DiHS/DRESS);
- Milder dermatoses with mucous membrane lesions (e.g., erythema multiforme).

Even minute amounts of the suspect drug can reactivate these reactions, and the response can then escalate even though no further drug is given.[116]

Inclusion of Placebo Doses

Inclusion of a placebo is strongly recommended to exclude false-positive reactions in patients with anxiety or other subjective reactions. Some patients experience unintentional anticipatory reactions (classic conditioning), particularly following a true allergic reaction or a frightening experience in association with drug treatment. These can often be elicited by placebo doses, thus reassuring the clinician and patient alike that the response is not due to the drug in question.

Challenge Protocols

The pace of the challenge and the degree of caution exercised depend upon the likelihood that the patient may be allergic, the patient's medical stability, and the clinician's experience and the level of comfort with the procedure.

Other considerations include:

1. Patients should *not* be premedicated with antihistamines or glucocorticoids because these agents may mask early signs of an allergic reaction.
2. Beta blockers taken for control of hypertension should be withheld for 24 hours before challenge, as these agents can interfere with the treatment of anaphylaxis with epinephrine, should that be not necessary. In contrast, beta blockers that are taken to control arrhythmias should not be withheld without consulting a cardiologist.

3. Patients with asthma, chronic obstructive lung disease, or other pulmonary diseases should have their pulmonary symptoms optimally controlled prior to undergoing the challenge.

For Immediate Reactions

If the previous reaction occurred less than 1 hour after drug administration and there is concern about a possible IgE-dependent reaction, then the challenge should be performed by an allergy expert and in a setting equipped to treat anaphylaxis.

1. The starting challenge dose should be low, typically between 1/10,000 and 1/1,000 of the therapeutic dose, depending on the severity of the past reaction. Using this strategy, any symptoms that are elicited should be mild.
2. The oral route is preferred when possible, since oral administration is generally associated with less severe symptoms compared with intravenous administration.
3. Tenfold increasing doses are administered every 30–60 minutes until the full therapeutic dose is reached. If subjective symptoms appear, the clinician can proceed more slowly by using threefold increases for one or two steps. Once the full therapeutic dose has been achieved without incident, continuous therapy should be begun immediately with appropriate monitoring.

For Delayed Reactions

Challenge schemes for simple delayed exanthema to drugs are usually performed either in the context of research (to document sensitivity) or at a time that the patient actively needs the drug. In the latter situation, the drug may be slowly increased, and the patient is instructed to contact the clinician immediately if any adverse events are noted.

For delayed or nonimmediate types of reactions, challenge procedures are less standardized and are based on the time course of the patient's reaction and the pharmacology of the drug involved.[116] The optimal approach is not known, and experts have differences in practice. In general, the time between doses should be long enough that delayed symptoms have time to develop before the next higher dose is administered. Some protocols may take days or even weeks.

An example of a challenge procedure for delayed reactions to cephalosporins involved administering doses at weekly intervals, starting with 1/100 of a usual dose on day 0, 1/10 of a dose on day 7, and a standard dose on day 14.[117] However, other studies have documented that some delayed reactions only develop after several days at a full therapeutic dose or in the presence of a concomitant viral infection.[118,119] Thus, there may be certain drug reactions that cannot be easily elicited with any challenge protocol.[120]

Negative Predictive Value of Challenge Procedures

If a patient tolerates a drug challenge, it is highly unlikely, but not impossible, that the drug will cause symptoms if taken again in the future. A small number of studies have examined the negative predictive value of challenges for immediate and delayed reactions. One study examined the negative predictive value of drug challenges in 203 children.[121] Of these, 163 of the children underwent allergy evaluation for immediate or delayed reactions. All were labeled as "not allergic to the drug" based on 175 negative drug challenges, consisting of one full dose of the drug. Re-evaluation after at least a 3-month interval showed that 91 (52%) of the 175 tested drugs were reported to have been used again: 65 children took the same antibiotic, 20 took the same NSAID, and 6 took other drugs. An immediate reaction was reported in 5 (5.5%) of these (four antibiotics, one NSAID). One patient developed an anaphylactic reaction and was skin test-positive upon repeat testing, suggesting either resensitization from the challenge or an error in the original skin testing. The remaining false-negative challenges were delayed reactions.

Other studies have described similar findings. Recurrent reactions in spite of negative prior challenges were reported in 7.6% of 118 adults re-exposed to the same beta-lactam antibiotics. All reactions were nonimmediate, and none was severe.[122]

Such studies demonstrate that single-dose challenge procedures have higher negative predictive values for immediate reactions than for delayed-onset reactions. Challenges may rarely result in resensitization, and thus a prior negative challenge is *not a guarantee* that the drug will be tolerated, especially regarding delayed reactions. In addition, patients with a recent anaphylactic drug reaction, even if allergy testing and challenge are negative, should be retreated only under medical surveillance.

OPTIONS FOR FUTURE TREATMENT

There are three options for future treatment in patients with a confirmed drug allergy:

- Administration of an unrelated medication.
- Careful administration of a related medication.
- Desensitization to the culprit drug.

Administration of an Unrelated Medication

The most straightforward option is administration of an unrelated medication that is safe and effective for the disorder in question. However, second-line therapies may confer their own risks, such as toxicities and higher costs.

Penicillin allergy illustrates the issues involved. Patients labeled penicillin allergic often receive non-beta-lactam antibiotics, which can be more expensive, associated with side effects, and in some cases, less efficacious.[123-126] Specifically, patients carrying the diagnosis of penicillin allergy are more likely to be treated with vancomycin or quinolones.[123,127-138] The use of these broad-spectrum antibiotics contributes to the development and spread of drug-resistant bacteria.[132-134] One study assessed various risk factors for the development of vancomycin-resistant *Enterococcus* (VRE) in a medical intensive care unit (MICU).[135] Among pre-MICU treatment with various classes of antibiotics, quinolones had the strongest association with subsequent development of VRE (odds ratio = 8.6), whereas treatment with penicillins/beta-lactamase inhibitors was not associated with developing VRE.[135] Some broad-spectrum antibiotics are also associated with *Clostridium difficile* infection. Thus, the use of alternative, unrelated medications is not without risk.

Administration of a Related Medication

The second alternative for drug-allergic patients is to receive a medication similar, but not identical to the offending drug.

The likelihood of cross-reactivity among similar drugs is partly dependent on the type of allergic reaction in question. As an example, a patient with a T-cell-mediated exanthema to amoxicillin is at low risk for reacting to a cephalosporin, whereas a patient with IgE-mediated anaphylaxis to amoxicillin is at some increased risk if given a cephalosporin. The related medication may be one for which skin testing is informative, or it can be initially given via graded challenge.

Desensitization to the Culprit Drug

The third option is desensitization to the culprit drug. Classical desensitization is predictably successful for type I, IgE-mediated allergy, although gradual dose escalation may be attempted with variable success to several other types of immunologic and nonimmunologic drug reactions.

Antibiotic desensitizations have been performed since the 1940s, initially with gradually increasing doses of penicillin concomitant with antihistamine and epinephrine injections.[136] However, it was not until the early 1980s when a safer desensitization protocol was developed by Sullivan et al., and most antibiotic desensitization protocols are quite similar to this (Table 29.4).[137] Oral desensitizations should be performed whenever possible, even before the parenteral use of the same antibiotic. The basic principle of an antibiotic desensitization is to start with about double the dose used to produce the positive skin test result that confirmed the presence of clinically significant amounts of antibiotic-specific IgE. This is generally about 1/10,000th of the final therapeutic dose, with doubling doses every 15 minutes. If a reaction occurs during the desensitization, treat the reaction, stabilize the patient, then repeat the dose that was last tolerated, and complete the desensitization. Desensitizations can be done even in pregnant patients.[138] Castells has developed a protocol using three different dilutions of a parenteral antibiotic starting with a 1:100 dilution, then a 1:10 dilution, and then the full concentration with advances in dosing made by increasing the rate of infusion[139] (Table 29.5). Adverse reactions to antibiotic drug desensitizations are generally less frequent, and no more severe, than to other desensitizations. They can be safely performed in an outpatient setting that routinely performs oral food challenges. Individuals performing antibiotic desensitizations need to be well trained and comfortable in the management of acute anaphylaxis. In one of the early studies by Sullivan et al. using oral penicillin desensitizations, about 30% had delayed-onset reactions, none had immediate or anaphylactic reactions.[137] Desensitization should be attempted only in the setting of well-documented IgE-mediated antibiotic allergy. Desensitizations are not clearly effective for T-cell-mediated reactions, such as benign delayed-onset rashes, and are contraindicated for more serious T-cell-mediated reactions.[123] Desensitizations are not possible for other nonimmunologically mediated reactions.[140]

It is critical to have continual exposure to the antibiotic after desensitization until the therapeutic course is completed. If more than five half-lives of the antibiotic expire without further dosing, then it will be necessary to repeat the desensitization. In certain settings, reactions can be noted with delayed redosing after as little as two half-lives, but reactions are also common in desensitized individuals even with continual dosing. In the setting of long-acting benzathine penicillin used for syphilis

Table 29.4: Penicillin oral desensitization protocol.

Step	*Penicillin V (units/mL)*	*Dose (mL)*	*Dose (units)*	*Cumulative dose*
1	1,000	0.1	100	100
2	1,000	0.2	200	300
3	1,000	0.4	400	700
4	1,000	0.8	800	1,500
5	1,000	1.6	1,600	3,100
6	1,000	3.2	3,200	6,300
7	1,000	6.4	6,400	12,700
8	10,000	1.2	12,000	24,700
9	10,000	2.4	24,000	48,700
10	10,000	4.8	48,000	96,700
11	80,000	1.0	80,000	176,000
12	80,000	2.0	160,000	336,700
13	80,000	4.0	320,000	656,700
14	80,000	8.0	640,000	1,296,700

Administer penicillin V orally every 15 minutes per step. Each dose can be diluted in 30 mL water for patient to ingest. Total time: 3 hours 45 minutes.

Table 29.5: Intravenous drug desensitization protocol.

Preparation of solutions

		Volume of diluent (e.g., 0.9% sodium chloride) (mL)		*Total amount to be injected in each solution (mg)*	*Final concentration (mg/mL)*
Solution 1		250		10	0.04
Solution 2		250		100	0.4
Solution 3		250		1000	4

Drug desensitization protocol

Step	*Solution*	*Rate (mL/h)*	*Time (min)*	*Administered dose (mg)*	*Cumulative dose (mg)*
1	1	2	15	0.02	0.02
2	1	5	15	0.05	0.07
3	1	10	15	0.1	0.17
4	1	20	15	0.2	0.37
5	2	5	15	0.5	0.87
6	2	10	15	1	1.9
7	2	20	15	2	3.9
8	2	40	15	4	7.9
9	3	10	15	10	18
10	3	20	15	20	38
11	3	40	15	40	78
12	3	80	15	80	158
13	3	160	15	160	318
14	3	320	15	320	638
15	3	640	9	362	1000

Total time = 219 minutes.

Full dose = 1000 mg.

therapy, patients appear to be capable of maintaining a desensitized state for as long as 3 weeks, and repeat desensitization is typically not needed.[137]

LONG-TERM MANAGEMENT OF PATIENTS PRONE TO DRUG ALLERGY

Once a drug allergy has been identified, the affected patient should be educated about avoidance and provided with a written list of the generic and brand names of the culprit drug, as well as possibly cross-reactive drugs. Patients with potentially severe reactions should carry wallet cards, wear identification jewelry, or register with a drug allergy information service.

As discussed previously, some individuals are vulnerable to allergic drug reactions as a result of genetic or metabolic abnormalities (e.g., multiple drug allergy syndrome), frequent and recurrent drug exposure (e.g., antibiotics in cystic fibrosis), or certain disease states related to immune dysfunction (e.g., HIV infection). In a drug allergy-prone population, pharmacotherapy requires special management to avoid adverse events and to prevent (to the degree possible) sensitization or resensitization.

Limit Antibiotic Use

Efforts should be made to limit unnecessary exposure to antibiotics. These include the diagnosis and treatment of underlying conditions that predispose to infections. As examples, rhinitis and asthma should be aggressively treated with glucocorticoid nasal sprays and inhalers to minimize sinopulmonary infections, and diabetes mellitus should be tightly controlled. Less commonly, undiagnosed immunodeficiency is present.

Age-appropriate Vaccinations

Should be administered and repeated at the recommended intervals. Avoidance of unnecessary exposures to contagious diseases may be helpful, especially in children and patients with immunodeficiency.

Proactive efforts to obtain culture data before initiating antibiotics can help to limit cumulative antibiotic exposure by avoiding treatment of viral infections and minimizing mid-treatment changes in antibiotic regimens. Enlisting the cooperation of the patient's other providers is important.

Consideration should be given to treating through mild cutaneous reactions, such as itching or mild rashes, especially early in therapy when an alternative antibiotic will usually be required. It is possible in delayed-onset exanthema. This is typically considered when alternative treatments are problematic, and an allergy specialist considers continued exposure to the drug to be of low risk. Ongoing vigilance for clinical and laboratory danger signs is necessary, and concomitant use of glucocorticoids (prednisone 0.5 mg/kg) may be required if the exanthem intensifies rather than improves.

Approach to Initiating New Drugs

In drug allergy-prone patients, new drugs should be started at lower than normal doses when feasible. Administration under medical observation is sometimes necessary.

Patients with past SJS/TEN and DRESS/DiHS should be taught about the earliest symptoms of these reactions, such as fever or mucosal irritation, and should know to stop medications immediately should these appear.

Many patients with prior DRESS/DiHS experience a period of drug intolerance during the weeks after the initial reaction, meaning that any new drug may exacerbate symptoms (exanthems, hepatitis), often without proof of a new sensitization. The symptoms may lead to the suspicion of a new drug allergy and further limit treatment. However, when the immune system is less activated (documented by circulating activated lymphocytes), the new drugs are again tolerated. This phenomenon has been termed a "flare-up" reaction.[141] However, some patients with prior DiHS/DRESS do develop genuine sensitizations to new compounds, and some develop multiple drug hypersensitivity.[141]

Patients with past IgE-mediated reactions to drugs should not be given premedications before gradual dose escalation of new drugs. Neither antihistamines nor glucocorticoids can prevent IgE-mediated anaphylaxis, and premedications may mask early symptoms and allow dosing to proceed more rapidly than advisable.

In contrast to the above scenarios, patients who have reacted with uncomplicated exanthemas, including mild urticaria, to a variety of different drugs may benefit from administration of an antihistamine when new drugs are initiated.

SUMMARY

Risk factors for developing drug allergies include past drug allergy, genetic factors, recurrent drug exposure, and certain diseases (e.g., HIV/AIDS). Individuals with two or more immunologic drug reactions to chemically unrelated medications are said to have "multiple drug allergy syndrome." Patients who develop signs/symptoms of drug allergy while receiving multiple medications simultaneously are best approached in a systematic manner. Evaluation involves a meticulous history of past and present drug reactions, additional information gathering from the medical record, and analysis of temporal patterns between drug administration and onset of symptoms. Once this information has been assembled, it is combined with knowledge about the types of allergic reactions most often caused by various classes of drugs, to identify potential culprit agents. Overall, objective testing for the diagnosis of drug allergy is limited. Skin testing is helpful for some medications that cause type I, immediate hypersensitivity reactions, although skin testing has been fully validated only for penicillin. In some cases, types II, III, and IV reactions can be evaluated with in vitro studies, although the majority of these tests are still investigational. Allergy to a drug can be excluded by performing a graded challenge. Graded challenge does *not* modify the allergic response to the drug or prevent recurrent reactions. Thus, challenges must be performed with caution and in a monitored setting, and patients who tolerate drug challenges prove that they are not allergic to that medication. There are three options for future treatment in patients with a confirmed drug allergy: administration of an unrelated medication, careful administration of a related medication, and desensitization to the culprit drug.

REFERENCES

1. Muszkat M. Interethnic differences in drug response: the contribution of genetic variability in beta adrenergic receptor and cytochrome P4502C9. Clin Pharmacol Ther. 2007;82:215.
2. Lennard L. Implementation of TPMT testing. Br J Clin Pharmacol. 2014;77:704.
3. Dern RJ, Beutler E, Alving AS. The hemolytic effect of primaquine V. Primaquine sensitivity as a manifestation of a multiple drug sensitivity. J Lab Clin Med. 1981;97:750.
4. Lennard L, Van Loon JA, Weinshilboum RM. Pharmacogenetics of acute azathioprine toxicity: relationship to thiopurine methyltransferase genetic polymorphism. Clin Pharmacol Ther. 1989;46:149.
5. Lazarou J, Pomeranz BH, Corey PN. Incidence of adverse drug reactions in hospitalized patients: a meta-analysis of prospective studies. JAMA. 1998;279:1200.
6. Pichler WJ. Delayed drug hypersensitivity reactions. Ann Intern Med. 2003;139:683.
7. Johansson SG, Bieber T, Dahl R, et al. Revised nomenclature for allergy for global use: Report of the Nomenclature Review Committee of the World Allergy Organization, October 2003. J Allergy Clin Immunol. 2004;113:832.
8. Ben m'rad M, Leclerc-Mercier S, Blanche P, et al. Drug-induced hypersensitivity syndrome: clinical and biologic disease patterns in 24 patients. Medicine (Baltimore). 2009;88:131.
9. Sachs B, Riegel S, Seebeck J, et al. Fluoroquinolone-associated anaphylaxis in spontaneous adverse drug reaction reports in Germany: differences in reporting rates between individual fluoroquinolones and occurrence after first-ever use. Drug Saf. 2006;29:1087.
10. Manfredi M, Severino M, Testi S, et al. Detection of specific IgE to quinolones. J Allergy Clin Immunol. 2004;113:155.
11. Schmid DA, Campi P, Pichler WJ. Hypersensitivity reactions to quinolones. Curr Pharm Des. 2006;12:3313.
12. Johansson SG, Florvaag E, Oman H, et al. National pholcodine consumption and prevalence of IgE-sensitization: a multicentre study. Allergy. 2010;65:498.
13. Birnbaum J, Vervloet D. Allergy to muscle relaxants. Clin Rev Allergy. 1991;9:281.
14. Florvaag E, Johansson SG. The pholcodine story. Immunol Allergy Clin North Am. 2009;29:419.
15. Chung CH, Mirakhur B, Chan E, et al. Cetuximab-induced anaphylaxis and IgE specific for galactose-alpha-1,3-galactose. N Engl J Med. 2008;358:1109.
16. Froehlich H, Verma R. Arthus reaction to recombinant hepatitis B virus vaccine. Clin Infect Dis. 2001;33:906.
17. Relyveld EH, Bizzini B, Gupta RK. Rational approaches to reduce adverse reactions in man to vaccines containing tetanus and diphtheria toxoids. Vaccine. 1998;16:1016.
18. Siegrist CA. Mechanisms underlying adverse reactions to vaccines. J Comp Pathol. 2007;137:S46.
19. Pichler WJ. Pharmacological interaction of drugs with antigen-specific immune receptors: the p-i concept. Curr Opin Allergy Clin Immunol. 2002;2:301.
20. Clark RA, Chong B, Mirchandani N, et al. The vast majority of CLA+ T cells are resident in normal skin. J Immunol. 2006;176:4431.
21. Schaerli P, Ebert L, Willimann K, et al. A skin-selective homing mechanism for human immune surveillance T cells. J Exp Med. 2004;199:1265.
22. Storrs FJ. Contact dermatitis caused by drugs. Immunol Allergy Clin North Am. 1991;11:509.
23. Pleasants RA, Walker TR, Samuelson WM. Allergic reactions to parenteral beta-lactam antibiotics in patients with cystic fibrosis. Chest. 1994;106:1124.
24. Illing PT, Vivian JP, Dudek NL, et al. Immune self-reactivity triggered by drug-modified HLA-peptide repertoire. Nature. 2012;486:554.
25. Hung SI, Chung WH, Liou LB, et al. HLA-B*5801 allele as a genetic marker for severe cutaneous adverse reactions caused by allopurinol. Proc Natl Acad Sci USA. 2005;102:4134.
26. Lonjou C, Borot N, Sekula P, et al. A European study of HLA-B in Stevens-Johnson syndrome and toxic epidermal necrolysis related to five high-risk drugs. Pharmacogenet Genomics. 2008;18:99.

27. Chung WH, Hung SI, Hong HS, et al. Medical genetics: a marker for Stevens-Johnson syndrome. Nature. 2004;428:486.
28. Ding WY, Lee CK, Choon SE. Cutaneous adverse drug reactions seen in a tertiary hospital in Johor, Malaysia. Int J Dermatol. 2010;49:834.
29. Locharernkul C, Loplumlert J, Limotai C, et al. Carbamazepine and phenytoin induced Stevens-Johnson syndrome is associated with HLA-B*1502 allele in Thai population. Epilepsia. 2008;49:2087.
30. Mehta TY, Prajapati LM, Mittal B, et al. Association of HLA-B*1502 allele and carbamazepine-induced Stevens-Johnson syndrome among Indians. Indian J Dermatol Venereol Leprol. 2009;75:579.
31. Ozeki T, Mushiroda T, Yowang A, et al. Genome-wide association study identifies HLA-A*3101 allele as a genetic risk factor for carbamazepine-induced cutaneous adverse drug reactions in Japanese population. Hum Mol Genet. 2011;20:1034.
32. McCormack M, Alfirevic A, Bourgeois S, et al. HLA-A*3101 and carbamazepine-induced hypersensitivity reactions in Europeans. N Engl J Med. 2011;364:1134.
33. Zhang FR, Liu H, Irwanto A, et al. HLA-B*13:01 and the dapsone hypersensitivity syndrome. N Engl J Med. 2013;369:1620.
34. Hershfield MS, Callaghan JT, Tassaneeyakul W, et al. Clinical pharmacogenetics implementation consortium guidelines for human leukocyte antigen-B genotype and allopurinol dosing. Clin Pharmacol Ther. 2013;93:153.
35. Spanou Z, Keller M, Britschgi M, et al. Involvement of drug-specific T cells in acute drug-induced interstitial nephritis. J Am Soc Nephrol. 2006;17:2919.
36. Klemola E. Hypersensitivity reactions to ampicillin in cytomegalovirus mononucleosis. Scand J Infect Dis. 1970;2:29.
37. Caubet JC, Kaiser L, Lemaître B, et al. The role of penicillin in benign skin rashes in childhood: a prospective study based on drug rechallenge. J Allergy Clin Immunol. 2011;127:218.
38. Stamp LK, Taylor WJ, Jones PB, et al. Starting dose is a risk factor for allopurinol hypersensitivity syndrome: a proposed safe starting dose of allopurinol. Arthritis Rheum. 2012;64:2529.
39. Yun J, Mattsson J, Schnyder K, et al. Allopurinol hypersensitivity is primarily mediated by dose-dependent oxypurinol-specific T cell response. Clin Exp Allergy. 2013;43:1246.
40. Messenheimer JA, Giorgi L, Risner ME. The tolerability of lamotrigine in children. Drug Saf. 2000;22:303.
41. Uetrecht J. Current trends in drug-induced autoimmunity. Autoimmun Rev. 2005;4:309.
42. Vergne P, Bertin P, Bonnet C, et al. Drug-induced rheumatic disorders: incidence, prevention and management. Drug Saf. 2000;23:279.
43. Gait RC, Affleck AG, Leach IH, Varma S. Perinuclear antineutrophilic cytoplasmic antibody-positive polyarteritis nodosa secondary to minocycline treatment for acne vulgaris. J Am Acad Dermatol. 2008;58:S123.
44. Li GC, Greenberg CS, Currie MS. Procainamide-induced lupus anticoagulants and thrombosis. South Med J. 1988;81:262.
45. Sheikhzadeh A, Schäfer U, Schnabel A. Drug-induced lupus erythematosus by amiodarone. Arch Intern Med. 2002;162:834.
46. Ozkaya E. Fixed drug eruption: state of the art. J Dtsch Dermatol Ges. 2008;6:181.
47. Mizukawa Y, Shiohara T. Fixed drug eruption: a prototypic disorder mediated by effector memory T cells. Curr Allergy Asthma Rep. 2009;9:71.
48. Shiohara T, Mizukawa Y. Fixed drug eruption: a disease mediated by self-inflicted responses of intraepidermal T cells. Eur J Dermatol. 2007;17:201.
49. Demoly P, Viola M, Rebelo Gomes E, Romano A. Epidemiology and causes of drug hypersensitivity. In: Pichler WJ, ed. Drug Hypersensitivity, Switzerland: Karger Basel, 2007:2.
50. Sullivan TJ, Remedios C, Ong MD, Gilliam LK. Studies of the multiple drug allergy syndrome. J Allergy Clin Immunol. 1989;83:270.
51. Moseley EK, Sullivan TJ. Allergic reactions to antimicrobial drugs in patients with a history of prior drug allergy. J Allergy Clin Immunol. 1991;87:226 (Abstract).
52. Asero R, Tedeschi A, Lorini M, et al. Sera from patients with multiple drug allergy syndrome contain circulating histamine-releasing factors. Int Arch Allergy Immunol. 2003;131:195.
53. Sullivan TJ. Management of patients allergic to antimicrobial drugs. Allergy Proc. 1991;12:361.
54. Kamada MM, Twarog F, Leung DY. Multiple antibiotic sensitivity in a pediatric population. Allergy Proc. 1991;12:347.
55. Gex-Collet C, Helbling A, Pichler WJ. Multiple drug hypersensitivity—proof of multiple drug hypersensitivity by patch and lymphocyte transformation tests. J Investig Allergol Clin Immunol. 2005;15:293.
56. Daubner B, Groux-Keller M, Hausmann OV, et al. Multiple drug hypersensitivity: normal Treg cell function but enhanced in vivo activation of drug-specific T cells. Allergy. 2012;67:58.
57. Moss RB, Babin S, Hsu YP, et al. Allergy to semisynthetic penicillins in cystic fibrosis. J Pediatr. 1984;104:460.
58. Avila PC, Kishiyama JL. Allergic manifestations in AIDS. Clin Rev Allergy Immunol. 1996-1997;14:433.
59. Kurtz KM, Beatty TL, Adkinson NF Jr. Evidence for familial aggregation of immunologic drug reactions. J Allergy Clin Immunol. 2000;105:184.
60. Chung WH, Hung SI, Chen YT. Human leukocyte antigens and drug hypersensitivity. Curr Opin Allergy Clin Immunol. 2007;7:317.
61. Chessman D, Kostenko L, Lethborg T, et al. Human leukocyte antigen class I-restricted activation of CD8+ T cells provides the immunogenetic basis of a systemic drug hypersensitivity. Immunity. 2008;28:822.
62. Wu Y, Farrell J, Pirmohamed M, et al. Generation and characterization of antigen-specific CD4+, CD8+, and

CD4+CD8+ T-cell clones from patients with carbamazepine hypersensitivity. J Allergy Clin Immunol. 2007;119:973.

63. Genin E, Chen DP, Hung SI, et al. HLA-A*31:01 and different types of carbamazepine-induced severe cutaneous adverse reactions: an international study and meta-analysis. Pharmacogenomics J. 2014;14:281.
64. Yun J, Marcaida MJ, Eriksson KK, et al. Oxypurinol directly and immediately activates the drug-specific T cells via the preferential use of HLA-B*58:01. J Immunol. 2014;192: 2984.
65. Mallal S, Nolan D, Witt C, et al. Association between presence of HLA-B*5701, HLA-DR7, and HLA-DQ3 and hypersensitivity to HIV-1 reverse-transcriptase inhibitor abacavir. Lancet. 2002;359:727.
66. Mallal S, Phillips E, Carosi G, et al. HLA-B*5701 screening for hypersensitivity to abacavir. N Engl J Med. 2008; 358:568.
67. Phillips E, Mallal S. Successful translation of pharmacogenetics into the clinic: the abacavir example. Mol Diagn Ther. 2009;13:1.
68. Daly AK, Donaldson PT, Bhatnagar P, et al. HLA-B*5701 genotype is a major determinant of drug-induced liver injury due to flucloxacillin. Nat Genet. 2009;41:816.
69. Pompeu YA, Stewart JD, Mallal S, et al. The structural basis of HLA-associated drug hypersensitivity syndromes. Immunol Rev. 2012;250:158.
70. Cameron SJ, Richmond J. Ampicillin hypersensitivity in lymphatic leukaemia. Scott Med J. 1971;16:425.
71. Kerns D, Shira JE, Go S, et al. Ampicillin rash in children. Relationship to penicillin allergy and infectious mononucleosis. Am J Dis Child. 1973;125:187.
72. Carr A, Swanson C, Penny R, Cooper DA. Clinical and laboratory markers of hypersensitivity to trimethoprim-sulfamethoxazole in patients with Pneumocystis carinii pneumonia and AIDS. J Infect Dis. 1993;167:180.
73. Daftarian MP, Filion LG, Cameron W, et al. Immune response to sulfamethoxazole in patients with AIDS. Clin Diagn Lab Immunol. 1995;2:199.
74. Rose EW, McCloskey WW. Glutathione in hypersensitivity to trimethoprim/sulfamethoxazole in patients with HIV infection. Ann Pharmacother. 1998;32:381.
75. Lanctôt KL, Ghajar BM, Shear NH, Naranjo CA. Improving the diagnosis of hypersensitivity reactions associated with sulfonamides. J Clin Pharmacol. 1994;34:1228.
76. Uetrecht JP. New concepts in immunology relevant to idiosyncratic drug reactions: the "danger hypothesis" and innate immune system. Chem Res Toxicol. 1999;12:387.
77. Idée JM, Pinès E, Prigent P, Corot C. Allergy-like reactions to iodinated contrast agents. A critical analysis. Fundam Clin Pharmacol. 2005;19:263.
78. Caubet JC, Kaiser L, Lemaître B, et al. The role of penicillin in benign skin rashes in childhood: a prospective study based on drug rechallenge. J Allergy Clin Immunol. 2011;127:218.
79. Adkinson NF Jr. Risk factors for drug allergy. J Allergy Clin Immunol. 1984;74:567.
80. Idsoe O, Guthe T, Willcox RR, de Weck AL. Nature and extent of penicillin side-reactions, with particular reference to fatalities from anaphylactic shock. Bull World Health Organ. 1968;38:159.
81. Kano Y, Hirahara K, Mitsuyama Y, et al. Utility of the lymphocyte transformation test in the diagnosis of drug sensitivity: dependence on its timing and the type of drug eruption. Allergy. 2007;62:1439.
82. Messaad D, Sahla H, Benahmed S, et al. Drug provocation tests in patients with a history suggesting an immediate drug hypersensitivity reaction. Ann Intern Med. 2004;140:1001.
83. Aberer W, Bircher A, Romano A, et al. Drug provocation testing in the diagnosis of drug hypersensitivity reactions: general considerations. Allergy. 2003;58:854.
84. Commins SP, Satinover SM, Hosen J, et al. Delayed anaphylaxis, angioedema, or urticaria after consumption of red meat in patients with IgE antibodies specific for galactose-alpha-1,3-galactose. J Allergy Clin Immunol. 2009;123:426.
85. Schwartz LB, Metcalfe DD, Miller JS, et al. Tryptase levels as an indicator of mast-cell activation in systemic anaphylaxis and mastocytosis. N Engl J Med. 1987;316:1622.
86. Empedrad R, Darter AL, Earl HS, Gruchalla RS. Nonirritating intradermal skin test concentrations for commonly prescribed antibiotics. J Allergy Clin Immunol. 2003;112:629.
87. Himly M, Jahn-Schmid B, Pittertschatscher K, et al. IgE-mediated immediate-type hypersensitivity to the pyrazolone drug propyphenazone. J Allergy Clin Immunol. 2003;111:882.
88. Adkinson NF Jr. Tests for immunological reactions to drugs and occupational allergens. In: Rose NR, Conway de Macario E, Folds JD, et al. eds. Manual of Clinical Laboratory Immunology. Washington, DC: American Society of Microbiology, 1997:893.
89. Manfredi M, Severino M, Testi S, et al. Detection of specific IgE to quinolones. J Allergy Clin Immunol. 2004;113:155.
90. Fontaine C, Mayorga C, Bousquet PJ, et al. Relevance of the determination of serum-specific IgE antibodies in the diagnosis of immediate beta-lactam allergy. Allergy. 2007;62:47.
91. Kleine-Tebbe J, Erdmann S, Knol EF, et al. Diagnostic tests based on human basophils: potentials, pitfalls and perspectives. Int Arch Allergy Immunol. 2006;141:79.
92. Ebo DG, Sainte-Laudy J, Bridts CH, et al. Flow-assisted allergy diagnosis: current applications and future perspectives. Allergy. 2006;61:1028.
93. Kvedariene V, Kamey S, Ryckwaert Y, et al. Diagnosis of neuromuscular blocking agent hypersensitivity reactions using cytofluorimetric analysis of basophils. Allergy. 2006;61:311.
94. Ebo DG, Bridts CH, Hagendorens MM, et al. Flow-assisted diagnostic management of anaphylaxis from rocuronium bromide. Allergy. 2006;61:935.
95. Sanz ML, Gamboa PM, Antépara I, et al. Flow cytometric basophil activation test by detection of CD63 expression

in patients with immediate-type reactions to betalactam antibiotics. Clin Exp Allergy. 2002;32:277.

96. Gamboa P, Sanz ML, Caballero MR, et al. The flow-cytometric determination of basophil activation induced by aspirin and other non-steroidal anti-inflammatory drugs (NSAIDs) is useful for in vitro diagnosis of the NSAID hypersensitivity syndrome. Clin Exp Allergy. 2004; 34:1448.
97. Gamboa PM, Sanz ML, Caballero MR, et al. Use of CD63 expression as a marker of in vitro basophil activation and leukotriene determination in metamizole allergic patients. Allergy. 2003;58:312.
98. Malbrán A, Yeyati E, Rey GL, Galassi N. Diclofenac induces basophil degranulation without increasing CD63 expression in sensitive patients. Clin Exp Immunol. 2007;147:99.
99. Sanz ML, Gamboa P, de Weck AL. A new combined test with flow cytometric basophil activation and determination of sulfidoleukotrienes is useful for in vitro diagnosis of hypersensitivity to aspirin and other nonsteroidal anti-inflammatory drugs. Int Arch Allergy Immunol. 2005; 136:58.
100. Yawalkar N, Pichler WJ. Immunohistology of drug-induced exanthema: clues to pathogenesis. Curr Opin Allergy Clin Immunol. 2001;1:299.
101. Romano A, Blanca M, Torres MJ, et al. Diagnosis of nonimmediate reactions to beta-lactam antibiotics. Allergy. 2004;59:1153.
102. Beeler A, Engler O, Gerber BO, Pichler WJ. Long-lasting reactivity and high frequency of drug-specific T cells after severe systemic drug hypersensitivity reactions. J Allergy Clin Immunol. 2006;117:455.
103. Barbaud A. Skin testing in delayed reactions to drugs. Immunol Allergy Clin North Am. 2009;29:517.
104. Wolkenstein P, Chosidow O, Fléchet ML, et al. Patch testing in severe cutaneous adverse drug reactions, including Stevens-Johnson syndrome and toxic epidermal necrolysis. Contact Dermatitis. 1996;35:234.
105. Barbaud A, Collet E, Milpied B, et al. A multicentre study to determine the value and safety of drug patch tests for the three main classes of severe cutaneous adverse drug reactions. Br J Dermatol. 2013;168:555.
106. Romano A, Quaratino D, Di Fonso M, et al. A diagnostic protocol for evaluating nonimmediate reactions to aminopenicillins. J Allergy Clin Immunol. 1999;103:1186.
107. Stejskal VD, Olin RG, Forsbeck M. The lymphocyte transformation test for diagnosis of drug-induced occupational allergy. J Allergy Clin Immunol. 1986;77:411.
108. Gruchalla RS, Sullivan TJ. In vivo and in vitro diagnosis of drug allergy. Immunol Allergy Clin North Am. 1991;11:595.
109. Nyfeler B, Pichler WJ. The lymphocyte transformation test for the diagnosis of drug allergy: sensitivity and specificity. Clin Exp Allergy. 1997;27:175.
110. Sachs B, Erdmann S, Malte Baron J, et al. Determination of interleukin-5 secretion from drug-specific activated ex vivo peripheral blood mononuclear cells as a test system for the in vitro detection of drug sensitization. Clin Exp Allergy. 2002;32:736.
111. Brugnolo F, Annunziato F, Sampognaro S, et al. Highly Th2-skewed cytokine profile of beta-lactam-specific T cells from nonatopic subjects with adverse drug reactions. J Immunol. 1999;163:1053.
112. Posadas SJ, Padial A, Torres MJ, et al. Delayed reactions to drugs show levels of perforin, granzyme B, and Fas-L to be related to disease severity. J Allergy Clin Immunol. 2002;109:155.
113. Zawodniak A, Lochmatter P, Yerly D, et al. In vitro detection of cytotoxic T and NK cells in peripheral blood of patients with various drug-induced skin diseases. Allergy. 2010;65:376.
114. Porebski G, Pecaric-Petkovic T, Groux-Keller M, et al. In vitro drug causality assessment in Stevens-Johnson syndrome—alternatives for lymphocyte transformation test. Clin Exp Allergy. 2013;43:1027.
115. Vaillant L, Camenen I, Lorette G. Patch testing with carbamazepine: reinduction of an exfoliative dermatitis. Arch Dermatol. 1989;125:299.
116. Scherer K, Brockow K, Aberer W, et al. Desensitization in delayed drug hypersensitivity reactions—an EAACI position paper of the Drug Allergy Interest Group. Allergy. 2013;68:844.
117. Romano A, Gaeta F, Valluzzi RL, et al. Diagnosing nonimmediate reactions to cephalosporins. J Allergy Clin Immunol. 2012;129:1166.
118. Borch JE, Bindslev-Jensen C. Full-course drug challenge test in the diagnosis of delayed allergic reactions to penicillin. Int Arch Allergy Immunol. 2011;155:271.
119. Blanca-López N, Zapatero L, Alonso E, et al. Skin testing and drug provocation in the diagnosis of nonimmediate reactions to aminopenicillins in children. Allergy. 2009;64:229.
120. Schnyder B, Pichler WJ. Nonimmediate drug allergy: diagnostic benefit of skin testing and practical approach. J Allergy Clin Immunol. 2012;129:1170.
121. Misirlioglu ED, Toyran M, Capanoglu M, et al. Negative predictive value of drug provocation tests in children. Pediatr Allergy Immunol. 2014;25:685.
122. Demoly P, Romano A, Botelho C, et al. Determining the negative predictive value of provocation tests with beta-lactams. Allergy. 2010;65:327.
123. MacLaughlin EJ, Saseen JJ, Malone DC. Costs of beta-lactam allergies: selection and costs of antibiotics for patients with a reported beta-lactam allergy. Arch Fam Med. 2000;9:722.
124. Borch JE, Andersen KE, Bindslev-Jensen C. The prevalence of suspected and challenge-verified penicillin allergy in a university hospital population. Basic Clin Pharmacol Toxicol. 2006;98:357.
125. Kraemer MJ, Caprye-Boos H, Berman HS. Increased use of medical services and antibiotics by children who claim a prior penicillin sensitivity. West J Med. 1987;146:697.
126. Loo VG, Poirier L, Miller MA, et al. A predominantly clonal multi-institutional outbreak of *Clostridium difficile*-associated diarrhea with high morbidity and mortality. N Engl J Med. 2005;353:2442.
127. Lee CE, Zembower TR, Fotis MA, et al. The incidence of antimicrobial allergies in hospitalized patients:

implications regarding prescribing patterns and emerging bacterial resistance. Arch Intern Med. 2000;160:2819.
128. Solensky R, Earl HS, Gruchalla RS. Clinical approach to penicillin-allergic patients: a survey. Ann Allergy Asthma Immunol. 2000;84:329.
129. Puchner TC Jr, Zacharisen MC. A survey of antibiotic prescribing and knowledge of penicillin allergy. Ann Allergy Asthma Immunol. 2002;88:24.
130. Kwan T, Lin F, Ngai B, Loeb M. Vancomycin use in 2 Ontario tertiary care hospitals: a survey. Clin Invest Med. 1999;22:256.
131. Cieslak PR, Strausbaugh LJ, Fleming DW, Ling JM. Vancomycin in Oregon: who's using it and why. Infect Control Hosp Epidemiol. 1999;20:557.
132. Bonafede M, Rice LB. Emerging antibiotic resistance. J Lab Clin Med. 1997;130:558.
133. Murray BE. Vancomycin-resistant enterococcal infections. N Engl J Med. 2000;342:710.
134. Rao GG. Risk factors for the spread of antibiotic-resistant bacteria. Drugs. 1998;55:323.
135. Martínez JA, Ruthazer R, Hansjosten K, et al. Role of environmental contamination as a risk factor for acquisition of vancomycin-resistant enterococci in patients treated in a medical intensive care unit. Arch Intern Med. 2003;163:1905.
136. Peck SM, Siegal S, Glick AW, et al. Clinical problems in penicillin sensitivity. JAMA. 1948;138:631-40.
137. Sullivan TJ, Yecies LD, Shatz GS, et al. Desensitization of patients allergic to penicillin using orally administered beta-lactam antibiotics. J Allergy Clin Immunol. 1982; 69:275-82.
138. Wendel GD Jr, Stark BJ, Jamison RB, et al. Penicillin allergy and desensitization in serious infections during pregnancy. N Engl J Med. 1985;312:1229-32.
139. Castells M. Rapid desensitization for hypersensitivity reactions to medications. Immunol Allergy Clin North Am. 2009;29:585-606.
140. Cernadas JR, Brockow K, Romano A, et al. General considerations on rapid desensitization for drug hypersensitivity—a consensus statement. Allergy. 2010; 65:1357-66.
141. Pichler WJ, Daubner B, Kawabata T. Drug hypersensitivity: flare-up reactions, cross-reactivity and multiple drug hypersensitivity. J Dermatol. 2011;38:216.

CHAPTER 30

Epidemiology of Food Allergy: Special Reference to Bronchial Asthma

Raj Kumar

Food hypersensitivity is estimated to be approximately 2% in adults and 8% in children.[1] The incidence of perceived adult food hypersensitivity varies (1.4–19.1%) largely across different countries.[2] Allergen sensitization varying in different countries may be the result of interaction of genetic factors, cultural and dietary habits, and/or exposure to new allergenic products early in life. Studies show higher prevalence of allergy to soy in Japan, peanut allergy in the United Kingdom, France, Switzerland, and North America, and sesame allergy in Israel.[3] Legumes are an important source of immunoglobulin E (IgE)-mediated reactions in Mediterranean and Asian countries.[4-6] Allergic diseases have increased worldwide, including Asian countries.[7,8]

Most of the world's population lives in Asia. However, not much published data about food allergy is available from this part of the world. This problem may be due to large population with diverse racial, cultural, and socioeconomic condition. Asia is also unique for its range of different cultures and eating habits. The most common cause of food-induced anaphylaxis in a cohort of children from Singapore is bird's nest (27%), followed by egg and milk (11% combined).[9]

The true prevalence of FA in the general population in Asia is uncertain. Estimates from Chinese studies range from 4.98% to 16.4%.[10,11] The latter percentage represented those diagnosed by skin prick test (SPT) and therefore reflects sensitization rather than true clinical allergy. In the late 1990s, a parent-reported questionnaire of children from Singapore estimated the prevalence of FA to be 4–5%.[12] A Korean study using a self-reported questionnaire in a huge cohort of children reported a lifetime prevalence of 10.9%.[13]

Similarly variable FA prevalence was noted in other Asian countries: as high as 5.5% in a cohort of Japanese children aged 18 years and as low as 1.2–1.7% in Israeli infants as assessed by detailed questionnaire and SPTs.[3] A cross-sectional study of 656 children of 6 months to 6 years of age in Thailand showed a prevalence of 6.25% FA in children less than 6 years based on a parent reported questionnaire survey versus the 0.45% established through SPT and food challenge.[14] This illustrates the discrepancy between reported and medically diagnosed allergy.

Recent studies in India show a considerable increase in the prevalence of bronchial asthma (8–15%)[15,16] when compared with the earlier report of <1%.[17] Many asthma and rhinitis patients may be suffering from food allergy but our knowledge about food hypersensitivity is limited to few studies carried out in the country.[18-20] These studies indicate that foods such as egg, milk, cereals, and legumes commonly induce IgE-mediated reaction in children and adult population.

Legumes are important causative agents of type I hypersensitivity in south Asia and Europe but such studies are lacking in Indian population. A study[21] investigated black gram sensitization in asthma and rhinitis patients and identifies immunoglobulin E (IgE)-binding proteins. Black gram induces IgE-mediated reactions in 1.7% of asthma and rhinitis patients and contains eight major IgE-binding components, of which six regained IgE reactivity after roasting. Black gram shares allergenicity with lentil and lima bean. A case[22] with definite history of allergy (asthma) was investigated using standard in vivo and in vitro tests. Double-blind oral challenge test with dehusked horse gram (pulses) showed severe pulmonary obstruction. Intradermal tests with seed extracts (pulses) revealed marked positive skin reactions. Further, ELISA with patient's serum showed significantly elevated IgE levels to various seed extracts compared to normal control. Immunoblotting with patient's serum showed 4–10

IgE-binding proteins with MWs 45, 38, 35, 30, 28, and 11 kDa to be common in the food extracts prepared from seeds of family leguminosae.

Sensitization to food varies in different countries reflecting a possible interaction of genetic factors, and cultural and dietary habits. Rice is a major food consumed worldwide and evaluated for IgE-mediated reactions. A study[23] was carried out to identify rice allergy in patients of rhinitis and asthma and to identify the allergenic proteins in raw and cooked rice. Of these, 20 (12.1%) patients demonstrated marked positive SPT and 13 patients showed significantly raised specific IgE to rice compared to normal controls. Double-blind, placebo-controlled food challenge (DBPCFC) confirmed rice allergy in 6/10 patients. Immunoblot with hypersensitive individual patient's sera showed 14–16, 33, 56, and 60 kDa proteins as major IgE-binding components in rice. Boiled rice retained four IgE-reactive proteins of 16, 23, 33, and 53 kDa. IgE-mediated rice allergy affects 0.8% (95% CI, 0.42–1.58) of asthma and rhinitis cases. The subjects with severe SPT reactions (4 mm or above) and specific IgE, 6.9 ng/mL to rice demonstrated positive blind food challenge with clinical symptoms.

Studies suggest the importance of total serum and specific IgE in clinical evaluation of allergic manifestations. Such studies are lacking in Indian subcontinent, though a large population suffer from bronchial asthma. In a study[24] the relevance of serum total and specific IgE was investigated in asthmatics with food sensitization. A total of 216 consecutive patients (mean age 31.9 years, SD 11.8) were screened by various diagnostic testing. Out of 216 patients, 172 were with elevated serum total IgE (201 to >800 IU/mL). Rice elicited marked positive SPT reactions in 24 (11%) asthma patients followed by black gram 22 (10%), lentil 21 (9.7%) and citrus fruits 20 (9.2%). Serum total IgE and specific IgE showed significant correlation, $p = 0.005$ and $p = 0.001$, respectively, with positive skin tests. Blind food challenges (DBPCFC) with rice and black gram confirmed food sensitization in 28–37% of cases. Hence, serum total IgE of 265 IU/mL or more with marked positive SPT (4 mm or more) can serve as a marker for atopy and food sensitization. Specific IgE, three times of normal controls, correlates well with positive DBPCFC and offers evidence for the cases of food allergy.

Studies have shown an association between food sensitivity, asthma, and/or other atopic disorders. But the knowledge about the true prevalence of food hypersensitivity in respiratory allergy patients is lacking in India. In a study,[25] the prevalence of food allergy in patients of asthma and rhinitis was investigated. Of 1860 patients (mean age 30 + 12 years) screened using standard questionnaire, 1097 (58.9%) gave history of food allergy. Of 470 patients (history positive) skin prick tested, 29.3% showed positive reactivity to at least one food, with rice (6.2%) as top sensitizers followed by black gram (5.9%), lentil (5.5%), and citrus fruits (5.3%). Patients with history of SPT positive reactions showed elevated specific IgE levels (0.98–79) IU/mL against respective food allergens than normal controls (0.60–0.80 IU/mL). Prick to prick test with fresh foods demonstrated more positive reactions than SPT with antigen extracts ($p = 0.0001$). Of 184 open food challenges (OFC), most of the positive OFCs were obtained with rice,[20] followed by citrus fruits,[14] banana,[10] and black gram.[6] Among blinded challenges on 45 individuals, 21 (47%) were assessed as positive. With DBPCFC as the end point, the prevalence of food sensitization was 1.1% [0.72–1.75 at 95% CI] in 1860 patients. We concluded that the perception of food-related symptoms is common among respiratory allergy patients. Self-reports could be confirmed in 21/470 (4.4%), resulting in an overall estimated prevalence of 1.1% [(0.72–1.75) at 95% CI] in respiratory allergy patients. The common offending foods are rice, black gram, citrus fruits, and banana.

Food allergies are the single most common cause of generalized anaphylaxis seen in the emergency department of hospital accounting for about one third of the cases. It is estimated that about 100 fatal cases of food-induced anaphylaxis occur in the United States each year. In addition to the cutaneous, respiratory, and gastrointestinal symptoms noted above, patients may have cardiovascular symptoms, including hypertension, vascular collapse, and cardiac dysrhythmia, presumably caused by massive mast cell mediator release. However, most of the food-induced anaphylactic reactions are not associated with increase in serum tryptase.

REFERENCES

1. Bruijneel-Koomen C, Ortolani C, Aas K, et al. Adverse reactions to foods. European academy of allergology and clinical immunology subcommittee. Allergy. 1995;50: 623-35.
2. Crespo JF, Rodriguez J. Food allergy in adulthood. Allergy. 2003;58:98-113.
3. Dalal I, Binson I, Reifen R, et al. Food allergy is a matter of geography after all: sesame as a major cause of severe IgE-mediated food allergic reactions among infants and young children in Israel. Allergy. 2002;57:362-5.

4. Ibáñez Sandín D, Martínez San Ireneo M, Marañón Lizana F, et al. Specific IgE determinations to crude and boiled lentil (Lens culinaris) extracts in lentil-sensitive children and controls. Allergy. 1999;54:1209-14.
5. Pascual CY, Fernandez-Crespo J, Sanchez-Pasor S, et al. Allergy to lentils in mediterranean pediatric patients. J Allergy Clin Immunol. 1999;103:154-8.
6. Sanchez-Monge R, Pascual CY, Diaz-Perales A, et al. Isolation and characterization of relevant allergens from boiled lentils. J Allergy Clin Immunol. 2000;106:955-61.
7. Harwanegg C, Hiller R. Protein microarray in diagnosing IgE-mediated diseases: spotting allergy at a molecular level. Expert Rev Mol Diagn. 2004;4:539-48.
8. Wang GWK, Leung TF. Asthma epidemiology and hygiene hypothesis in Asia. Allergy Clin Immunol Int. 2004;16:155-60.
9. Goh DL, Lau YN, Chew FT, et al. Pattern of food-induced anaphylaxis in children of an Asian community. Allergy. 1999;54:84-6.
10. Wang Z. An allergy prevalence survey in population of 10,144 people. Chin Epidemiol J. 1990;11:100-2.
11. Kim JS, Ouyang F, Pongracic JA, et al. Dissociation between the prevalence of atopy and allergic disease in rural China among children and adults. J Allergy Clin Immunol. 2008;122:929-35.
12. Lee BW, Chew FT, Goh DYT. Changing prevalence of childhood allergic diseases in Singapore. In: 5th West-Pacific Allergy Symposium & 7th Korea-Japan Joint Allergy Symposium; 11-14 June, 1997; Seoul, South Korea; 1997:17-22.
13. Lee SI, Shin MH, Lee HB, et al. Prevalence of symptoms of asthma and other allergic disease in Korean children: a nationwide questionnaire survey. J Korean Med Sci. 2001;16:155-64.
14. Santadusit S, Atthapaisalsarudee S, Vichyanond P. Prevalence of adverse food reactions and food allergy among Thai children. J Med Assoc Thai. 2005;88:27-32.
15. Chhabra SK, Gupta CK, Chhabra P, Rajpal S. Prevalence of bronchial asthma in school children in Delhi. J Asthma. 1998;35:291-6.
16. Gaur SN, Sanjay R, Ashish R. Prevalence of bronchial asthma and allergic rhinitis among school children in Delhi. Intern Med J Thai. 2004;20:8-13.
17. Vishwanathan R. Definition incidence, etiology and natural history of asthma. Ind J Chest Dis. 1964;6:108-24.
18. Patil SP, Niphadkar PV, Bapat MM. Chickpea: a major food allergen in the Indian subcontinent and its clinical and immunochemical correlation. Ann Allergy Asthma Immnuol. 2001;87:140-5.
19. Parihar H, Kumar L, Puri Kumar V. The incidence of allergic diseases and feeding patterns in children up to 2 years of age. Indian J Paediatr. 1984;51:7-12.
20. Sharman J, Kumar L, Singh S. Allergenicity of common foods restricted in respiratory allergy. Indian J Paediatr. 2000;67:713-20.
21. Kumar D, Kumar R, Sridhara S, et al. Sensitization to black gram in patients with bronchial asthma and rhinitis: clinical evaluation and characterization of allergens. Allergy. 2006;61:104-10.
22. Kumar R, Sridhara S, Verma J, et al. Clinico-immunologic studies on allergy to pulses—A case report. Indian J Allergy Appl Immunol. 2000;14:15-20.
23. Kumar R, Srivastava P, Kumari D, et al. Rice (Oryza sativa) allergy in rhinitis and asthma patients: a clinico-immunological study. Immunobiology. 2007;212:141-7.
24. Kumar R, Singh BP, Srivastava P, et al. Relevance of serum IgE estimation in allergic bronchial asthma with special reference to food allergy. Asian Pac J Allergy Immunol. 2006;24:191-9.
25. Kumar R, Dolly K, Prakriti S, et al. Prevalence of food allergy and its impact on bronchial asthma and rhinitis patients. Allergy. 2007;62:167-551.

CHAPTER 31

Food Allergy: Diagnosis and Treatment

PC Kathuria

INTRODUCTION

Over the last two decades, food allergy has increased in prevalence and severity in the industrialized countries and is frequently the first manifestation of allergic disorders. There is a discrepancy between the public perception of reactions to food additives state as affecting 7.4% of the population but reactions confirmed by double-blind, placebo-controlled testing prevalence figures between 0.01 and 0.23% (Young et al. 1987)[1] in children. Food allergies are the single most common cause of anaphylaxis and this problem may account for 120–150 deaths per year. Food allergies may affect up to 8% of the children less than 3 years of age and 1–2% of the general population. The confirmed prevalence of food allergy and food intolerance is 0.8–2.4%, while food additive is 0.01–0.23%. The incidence in young children is 1.3%, while in adult is 0.3%.[2]

- *Food hypersensitivity*: All the immunological-mediated adverse reactions to food (IgE and Non- IgE mediated). There is a specific form of food allergy protein that activates the immune system, which sets off a chain of reaction including the release of antibodies.
- *Food intolerance*: Are the non-immunological-mediated reactions to foods involve the body metabolism. The possible mechanisms are as follows:
  - Mucosal enzyme deficiencies—lactase deficiency in lactose intolerance.
  - Systemic enzyme deficiency, e.g., phenylalanine-hydroxyl deficiency in phenylketonuria and fructose-1-phosphate deficiency in fructose intolerance.
  - Direct, toxin, or chemical intolerance.
- *Food aversion*: Suspected, psychologically often self-diagnosed by affected individuals or parent.[3,4]

Q. What makes food allergic?[2] Food proteins which are water-soluble glycoproteins with molecular weights of 10–70 kDa and stable to heat and digestive enzymes tend to be responsible for most allergic reactions. The protein family database lists 7,677 different families of proteins, all known plant food allergens are present in only 20 families, representing 0.25% of the total number of families. The most important of these families are family-10 of the pathogenesis-related (**PR-10**) proteins and the ***cupin family of proteins***. These proteins are quite conserved, and cupin derivatives can be found in bacteria, plant, and animals.

Most plant food allergens belong to only four structural families which determine or promote allergic properties. Allergens from the same species with greater than 67% sequence identity have been defined by the Allergen Nomenclature Committee as isoallergens.

These four families of plant food allergen are as follows:

1. *Cereal prolamin superfamily*: It is composed of the following:
   - Cereal storage proteins (e.g., the ω-5 gliadin allergen of wheat).
   - *Lipid transfer proteins (LTPs)*: These are a family of stable proteins that resist heating and enzymatic digestion and may give systemic reactions. It is present in the Rosaceae family, tree nuts, peanuts, maize, mustards, asparagus, grapes, mulberry, cabbage, dates, orange, fig, kiwi, lupine, fennel, celery, tomato, eggplant, lettuce, chestnut, and pineapple.

Lipid proteins Prup 3 and Zea m 14 are present in peach and corn, respectively.
   - 2 S storage albumins (e.g., Bere 1 from Brazil nut)
   - Inhibitors of trypsin and alpha amylase.
2. *Cupins*: Allergenic members of the cupin family include the vicillins (major allergens from peanut, soya been, lentil, pea, walnut, cashew, and sesame seed) and the legumes (peanut, soybean, hazelnut, walnut, almond, Brazil nut, cashew, and coconut). It also includes 7S and 11S globulin storage proteins of seeds to which many allergens belong, notably Arah 1, Arah 3, and Arah 4 from peanuts.
3. *Bet V1 related*: It is a homologus of the major birch pollen allergen Bet V1 (such as Mald 1 in apple and Apig1 in celery).
4. *Profilins*: These are proteins usually unstable to heat and acid, present in pollens and plant foods. They may induce local reactions in the oropharyngeal mucosa when exposed to fruit and or vegetable profilins. There is a h/o allergy to melon, watermelon, tomato, banana, pineapple, and orange.

The majority of animal food allergen can be classified into three protein groups as follows:
1. Caseins
2. EF-hand proteins (primarily parvalbumin)
3. Tropomyosins

DIAGNOSIS OF FOOD ALLERGY

The following are factors that are useful for the diagnosis of food allergy:
- Clinical food history[2,3]
- Skin tests and specific IgE
- Oral food challenge (OFC)
- Component-resolved diagnosis (CRD)
- Basophil activation tests (BAT).

Clinical Food History

Four ways of presentation are as follows:
1. "Whenever I eat a nut, I get swollen lips hives, then itchy spots, and I sometimes vomit."
2. "I cannot eat nuts" (reason vague or based on a single episode long ago).
3. "I wonder if this rash could be caused by something in my diet."
4. I have given up eating nuts because the lady in the health food shop says, I must be allergic to them."

Questions
- What are the ill effects of food?
- Are there any local or generalized symptoms by food?
- The effect of food on the severity of itchiness or worsening of symptoms?
- What are the offending foods?
   - Foods of animal origin, e.g. milk, egg, fish, meat, poultry, and seafoods.
   - Foods of vegetable origin, e.g. nuts and seeds, fruits and vegetables, herbs and spices, grain products, drinks such as wine, bear, tea, and cola.

Signs and Symptoms of Food-induced Allergic Reactions in Various Target Organs (Fig. 31.1)

Skin: Urticaria/angioedema flushing, erythematous pruritic rash, and atopic dermatitis.[4]
Gastrointestinal tract: Pruritus and/or swelling of the lips, tongue, or oral mucosa; nausea, abdominal cramps, colic vomiting, or reflux diarrhea.
Respiratory tract: Nasal congestion, rhinorrhea, pruritus/sneezing, laryngeal edema, staccato cough and/or dyspnea, and wheezing/cough.
Cardiovascular: Hypotension/shock, dizziness.
Other: Cramping back pain (uterine contraction feeling of "impending doom").

Skin Tests and Specific IgE

Panel of Food Items for Testing

1. The well-known food allergens of both animal and vegetable origin (Fig. 31.2).[4-6]

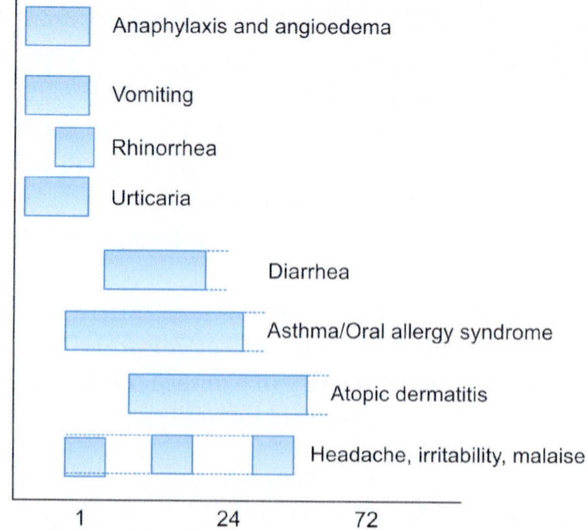

Fig. 31.1: Time (hours) course of symptoms of food allergy and intolerance.[3,4]

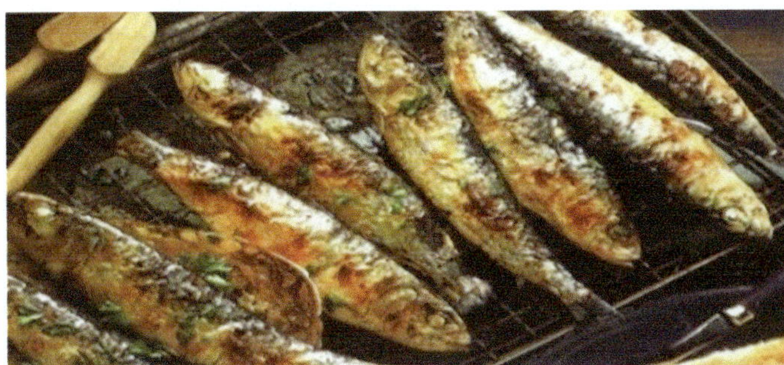

Fig. 31.2: Fried Fish

Milk	Peanut	Nuts
Egg	Soy	Apple
Fish	Wheat	Celery
Meat		Potato
Seafood (shrimp)		Para pollen allergens

2. The food families showing extensive cross sensitivity: For example, Papilonaceae—pea, black gram and ground nut; Solanaceae—e.g., —potato, brinjal and tomato.
3. Food items that may serve as "alimentary alternative" are as follows:
   - Rosaceae—citrus, banana, grape, melon.
   - Umbelliferae, Compositae, Liliaceae, Cruciferae, and Chenopodiaceae.
4. The food item the patient regards as (possibly) harmful.

Determination of SPT and RAST Depends

Determination of SPT and RAST depends on the following:

1. Technical performance
2. Allergen quality
3. Patient sample (quality)
4. Cross-reactivity.

The skin test and RAST positivity should be interpreted with care.[7-9] The presence of IgE antibodies to a food does not mean that the patient is clinically allergic to it. Many atopic people have IgE antibodies but no symptoms, so positive results must be interpreted in conjunction with a careful history. Food should not be restricted on the basis of a positive result, if no clinical symptoms exist. On the other hand, a negative skin test or RAST result is a good evidence that shows a reaction to food is not mediated by IgE but it does not exclude sensitivity mediated by non-IgE mechanism. It is to be noted that IgE-ab to foods appear during infancy and disappear during childhood, whereas IgE-ab to inhalants appear later and in increasing frequency from 2 years of age. Patients presenting symptoms of food allergy and low IgE levels have a higher probability of obtaining resolution of their allergy after several years, while patients with high food-specific IgE levels (three times or more) have a low probability of outgrowing their hypersensitivity to these foods even after 5 years. It is therefore useful to perform follow-up food-specific IgE assays in order to determine the optimal time for a repeat challenge test.

Double-blind, placebo-controlled food challenges (DBPCFC) is the only confirmatory test in adults and children, while in infants, open challenges may be sufficient. But in practice, it is difficult to perform DBPCFC, as it is time-consuming and potentially dangerous, moreover, it needs hospitalization and intensive surveillance. So we try to base the diagnosis by one or more allergy tests, e.g., skin prick tests (SPT) and specific IgE (RAST). These two tests have demonstrated a sufficiently high sensitivity and specificity to justify their use in daily clinical practice. This is at least true for most common allergens. One of the major problems with SPT and RAST is the lack of standardized extracts used in the tests. Allergenic activity is lost during the processing of the allergen, then Prick-Prick tests, means pricking the needle in the unprocessed foods and then pricking on the skin specifically of fresh vegetables, is more potent than commercial extracts. A h/o of anaphylactic reactions clearly related to a specific food is a relative contraindication to provocation and most patients are associated with positive SPT and RAST. SPT is also useful in identifying the allergic cause of idiopathic recurrent and acute urticaria. The syndrome of fruit/tree pollen sensitivity is a special case, in that the history and skin tests are so specific as to make provocation probably superfluous. The patients are adults with a history of seasonal tree pollen rhinitis and asthma, who suddenly develop immediate oropharyngeal reactions (OAS) to fresh fruits. They suffer similar reactions to other fruits and often to raw potatoes, carrots, etc. Here, SPT to standard tree pollen extracts are positive but to commercial food extracts negative, but prick–prick test is more informative. Allergist should have knowledge of botanically related foods before interpretation of SPT and RAST for example. If SPT is positive (peanuts), then it will be also positive to soya bean, green bean, pea, etc, but if we do DBPCFC with these cross-reactive foods, it will be negative.

Food Challenge

The double-blind, placebo-controlled food challenge has been labeled as the "gold standard" for the diagnosis of food allergies.[10-12] DBPCFC has proven to be the most accurate means of diagnosing food allergies, rare false negative (1.8%) and false positive (0.5%) (e.g., ch. urticaria, atopic dermatitis, occupational br. asthma, etc.). It should be conducted in clinic or hospital setting, especially if an IgE-mediated reaction is suspected, and only if trained personnel and equipment for treating systemic anaphylaxis are present. If life-threatening anaphylaxis is suspected and the causative antigen cannot be conclusively determined by history, a challenge should be conducted in the intensive care unit of a center frequently dealing with food-allergic reactions. The selection of foods to be taken in DBPCFC is generally based on history and/or skin test (RAST) results but before undertaking DBPCFC, one should consider several factors as follows:

- Eliminate suspected food for 14 days before the challenge.
- Discontinue antihistamine: Minimize other medications.
- Administer challenge to the patient on an empty stomach.
- An equal number of food and placebo challenges need to be administered randomized by non-interested party (Dietician).
- Lyophilized foods are blinded in liquid or capsules.
- Administer 10 gm. Over 1 hour, Ist dose $\leq$ 500 mg.
- Utilize a standardized scoring system.
- The length of the observation period expands on type of reactions being studied.
- Appropriate equipment should be available to treat systemic anaphylaxis.
- All negative challenges must be confirmed by an open feeding under observation.

The food challenge is administered in the fasting state; starting with a dose unlikely to provoke symptoms (125–500 mg of lyophilized food) the dose is then doubled every 15–60 minutes depending on the type of reaction suspected. After the patient has tolerated 10 g. Of lyophilized food blinded in capsules or liquid, clinical reactivity is generally ruled out. If the blinded challenge is negative, however, it must be confirmed by an open feeding under observation to rule out rare false-negative challenges. An equal number of food-antigen and placebo-challenge are necessary, to control the potential confounding factors. The order of administration should be randomized by a non-interested third party (e.g., dietician) a standardized scoring system should be utilized for all challenges. The time of observation depends on the type of reaction suspected (e.g., generally up to 2 hours. for IgE-mediated reaction and up to 4–8 hours for mild induced enterocollitis). Results of blinded challenges for objective signs and symptoms are rarely equivocal but can be made more objective by monitoring a variety of laboratory parameters (such as plasma histamine, pulmonary function tests and nasal airway resistance).

Elimination Diets

- The meat least likely to cause reactions is *lamb*.[13]
- The least antigenic cereal is *rice*.
- Vegetables: Peeled potatoes and lettuce.
- Fruits: Pears (peeled).
- Fat: A refined vegetable seed oil, e.g., (cold processed) sunflower or safflower.
- Drink: Water and sugar.
  If the diet continues for more than a week then uncolored multivitamin supplement should be taken. Other foods are included in some elimination diets, depending on the type of reaction and the suspected ingredients.

Component-resolved Diagnosis (CRD)

The SPT or serum IgE assesses the presence of IgE to bind the whole allergen protein sequence and therefore rely on the crude allergen extract.[3,14,15] In component testing, the extract identifies and quantifies IgE directed against specified protein components of each allergen such as omega 5 gliadin in wheat-dependent, exercise-induced anaphylaxis or Arah 1, 2, 3, 8, and 9 in peanut allergy. Arah 1, Arah 2, and Arah 3 appear to be associated with a higher likelihood of true clinical allergy, whereas reactivity to Arah 8 is associated with cross-sensitization to birch pollen and less likely to be associated with significant clinical allergy. Arah 9 is a member of the heat stable LTP and is also related to cross and co-sensitization with similar allergen. Here a large number of recombinant and purified components are assayed simultaneously for fruits and vegetables with oral allergy syndromes. Similarly, Ovamucoid has been associated with clinical allergy and severity of reaction to extensively heated egg products such as baked cakes and muffins in egg. This will improve the ability to prognostic and reduce the need for OFC.

Basophil Activation Test

Basophil activation test (BAT) is useful and complement to provocation, Sp IgE, and other skin allergy tests.[3] Provocation testing has been considered as the gold standard for allergic diagnosis; however, it is as fluctuating as the gold price. It can be and was recently shown to have inferior test capabilities when compared to BAT. BAT can be useful to distinguish the primary sensitizer from a cross-reactive allergen as sensitivity toward the primary sensitizer is higher. BAT is useful to confirm reactivity in patients who have a clinical history but are negative in other confirmatory test. BAT is useful in the diagnosis of food allergy, be it a primary sensitizer or cross-reactive symptoms. BAT has better sensitivity and NPV than IgE and SPT. BAT showed 100%, specificity, 83.3% sensuality, 100% PPV, 90.2% NPV, and 93.4% accuracy and was superior to SPT, Sp IgE, and CRD. BAT discriminates between allergy and tolerance in peanut-sensitized children. BAT is useful for distinguishing reactivity to cooked and raw allergen and to determine where a food challenge is required. It is an in vitro assay in which the expression of activation markers on the surface of basophils is evaluated by using flow cytometry after stimulation with food allergens. It can be performed using 1 mL of blood. Without requiring cell separation BAT was expressed as percentage of CD63 basophiles and as the stimulation index of the mean fluorescence and intensity (MFI) of CD203c.

MANAGEMENT OF FOOD ALLERGY

The optimal management of food allergy consists of multidisciplinary and multifaceted approach which encompasses the treatment of acute episodes of the disease, identification of patients at risk of severe reaction, and long-term management strategy in order to minimize the recurrences of reactions and improve quality of life.[15-19] For detailed guidance on the emergency management of anaphylaxis, readers are referred to EAACI Anaphylaxis Guidelines.[16] The "standard of care" for food allergy consists of educating patients and caregivers how to avoid food allergens and arming them with medications to treat accidental ingestions. Food allergic patients with asthma or a history of a previous severe reaction (peanuts, Nut, seeds, or seafood) should be given, and self-injectable epinephrine. However, given the continued high rate of severe food allergic reactions, it is clear that the current "standard of care" is inadequate.

Acute Management

The patient at risk of severe reactions should be properly and timely identified, and adrenaline should be immediately administered for cardiovascular symptoms and/or respiratory symptoms such as altered voice, stridor, or bronchospasm that are thought to be induced by food allergy. Short-acting beta agonist should be included in the management plan for all patients with coexisting asthma and should be administered for bronchospasm after adrenaline has been administered. Glucocorticosteroid may be given with reactions to possibly prevent late-phase respiratory symptoms (self-administered if traveling far from medical care, otherwise in emergency center).

Long-term Management Strategy

Elimination Diet

Appropriate dietary avoidance is the key treatment in the management of food allergy. Patient with food allergy who are on long-term elimination diets should have access to appropriate dietetic counseling, ideally by a dietician with competencies in food allergy, and regular monitoring of growth (in children). Extensively, hydrolyzed cow's milk formulas with documented hypoallergenicity can be recommended as first choice for the treatment of cow's milk allergy, especially in infants and young children. Amino acid formulas can also be recommended especially for the subgroup of patient with more severe symptoms. Soya formulas should not be recommended before 6 months of age and at any age in the presence of gastrointestinal symptoms. From 6 to 12 months, it can be considered on a case-by-case basis.

Currently, probiotic supplements cannot be recommended for the management of food allergy.

Education and Risk Assessment

All patients with food allergy require a management plan with appropriate education for the patient, caregiver, including school. Education should cover allergen avoidance, symptoms recognition, indication for specific treatment, and administration of specific medication. Absolute indication with adrenaline autoinjector includes previous anaphylaxis to any food, food allergy associated with persistence or severe asthma, and exercise-induced food dependent anaphylaxis. Relative indications for adrenaline auto-injector with food allergy include the following:

- Food allergy that is likely to be persistent.
- Mild-to-moderate allergic reaction to peanuts and/or tree nuts.
- Specific high-risk group, e.g., adolescents, young adult male, and poor access to medical care.

Specific Immunotherapy

Food allergen-specific immunotherapy for primary food allergy is a promising immunomodulatory treatment approach, but it is associated with the risk of adverse reaction, including anaphylaxis; it is therefore not currently recommended for routine clinical use.

For patient with respiratory or other allergic symptoms to inhalant allergens, it may also cause cross-reactive food allergy; specific immunotherapy is only recommended for the treatment of respiratory symptoms, but not for the cross-reactive food allergy.

Anti-IgE

The use of anti-IgE alone or in combination with specific immunotherapy is currently not recommended for the treatment of food allergy although it represents a promising treatment modality.

Challenges at Regular Interval to Assess Achievements of Tolerance

Oral food challenge should be performed at regular intervals, as appropriate for the specific food and patient's history, in order to assess achievement of tolerance.

Specific IgE testing (in vitro and skin prick test) has limited value in guiding adequately the timing of the OFCs for the development of tolerance.

Cofactors

In food allergy reactions, the potential augmenting role of cofactors [e.g., exercise, NSAID (Nonsteroidal Anti-inflammatory drugs), omeprazole, alcohol intake] should be assessed in a structured history.

In allergic reaction occurring after exercise, NSAID, or alcohol intake, an underlying allergy to food consumed in the previous hours should be assessed (especially gliadin sensitization or lipid-transfer proteins in Southern Europe).

SUMMARY

Oral Food Challenge (OFC) is a gold standard for food allergy but it is laborious, time-consuming, and risky. Therefore, in clinical practice the diagnosis of food allergy is based on the combination of a history together with in vivo or in vitro measurement of sensitization. In order to improve the utility of SPT and Sp IgE, diagnostic decision cutoff points values have been determined still there is a large immunological gray area between 95% PPV and 95% NPV cutoff for SPT, Sp IgE, CRD, e.g., to situation in which SPT cannot be interpreted because of a negative histamine control or in which Sp IgE cannot be interpreted in the light of a high polyclonal IgE production or indeed, when an FC is also inconclusive and also carries the risk of causing an acute allergic reaction. If we perform BAT, it has major effect in reducing the number of OFCs. It has been found that performing BAT after SPT or CRD allows a 97% reduction in the number of OFCs. The total number of OFCs was significantly reduced by 64% (SPT-BAT) or 69% (CRD-BAT) compared with SPT and specific IgE. So SPT followed by BAT is better than CRD followed by BAT for practical reasons as SPT provides immediate results. While, CRD followed by BAT requires two times separate blood collections. To conclude, among SPT, specific IgE, CRD, and BAT test, BAT has been the best diagnostic profile and needs further studies whether BAT can be added to the OFC as an in vitro gold standard test.

The most important point for a caregiver to make with patients/patents is that patient with food allergy must learn to "live in the world". Liberalization of allergen avoidance diets can improve not only the quality of life of the patients with food allergy, but also may hasten their tolerance acquisition. Over the next few decades, it is likely that immunotherapy for food allergy will become a standard clinical tool with us for adjuvant co-administration, will lead to long-term sustained tolerance, and will provide high-quality evidence for both diagnosis and management of food allergy.

REFERENCES

1. Young E, Patel S, Stoneham M. The prevalence of reaction to food additives in a survey population. JR Coll Physicians Lond. 1987;21:241-7.
2. Novembre E, Veneruso G, Sabatini C, et al. Incidence of asthma caused by food allergy in childhood. Pediatr Med Chir. 1987;9:399-404.
3. Muraro A, Agache I, Clark A, et al. EAACI food allergy and anaphylaxis guidelines: managing patients with food allergy in the community. Allergy. 2014;69:1046-57.
4. Exl BM, Muller-Teicher G, Vandenplas Y, et al. Preventive possibilities within the context of cow's milk allergy. Allergy Clin Immunol Int. 2000;12(2):68-7.
5. Ortolani C, ed. Atlas on mechanisms in adverse reactions to food. Allergy. 1995;50(Suppl 20):5-81.
6. May CD, Book SA. Adverse reactions to food due to hypersensitivity. Middleton E, Reed Cr. Eds Allergy. Principles & Practices. St. Louis: C.V. Mostby Co; 1978.
7. Kathuria PC. Food allergy. Ind J Allergy Appl Immunol. 1996;87-8.

8. Eigenmann PA, Sampson HA. Interpreting skin prick tests in the evaluation of food allergy in children. Pediatr Allergy Immunol. 1998;9(4):186-91.
9. Brostofe J, Stephen T. Food allergy & intolerance. Textbook of Food Allergy & Intolerance. 1987;59:985-93.
10. Bindslev-Jensen C, et al. In: Johansson SGO, ed. Techniques in Diagnosis of Food Hypersensitivity Progress in Allergy & Clinical Immunology. Vol 3. Stockholm; 1995:268-74.
11. Allergy Practice Forum. Clinical diagnosis in food allergy. Clin Exp Allergy. 1989;19:83-5.
12. Van Ree R, Akkerdaas JH, van Leeuwen WA, et al. New perspectives for diagnosis of food allergy. ACI Int. 2000;12(1):7-12.
13. Nekam K. Management of food allergy. Allergy. 1998;53: 122-4.
14. Sampson HA, Aceves S, Allan Bock S, et al. Food allergy: a practice parameter update. J Allergy Clin Immunol. 2014;134(5):1016-25.e43.
15. Sampson HA. Food allergy diagnosis & management. J Allergy Clin Immunol. 1999;103(6):981-9.
16. Golbert TM. Food allergy textbook of allergic diseases diagnosis management. Edi. Patterson. 1993;14:353-78.
17. Onorato J, Merland N, Terral C, Michel FB, Bousquet J. Placebo-controlled, double-blind food challenge in asthma. J Allergy Clin Immunol. 1986;78:1139-46.
18. Turner PJ, Campbell DE. What's new in the diagnosis and management of food allergy in children? Asia Pac Allergy. 2013;3:88-95.
19. Food Allergies: The Basics, Rudolf Valenta, et al., Gastroenterology Vol. 148, No.6, 2015;148:1120-11631.

CHAPTER 32

Evaluating Potential Allergenicity of Genetically Modified Food Crops

Ankita Mishra, Naveen Arora

BACKGROUND

Genetically modified (GM) food crops developed by the recombinant DNA (r-DNA) technology aim at improving food quantity and quality. Transgenic proteins expressed by GM crops improve crop characteristics like nutritional value, taste, and texture and endow the host plant with resistance against fungus, pests, and insects. With the advancements in the field of agricultural biotechnology, the number of GM varieties ready for commercialization is increasing in proportion with the area under GM crop cultivation and the number of countries consuming GM crops. However, prior to the release of a GM crop in the market, it must pass through rigorous safety evaluation tests to ensure its safety for feed, fodder, and the environment. In the past few decades, several international regulatory authorities have defined guidelines for the safety assessment of transgenic food products. These protocols have been modified from time to time, and efforts are underway to ensure the complete safety of the consumers. FAO/WHO (2001) and Codex (2003) guidelines for the safety assessment of GM foods are the most widely accepted among all of the available guidelines. Safety evaluation studies do not rely on a single parameter, therefore, we take into account results from different tests to define the safety of a GM crop on a relative scale.

INTRODUCTION

Recent advances in the field of r-DNA technology and improved agricultural equipment have paved the way for large-scale cultivation of genetically modified (GM) crops. Molecular biology methods are very precise and aim at introducing only one or, at most, a few well-defined genes, rather than inserting parts of chromosomes as in traditional plant breeding. To date, over 30 million hectares of transgenic crops are being grown for human consumption. These are high-yielding varieties resistant to pathogen attack and tolerant to environmental imbalances like drought, cold, and salinity.[1,2] Transgenes expressed in GM crops encode for proteins foreign to the wild-type varieties. These proteins must be evaluated for their potency to act as novel allergens, before using GM crops as feed or fodder. Transgenic proteins expressed in host plants may share homology with the host plant proteins, or these may share identity with the reported food allergens.[3,4] Therefore, prior to the release of GM crops in the consumer market, it is essential to conduct safety assessment of the GM crops and/or transgenic proteins.[5-7] Along with this, GM food labeling should also be made mandatory for all new and existing varieties.

Food allergy is defined as an adverse health effect arising from a hypersensitivity reaction induced upon exposure to a particular food allergen that occurs reproducibly on subsequent exposures. Type 1 hypersensitivity food allergic reactions are characterized by the activation of mast cells and basophils and result in histamine release followed by synthesis of other inflammatory molecules like leukotrienes, prostaglandins, cytokines, etc. These events manifest into severe allergic symptoms like eczema, hives, allergic rhinitis, asthma, and gastrointestinal (GI) tract allergies. Food allergy is reported by individuals of all age groups; however, the current prevalence reported is 10% of children and 6% of the adults in the Western countries.[8] In general population, self-reported prevalence of food allergy is 5% in Korea, 3.5% in France, and 22.2% in Australia.[9] Food allergy is a major health issue, and food-related allergic reactions can often be life-threatening like food-induced anaphylaxis.[10]

Food allergic reactions may be IgE-mediated, non-IgE-mediated, both IgE- and non-IgE mediated, or cell-mediated immune reactions, induced upon exposure to the allergenic food.

In Europe and most of the Western countries, 90% of the food allergic reactions are elicited due to exposure to one or more of the following commodities: milk, egg, wheat, soy, peanut, tree nut, shellfish, and fish.[11] However, the prevalence of food allergy is greatly influenced by age and dietary habits.

REGULATORY GUIDELINES FOR SAFETY ASSESSMENT OF TRANSGENIC PROTEINS

Protocols commonly used for safety assessment of GM food crops are drafted in compliance with internationally acclaimed guidelines released by the Organization for Economic Cooperation and Development (OECD),[12] Food and Agriculture Organization (FAO) of the United Nations/World Health Organization (WHO),[13] and the Codex Alimentarius Commission (Codex, 2003).[14]

For the first time, when the need to evaluate the safety of the GM crop was felt, it was compared to its native counterparts. The aim was to identify the differences between the two types of varieties (GM/non-GM), and whether the differences would account for any unintended allergies. Later, FAO and WHO in 1991 in a joint consultation proposed the idea of substantial equivalence (SE), and later in 1993 OECD further elaborated on the principles of "SE".[12] Joint FAO/WHO Expert Consultation on "Safety Aspects of Genetically Modified Foods of Plant Origin" proposed the usefulness of the concept of SE and concluded that "there were presently no alternative strategies that would provide a better assurance of safety of GM foods than the appropriate use of the concept of SE" measures whether the GM variety is safe as its traditional counterpart, if such counterpart exists or to an earlier approved variety. SE is evaluated on a scale of three, where one (1) refers to "complete", two (2) means "partial", and three (3) stands for "not at all". SE (1) implies that the GM food is similar to the native counterpart; (2) SE explains that GM food is substantially equivalent except for the inserted gene; and (3) "not at all" means that the GM food is not at all equivalent to its counterpart and a thorough evaluation of the transgenic food is mandatory.[15] However, the comparison of the GM and non-GM varieties is bound by certain limitations; like both the varieties should be grown under similar environmental conditions, and the choice of the statistical designs for field trials should be similar for both the varieties. A detailed safety assessment strategy involves a step-by-step evaluation of the transgenes expressed in the host plant.[16,17]

Most commonly used safety assessment protocols primarily evaluate the source of the transgenes, followed by bioinformatic studies to compare the transgenic protein sequences with the reported allergens. Depending on the results obtained for the preliminary tests, the transgenic protein is assessed for pepsin resistance (simulated gastric fluid digestion), thermal stability, and IgE binding with food allergic patients' sera (serum screening by ELISA).[18,19]

As per the decision tree approach proposed by FAO/WHO (2001) (Fig. 32.1), the weight of evidence approach by Codex (2003)[14] and guidelines given by ICMR (2008)[20] below are mentioned some of the parameters to be assessed for safety testing of GM crops:

Source of the Gene

Use of recombinant DNA technology for the development of GM food crops involves transfer of genes from a wide variety of organisms (donors). However, the conventional breeding programs involved crossing between closely related species or genera. Therefore, regulatory bodies have laid emphasis on evaluating the source of the transgene, because diversity in selection of the donor species may account for unforeseen allergenicity. Nordlee and group in 1996 reported that transgenic soybeans expressing 2S albumin (major allergen) protein from Brazil nut displayed allergenic properties. And this was one of the landmark studies emphasizing on the importance of evaluating the source of the transgene for developing GM food crops. Depending on the information available, transgene donors have been categorized as allergic/nonallergic or moderately allergic. Events where the GM food crops contain genes from sources with known allergenic properties, rigorous in vitro and in vivo safety testing procedures are employed to ensure safety of the GM product.[21]

In Silico Sequence Homology Studies

Allergens are proteins recognized by the immune system, and specific antibodies are generated in response to different proteins. Although, the human diet comprises several different types of proteins, but allergic reactions

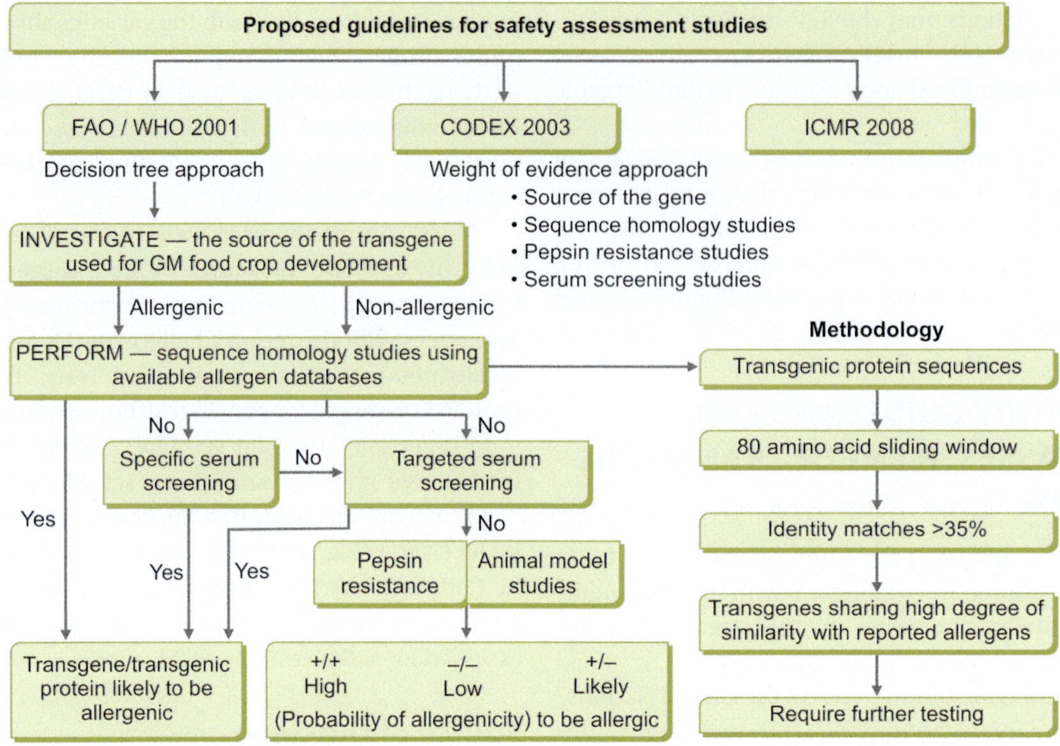

Fig. 32.1: Safety assessment guidelines used for GM food testing.

are elicited only for some specific proteins in predisposed individuals. Hence, it is interesting to know what renders the proteins as allergic/nonallergic. The presence of epitopes on the proteins accounts for allergenicity. Epitopes may be linear and/or conformational; these may be on the surface or cryptic. Therefore, in order to evaluate the allergenic potential of a novel protein, it is important to investigate epitopic regions on the protein structure.

Previous studies have reported that proteins sharing similarity among the primary and tertiary structures may also share cross-reactive epitopes.[22] And, these findings have formed the basis, for sequence homology studies, to be used for assessing potential allergenicity of novel proteins. A sequence homology study involves comparison of the primary amino acid sequence, of the novel protein with that of the reported allergens. BLAST[23] and FASTA[24] are the most commonly used alignment algorithms available online for bioinformatic studies. Both the algorithms predict functional similarity and clinically relevant cross-reactivity, on the basis of sequence similarity among proteins. Therefore, FAO/WHO (2001) and Codex (2003) proposed that greater than 35% identity over any stretch of 80 amino acids, between the GM protein and any reported allergen, depicts that the GM protein may act as an allergen and should be subjected to rigorous testing.[25,26]

Hileman and coworkers in 2002 reported that if proteins display significant linear sequence similarity, they may share three-dimensional structural motifs and cross-reactive epitopes.[27] Hence, high degree of similarity among protein sequences, i.e., transgenic protein and reported allergens, requires IgE serum screening studies, to further validate the safety of the protein in question.[28,29] Several allergen databases like Food Allergy Research and Resource Program (FARRP), Structural Database of Allergenic Protein (SDAP),[30] AlgPred,[31] EVALLER,[32] etc., are available online for homology studies.

Pepsin Resistance, in Vitro Digestibility Assay, and Thermal Stability

The FAO/WHO (2001), Codex Alimentarius (2003), and ICMR (2008) have proposed that transgenic proteins should be assessed for simulated gastric fluid (SGF)/intestinal fluid (SIF) digestibility and thermal stability before use in crop development. Thermal stability of food proteins is evaluated over a broad temperature range, i.e., 25–95°C for up to 60 minutes.[16] While SGF/SIF tests are designed to mimic the physiological conditions of gastric digestion and evaluate the allergenic potential of foreign proteins.

Several studies suggest that a correlation exists between the potential of a protein to act as an allergen and its resistance to SIF digestion, pepsin degradation, and thermal stability.[33] For example, food allergens that sensitize through the oral route demonstrate stability during gastric and/or intestinal digestion under physiological conditions.[34-36] Since, most of the foods are cooked (boiled, fried, roasted, baked, etc.) before consumption, therefore, heat labile proteins might not elicit allergic reactions, due to lack of potential epitopes. However, the reverse might be true for heat-stable proteins, as these might possess intact epitopic regions.

In addition, numerous reports have also demonstrated that this correlation is not an absolute parameter, and several proteins act differently, i.e., proteins resistant to pepsin degradation or stable at high temperatures might not be allergenic on interaction with the gut lining, while heat and/or pepsin labile proteins may act as allergens.[37-39]

Some of the commonly used food-processing techniques like refrigeration/freezing, canning, dehydration, freeze drying, pickling (salting), pasteurizing, fermentation, moist or dry heating,[40] etc., disrupts the 3D conformation of some of the food proteins. And this in turn affects the overall allergenicity of the foods,[41] due to loss of conformational epitopes, activation of new epitopes, or improving accessibility of cryptic epitopes.[42] However, sometimes, the processing methods may reduce antigenicity of the food proteins, for example, γ-irradiation has been reported to reduce the antigenicity of ovalbumin, bovine serum albumin, milk protein, and shrimp tropomyosin.[22,43,44]

IgE Serum Screening Studies

The "decision tree" and "weight of evidence" approaches proposed by FAO/WHO (2001) and Codex (2003), respectively, involve IgE serum screening studies for the safety assessment of transgenic proteins. If the transgenic proteins do not share significant sequence homology with any of the reported allergens, under such circumstances random serum screening studies might not be of any use. However, serum screening should be performed for proteins showing greater than 35% homology with the reported allergens. Two types of serum screening studies may be performed depending on the requirement,[45] i.e., specific or targeted serum screening.

- In case if the transgene is obtained from an allergic source, or the transgene shares homology with any of the reported allergens, specific serum screening is recommended by FAO/WHO (2001). Specific serum screening studies evaluate the IgE-binding potential of the transgenic protein, by ELISA, using patients' sera from individuals allergic to the source of the transgenic protein and/or individuals allergic to other sources sharing cross-reactive epitopes with the source of the transgenic protein. These findings will assess whether the allergen-specific IgE antibodies present in patients' sera react with the epitopes present on the novel proteins.[46]
- While targeted serum screening involves evaluating the IgE-binding potential of the transgenic protein by ELISA, using sera from individuals allergic to a broad range of allergens. For targeted serum screening studies, a wide range of allergen groups are taken into consideration, because the information in context to the source of transgene is limited (Table 32.1).

The major concern for conducting IgE serum-screening studies is lack of proper documentation of the serum donor and his/her clinical history.[47] If experiments demand the use of pooled serum, it is important to

Table 32.1: Information related to targeted serum screening studies, with reference to the type of transgene used and the appropriate sera sample required for the IgE screening.

Source of transgene	*Serum from individuals allergic to the following sources, for targeted serum screening studies*	
	Source	Examples
Monocot	Monocot allergens	Grass, rice, asparagus, onion, etc.
Dicot	Dicot allergens	Tree pollens, weed pollens, celery, peanuts, tree nuts, etc.
Fungi	Fungal allergens	*Alternaria*, *Cladosporium*, *Trichophyton*, etc.
Invertebrate	Invertebrate allergens	Mites, cockroaches, shrimps, chironomids, etc.
Vertebrate	Vertebrate allergens	Mammalian pets, laboratory animals, cow's milk, fish, egg white and chicken egg yolk/serum proteins, etc.

characterize individual serum samples before use. This will limit a sample from dominating over others and diluting the antibodies present in low abundance.[47] However, the gold standard method for food allergy testing till date remains—a positive response to oral food challenge, but is not commonly used for practical and ethical reasons.

Animal Model Studies

As per the FAO/WHO (2001) decision tree approach, the allergenic potential of transgenic proteins should be investigated by animal model studies, on obtaining positive results from IgE serum screening studies. Different animal models may be used for safety assessment studies like mice, rats, guinea pigs, atopic dogs, or neonatal swine.[48-50] For safety testing of transgenic proteins, food allergic conditions are developed in animal models by administering well-known allergens like ovalbumin, peanut allergens, etc. Followed by the administration of the transgenic proteins in varying concentrations (ranging from optimum to high) via different routes of sensitization like skin, oral, nasal, intraperitoneal, etc., symptoms are scored as per the immunization protocols. These models evaluate the allergic potency of the transgenic proteins on the basis of IgE production, Th-2 cytokine release, and clinical responses on re-exposure. Although, these studies have the potential to predict allergenicity of foreign proteins, however, these are only sensitization models and do not reflect all aspects of food allergies in humans.

Among the various animal models available, murine models are the most commonly used for food allergy-related studies. In addition to the numerous advantages associated with the use of murine models, a major drawback is that animals develop oral tolerance to the ingested protein and do not show allergic symptoms. However, oral tolerance can be avoided by the use of adjuvants like cholera toxin, etc.

Therefore, depending on the available scientific information, further studies are necessary to develop better animal models with improved immunization protocols, capable of predicting potential allergenicity of transgenic proteins, and imitating human food allergy conditions.

SUMMARY

Genetically modified crops are engineered with specific transgenes incorporated in the genome, to endow the host plant with enhanced characteristics like disease resistance, improved yield, biotic and abiotic stress tolerance, etc. Although classical breeding also aims at improving the crop characteristics by incorporating beneficial genes, however, the methodology followed is labor-intensive and time-taking. GM crops possess an edge over other conventionally developed varieties, but concern is raised against the safety of the foreign gene used for GM crop development.

Therefore, regulatory bodies have released guidelines for safety assessment of GM food crops. The foreign gene and/or the transgenic protein should be assessed for intended and unintended effects, immediate and long-term effects via animal model studies, etc. The current protocols used for allergenicity assessment of GM food crops are not completely predictive of the safety of the foreign proteins. Consequently, further refinement is required based on scientific research and findings. Future protocols should not only target safety assessment of foreign proteins, instead should also focus on limiting the use of allergenic components in development of GM crops.

Some of the nongovernment organizations and environmentalists hold an opinion that until there are validated and accepted methods for detection of potential allergenicity, there should be no further approvals of GM crops and foods, and existing approvals should be suspended. Rather than simply increasing the use of animal testing, which will not necessarily reflect human allergic reactions, there is a need to question the actual need for a GMO before the testing phase is reached. The need for the product must justify both the expense and the ethical issues involved in its testing.

REFERENCES

1. Huang J, Hu R, Rozelle S, Pray C. Insect-resistant GM Rice in farmers' fields: assessing productivity and health effects in China. Science. 2005;308:688-90.
2. Raman R. The impact of Genetically Modified (GM) crops in modern agriculture: a review. GM Crops Food. 2017;8(4):195-208.
3. Eizaguirre M, Albajes R, López C, et al. Six years after the commercial introduction of Bt maize in Spain: field evaluation, impact and future prospects. Transgenic Res. 2006;15:1-12.
4. Romeis J, Meissle M, Bigler, F. Transgenic crops expressing Bacillus thuringiensis toxins and biological control. Nat Biotechnol. 2006;24:63-71.
5. Singh AK, Singh BP, Prasad GB, et al. Safety assessment of bacterial choline oxidase protein introduced in transgenic crops for tolerance against abiotic stress. J Agric Food Chem. 2008;56:12099-104.

6. Lu M, Jin Y, Ballmer-Weber B, Goodman RE. A comparative study of human IgE binding to proteins of a genetically modified (GM) soybean and six non-GM soybeans grown in multiple locations. Food Chem Toxicol. 2018;12:216-23.
7. Andrew J, Ismail NW, Djama, M. An overview of genetically modified crop governance, issues and challenges in Malaysia. J Sci Food Agric. 2018;98:12-7.
8. Sicherer SH, Sampson HA. Food allergy: a review and update on epidemiology, pathogenesis, diagnosis, prevention, and management. J Allergy Clin Immunol. 2018;141(1):41-58.
9. Falcão H, Lunet N, Lopes C, Barros H. Food hypersensitivity in Portuguese adults. Eur J Clin Nutr. 2004;58:1621-5.
10. Allen KJ, Koplin JJ. The epidemiology of IgE-mediated food allergy and anaphylaxis. Immunol Allergy Clin North Am. 2012;32:35-50.
11. Sampson HA. Food allergy. Part 1: Immunopathogenesis and clinical disorders. J Allergy Clin Immunol. 1999;103: 717-28.
12. OECD. Safety evaluation of foods derived by modern biotechnology—concepts and principles. http://www.agbios.com/docroot/articles/oecd_fsafety_1993.pdf, 1993.
13. FAO/WHO. Evaluation of allergenicity of genetically modified foods. Report of a Joint FAO/WHO Expert Consultation on Foods Derived from Biotechnology, Food and Agriculture Organization of the United Nations/World Health Organization, Rome, Italy. January 22-5;2001.
14. Codex, Alinorm 03/34: Joint FAO/WHO Food Standard Programme, Codex Alimentarius Commission, Appendix III, Guideline for the conduct of food safety assessment of foods derived from recombinant-DNA plants (CAC/GL 45-2003), 25th Session, Rome, Italy, June 30-July 5; 2003:47-60.
15. Kuiper HA, Kleter GA, Noteborn HP, Kok EJ. Substantial equivalence*/an appropriate paradigm for the safety assessment of genetically modified foods. Toxicology. 2002;181-182:427-31.
16. Metcalfe DD, Astwood JD, Townsend R, et al. Assessment of the allergenic potential of foods derived from genetically engineered crop plants. Crit Rev Food Sci Nutr. 1996;36(Suppl):S165-86.
17. Panda R, Ariyarathna H, Amnuaycheewa P. Challenges in testing genetically modified crops for potential increases in endogenous allergen expression for safety. Allergy. 2013;68:142-51.
18. Mishra A, Sharma P, Goel C, et al. Allergenicity assessment of genetically modified foods. Int J Integr Biol. 2010;10:1-8.
19. Arora N, Mishra A. Safety assessment of genetically modified food crops. Indian J Allergy Asthma Immunol. 2011;25(2):53-60.
20. Indian Council of Medical Research. Indian guidelines on assessing GM crops. http://igmoris.nic.in/files%5CCoverpage.pdf; 2008.
21. Nordlee JA, Taylor SL, Townsend JA, et al. Identification of a Brazil-nut allergen in transgenic soybeans. N Engl J Med. 1996;334(11):688-92.
22. Byun MW, Lee JW, Yook HS, et al. Application of gamma irradiation for inhibition of food allergy. Radiat Phys Chem. 2002;63:369-70.
23. Altschul SF, Madden TL, Schäffer AA. Gapped BLAST and PSIBLAST: a new generation of protein database search programs. Nucleic Acids Res. 1997;25:3389-402.
24. Pearson WR, Lipman DJ. Improved tools for biological sequence comparison. Proc Natl Acad Sci USA. 1988; 85(8):2444-8.
25. Mishra A, Arora N. Allergenicity assessment of transgenic wheat lines in silico. Methods Mol Biol. 2017;1679:97-111.
26. Compton J, Fanning JB, Nickel, AS. Genetically modified products and food allergy: beliefs, evidence, and opportunity. Ann Allergy Asthma Immunol. 2017;119(3): 198-9.
27. Hileman RE, Silvanovich A, Goodman RE. Bioinformatic methods for allergenicity assessment using a comprehensive allergen database. Int Arch Allergy Immunol. 2002;128(4):280-91.
28. Goodman RE, Hefle SL. Gaining perspective on the allergenicity assessment of genetically modified food crops. Exp Rev Clin Immunol. 2005;1(4):561-78.
29. Mishra A, Gaur SN, Singh BP, Arora N. In silico assessment of the potential allergenicity of transgenes used for the development of GM food crops. Food Chem Toxicol. 2012;50(5):1334-9.
30. Ivanciuc O, Schein CH, Braun W. SDAP: database and computational tools for allergenic proteins. Nucleic Acids Res. 2003;31(1):359-62.
31. Saha S, Raghava GP. AlgPred: Prediction of allergenic proteins and mapping of IgE epitopes. Nucleic Acids Res. 2006;34:W202-9.
32. Barrio AM, Soeria-Atmadja D, Nistér A, et al. EVALLER: a web server for in silico assessment of potential protein allergenicity. Nucleic Acids Res. 2007;35(Web Server issue):W694-700.
33. Mishra A, Gaur SN, Lavasa S, Arora N. In vitro assessment of allergenicity features and localization of probable IgE-binding regions. Food Chem Toxicol. 2015;84:181-7.
34. Singh AK, Mehta AK, Sridhara S. Allergenicity assessment of transgenic mustard (*Brassica juncea*) expressing bacterial codA gene. Allergy. 2006;61:491-7.
35. Taylor SL, Lemanske RF Jr, Bush RK, Busse WW. Food allergens: structure and immunologic properties. Ann. Allergy. 1987;59:93-9.
36. Astwood JD, Leach JN, Fuchs RL. Stability of food allergens to digestion in vitro. Nat Biotechnol. 1996;14:1269-73.
37. Bannon GA, Goodman RE, Leach JN, et al. Digestive stability in the context of assessing the potential allergenicity of food proteins. Comments Toxicol. 2002;8:271-85.
38. Fu TJ. Digestion stability as a criterion for protein allergenicity assessment. Ann NY Acad Sci. 2002;964:99-110.
39. Fu TJ, Abbott UR, Hatzos C. Digestibility of food allergens and nonallergenic proteins in simulated gastric fluid and simulated intestinal fluid—a comparative study. J Agric Food Chem. 2002;50(24):7154-60.

40. Sathe SK, Teuber SS, Roux KH. Effects of food processing on the stability of food allergens. Biotechnol Adv. 2005;23:423-9.
41. Besler M, Steinhart H, Paschke A. Allergens of animal origin: stability and allergenicity of processed foods. Int Symp on Food Allergens. 2000;2(4):171-84, http://www.food-allergens.de.
42. Hefle SL. Impact of processing on food allergens. Adv Exp Med Biol. 1999;459:107-19.
43. Kume T, Matsuda T. Changes in structural and antigenic properties of proteins by radiation. Radiat Phys Chem. 1995;46:225-31.
44. Lee JW, Kim JH, Yook HS, et al. Effects of gamma radiation on the allergenic and antigenic properties of milk proteins. J Food Prot. 2001;64:272-6.
45. Poulsen LK. Allergy assessment of foods or ingredients derived from biotechnology, gene modified organism, or novel foods. Mol Nutr Food Res. 2004;48:413-23.
46. Taylor SL, Hefle SL. Genetically engineered foods: Implications for food allergy. Curr Opin Allergy Clin Immunol. 2002;2(3):249-52.
47. Goodman RE. Performing IgE serum testing due to bioinformatics matches in the allergenicity assessment of GM crops. Food Chem Toxicol. 2008;46:S24-34.
48. Penninks AH, Knippels LM. Determination of protein allergenicity: studies in rats. Toxicol Lett. 2001;120 (1-3):171-80.
49. Van Gramberg JL, de Veer MJ, O'Hehir RE, et al. Use of animal models to investigate major allergens associated with food allergy. J Allergy (Cairo). 2013;2013: 635-95.
50. Bøgh KL, van Bilsen J, Głogowski R, et al. Current challenges facing the assessment of the allergenic capacity of food allergens in animal models. Clin Transl Allergy. 2016;6:21.

CHAPTER 33

Insects as Source of Inhalant Allergens

MK Agarwal, Shashi Chawla

INTRODUCTION

The etiologic significance of various airborne particles in type I allergy of respiratory system was first demonstrated by Sir Charles Harrison Blackley in 1873. Subsequent clinical studies established significance of these bioparticles derived from pollen, fungi, animal danders, etc. as inhalant allergens. Besides these, emanations and detritus of insects may also induce allergic response in susceptible individuals. The estimated number of insect species in the world ranges from 625,000 to 1,500,000. However, very few studies are available on the etiologic significance of insects in type I respiratory disorders. Till 1956, most of the studies were case reports only. Feinberg (1956), Perlman (1961, 1965), and Osgood (1957) were among the early workers who undertook systematic studies on the subject.[1] They performed skin tests with insect whole body extracts (WBEs) on patients suffering with asthma, rhinitis, dermatitis, and conjunctivitis, and also on nonallergic healthy volunteers (NHVs). They observed a larger number of positive skin reactions in allergic subjects than in NHVs. Their results suggested that the incidence of respiratory allergy to insects was much higher than that to pollen, fungal, and other allergens. Bellas (1982) implicated insect species from at least 12 orders in type I respiratory allergic disorders.[2] However, many of these reports are case histories, and thus provide little information on the nature of sensitizing insect components or on the mechanisms underlying the adverse reactions.

The insects release scales and other emanations on flying and detritus on death, which may become airborne and trigger allergic response on genetically predisposed individuals (Fig. 33.1). Yet, the role of insect-derived material as inhalant allergens did not get adequate attention for a long time. The reasons for ignoring the role of insects in nasobronchial allergy were (i) difficulty in their identification, (ii) their varying diurnal and seasonal patterns, and (iii) inability to detect atmospheric dispersion of insect emanations. However, the most important reason was the inability to demonstrate and quantify the presence of insect-derived allergens in respirable-size particles in the air. In 1981, Agarwal et al. developed an immunochemical technique, which proved to be an important tool to not only demonstrate the presence of various allergens in the air (including amorphous allergens such as insect emanations and debris) but also quantify all these aeroallergens.[3] Since then comprehensive, systematic studies have been conducted on the role of insects as source of inhalant allergens. The technique involves the collection of airborne particles by sucking the air through a filter sheet (mounted on an air suction sampler) and elution of the particles trapped on these filters. These elutions were used in RAST/ELISA inhibition assays, using solid-phase insect allergens, to quantify different airborne insect allergens. The aeroprevalence of various insects studied using this technique is described later.

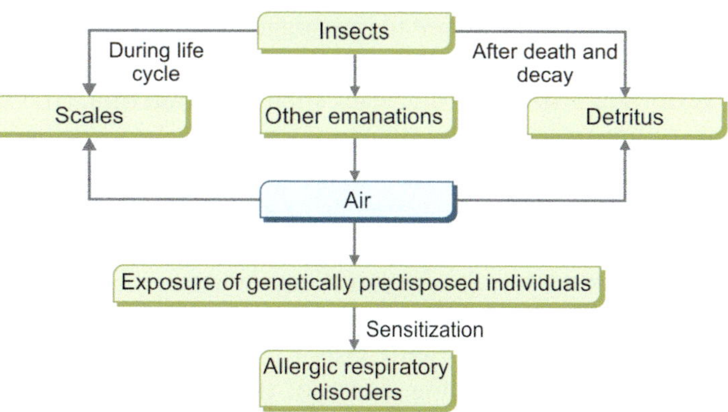

Fig. 33.1: Insect emanations and debris can serve as source of inhalant allergens.

The prevalence and severity of respiratory allergies is on the rise in most of the countries due to pollution, changes in climatic conditions, etc. It is a well-established fact that respiratory allergy is a local problem. Depending on the local flora and fauna, aeroallergens differ from place to place both qualitatively and quantitatively. Thus, for proper diagnosis and treatment of respiratory allergy, patients of a particular geographical area, regular monitoring of various local allergens, and study of their prevalence and seasonal distribution are important. In India, the field of research in respiratory allergy remained unexplored for a long time as allergy was considered to be a malady confined only to the temperate regions of the world. However, studies conducted in the last few decades in India have found the incidence of type I respiratory allergic disorders in our country to be quite high. In India, research on aeroallergens was initiated in the 1960s. Initial studies were mainly confined to study the allergenic significance of pollen, fungal spores, animal danders, and dust allergens. Like other countries, the role of insects as source of inhalant allergens in India also remained a subject of debate. The research on the identification of causative insect allergens in patients with bronchonasal disorders and their treatment by immunotherapy was initiated by Shivpuri, Agarwal et al. in 1969 at the Vallabhbhai Patel Chest Institute, Delhi.[4] Since then, extensive research has been conducted on the subject, and lots of information have been generated.

INSECT-DERIVED INHALANT ALLERGENS IN INDIA

1969–1980: Phase of Preliminary Studies

During initial phase from 1969 to 1985, a few preliminary studies were undertaken to investigate the role of insects as inhalant allergens. All these studies were based only on various in vivo diagnostic tests, such as intradermal (ID) test, Prausnitz-Kustner (PK) test, bronchial provocation test (BPT), and conjunctival test. However, no in vitro test was used to detect the presence of insect-specific IgE in the sera of patients. Shivpuri et al. (1969) published the first report on the role of insect allergens in nasobronchial allergy.[4] WBEs of 16 common insects of Delhi area were tested on 507 patients with nasobronchial disorders and 16 NHVs. On ID testing, 34.9% of the patients elicited positive (1+ to 4+) reactions, with 17.6% being markedly positive (2+ to 4+). In NHVs, such reactions were obtained only in 4.5% and 0.7% cases, respectively. The 2+ to 4+ skin reactions in patients varied from 5.5% with honeybee (*Apis indica*) to 29.7% with ladybird beetle, *Coccinella septempunctata* (Table 33.1). The positive skin tests were confirmed by performing other in vivo tests namely PK test, BPT, and conjunctival test. A direct association was found between the intensity of positive ID reactions and positivity rate of BPT, conjunctival test, and PK test. In 1971, same group reported the results of another study using 22 insect WBEs.[5] Of the 11,269 ID tests performed with these extracts on 1,078 patients having nasobronchial allergy, 19.6% showed 2+ to 4+ ID reactions, varying from 6.9% with khapra beetle (*Trogoderma granarium*) to 30.7% with red pumpkin beetle (*Aulacophora foveicollis*) extracts as against 3.9% in NHVs (Table 33.1). Of the other in vivo tests on the patients showing different grades of positive skin reactions (1+ to 4+), 55% BPT, 59.8% conjunctival test, and 82.1% PK test were found to be positive (Table 33.2). All these tests were uniformly negative on patients showing negative ID reactions as well as on NHVs.

Shali, Agarwal and Shivpuri (1970) also reported the presence of some sex-specific allergens and antigens in cockroach (*Periplaneta americana*).[6] Of the 410 patients tested, 37% (152) patients showed positive response to both the extracts, whereas 13.4% and 10.7% elicited positive response exclusively to female and male cockroach WBEs, respectively. In accordance with the results of ID tests, BPTs, conjunctival test, and PK test on patients were positive to either both or only one (any one) of the two WBEs. Four patients eliciting positive ID response to both the extracts were administered immunotherapy with only one of these extracts. On retesting, after 10–18 months of immunotherapy, the cutaneous reactivity reduced significantly with the putative extract while it remained unaltered to the other extract. These results supported the presence of sex-specific allergens in cockroach.

Saha et al. (1977)[7] successfully used monkey ileum sensitization test for demonstrating the presence of insect-specific regains in the sera of patients with allergic bronchial asthma. During this time, some more studies on insect allergy based only on ID tests were reported from different parts of India.[8-11] A high incidence of 2+ to 4+ reactions to insect allergens (29.5%) was reported in one such study from Andhra Pradesh, and no correlation was found between house dust and cockroach allergy.[8]

Table 33.1: Intradermal test results with insect whole blood extracts on patients and nonallergic healthy volunteers (NHVs) reported in different studies.

Study		*Patients*			*NHVs*		
		*TTD**	*1+ to 4+*	*2+ to 4+*	*TTD**	*1+ to 4+*	*2+†*
Shivpuri et al. (1969)	No.	5,101	1,780	897	288	13	2
	%		34.9	17.6		4.5	0.7
Shivpuri et al. (1969)	No.	11,269	4,327	2,209	725	98	29
	%		38.4	19.6		13.5	3.9
Chaudhry (1988)	No.	2,929	1,356	701	600	67	12
	%		46.3	23.9		11.2	2
Gupta et al. (1990)	No.	892	247	92	240	17	0
	%		27.7	10.2		7.1	0
Jhamb et al. (1992)	No.	2,508	1,467	1,006	1,000	21	0
	%		58.5	40.1		2.1	0

*Total tests done.
†None of the NHVs showed a 3+ or 4+ reactions.

Table 33.2: Results of various in vivo tests with insect whole body extracts on patients showing different grades of ID responses in different studies.

		Bronchial provocation test			*Conjunctival test*			*Prausnitz–Kustner test*		
	ID	*TTD*	*Positive*		*TTD*	*Positive*		*TTD*	*Positive*	
Study	*response*		*No.*	*%*		*No.*	*%*		*No.*	*%*
Shivpuri et al. (1969)	1+	11	2	18.2	14	1	7.1	1	0	0.0
	2+	34	21	61.8	49	17	34.7	16	16	100
	3+	35	27	77.1	48	37	77.1	27	25	92.6
	4+	22	17	77.3	33	30	90.9	24	24	100
	1+ to 4+	102	67	65.7	144	85	59.0	68	65	95.6
	2+ to 4+	91	65	71.4	130	84	64.6	67	67	97.0
Shivpuri et al. (1971)	1+	17	3	17.6	17	1	6.0	3	0	0.0
	2+	61	27	44.3	60	25	41.7	40	31	77.5
	3+	54	36	66.7	56	42	75.0	41	36	87.8
	4+	28	22	78.6	36	33	91.7	28	25	89.3
	1+ to 4+	160	88	55.0	169	101	59.8	112	92	82.1
	2+ to 4+	143	85	59.4	152	100	65.8	109	92	84.4

None of these tests were positive in NHVs and patients eliciting negative intradermal response.
ID, intradermal.

In brief, studies undertaken during 1969–1980 suggested that (1) insects played an important role in the etiology of respiratory allergic disorders, (2) the two sexes of the cockroach possessed some shared and a few sex-specific allergenic components, and (3) there was an urgent need to develop an in vitro method for enumeration of insect allergen-specific IgE in the serum of patients.

Studies Conducted in 1980 Onward: Phase of Comprehensive, Systematic Studies

In 1980, Shivpuri observed a high frequency of 3+ and 4+ ID reactions with 22 insect WBEs on patients.[12] Based on these results, he shortlisted only six insects to be clinically important: mosquito, ant, light moth, rice weevil, cockroach, and wheat beetle. He recommended that other insect extracts should not be tested on patients as these were producing false-positive skin reactions due to the presence of some irritants or histamine-releasing substances. However, he did not use any control group of NHVs in this study to substantiate his observations. To address this problem of high frequency of 3+ and 4+ reactions with insect WBEs, Gaur et al. (1985) performed ID tests with 19 insect WBEs in 10-fold serial dilutions (1:500, 1:5,000, 1:50,000 w/v) on 30 patients suffering with nasobronchial allergy and also on 10 NHVs.[13] On an average, 32.5% markedly positive reactions (2+ to 4+) were observed in the patients with 1:500 w/v dilution as against 4.2% in the NHVs. None of the NHVs showed a 3+ or 4+ skin response to any of the three test dilution of the insect's WBE. These results did not support the observations of Shivpuri (1980). It was recommended that 1:500 w/v dilution was appropriate for routine ID testing and that the significantly positive cutaneous reactions should be retested on the same day, preferably in serial dilutions.

One common observation from the abovementioned studies was that all the test insect extracts elicited a high percentage of markedly positive (2+ to 4+) ID reactions in the patients with nasobronchial disorders. However, there were several lacunae in these studies which are as follows:

- In some studies, the insects were investigated only on the basis of their vernacular names. The vernacular names of several insects may be the same while their genera, species, and allergenic properties may differ.
- The WBEs were prepared by killing and then drying the insects at 40°C. This might have denatured some thermolabile allergenic components of insect WBEs.
- The results of these studies were based only on in vivo tests, mostly skin tests. No attempts were made to enumerate the circulating insect allergen-specific IgE levels.
- The presence of airborne insect-derived particles was not demonstrated. Hence, patient's exposure to insect aeroallergens could not be substantiated.

Therefore, a series of comprehensive, systematic studies were undertaken on this subject at VP Chest Institute, University of Delhi. The insects studied were zoologically identified, the method for the preparation of WBEs was modified, and insect WBE-specific IgE levels were estimated in the serum of patients. Besides, the presence of small-sized insect-derived allergenic particles in the air was studied, and attempts were made to identify and characterize allergenic and antigenic components of various insect WBEs.

Allergenic Significance of Insects

The first and the foremost prerequisite for studying the etiologic significance of insects as inhalant allergens was to modify the method of allergen extract preparation. For this purpose, the WBEs of various insects were prepared by both the conventional and modified methods. The conventional method involved killing and drying of insects at 40°C, defatting in solvent ether, extraction in phosphate-buffered saline, and dialysis.[5] The modified method involved rapid killing in liquid nitrogen, drying by lyophilization, defatting, extraction in 100 mM ammonium bicarbonate (NH_4HCO_3), dialysis, and lyophilization.[14] The extracts prepared by the modified method gave similar, if not higher, percentage of 2+ to 4+ ID reactions in patients compared to the extracts prepared by the conventional method. The prevalence of positive ID tests in NHVs was very low with the WBEs prepared by both the methods. Hence, subsequent studies were conducted with WBEs prepared by the modified method.

Chaudhry (1988) conducted systematic study on the clinicoimmunologic properties of nine zoologically identified insects including cockroaches (male and female), housefly, locust (male and female), mosquitoes, and moths.[14] The results of 2,929 ID tests on 350 patients and 600 ID tests on 52 controls with these extracts (1:500 w/v) showed that 23.9% (n = 701) reactions in the patients were significantly positive, 6.7% being 3+ or 4+ ID responses (Table 33.1). The 2+ to 4+ ID responses ranged from 12.0% with *Heliothis armigera* (a moth) to 31.0% with *Anopheles stephensi* (mosquito) WBEs. In healthy controls, there were no 3+ and 4+ skin responses, and only 2.0% of the tests turned out to be positive (1+ and 2+). The specificity of intradermal reactions to some insect allergens (*P. americana* male and female, and *A. stephensi*) was confirmed by performing RASTs for estimating the circulating insect allergen-specific IgE in the sera of patients showing different grades of ID responses. Elevated levels of allergen-specific IgE were observed in 89.4% and 95.0% of the sera from patients eliciting 1+ to 4+ and 2+ to 4+ cutaneous responses to allergens, respectively. Both RAST positivity and average RAST ratio increased with the increase in skin response to various insect WBEs. The sera from NHVs and patients eliciting negative ID response to insect WBEs were RAST negative (Table 33.3).

Table 33.3: Summarized RAST results with the sera of patients showing different grades of skin response to insect whole blood extracts.

Study	*Intradermal response*	*TTD*	*Positive RAST No.*	*%*	*Average RAST ratio*
Chaudhry (1988)	−ve	11	1	9.1	2.33
	1+ to 4+	47	42	89.4	14.82
	2+ to 4+	39	37	95.0	16.60
Jhamb et al. (1992)	−ve	40	0	0.0	1.14
	1+ to 4+	794	578	72.9	7.70
	2+ to 4+	626	501	80.0	9.04

In 1990, Gupta et al. tested WBEs of 13 common insects from Delhi, India, on 75 asthmatics.[15] These extracts produced 10.2% 2+ to 4+ responses on intradermal testing in patients as against none in control group. BPTs on patients giving positive ID tests with the insect WBEs were positivity 61.5% of the cases. Similarly, RASTs were positivity 87.5% of the sera tested from patients with positive ID responses to insect extracts. These results established the role of insects as source of inhalant allergens in asthmatics in India. In addition, the authors also analyzed the skin reactivity of the patients with their clinical characteristics. It was found that the skin positivity (1+ to 4+) to insect WBEs was significantly higher ($p < 0.01$) in asthmatics (i) at an early age of the onset of the disease (<20 years), (ii) having seasonal periodicity of asthma, (iii) in the presence of an associated allergic disorders such as allergic rhinitis and eczema, and (iv) with positive family history of allergic disorders. The cutaneous response to insect allergens was not affected by the duration of the disease. These results showed that ID test positivity to insects has a significant bearing on the clinical characteristics of these patients.

In 1992, in another study, the total skin test positivity (1+ to 4+) in the patients with nasobronchial disorders using the insect WBEs turned out to be 58.4%. Of these, 40.1% were 2+ to 4+ reactions.[16] None of the NHVs elicited positive response to these extracts establishing the specificity of significantly positive ID reactions. Sera of patients showing 2+ to 4+ cutaneous reactions exhibited 80.0% RAST positivity. Further, each extract produced dose-related inhibition of homologous RASTs giving evidence for specificity of the RAST assays.

Studies conducted after 2000 used skin prick tests (SPTs) instead of ID tests.[17,18] One such study reported average SPT positivity as 27.2%, with various insect WBEs of 1:20 w/v dilution. Insect allergen-specific IgEs

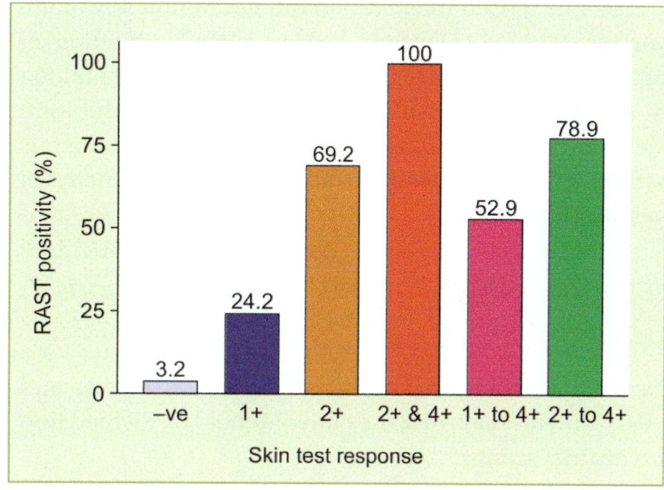

Fig. 33.2: Bar chart showing correlation between skin prick test response and RAST positivity.

were demonstrated by RAST in the sera of 52.9% patients showing various grades of positive SPT response (1+ to 4+). Sera of patients showing 2+ to 4+ SPT response exhibited 78.4% RAST positivity while those with 3+ and 4+ responses were 100% RAST positive. However, 3.2% positive RASTs were also obtained with the sera of patients showing negative cutaneous response to the WBEs, suggesting the presence of a few false-negative SPT response (Fig. 33.2).

The results of all these studies conclusively established the etiologic significance of insect WBEs in nasobronchial disorders in India. Both the frequency and the intensity of positive skin responses to insect WBEs were found to be very high compared to pollen, fungal, and animal dander allergens.

Aeroprevalence of Insect-derived Allergens

Using the immunochemical technique, aeroallergens derived from mosquito, butterfly, housefly, and sugarcane leafhopper were quantified in the air of Delhi area.

Seasonal variations were observed in the amount of these airborne allergens, which varied from insect to insect.[18,19] Figure 33.3 depicts a graphical representation of varying amounts of airborne allergens derived from mosquito, *Culex quinquefasciatus*, over a year from September 2004 to August 2005 (Table 33.4). The specificity of the immunochemical technique was checked by (i) using unexposed filter elution as negative control in each RAST and (ii) performing ELISA inhibition assays with varying amounts of a pool of filter elutions of the air samples exhibiting high concentration of the allergen being quantified.

The unexposed filter elution did not inhibit any of the four insect RASTs. Further, a dose-related inhibition of sugarcane leafhopper and butterfly RASTs was obtained by the pooled atmospheric elutions. These inhibition lines were parallel to those obtained with the homologous extracts.[16,19] These results established the specificity of these RAST assays.

Heterogeneity of Patients' Immune Response to Insect WBEs

Jhamb et al.[19] observed that on the basis of ID tests and RASTs with insect WBEs, the patients could be divided into two distinct groups:

- Group 1: Patients who were selectively positive to a limited number of insect WBEs.
- Group 2: Those positive to most of the insect extracts.

These results suggested that the immune responses against insect allergens varied in different patients. This heterogeneity in immune response was further investigated by performing inhibition of cricket RAST with two separate anti-cricket sera pools prepared from the abovementioned two groups (groups 1 and 2) of patients. The inhibition lines produced in the two systems varied in both their positions and slopes, suggesting that there was heterogeneity in patients' immune response to insect WBEs.

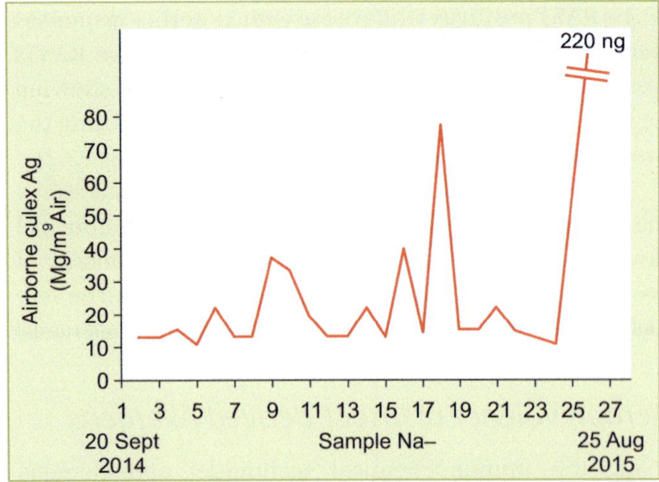

Fig. 33.3: Graph showing seasonal variation in immunochemically quantified airborne mosquito allergen (*Culex* sp.) in different months.

Table 33.4: Results of immunochemical quantitation of insect-derived aeroallergens.

Insect aeroallergen		
	Range of allergen content (ηg/m³)	*Peak season(s)*
Mosquito	0–220	April–May, July
Housefly	0–58	Not available
Butterfly	0–176	Jan–Feb, May–June, Aug–Sept
Moth	0–220	Jan–Feb, Aug–Dec

Immunoblot experiments using WBEs of mosquito (*Cq*) and cockroach performed with the sera of patient to study the heterogeneity in patients' immune response to different allergenic components of these insect allergens (Figs. 33.4A and B).[17,18,20]

These immunoblots revealed several IgE-stained bands with each patient's serum indicating that each serum contained IgE antibodies against multiple allergenic components of the insect WBE (Figs. 33.4A to C). The profile of these stained bands varied from patient to patient suggesting that sensitivity to different allergenic components varied from patient to patient. In other words, there was a gross heterogeneity of immune response in patients hypersensitive to these two insect extracts.

Shared or Specific Allergenic and Antigenic Components among Insect WBEs

Comprehensive studies were undertaken to study the presence of cross-reacting and/or specific allergenic and antigenic components among different insect WBEs. Since mosquitoes and cockroaches are among the most common insects in the environment of Delhi area, their extracts were evaluated for the presence of shared or species-specific allergenic components.[14,18,20,21] Three prevalent species of mosquitoes studied were *Aedes aegypti (Aa)*, *A. stephensi (As)*, and *C. quinquefasciatus (Cq)*. The two species of cockroaches investigated were *P. americana (Pa)* and *Blattella germanica (Bg)*.

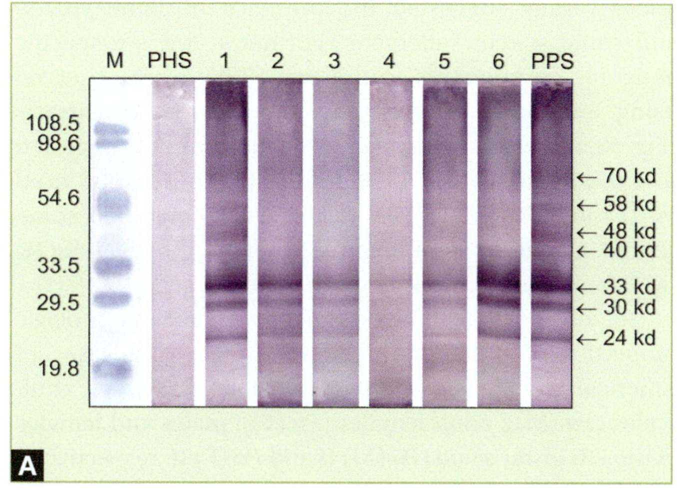

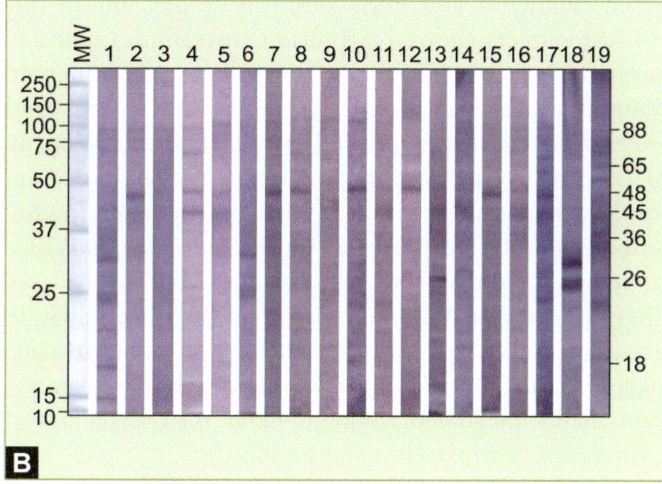

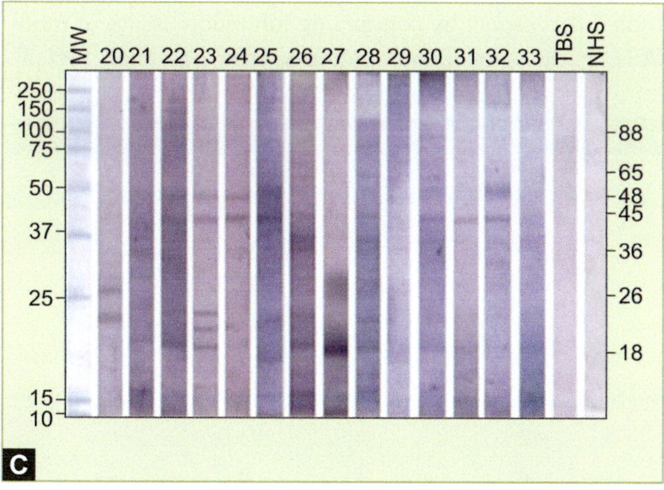

Figs. 33.4A to C: IgE western blots of (A) mosquito and (B) cockroach male extract with pooled patient's serum (PPS) and serum of each of 6 and 32 patients, respectively, exhibiting heterogeneity of immune response.

Allergens in different genera of mosquitoes: On skin testing with *Aa* and *As* WBEs on 26 patients who were SPT positive to *Cq* extract, 73.1% (19) of them elicited positive responses to both the heterologous extracts and 3 each to *Aa* or *As* extract only. Remaining one patient had exclusively positive results to *Cq* WBE. These results suggested the presence of cross-reacting allergens in the three species of mosquitoes.[14] This observation was further supported by the results of RAST inhibition and immunoblot experiments.[20] In *Cq* RASTs, homologous (*Cq*) as well as the two heterologous mosquito WBEs (*Aa and As*) produced dose-related inhibition. Slopes of the inhibition lines obtained with the two heterologous extracts were not significantly different from those of the homologous extract ($p > 0.05$). There was no much difference in the quantity of the three mosquito WBEs required for 50% inhibition of *Cq* RASTs (1.08 mg for *Cq*, 0.97 mg for *Aa*, and 1.4 mg for *As*). However, no significant inhibition of *Cq* ELISA was produced by eight non-related allergen extracts.

In immunoblot experiments using pooled patient's serum for *Cq* and the three mosquito extracts, two IgE-binding major allergenic proteins of *Cq* extract (30 and 33 kDa) were also detected in *Aa* and *As* WBEs (Fig. 33.5). When PPS (*Cq*) was incubated with homologous solid-phase allergen, the supernatant failed to show any IgE-binding proteins in immunoblots with the three mosquito WBEs. These results provided evidence that 30 and 33 kDa proteins were shared among the three mosquito WBEs.[20]

Allergens in different genera of cockroaches: A systematic study on the presence of shared and specific allergenic components in different genera of cockroaches was conducted by Chaudhry (1988).[14] On ID testing on patients, the WBEs of *Pa* (F), *Pa* (M), *Bg* (F), and *Bg* (M) produced 30.2%, 26.2%, 16.2%, and 26.4% 2+ to 4+ skin reactions, respectively. When compared, the ID test results of *Pa* (F) with *Bg* (F) and *Bg* (M) with *Pa* (M); with *Bg* (F) and *Bg* (F), there were many patients who showed positive response to both the extracts and some who were positive to only one of the two extracts compared (Table 33.5). These results suggested that both shared as well as genera-specific allergenic components were present in cockroaches also. This observation was supported by the inhibition of *Pa* (F) RAST with different cockroach WBEs. Even though both the homologous as well as heterologous extracts produced dose-related inhibition, only 2.5 µg of the homologous WBE produced 50% inhibition while much higher dose (40 µg) of the heterologous WBEs was required to get similar inhibition. These results indicated

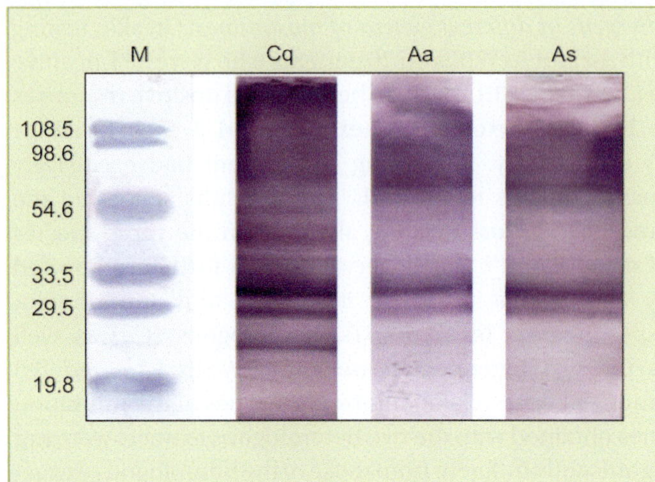

Fig. 33.5: Immunoblot of the whole blood extracts of three species of mosquitoes with pooled patient serum against *Cq*.

that the quantity of shared allergenic component(s) was much less in heterologous extract.

Allergens and antigens in different maturation stages and sexes of cockroaches: The presence of unique allergenic components among the cockroach male and female extracts was initially suggested by Shali et al. in 1969.[6] However, Chaudhry et al. (1990) investigated this subject in detail.[22] Of the 170 subjects skin tested with *Pa* (F) and *Pa* (M) WBEs, 52 showed markedly positive reactions to only one (n = 32; 22 to *Pa* female, 10 to *Pa* male) or both (n = 20; 13 showed identical, and seven varying grades of ID positivity) the extracts tested. On RAST inhibition, both the extracts produced dose-related inhibition of *Pa* male as well as *Pa* female RASTs. However, the slopes and position of inhibition curves were different (Fig. 33.3). These results suggested the presence of some shared and some specific allergens. Further, a few sex-specific antigenic components in the two WBEs were observed using antibodies to *Pa* male and *Pa* female extracts (Fig. 33.4). Results of partial purification studies suggested that the fractions *Pa* (F) Ill and *Pa* (M) m isolated from *Pa* (F) and *Pa* (M) WBEs, respectively, contained some shared allergenic components, whereas the fraction *Pa* (M) I had unique components of male extract.

Jhamb et al. (1992) investigated the clinicoimmunologic properties of different maturation stages and sexes of American cockroach (*Periplaneta americana*), i.e., adult males (*Pa* (M)); adult females (*Pa* (F)); males and females of the 7th instar stage (*Pa* (M) II and *Pa* (F) II, respectively) and the 2nd instar insects (*Pa* nymph).[16] Statistical analysis of the cutaneous and RAST positivity to any one of the two test extracts showed significant correlation in all the comparisons, the best correlations being in different maturation stages ($r > 0.69$). *Pa* (F) as well as the four heterologous extracts produced dose-related inhibition of *Pa* (F) RAST. However, the inhibition curves varied in positions and slopes. In TDIEP experiments using rabbit antibodies to *Pa* (M) and *Pa* (F), the homologous WBEs produced 20 and 32 precipitin peaks, respectively. The other heterologous WBFs also produced a large number of precipitin peaks with these rabbit antibodies. All these results suggested that a large number of allergenic and antigenic components are shared among different maturation stages and sexes of *Pa* while a few may be specific.

Allergens of different genera of insects: Gupta S further studied this aspect by conducting inhibition assays of moth RAST using sera of four patients, who had high SPT as

Table 33.5: ID test results with Pa (F) and Bg (F) and (M) WBEs on respiratory allergy patients.

Patients showing positive reactions	Pa *(F) vs.* Bg *(M) (*n = *140)*		Pa *(F) vs.* Bg *(F)* (n = *166)*	
	No.	*%*	*No.*	*%*
To only one extract	35	68.6	34	68.0
P. americana	20	39.2	26	52.0
B. germanica	15	29.4	8	16.0
To both the extracts	16	31.4	16	32.0
Identical	7	13.7	12	24.0
Nonidentical	9	17.6	4	8.0
Total	51		50	

*Similar results were obtained on comparison of ID test results of *Pa* (M) WBE with those of *Bg* (M) and *Bg* (F) extracts.
ID, intradermal; WBE, whole blood extracts.

well as RAST positivity to moth extract.[17] Besides, all these patients were SPT and RAST positive to varying number of other WBEs of housefly, cockroach male, and cockroach female. The results obtained are summarized as follows:

- Only homologous extract and none of the three heterologous extracts produced significant inhibition of moth RAST with the serum of a patient (SG-34) who was exclusively positive to moth WBE.
- All the three heterologous insect extracts including housefly failed to produce significant inhibition using the serum of patient SG-28 (positive to moth and housefly).
- With the serum of patient SG-172 (positive to moth, housefly, and cockroach male), significant dose-related inhibition was produced only by moth and housefly WBEs, and
- Using the serum of another patient SG-35, who was highly allergic to all the four WBEs, homologous as well as all the three heterologous WBEs produced significant dose-related inhibition.

The results of the above inhibition assays of moth RAST performed with the sera of four patients suggested that (i) patient SG-34 is allergic to some specific allergenic components of the moth extract, (ii) patient SG-28 may have sensitivity to some specific allergenic components in the two insects: moth and housefly, (iii) patient SG-172 is likely to be allergic to some shared allergenic components of moth and housefly and also to some specific component of cockroach (male) extract, and (iv) patient SG-35 was hypersensitive to some cross-reacting allergenic components present in all the four insect extracts. These results indicate the need for proper evaluation of each patient before immunotherapy.

Stability of Insect WBEs

The biological activity of an extract depends on its extraction procedure (discussed earlier) and storage conditions. Since each extract has its own biochemical composition, the optimum conditions required for proper storage of various allergen extracts would vary. In 1990, for the first time in India, an attempt was made to study the stability of lyophilized insect WBEs when stored at different temperatures. The cockroach female extract was found to be biologically active at 4°, 37°, and 56°C for 15 months. It was recommended that in lyophilized form it need not be stored at –20°C or 4°C. Instead, it can be kept at room temperature for at least 15 months. The housefly extract, on the other hand, retained its allergenic activity for 12 months when stored at 4°C and lost it rapidly at 37°C and 56°C.[16]

Immunotherapy with Insect Allergen Extracts

Eighty-five patients of asthma or rhinitis or both completed a double-blind placebo-controlled trial of mix and single allergen immunotherapy (IT) for 1 year.[23] There were two groups: (i) active allergen IT ($n = 61$) with three subgroups single insect extract (cockroach, housefly, or mosquito) and mix allergen IT (two or three insect extracts) and (ii) placebo ($n = 38$). The active allergen IT group patients showed a significant improvement compared to baseline values ($p < 0.05$) and placebo group patients ($p < 0.05$) with regard to symptom scores, FEV_1 values, and immunological parameters (IgG4). No significant difference was found between mixed and single IT group patients for changes in clinical and immunological parameters. Positive correlation was observed between increase in IgG4 and clinical improvement. The changes in the abovementioned parameters in the placebo group were nonsignificant after 1 year of treatment. IT with two to three mix extracts from the same allergen group is effective for insect hypersensitivity.

In brief, the results of the abovementioned clinico-immunologic and immunochemical studies have revealed that insects constitute the most important group of inhalant allergens. They contribute substantial amount of clinically important allergens to air. There is heterogeneity of immune response in patients with respiratory allergic disorders to different allergenic components of various WBEs. Some patients exhibit allergy to a large number of insects, whereas others show allergy to a limited number of insects. Insects contain both cross-reacting as well as unique allergenic components in different genera, species, sexes, and maturation stages. Shelf life of each insect WBE varies and needs to be worked out. Even though immunotherapy seems to be effective for insect allergy, the development of standardized extracts without any batch-to-batch or manufacturer-to-manufacturer variations is need of the hour. Thus, the quest for further research in the field of insect-derived allergens needs to be continued.

REFERENCES

1. Agarwal MK, Chawla S. Etiologic significance of environmental insects in IgE mediated naso-bronchial disorders in India: an over view. In: Proceedings of 2nd International Symposium on Molecular Medicine. Baroda, India; January 20-23, 2002:121-40.

2. Bellas TE. Insects as a cause of inhalant allergens: a bibliography. CSIRO Division of Entomology Report No. 25, 1982.
3. Agarwal MK, Yunginger JW, Swanson MC, Reed CE. An immunochemical method to measure atmospheric allergens. J Allergy Clin Immunol. 1981;68:194-200.
4. Shivpuri DN, Shali PL, Bhatnagar PL, Agarwal MK. Studies on insect allergy in Delhi. Asp Allergy Appl Immunol. 1969;II:81-90.
5. Shivpuri DN, Shali PL, Agarwal MK, et al. Insect allergy in India. Ann Allergy. 1971;29:588-97.
6. Shali PL, Agarwal MK, Shivpuri DN. Sex specific antigens in insects. Asp Allergy Appl Immunol. 1970;III:77-84.
7. Saha K, Shali PL, Shivpuri DN. Arthropod allergy in Delhi. Detection of insect specific regains in the serum of insect sensitive bronchial asthma patients. Indian J Med Res. 1977;66:487-97.
8. Acharya PJ. Allergy to house dust, mite and cockroach. Comparison of skin test results. Asp Allergy Appl Immunol. 1978;X:79-84.
9. Acharya PJ. Skin test response to some inhalant allergens in patients of nasobronchial allergy from Andhra Pradesh. Asp Allergy Appl Immunol. 1980;13:14-8.
10. Ghosh P, Guha TK, Lahiri SC. Allergen skin tests on respiratory allergy patients in Calcutta (a preliminary report). Asp Allergy Appl Immunol. 1974;7:41-5.
11. Shanker A, Jain PC, Kumar U. A study of identification of offending allergens in patients of bronchial asthma in Gwalior attending J J Group of Hospitals. Indian J Chest Dis All Sci. 1979;21:166-73.
12. Shivpuri DN. Clinically important pollen, fungal and insect allergens for nasobronchial allergy patients in India. Asp Allergy Appl Immunol. 1980;XIII:19-23.
13. Gaur SN, Kapoor M, Garg DC, Agarwal MK. Etiologic significance of insects in nasobronchial allergy. Asp Allergy Appl Immunol. 1985;XVIII:19-27.
14. Chaudhry S. Clinico-immunologic studies on the significance of insects as inhalant allergens in respiratory allergic disorders [Ph.D. thesis]. New Delhi: University of Delhi; 1988.
15. Gupta S, Jain S, Chaudhry S, Agarwal MK. Role of insects as inhalant allergens in bronchial asthma with special reference to the clinical characteristics of patients. Clin Exp Allergy. 1990;20:519-24.
16. Jhamb S. Sudies on the allergen-specific immune response in Type-I hypersensitivity of respiratory system including observations on the etiologic role of influenza virus [Ph.D. thesis]. New Delhi: University of Delhi; 1988.
17. Gupta S. Studies on the heterogeneity of the immune response to insects in patients with IgE-mediated Type-I allergic respiratory diseases and their allergenic and antigenic relationship [Ph.D. thesis]. New Delhi: University of Delhi; 1988.
18. Kausar MA. Clinicoimmunologic and biochemical studies on mosquitoes as sources of allergens [Ph.D. thesis]. New Delhi: University of Delhi; 1988.
19. Jhamb S, Jain SK, Chhabra SK, et al. Insects as inhalant allergens: studies on allergenic and antigenic properties, their aerosolization and heterogeneous immune response in patients. Indian J Allergy Appl Immunol. 1992;6:7-14.
20. Kausar MA, Vijayan VK, Bansal SK, et al. Mosquitoes as sources of inhalant allergens: clinicoimmunologic and biochemical studies. J Allergy Clin Immunol. 2007;120: 1219-21.
21. Agarwal MK, Chaudhry S, Jhamb S, et al. Etiologic significance of mosquito (*Anopheles stephensi*) in respiratory allergy in India. Ann Allergy. 1991;67: 598-602.
22. Chaudhry S, Jhamb S, Chauhan UPS, et al. Shared and specific allergenic and antigenic components in the two sexes of American cockroach-*Peripaneta americana*. Clin Exp Allergy. 1990;20:59-65.
23. Srivastava D, Singh BP, Arora N, Gaur SN. Clinico-immunologic study on immunotherapy with mixed and single insect allergens. J Clin Immunol. 2009;29:665-73.

CHAPTER 34

Latex Allergy

PA Mahesh

HISTORY AND INTRODUCTION

Latex was in common use as early as 1600 BC, and the first surgical gloves were developed in the early 19th century.[1] The first possible report of allergic reactions to latex was reported in 1927 in Germany by Stern and included two cases with urticaria and laryngeal edema and the delayed contact reactions in 1933. But the prevalence of latex allergies dramatically increased in the 1980s onwards after greater use of latex gloves in most medical procedures, and universal precautions were advised.[1] The first report of anaphylaxis to latex was reported in 1984 to surgical gloves.

Sensitization to latex was demonstrated to be quite high with >6% of hospital employees in the surgical department being sensitized to latex when compared to 1.6% in other departments. Association with atopy was confirmed when it was observed that 67% of patients sensitized to latex were also sensitized to other allergens.[1] Slater reported latex-induced anaphylaxis in children with spina bifida undergoing multiple surgeries as part of their treatment in 1989.[1] Cross-reactivity between latex and foods was identified in 1989 and cross-reactivity to fruits was recognized in 1991.[1] The latex balloons in enema catheters led to severe anaphylactic reactions including a fatal reaction and was reported in 1991.[1] One of the key allergens in latex was the rubber elongation factor and was identified by Czuppon in 1993. Since then another 10 allergens have been recognized.[1]

A sudden surge of latex allergy cases was reported in the late 1980s. Though there is no conclusive proof, some of the key reasons hypothesized for this are better recognition of these latex allergy cases, which were not diagnosed earlier, a phenomenon called ascertainment bias, since the clinical characteristics and the diagnostic protocols were in place.[1] The advent of AIDS and the implementation of universal precautions contributed to the extensive use of latex gloves for all the medical procedures and care of patients. The sudden increase in exposure may have led to an increase in the number of cases.[1] Due to the sudden rise in demand for gloves, the manufacturing process that would reduce the allergen content in the gloves may have been circumvented leading to increased allergen exposure.[1] Also, the manufacturing of the latex gloves moved from manufacturing countries to countries that produced latex. Due to this, the time taken from collection of raw latex from rubber trees in ammonia-containing plastic containers and manufacture of gloves took as short as 4–6 weeks. Normally, when shipped to other countries in ocean tankers, during which the ammonia would denature the latex proteins during transit would take many months leading to reduced allergen content in the gloves.[1] Also, the selective cultivation of high-latex-yielding trees increased automatically the allergen content in the latex collected, and the use of chemicals to increase the yield such as ethanol may alter the latex protein structure, making them more allergenic.[1]

EPIDEMIOLOGY OF LATEX ALLERGY

Its barrier properties and elasticity makes natural rubber latex very attractive for use in medical procedures. More than 20 billion pairs of gloves are used in one year in the USA alone.[2] Latex allergy prevalence in various studies shows a large variability.[3] Lack of use of similar diagnostic criteria, standardization of Skin Prick Test or Radioallergosorbent test used for diagnosis and bias in selection of subjects may contribute to these differences. The prevalence of latex allergy varied from 0% to 30% with most studies in the range of 5% to 17%.[3] However, a systematic review was not able to identify the reasons for this large variation.[3] Most studies were cross-sectional and did not have adequate controls, which has significant drawbacks. Two seminal prospective cohort studies add significantly to our understanding. Sussman found no difference between the incidences of latex sensitization in users of either powdered or nonpowdered latex gloves, which was 1% in both the groups.[4] Gautrin observed that the incidence of latex allergy was 2.5% per year among dental hygiene apprentices when compared to two other apprentice groups.[5] Many studies did not assess environmental exposure adequately and therefore there are difficulties to understand the risk factors for sensitization.[3]

In children with spina bifida, the prevalence of sensitization to latex as well as clinical latex allergy increases with early and frequent exposures to latex allergen.[2] The studies by Baur observed that all the subjects with latex sensitization and clinically symptomatic allergies occurred with a threshold ambient aerosol exposure of 0.6 ng/m^3.[6] But this finding has not been replicated in other studies, which have observed levels varying from 5 to 83 ng/m^3 in summer and 40 to 616 ng/m^3 in winter but did not observe differences in levels of sensitization according to thresholds of exposure.[3]

As with other allergens, the development of latex sensitization and allergy is likely to be due to a complex interplay of genetic and environmental factors, which are yet to be understood. It was observed by Gabarant in a meta-analysis that the duration of exposure to latex as elucidated by time spent in health care, time spent wearing gloves, frequency of exposure, use of powdered or nonpowdered latex gloves, job categories, and the ambient threshold of exposure to latex did not correlate significantly with the latex allergy.[3] But this review was criticized later for its interpretation of the study findings.[7]

The second systematic review in 2006 addressed earlier drawbacks and confirmed that the healthcare workers were indeed at a higher risk for latex allergy. This review by Bousquet observed that the healthcare workers exposed to latex had a prevalence of latex allergy of 4.3% when compared to 1.3% in the general population.[7] Skin prick test positivity for latex was found to be 2.1–3.7% in the general population and 6.9–7.8% among healthcare workers. The odds of various manifestations of latex allergy were higher among healthcare workers: hand dermatitis (2.4), asthma or wheezing (1.5), and rhinoconjunctivitis (2.7).[7] It is possible that these values would also be an underestimate of the true prevalence of latex allergy, since symptomatic subjects who would be really troubled by latex allergy may have moved to other jobs (the healthy worker effect).[7]

GENETICS AND LATEX ALLERGY

One of the studies evaluated the linkage of HLA with latex allergy and latex sensitization in healthcare workers and children with spina bifida and the general population. The study observed a significant association between HLA-DQ8 and the HLA-DQ8-DR4 haplotype with latex allergy, specifically IgE to heve in in healthcare workers.[8]

DIAGNOSIS OF LATEX ALLERGY

It is important to confirm the sensitivity to natural rubber latex through standardized diagnostic methods. The first step in identifying a subject with latex allergy is via a good history. The details of the relevant history are listed in Box 34.1. Atopy is an important risk factor for latex allergy and a detailed history is necessary to confirm previous atopy. Repetitive exposures to natural latex products increase the risk of developing latex allergy in susceptible individuals. The frequency of use of powdered gloves and duration of use are important considerations for a healthcare worker, whereas the frequency of undergoing repeated surgeries is important in a patient with suspected latex allergy.[9] Type I hypersensitivity reactions tend to occur early generally within minutes of exposure, whereas type IV reactions tend to occur many hours or days after the exposure. Type IV reactions also tend to be localized to the skin area that has come in contact with latex and not in other areas or other organ systems. Type I reactions to latex can be similar to a systemic reaction to foods or drugs and include sudden itching of the eyes, nose, throat, with or without swelling of the throat or tongue, urticarial rashes on the skin, and angioedema. This can be associated with severe organ involvement such as wheezing, bronchospasm, cyanosis, tachypnea or respiratory arrest (respiratory), tachycardia, hypotension, arrhythmias, cardiac arrest (cardiac), vomiting, diarrhea, abdominal cramps (GIT), anxiety, and loss of consciousness (CNS) among others.[9]

The second is to confirm the presence of IgE antibodies to latex via the serological tests or an SPT. Unlike most other allergens, the serological tests are preferred over SPT for latex allergy in the diagnostic algorithm. The reason for it is the high prevalence of severe adverse reactions on SPT with the latex allergen, which can sometimes induce anaphylaxis on skin prick testing. Whereas the incidence of severe adverse reactions such as systemic reactions, hypotension and anaphylaxis on SPT for other allergens in patients with asthma, and allergic rhinitis is around 0.04%, for latex allergens it is 8.4% with a high rate of anaphylaxis.[9] One of the patients had a systemic reaction to a 1:1,00,000 dilution of a latex glove extract.[9] Therefore, SPT for latex allergens must always be performed with caution with physician in attendance ready to handle anaphylaxis.

The prick testing solution contains Hev b1,3,5 and 6 but not Hev b8. Hev b8 is involved with very mild reactions mainly oral allergy syndrome on consumption of foods. Many patients show a positive reaction to ImmunoCAP for Latex, but test negative on SPT and is due to sensitization to Hev b8. This protein (Hev b8) also cross-reacts with complex carbohydrate determinants (CCD).[10] The diagnosis of clinically important latex allergy and differentiating from latex sensitization is important to prevent serious reactions and prevent mortality. The recent development of a microarray based on ISAC-chip platform is a useful tool in this regard.[10]

Key points to be elicited on the clinical history of a suspected latex allergy subject are as follows:

1. General atopic history—allergic rhinoconjunctivitis, atopic dermatitis, food allergy, asthma.
2. Is there an exposure to latex/natural rubber products?
3. Temporal relationship of latex exposure and onset of symptoms.
4. Are the types of symptoms suggestive of latex allergy?
5. What is the severity of reactions and how long does it last?

The third step is to confirm clinical sensitivity with a provocation test, which could be a workplace exposure test or a challenge in a controlled chamber. A glove use test is also sometimes used. A glove test has been used in different variations. In the simplest version, the subject wears a latex glove for 15–60 minutes and their skin is observed for erythema, pruritus, rash, and nasal and bronchial symptoms. Nonlatex gloves are used as controls. Other variations include wearing the gloves for 2 hours for consecutive 3 days, wearing a latex powdered glove on the one hand and a latex glove washed in saline for 48 hours as control on the other hand, wearing sequentially only a finger of a glove and then the whole glove. Wearing a glove after skin puncture on the volar aspect of the hand to increase absorption of latex allergens through the skin and rubbing the punctured area over the glove while the subject was wearing a vapor mask and ocular goggles to prevent exposure through the respiratory tract or conjunctiva.[9] All of these have a lot of drawbacks including difficulty to mask the latex gloves from nonlatex gloves, difficulties in standardizing and validating the readings of the tests, inability to assess the latex load in these gloves, and many of the results from these studies were not reproducible.[9]

A challenge testing was developed which involved sequential exposure to vinyl gloves, low-latex gloves, and five increasing exposures to high-latex gloves by Laoprasert. After each exposure, symptoms and lung functions were monitored for 60 minutes. It was possible during this exposure to semiquantitatively measure the amount of latex the subject was exposed to.[9] Another method of exposure was the use of a hooded exposure chamber by Kurtz using latex allergen-associated cornstarch from powdered latex gloves. The number of latex particles as well as the particle size can be monitored in the chamber using a laser particle counter continuously. This chamber could mask the exposure either to plain cornstarch or cornstarch-associated latex particles and accurately measures latex exposure and was the first mechanism where this was possible. However, the setting up of such an exposure chamber is expensive.[9]

ALLERGENS IN NATURAL RUBBER LATEX

Latex is a mixture of many proteins that may be clinically important allergens. The common proteins are listed in Table 34.1.[11] Hev b5 and Hev b6 are most important in healthcare

Table 34.1: Natural rubber latex proteins.

Hev b1	Rubber elongation factor
Hev b2	Beta 1,3 glucanase
Hev b3	Small rubber particle protein
Hev b4	Microhelix component
Hev b5	Acidic latex component
Hev b6	Preprotein C(6.01), mature Hevein (6.02)
Hev b7	Patatin-like protein
Hev b8	Latex profilin
Hev b9	Latex enolase
Hev b10	Manganese superoxide dismutase
Hev b11	Class I chitinases
Hev b12	Lipid transfer protein
Hev b13	Latex esterase
Hev b14	Hevamine—also a Latex chitinase

workers and in patients with respiratory symptoms and to a lesser extent in patients with spina bifida. Hev b9 is important only in healthcare workers. Spina bifida patients mainly show reactivity to Hev b1 and Hev b3 and Hev b8, a profillin is important in latex fruit syndromes.[10] The most serious reaction of an intra-operative anaphylaxis is usually seen with sensitization to Hev b6.

CROSS-REACTIVITY TO OTHER FOODS (LATEX-FRUIT SYNDROME)

Latex is known to cross-react with various foods such as banana, kiwi, potato, chestnut, avocado, papaya, melon, peach, chestnut, cucumber, bell pepper, and figs. Structural similarities between latex allergens and plant food allergens are responsible for these cross-reactive allergies. Patients with latex allergy will have clinical cross-reactivity to one of the above foods in at least 35% of the cases and patients with food allergies will have cross-reactivity to latex in 11% of the cases.[12]

MANAGEMENT

The key management issues would revolve around prevention of new sensitization and handling patients/ subjects already sensitized to latex in the long-term (Box 34.1). and managing the acute reaction in the short-term.[13] The acute reaction is to be managed according to standard guidelines depending on the reaction. An acute asthma episode has to be managed according to the guidelines for handling an acute asthma or an anaphylaxis with adrenaline along with other supportive measures. It is important to give these patients treatment using latex-free material in a latex-free environment. The patients after recovery must be advised to carry epinephrine for injection with them and to avoid contact with latex.

BOX 34.1: Summary of management strategies for latex allergy.

a. Confirm diagnosis of latex allergy using validated methods.
b. Justify stopping the further use of latex in the workplace.
c. Confirm presence of impairment and disability due to latex allergy.
d. Inform employer and discuss ways to avoid latex in work place.
e. Advice worker to seek workplace compensation and change work.

Common household items that may contain latex include diapers, condoms, rubber bands, shoes and slippers, gloves, elastic hair and other bands, balloons, adhesives, rubber mats, rubber handles and toys, baby bottles and nipples, pacifiers, contraceptive diaphragms, rubber in kitchen utensils, etc.[13] The healthcare worker needs to be aware to educate the patients as well as other healthcare workers that many of the medical equipment contain latex including various catheters like Foley's catheter, syringes, ventilator tubings and ambu bags, endotracheal tubes, Ryle's tube, drain tubes, rubber stoppers of injection vials, many shunt tubes such as ventriculoperitoneal shunts, slippers, masks used for nebulization or non-invasive ventilation, tourniquets, elastic bandages, stethoscope tubes, etc.[13]

Avoidance of Exposure to the Latex

Patients once diagnosed must be careful about modifying their lifestyle to avoid exposure to latex as much as possible. It is considered almost impossible to avoid exposure to latex due to its widespread use in the community. Most subjects, however, do tolerate everyday exposure to these rubber-containing objects.[13] Patients are given a medical bracelet that informs healthcare workers about their latex allergy and it must be carefully documented during every admission to avoid inadvertent exposure to latex in the hospital. A list of common latex containing objects needs to be given to the subjects along with the alternatives.

Recommendations for the Use of Natural Rubber Latex Gloves

The American College of Allergy Asthma and Immunology gave the guidelines for the use of natural rubber latex gloves in 1997.[2] It is generally agreed that most of the purchasers of the gloves would not have data on the levels of antigens present in these gloves. The key points[2] were:

1. There should be a restriction on the use of latex gloves in the hospitals. Workers not handling contaminated fluids such as food handlers and other personnel should be strongly discouraged.
2. The examination gloves to be used should be non-powdered and non-sterile (non-powdered means less than 2 mg donning powder per glove).
3. Powder-free sterile natural rubber latex gloves should be recommended for use. Sterile NRL gloves rarely cause problems in healthy individuals and therefore can be safely used. If a hospital wishes to

use low-protein powdered latex gloves, they should institute a mechanism for continuous monitoring of latex sensitization and clinical latex allergy.

There is a progressive effort to replace powdered latex gloves as well as development of other synthetic alternatives for latex. Studies have shown that healthcare workers with latex allergy had complete resolution of their symptoms when they switched to non-NRL gloves. The two options in the management of subjects with latex allergy are either to shift the subject to an area in the healthcare facility to an area where there is no exposure to the latex allergen. For example, an OT nurse or an ICU nurse could be shifted to the OPD where gloves are not used. The other more expensive option is to make the present work area latex free, which is more difficult. It is important to confirm the diagnosis of latex allergy since it will significantly affect the options for future work for the healthcare worker and, in most cases, lead to reduced earnings.

Latex Substitutes

For most of the devices latex substitutes are available. The most important source of exposure is the latex gloves and these can be substituted by vinyl material, neoprene, Nitryl (acrylonitrile butadiene) or silicone material. Of these materials nitryl gloves are equivalent to latex in acting as a barrier to infections. As a surgical barrier the other group of materials that are useful are the neoprenes (elastiprene, butadiene, polychloroprene, polyisoprene), which are synthetic materials.[13] Further details on the latex substitutes available are given in the following online resources: www.latexallergyresources.org, www.latexallergy.ndo.co.uk

Immunotherapy for Latex Allergy

Studies have evaluated for efficacy and safety of both oral and parenteral immunotherapy for latex allergy. Studies have demonstrated reduction of clinical sensitivity to latex after immunotherapy. However, at present the adverse reactions are too high and too severe to recommend routine use and should be tried only under careful supervision.[13]

OMALIZUMAB IN HEALTHCARE WORKERS WITH LATEX ALLERGY

The humanized monoclonal antibody omalizumab has been shown to be effective in patients with allergic asthma and rhinitis. One of the double-blind randomized controlled study observed significant beneficial effects in healthcare workers with latex allergy over a period of 16 weeks. Most patients who were on omalizumab did well except a couple who had local side effects such as swelling or itching.[14]

LONG-TERM OUTCOMES OF PATIENTS WITH LATEX ALLERGY

For cases with occupational asthma, the maximum improvement in lung functions may take as much as 5 years after cessation of exposure and therefore continuous monitoring is essential even after cessation to exposure.[15] Studies have shown that majority of patients do well when the exposure ceases either with the introduction of non-latex gloves or change in occupation. Contact urticaria due to latex allergy resolves completely and patients with occupational asthma due to latex allergy also do well on cessation of exposure.[15] Patients with anaphylaxis will need to change their jobs. Most patients with latex allergy have shown a reduction in their annual incomes due to change of their jobs or work profiles.[15]

REFERENCES

1. Ownby DR. A history of latex allergy. J Allergy Clin Immunol. 2002;110:S27-32.
2. Charous BL, Blanco C, Tarlo S, et al. Natural rubber latex allergy after 12 years: recommendations and perspectives. J Allergy Clin Immunol. 2002;109:31-4.
3. Garabrant DH, Schweitzer S. Epidemiology of latex sensitization and allergies in health care workers. J Allergy Clin Immunol. 2002;110:S82-95.
4. Sussman GL, Liss GM, Deal K, et al. Incidence of latex sensitization among latex glove users. J Allergy Clin Immunol. 1998;101:171-8.
5. Gautrin D, Ghezzo H, Infante-Rivard C, Malo JL. Incidence and determinants of IgE-mediated sensitization in apprentices. A prospective study. Am J Respir Crit Care Med. 2000; 162:1222-8.
6. Baur X, Chen Z, Allmers H. Can a threshold limit value for natural rubber latex airborne allergens be defined? J Allergy Clin Immunol. 1998;101:24-7.
7. Bousquet J, Flahault A, Vandenplas O, et al. Natural rubber latex allergy among health care workers: a systematic review of the evidence. J Allergy Clin Immunol. 2006;118: 447-54.
8. Rihs HP, Chen Z, Rueff F, et al. HLA-DQ8 and the HLA-DQ8-DR4 haplotype are positively associated with the hevein-specific IgE immune response in health care workers with latex allergy. J Allergy Clin Immunol. 2002;110: 507-14.

9. Hamilton RG, Peterson EL, Ownby DR. Clinical and laboratory-based methods in the diagnosis of natural rubber latex allergy. J Allergy Clin Immunol. 2002;110: S47-56.
10. Schuler S, Ferrari G, Schmid-Grendelmeier P, Harr T. Microarray-based component-resolved diagnosis of latex allergy: isolated IgE-mediated sensitization to latex profillin Hev b8 may act as confounder. Clin Transl Allergy. 2013;3:11.
11. Poley GE Jr, Slater JE. Latex allergy. J Allergy Clin Immunol. 2000;105:1054-62.
12. Sicherer SH. Clinical implications of cross-reactive food allergens. J Allergy Clin Immunol. 2001;108:881-90.
13. Cabanes N, Igea JM, de la Hoz B, et al. Latex allergy: position paper. J Investig Allergol Clin Immunol. 2012;22:313-30; quiz follow 330.
14. Leynadier F, Doudou O, Gaouar H, et al. Effect of omalizumab in health care workers with occupational latex allergy. J Allergy Clin Immunol. 2004;113:360-1.
15. Bernstein DI. Management of natural rubber latex allergy. J Allergy Clin Immunol. 2002;110:S111-6.

CHAPTER 35

Human Seminal Plasma Allergy

Ashok Shah

INTRODUCTION

Human seminal plasma allergy (HSPA) in women is a rare phenomenon. It was first described by the Dutch gynecologist Specken[1] in 1958, but the first report in the English literature was published in 1967 by Halpern and colleagues[2] from France. Since then, sporadic cases have documented the existence of this little-known disorder. The first case from India and the Asian continent was reported by us in 1988,[3] and subsequently we presented two more patients.[4] In 2004, we reviewed 80 documented patients of this unusual syndrome.[5] Since then, 25 more such subjects have been published.

DEFINITION

Sensitization to seminal fluid proteins causes HSPA. The allergic manifestations, which range from local pruritus to life-threatening anaphylaxis, can occur during or after coitus. This is mediated by the classical IgE-mediated pathophysiological mechanism.

CLINICAL PROFILE

The HSPA can present with either systemic or local symptoms or both. The systemic features, which occurred in more than two-thirds of the patients,[5] include pruritus, urticaria, angioedema, chest tightness, cough, breathlessness, wheezing, nasal symptoms (sneezing and rhinorrhea), and dizziness. Anaphylaxis leading to collapse and loss of consciousness, thereby requiring emergency room visits, has also been reported. Local manifestations, viz. vulvar and vaginal itching, burning, redness, swelling, and pain often precede or occur simultaneously with the systemic syndrome. These were described in more than half of the subjects.[5] Four cases, i.e., mother and her three daughters of the same family, are presented with recurrent "allergic seminal vulvovaginitis" without systemic symptoms.[6] One patient developed fixed cutaneous eruptions in the form of erythematous macular lesions within 2–48 hours of intercourse.[7]

The symptoms can occur during or soon after coitus. A gradual worsening over a few hours was noted in some patients. A reduction in the time of onset of symptoms during repeated attacks was also observed.[5] An increase in the severity of systemic or local symptoms was also recorded. Progression from local to systemic manifestations over the course of time was observed in the first Indian patient described by us.[3] In another patient, systemic and local symptoms occurred at different time durations after intercourse.[8] Spontaneous regression of symptoms was seen in a majority of the patients. Mitigation of symptoms after a shower was also reported in four patients.[6,9,10]

Initial Occurrence of Symptoms

Seminal allergy has been reported after the first intercourse in a large number of patients, although it can occur at any time. In more than half of the patients, symptoms of HSPA occurred for the first time in the age group of 20–30 years. However, the index case, reported by Specken,[1] was a 65-year-old woman who developed generalized urticaria after intercourse. Skin testing with human seminal plasma was found to be positive. Another patient first noticed local reactions when her partner stopped using a condom after her menopause.[11] Our review[5] of 80 patients showed that HSPA occurred at the time of the first intercourse in 41% of patients.

Some women developed reactions with multiple sexual partners,[5] but one patient had symptoms with her second husband only.[12] A severe generalized systemic reaction after topical contact with seminal fluid has also been described in one patient, who had never had intercourse.[13] The first episode of HSPA has also occurred on resuming intercourse after a time gap. This gap was attributable to pregnancy in four patients,[14-17] and to insertion of an intrauterine device,[18] partial prostatectomy in the male partner[19], and hysterectomy[20], one in each patient.

Relation with Atopy and Infertility

Most patients have a strong atopic background. A personal or family history of asthma, allergic rhinoconjunctivitis, or atopic dermatitis was elicited in a majority of the patients. A positive family history of allergy to foodstuffs was also present. However, an atopic background was not only seen in many patients with local symptoms, but also in the patient in whom the reaction was limited to cutaneous eruptions.[7] Infertility has been observed in a majority of the patients with HSPA.[5] Inability to conceive in such patients was earlier regarded as an important clue for achieving the diagnosis. Later on, the successful induction of pregnancy by artificial insemination of spermatozoa,[21,22] and also by conceiving spontaneously after treatment for HSPA[23] was demonstrated.

IMMUNOLOGICAL MECHANISM

The classical IgE-mediated pathophysiological mechanism is responsible for the features of HSPA. Reaginic humoral antibodies are produced against an antigen present in the seminal plasma. The antigen reacts with these IgE antibodies, which are bound to mast cells or circulating basophils, leading to degranulation of mast cells. This results in the release of vasoactive amines including histamine, which mediate the hypersensitivity reactions. Cell-mediated immunity (type IV hypersensitivity) has also been implicated in recurrent allergic vulvovaginitis.[16]

Halpern and colleagues[2] separated the protein constituents of the seminal fluid by zone electrophoresis and identified the sensitizing antigen as a basic sialic acid-rich glycoprotein. A few years later, Levine et al.[24] fractionated the seminal plasma using column chromatography and isolated a protein fraction of 20–30 kDa. Subsequently, positive skin reactions have been elicited with antigen proteins of molecular weights ranging from 12,000 to 75,000 Da.[5] It has been demonstrated that the prostatic secretion is the source of this allergen.[14,24] However, one patient also had a positive skin test to spermatozoa extract.[16]

DIAGNOSIS

The diagnosis must be confirmed by demonstration of sensitization to seminal fluid proteins by in vivo and in vitro immunologic methods. Characteristic symptoms which occur in relation to coitus and can be prevented by condom usage or coitus interruptus point toward a definitive diagnosis.

In vivo skin tests include prick tests and intradermal tests, which are usually done on the volar surface of the arms. Fresh semen from the patient's partner is used to prepare the seminal plasma antigen (SPA). These tests are performed on the patient in serial dilutions of the SPA along with a negative control (buffered saline) and a positive control (histamine 100 µg/mL) and graded. Pooled donor semen can also be used for the skin tests after excluding diseases spread through body fluids. The in vitro tests comprise demonstration of high total serum IgE levels and elevated specific IgE antibodies to seminal plasma. The semen-specific IgE antibodies are measured by the radioallergosorbent test (RAST) or by enzyme-linked immunosorbent assay.

DIFFERENTIAL DIAGNOSIS

In women, HSPA needs to be distinguished from other types of asthmatic attacks that occur after coitus.[25,26] These include postcoital asthma[27] and condom-induced asthma.[28,29] Postcoital asthma and rhinitis, also called "sexercise-induced asthma"[30] and "honeymoon rhinitis"[31] respectively, can be seen in both males and females. The symptoms in these patients are usually due to sexual excitement. Asthma can also be caused by condom usage.[28] This is due to latex allergy, and can occur in both males and females. Two cases of HSPA with concurrent latex allergy have been reported.[32,33]

The local forms may often be misdiagnosed as vulvovaginitis.[34] Allergens such as pollens, and chemicals present in soaps, perfumes, nail polish, and contraceptive spermicides can cause allergic vulvovaginitis.[35] Symptoms due to transfer of allergens present in the seminal fluid may simulate HSPA. Such allergic reactions have been described with vinblastine,[36] walnuts,[37] thioridazine,[38] and penicillin.[39]

TREATMENT

Allergen avoidance is the mainstay of management. Exposure to seminal fluid can be avoided by abstinence or coitus interruptus, but this is rarely acceptable. Usage of condoms is the most widely advocated method but in case the female patient is latex-sensitive,[32] condoms made of material other than latex should be used.

As in other forms of atopy, desensitization should be contemplated. Variable success has been reported with the conventional method of immunotherapy. The first attempt was by Halpern et al.[2] but this was unsuccessful. On their patient's request, Mathias et al.[15] tried immunotherapy using serial dilutions of the husband's seminal plasma. Although immunotherapy attenuated the severity of the reaction, the objective parameters including RAST remained elevated.

In a series of 13 patients described by Drouet and colleagues,[40] immunotherapy was not successful in three patients with local reactions; while five out of six patients who had systemic manifestations were successfully treated by immunotherapy. Subsequently, "rush" immunotherapy has been performed by both the subcutaneous and the intravaginal route with near total success achieved in 11 patients.[5] Successful pregnancy after immunotherapy was also recorded.[41,42]

CONCLUSION

Human seminal plasma allergy is difficult to recognize, especially the local forms. A high index of suspicion is required as HSPA may easily be overlooked due to patient embarrassment and lack of physician awareness.[43,44]

REFERENCES

1. Specken JLH. Een merkwaardig geval van allergie in de gynaecologie. Ned Tjidschr Verloskd Gynaecol. 1958;58:314-8.
2. Halpern BN, Ky T, Robert B. Clinical and immunological study of an exceptional case of reaginic type sensitization to human seminal fluid. Immunology. 1967;12:247-58.
3. Shah A, Sethi S, Agarwal MK. Human seminal plasma allergy in India. J Asthma. 1988;25:137-40.
4. Shah A, Panjabi C, Singh AB. Asthma caused by human seminal plasma allergy. J Asthma. 2003;40:125-9.
5. Shah A, Panjabi C. Human seminal plasma allergy: a review of a rare phenomenon. Clin Exp Allergy. 2004;34:827-38.
6. Chang TW Familial allergic seminal vulvovaginitis. Am J Obstet Gynecol. 1976;126:442-4.
7. Best CL, Walters C, Adelman DC. Fixed cutaneous eruptions to seminal-plasma challenge: a case report. Fertil Steril. 1988;50:532-4.
8. Mike N, Bird G, Asquith P. A new manifestation of seminal fluid hypersensitivity. QJ Med. 1990;75:371-6.
9. Matloff SM. Local intravaginal desensitization to seminal fluid. J Allergy Clin Immunol. 1993;91:1230-1.
10. Ludman BG. Human seminal plasma protein allergy: a diagnosis rarely considered. JOGNN. 1999;28:359-63.
11. Kroon S. Allergy to human seminal plasma: a presentation of six cases. Acta Dermatovener (Stockholm). 1980;60:436-9.
12. Frankland AW, Parish WE. Anaphylactic sensitivity to human seminal fluid. Clin Allergy. 1974;4:249-53.
13. Ohman JL Jr., Malkiel S, Lewis S, Lorusso JR. Allergy to human seminal fluid: characterization of the allergen and experience with immunotherapy. J Allergy Clin Immunol. 1990;85:103-7.
14. Voorhorst R. Female allergy to seminal fluid. Ann Allergy. 1978;40:252.
15. Mathias CGT, Frick OL, Caldwell TM, et al. Immediate hypersensitivity to seminal fluid and atopic dermatitis. Arch Dermatol. 1980;116:209-12.
16. Bernstein IL, Englander BE, Gallagher JS, et al. Localized and systemic hypersensitivity reactions to human seminal fluid. Ann Intern Med. 1981;94:459-65.
17. Bernstein IL, Gallagher JS, Friedman SA, et al. Standardized immunotherapy protocol for IgE-mediated anaphylaxis to human seminal plasma. Contr Gynec Obstet. 1985;14:151-9.
18. Reunala T, Koskimies AI, Björksten F, et al. Immunoglobulin E-mediated severe allergy to human seminal plasma. Fertil Steril. 1977;28:832-5.
19. Mumford DM, Haywood TJ, Daily LJ Jr., et al. Female allergy to seminal plasma—A case report. Ann Allergy. 1978;40:40-3.
20. Friedman SA, Bernstein IL, Enrione M, Marcus ZH. Successful long-term immunotherapy for human seminal plasma anaphylaxis. JAMA. 1984;251:2684-7.
21. Shapiro SS, Kooistra JB, Schwartz D, et al. Induction of pregnancy in a woman with seminal plasma allergy. Fertil Steril. 1981;36:405-7.
22. Iwahashi K, Miyazaki T, Kuji N, Yoshimura Y. Successful pregnancy in a woman with a human seminal plasma allergy. A case report. J Reprod Med. 1999;44:391-3.
23. Park JW, Ko SH, Kim CW, et al. Seminal plasma anaphylaxis: successful pregnancy after intravaginal desensitization and immunodetection of allergens. Allergy. 1999;54:990-3.
24. Levine BB, Siraganian RP, Schenkein I. Allergy to human seminal plasma. N Engl J Med. 1973;288:894-6.
25. Shah A. Editorial—Asthma and sex. Indian J Chest Dis Allied Sci. 2001;43:135-7.
26. Shah A, Panjabi C. Asthma, hypersensitivity, and coitus. Am J Respir Crit Care Med. 2004;170:1135.
27. Shah A, Sircar M. Postcoital asthma and rhinitis. Chest. 1991;100:1039-41.
28. Turjanmaa K, Reunala T. Condoms as a source of latex allergen and cause of contact urticaria. Contact Dermatitis. 1989;20:360-4.
29. Shah A. Coitus-induced asthma or condom-induced asthma? Chest. 1992;102:327-8.

30. Symington IS, Kerr JW. Sexercise-induced asthma. Lancet. 1976;2:693.
31. Mackay IS. Rhinitis and sinusitis. Br J Dis Chest. 1988;82: 1-8.
32. Kint B, Degreef H, Dooms-Goossens A. Combined allergy to human seminal plasma and latex: case report and review of literature. Contact Dermatitis. 1994;30:7-11.
33. Yocum MW, Jones RT, Yunginger JW. Concurrent sensitization to natural rubber latex and human seminal fluid. J Allergy Clin Immunol. 1996;98:1135-6.
34. Jones WR. Allergy to coitus. Aust N Z J Obstet Gynaecol. 1991;31:137-41.
35. Moraes PSA, Taketomi EA. Allergic vulvovaginitis. Ann Allergy Asthma Immunol. 2000;85:253-67.
36. Paladine WJ, Cunningham TJ, Donavan MA, Dumper CW. Possible sensitivity to vinblastine in prostatic or seminal fluid. N Engl J Med. 1975;292:52.
37. Haddad ZH. Clearer picture of food allergens is still needed. Perspect Allergy. 1978;1:2-3.
38. Sell MB. Sensitization to thioridazine through sexual intercourse. Am J Psychiatry. 1985:142:271-2.
39. Green RL, Green MA. Postcoital urticaria in a penicillin-sensitive patient. JAMA. 1985;254:531.
40. Drouet M, Sabbah A, Hassoun S. Thirteen cases of allergy to human seminal plasma. Allergy. 1997;52:112-4.
41. Bernstein JA, Herd ZA, Bernstein DI, et al. Evaluation and treatment of localized vaginal immunoglobulin E-mediated hypersensitivity to human seminal plasma. Obstet Gynecol. 1993;82:667-73.
42. De Cuyper C, Bogaerts Y, Vandekerckhove F. Intravaginal desensitization and successful pregnancy in a woman with seminal fluid allergy. J Allergy Clin Immunol. 1996;97: 1427-28.
43. Shah A, Agarwal MK. Human seminal plasma allergy as a cause of postcoital asthma. Eur Respir J. 1988;1:972.
44. Shah A. Human seminal plasma allergy. In: Prasad R, ed. Advances in Allergy and Asthma. Lucknow, India: Shivam Publications, 2000:156-8.

CHAPTER 36

Aspirin Allergy

Kiran Vishnu Narayan

INTRODUCTION

Nonsteroidal anti-inflammatory drugs (NSAIDs) include a dozen of compounds with similar anti-inflammatory activity used primarily for the treatment of chronic inflammatory disorders, pain, and fever.[1] The prototype aspirin has been the most widely used, being ubiquitous in prescriptions for ischemic heart disease and ischemic cerebrovascular accidents. Side effects of these drugs vary from mild skin rashes or gastritis to even life-threatening anaphylaxis.

The NSAIDs primarily inhibit the cyclooxygenase (COX)-mediated arachidonic acid pathway, inhibiting prostaglandins, prostacyclins, and thromboxane synthesis. As a result, the arachidonic acid is redirected into the lipoxygenase pathway resulting in increased levels of leukotrienes. Depending on the preferential isoform inhibition, NSAIDs may be either COX-1 or COX-2. Most of the "classical" NSAIDs (e.g., aspirin, naproxen, diclofenac) predominantly inhibit COX-1 and to a lesser extent COX-2. The COX-1 inhibitors affect the formation of protective prostanoids in the gastrointestinal tract. The selective COX-2 inhibitors (celecoxib, rofecoxib) inhibit the inflammatory prostanoids strongly but affect the formation of protective prostanoids to a mild extent. AERD is primarily due to the COX-1 inhibition.

Cross-reactivity among NSAIDs has been explained by Szczeklik et al. in 1975. He showed that some of the skin and respiratory hypersensitivity reactions could be explained by the inhibition of prostaglandins. Majority of the hypersensitivity reactions seen with NSAIDs are due to COX-1 inhibition and are not due to immunological mechanisms. Some of the NSAIDs have different chemical structures and these may act as antigens, thereby causing the immune system to respond by producing drug-specific antibodies.[2]

TYPES OF NSAID REACTIONS

The NSAID ingestion can give rise to both allergic and nonallergic (previously called as pseudoallergic or idiosyncratic) reactions, which occur within minutes to hours of ingestion. Allergic reactions occur due to an abnormal immunological response to the consumed drug. To describe a reaction as allergic hypersensitivity or drug allergy, a definite immunological mechanism has to be demonstrated, e.g., demonstration of drug-specific antibodies. Allergic reactions can be further classified into IgE and non-IgE Keep or T-cell-mediated hypersensitivity reactions. Nonallergic reactions are nonimmunological reactions occurring due to alterations in biochemical pathways upon which NSAIDs inhibited the prostaglandin pathway and therefore increased the production of leukotrienes.

Stevenson et al. proposed the first classification of acute NSAID hypersensitivity based on the various clinical patterns and the underlying pathogenetic mechanisms.[3] More recently, the European Academy of Allergy and Clinical Immunology (EAACI) "Task Force on NSAID Hypersensitivity" presented a new and updated classification for acute and delayed NSAID-induced hypersensitivity reactions. They classify reactions into allergic or selective and nonallergic or cross-reactive.[4,5] Drug hypersensitivity reactions to NSAID may manifest with symptoms of the respiratory, skin, abdominal, neurological systems, or even as anaphylaxis. The presentation may appear at different times after the time of drug intake. The reactions are classified as selective or allergic, when the patient reacts only to a specific drug or a drug with the same biochemical structure. The selective reactions which may be either IgE or non-IgE (T-cell)-mediated are due to an immunologically mediated reaction to the suspected drug. Cross-reactive reactions occur when the person may react to several NSAID drugs which are chemically unrelated. Cross-reactivity to several NSAIDs occurs due to the common property of inhibition of COX enzymes.[6]

The selective (allergic) reactions include the following:

1. Single NSAID-induced urticaria/angioedema/anaphylaxis (SNIUAA).
2. NSAID-induced delayed hypersensitivity reaction (NIDHR).

The nonselective (cross-reactive) reactions include the following:

1. NSAID-exacerbated respiratory disease (NERD).
2. NSAID-exacerbated cutaneous disease (NECD).
3. NSAID-induced urticaria/angioedema (NIUA).

Selective Reactions

1. Single NSAID-induced urticaria/angioedema/anaphylaxis (SNIUAA)
   These occur in patients without a history of asthma or chronic urticaria. This is a Type 1 Immediate hypersensitivity reaction (usually within an hour) occurring to a single drug and manifests as urticaria, angioedema, laryngeal edema, and/or anaphylaxis. Other chemically non-related drugs are tolerated.
2. NSAID-induced delayed hypersensitivity reaction (NIDHR)
   As it is a *delayed* hypersensitivity reaction, manifestations occur after 24 hours of consumption of the NSAID. The underlying immunological mechanism is presumed to be stimulation of drug-specific CD4+ and CD8+ T cells through their T-cell receptors. It presents with cutaneous symptoms (exanthems/fixed drug eruptions/severe cutaneous reaction), or organ involvement in the form of pulmonary (wheezing) or renal involvement.

Nonselective (Cross-reactive) reactions

1. NSAID-exacerbated respiratory disease (NERD)
   The classically described AERD/Samters triad/Widal syndrome belongs to this group. This is a nonallergic reaction occurring in patients with the underlying chronic rhinosinusitis and nasal polyposis and/or asthma. It manifests with both the upper and lower respiratory symptoms of rhinorrhea, nasal congestion, bronchial obstruction, and dyspnea. NSAID hypersensitivity in these patients is a risk factor for severe asthma or near-fatal asthma. People with AERD are not only sensitive to aspirin but also showed cross-sensitivity to other NSAIDs like ibuprofen, naproxen, and diclofenac. The rates of sensitivity were 98% for ibuprofen, 100% for naproxen, and 93% for diclofenac in a study but only 7% were sensitive to acetaminophen, and reactions tend to be less severe compared with other NSAIDs.[7,8]
2. NSAID-exacerbated cutaneous disease (NECD)
   This occurs in patients with a history of chronic idiopathic urticaria. Cutaneous manifestations of wheals and/or angioedema are exacerbated on NSAID consumption. It is described with aspirin as aspirin-induced urticaria or aspirin-exacerbated cutaneous disease or Pseudo-Samter's syndrome.
3. NSAID-induced urticaria/angioedema (NIUA)
   As the name suggests, the suspected drug induces the development of wheals and/or angioedema in persons without any history of urticaria. Symptoms are induced by at least two NSAIDs with a different chemical structure.

The description of all NSAID-induced reactions is beyond the realm of this chapter. From an allergy and immunological point of view, nonselective reactions are more commonly seen. The classical conditions of AERD and aspirin-induced cutaneous reactions will be described in detail here.

Epidemiology and Types

Aspirin-exacerbated Respiratory Disease

As the name suggests, it is a disease exacerbated by the use of aspirin. As mentioned previously, there is evidence of cross-reaction with other COX-1 NSAIDs.[9] AERD affects 0.3–0.9% of the general population. The prevalence increases in the asthmatic population to 10–20% and 30–40% in asthmatics with nasal polyposis. Though, AERD has been considered rare in children, the prevalence is around 5% when children are subject to oral provocation testing.[10] Three large population-based surveys of AERD were published from Finland, Poland, and Australia. The prevalence described was 4.3%, 8.8%, and 10.5% in Poland, Finland, and Australia, respectively.[11-13] A 2014 meta-analysis showed that the prevalence of AERD was almost 7% among asthmatics. The prevalence is higher with 14%, 10%, and 9% among patients with severe asthma, nasal polyps, and chronic rhinosinusitis, respectively.[14]

Among 300 patients with AERD seen during a period of 6 years, 171 (57%) patients were females with nasal polyposis or asthma appearing at an average age of 34 years.[15] In a European multicentric study which analyzed 500 patients from 16 centers, persistent rhinitis appeared at a mean age of 30 years followed by asthma, aspirin/NSAID-induced respiratory reactions, and finally nasal polyps. Here also females outnumbered males, had an earlier onset, and had more severe disease. Atopy was seen in one-third of patients and a family history of AERD in 6% cases.[16]

The clinical setting which arouses a suspicion of AERD is when an uncontrolled asthmatic presents with relentless nasal polyps formation with pansinusitis on imaging. A study done among 300 AERD patients showed that almost 99% had evidence of pansinusitis on Sinus X-rays or CT paranasal sinuses.[17] Most aspirin-tolerant patients with nasal polyps and pansinusitis have IgE-mediated rhinitis usually to dust mites. Remaining patients have intrinsic rhinosinusitis and asthma of unknown cause.

A recent study conducted to assess comorbidities among 414 AERD patients compared with 338 asthmatic control patients found that, after adjusting for age, sex, smoking, obesity, hyperlipidemia, and hypertension, coronary artery disease and congestive heart failure were associated significantly with AERD (OR 4.63; 95% CI 1.61–13.31). The range of 95% CI could decrease the power of the study, and the authors conclude that large prospective studies would be required to assess whether a definite association exists for AERD and coronary artery disease and congestive heart failure.[18]

Chronic Idiopathic Urticaria

A subpopulation of patients (one third to two thirds of patients) with chronic idiopathic urticaria tend to develop flares of urticaria when exposed to aspirin or NSAID. The more active the urticaria, the more likely that the drug will cause an acute flare. The prevalence of aspirin-induced flares in patients with chronic idiopathic urticaria has found to be around 21–30%, and the majority of patients (80%) with active chronic urticaria will develop flares on aspirin challenge.[19-21] Avoidance of the drug does not change the course of illness other than to reduce the acute flares. These reactions also tend to occur more in adulthood and in young females. Cutaneous reactions to aspirin have been documented to occur more frequently in atopic individuals.[22,23]

PATHOGENESIS OF NSAID-INDUCED REACTIONS

Membrane phospholipids are cleaved by phospholipase A2 to arachidonic acid, which are metabolized by cyclooxygenase enzyme into prostanoids (prostaglandins, prostacyclin, and thromboxane) and by lipoxygenase enzyme into lipoxins and leukotrienes, all of which are involved in the genesis of inflammation (Fig. 36.1).

As described previously, NSAID-induced reactions may be allergic and nonallergic. NSAIDs block the synthesis of prostanoids by inhibiting cyclooxygenase. The cyclooxygenase enzyme was previously called as prostaglandin G/H-synthase, and it exists as two isoforms (COX-1 and COX-2). COX-1 is constitutively expressed in most mammalian cells including respiratory, renal, and gut epithelial cells as well as most inflammatory cells, leading to the production of prostanoids (prostaglandin, prostacyclin or PGI2, thromboxane). The prostanoids help in maintaining platelet aggregation, normal renal function, and gastric mucosal integrity. In contrast, enzyme COX-2 is highly inducible by proinflammatory mediators (cytokines, growth factors) that are released from sites of tissue injury. So, COX-2 is concentrated in inflammatory cells. Aspirin is a nonspecific COX inhibitor with potent inhibition of COX-1 more than COX-2. The alternate pathway for

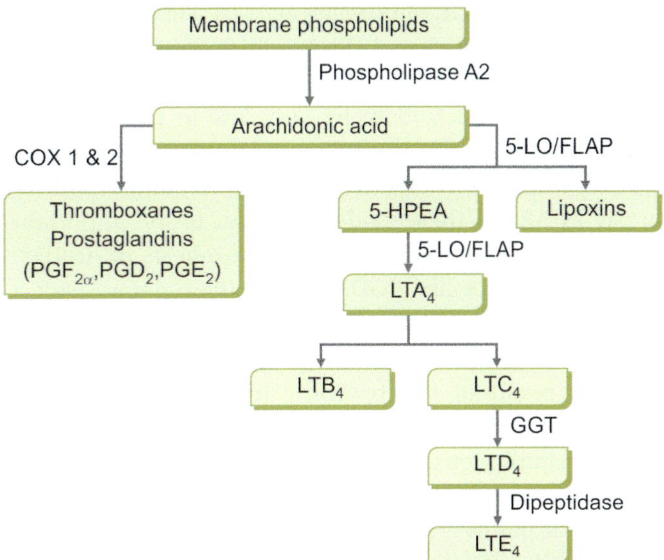

Fig. 36.1: Arachidonic acid pathway involving the cyclooxygenase and lipoxygenase enzymes. 5-LO, 5-lipoxygenase; FLAP, 5-lipoxygenase-activating protein; 5-HPEA, 5-hydroperoxyeicosatetraenoic acid; GGT, gamma-glutamyl transpeptidase; PG, prostaglandins; LT, leukotrienes.

arachidonic acid metabolism is the lipoxygenase pathway (LOX pathway) by the enzyme 5-lipoxygenase. The end products of the LOX pathway include various cysteinyl and noncysteinyl leukotrienes like LTB_4, LTC_4, LTD_4, and LTE_4. These proinflammatory mediators which are synthesized mainly by mast cells and also by eosinophils and platelets produce upper airway congestion, mucus hypersecretion, airway edema, and potent bronchoconstriction.[24,25]

Pathogenesis in AERD

Patients with AERD have a baseline dysregulation of arachidonic acid metabolism, in which there is an increased production of leukotrienes with reduction in prostaglandins. This increased production occurs both in the nasal as well as airway mucosa, causing the symptoms of nasal congestion and bronchospasm.

Low concentrations of aspirin inhibit COX-1 in AERD patients, thereby reducing PGE_2. PGE_2 is anti-inflammatory by inhibiting the lipoxygenase pathway and leukotriene production. They also produce bronchodilation. In AERD, there is a decreased production of PGE_2, which also removes the inhibitory effect on leukotriene production. The PGE_2 levels in AERD are lower at baseline and fall when challenged with COX-1 inhibitors. This has been substantiated in studies where inhaled PGE_2 was found to prevent the COX-1-induced inflammation and increased leukotriene production.[26-28] PGE_2 normally acts by suppressing the activity of protein kinase-A (PKA), which therefore reduces the leukotriene production. The PKA activity in white blood cells (WBC) was found to be very low in patients with AERD compared with controls.[29] In addition, the number of PGE_2 receptors are reduced in the nasal and bronchial airway in AERD. These evidences point to the important role of PGE_2 homeostasis in the pathogenesis of AERD.[30] Other metabolites like PGD_2 are proinflammatory with a bronchoconstricting effect. Increased levels of PGD_2 are found at baseline and also after challenge with aspirin.[31-33]

As a result of the baseline, increased leukotriene production already present in AERD and loss of PGE_2-mediated inhibition on 5-lipoxygenase, an overproduction of leukotrienes occur. As LTE_4 is the terminal product in the leukotriene pathway (see Fig. 36.1), urinary concentrations of LTE_4 will reflect systemic synthesis of leukotrienes. In fact baseline levels of LTE_4 have found to predict the severity of subsequent aspirin-induced lower respiratory reactions.[34,35] Christie and Smith et al. reported elevated baseline levels of LTE_4 and thromboxanes in the urine of AERD patients compared with normal controls and with aspirin-tolerant asthmatics.[36,37] Subsequent investigations have confirmed the findings that the levels of LTE_4 in urine samples were elevated before any exposure to aspirin.[38,39] High baseline levels of LTE_4 were associated with severe asthmatic reactions, and FEV_1 (forced expiratory volume in first second) fell by more than 30% on exposure to aspirin, whereas low baseline levels were associated with only mild naso-ocular reactions.[40]

Also, a high level of thromboxanes denotes an increased systemic synthesis of COX products. In vivo evidence of an increased synthesis of prostanoids and leukotrienes has been found in AERD asthmatics, even before exposure to aspirin. In addition to the increased generation of leukotrienes, AERD patients generate less of the anti-inflammatory lipid mediators, lipoxins, and 15-epimer lipoxins which are also part of the lipoxygenase pathway.[41] A study comparing the levels of lipoxins after stimulation of blood with calcium ionophore in normal subjects, aspirin-tolerant asthmatics, and AERD patients found that the latter generated very low levels of lipoxins. In this study, pretreating the whole blood samples of patients with aspirin led to an increased lipoxin production in aspirin-tolerant asthmatics but not in cells of AERD patients.[42] Lipoxins are anti-inflammatory substances, and reduced generation of lipoxins is seen in AERD patients.

Aspirin-induced reactions require an inhibition of COX-1 enzyme. So, selective COX-2 inhibitors fail to induce reactions. COX-1 enzymes vary between AERD asthmatics and aspirin-tolerant asthma controls in function and expression. In vitro studies of peripheral blood monocytes taken from AERD patients during aspirin-induced reactions showed that inhibition of COX-1 enzymes could occur at low doses like 60 mg. In contrast, COX-1 inhibition in aspirin-tolerant asthmatics and normal volunteers required 325–650 mg of aspirin.[43] This explains the difficulty in initiating aspirin at an antiplatelet dosage (low dose) for AERD patients with concurrent ischemic heart disease or neurological disease. Even a low dose would cause exacerbation of upper and lower airway symptoms in AERD.

Inflammatory Cells in AERD

The upper and lower airways in patients with AERD have mast cells, which are activated and degranulate during aspirin challenge. An increase in histamine, mast cell tryptase, and PGD_2 levels is seen consequent to this. Antihistamines have found to reduce the development of reaction in these cases. Studies in the nasal and lung tissue of AERD patients have shown that eosinophils and activated mast cells, which overexpress the enzyme LTC_4 synthase are disproportionately increased.[44] This results in an increased production of leukotrienes and inflammation. In a study by Yamashita et al., immunohistochemical staining of polyp tissue from AERD patients showed numerous eosinophils and degranulated mast cells.[45] A study by Cowburn et al. found high concentrations of tryptase, histamine, and LTC_4 in nasal secretions after oral aspirin challenges. These mediators which are preformed mediators of mast cells substantiate its role in the development of AERD.[46,47] Similar findings have been seen in lower airway samples also. Bronchial biopsies from AERD patients have also shown increased eosinophils and mast cells. In a study by Nasser et al., endobronchial challenge with aspirin lysine produced a decrease in the number of mast cells (indicating degranulation) and an increase in numbers of activated eosinophils.[48] Sladek et al. estimated (BAL) levels of these mediators in AERD patients before and after aspirin challenge. There was an increased concentration of eosinophilic cationic protein, LTC_4, histamine, and decreased concentrations of thromboxane. The increased recruitment of eosinophils is also supported by a delayed apoptosis in AERD patients, thereby maintaining a persistent inflammatory state.[46,49]

So, the inflammatory process occurring in the mucus membranes and submucosal bronchial tissues is reflected also in the nose and paranasal sinus membranes. The exact reason behind the initiation and persistence of the inflammatory stimuli is still under study. As mentioned previously, other cells like polymorphonuclear leukocytes may be the source of lipoxins, and they may also be involved in the pathogenesis of AERD. An abnormally increased numbers of platelets and leukocytes in both the nasal tissue and peripheral blood have been seen in studies. The platelets and leukocytes act synergistically to produce elevated levels of proinflammatory leukotrienes. The leukocytes in AERD patients have shown to overexpress leukotriene receptors for cysteinyl leukotrienes. Therefore, drugs like leukotriene receptor antagonists or leukotriene synthesis inhibitors blunt the bronchospasm and nasal congestion by blocking the leukotriene pathway.[50,51]

Epithelial Cells in AERD

Epithelial cells from nasal polyps of AERD patients have been found to produce less amounts of PGE2 compared to aspirin-tolerant asthmatics in a study conducted by Kowalski et al. in cultured epithelial cells. In this study after addition of aspirin compounds, epithelial cells of AERD patients were found to produce increased amounts of leukotriene pathway products, with very low levels of PGE2. Because PGE2 levels were lower at baseline in AERD patients compared to controls, aspirin further reduced these levels, and this resulted in unopposed levels of leukotrienes as explained in the pathogenesis above.[52] Since epithelial cells are higher in number compared to inflammatory cells, the reduced synthesis of PGE2 is an important defect in the pathogenesis of aspirin-induced respiratory reactions.

APPROACH TO DIAGNOSIS OF ASPIRIN-INDUCED HYPERSENSITIVITY

A good clinical history, physical examination of a patient, and, if possible and appropriate, in vitro or in vivo tests, followed by drug challenge, are useful in identifying NSAID-induced drug reactions. If drug reaction occurs, the history should focus on determining the possible medication, the type of drug reaction, the time between consumption and development of symptoms, disappearance of symptoms on drug withdrawal, and history of previous reactions to drugs. History of any systemic illness present during the drug consumption which may have mimicked the drug reaction should be asked. For example, asthma attacks, asthma precipitated by infections, menstruation, etc. may itself be responsible for symptoms which are difficult to differentiate from NSAID-induced reactions. If available, prescription papers documenting drug allergy and name of suspected drug with dose should be seeked. Assessment of comorbidities like rhinosinusitis, nasal polyposis, asthma, and chronic urticaria should also be done.

NSAID/aspirin-induced drug reactions consist of one or more of the following:

1. *Naso-ocular*: These are usually the initial manifestations and may mimick an upper respiratory infection. This includes nasal congestion, rhinorrhea, periorbital puffiness, and/or conjunctival suffusion.
2. *Asthmatic symptoms*: Mimicks an asthma attack with chest tightness, cough wheezing, and dyspnea. Objectively, there is a marked fall in FEV1.
3. *Systemic*: Severe reactions may also manifest with facial flushing, laryngospasm, abdominal cramps, epigastric pain, and hypotension. Severe reactions may be difficult to distinguish from anaphylaxis.

If the patient gives a history of NSAID reaction, an attempt should be made to find out if there is any reaction to other COX-1 inhibitors. If cross-reactions are present, this will help in ruling out an immunologically mediated (IgE or T cell) reaction to a single NSAID. Since NSAID reactions are acquired, a history of NSAID consumption without any manifest side effects may be present. Also many patients who have reactions and are accustomed to it will not report it. Some may also have avoided NSAID/ aspirin for years. So, the history alone cannot make a correct diagnosis, and therefore requires a drug challenge testing as described later.

APPROACH TO AERD

The description of this entity dates back to the year 1902 when aspirin was introduced into clinical ractice and sensitivity in an asthmatic was described. The Samters triad was named after Dr Samter, and Dr Beer noticed a triad of asthma, nasal polyps, and aspirin sensitivity in patients.[53] The prevalence of AERD is likely underestimated in the literature, partly because of the difficulty in establishing the diagnosis when relying on patient history alone. But the clinical history will help in determining appropriate tests. The diagnosis is suspected when an adult asthmatic with chronic rhinosinusitis presents with an acute exacerbation of both upper and lower respiratory tract symptoms after the ingestion of aspirin or a COX-1 NSAID. It rarely affects children and adolescents. The full components of the triad usually develop slowly over a period of years, though a rapid progression of rhinosinusitis to full-blown asthma has also been documented. A strong suspicion for AERD should be kept in asthmatics with poor control and history of nasal polyposis/polypectomies. Overall, AERD patients between 36% and 96% are affected with polyps.[54]

Patients typically present with nasal congestion, rhinitis with chronic rhinorrhea, and reduced smell which finally progresses to pansinusitis and eventually polyposis.[55] The majority of the patients develop nasal symptoms at the onset. They frequently undergo multiple sinus surgeries/ polypectomies before diagnosis. Individuals may also develop facial deformation due to the increased pressure of polyps on the sinonasal bones. As the persistent nasal symptoms progress and worsen, it gradually involves the lower airways, and a diagnosis of asthma can also be made. The asthma progresses and persists regardless of environmental exposures. Somewhere during this march, aspirin/NSAID sensitivity appears. Ironically, the upper respiratory symptoms and asthma aggravate over time even with NSAID avoidance.[8,12,15,54]

But all patients do not have severe asthma, and many patients have only an upper respiratory involvement in the form of chronic rhinosinusitis and nasal polyposis. Rarely, a history of aspirin or a COX-1 inhibitor consumption with intolerance is obtained with asthma presenting late. As observed in the European network of aspirin-induced asthma, the majority of patients will be females. Females also tend to have an earlier onset and more severe type of disease. Around 30–70% of patients with AERD are atopic, and some of these patients have high levels of specific immunoglobulin E antibodies to allergens usually dust mites.[16] Peripheral blood eosinophilia is seen in around 50% of AERD patients. Another clinical association observed was a reaction to alcohol ingestion. In a study, AERD patients reported upper and lower respiratory symptoms in response to consumption of alcohol or alcoholic beverages.[56]

The diagnosis cannot be confirmed with a clinical history and examination alone as approximately two thirds of patients with an identical clinical picture never react to aspirin/NSAIDs. So, the absence of a history of an aspirin reaction does not exclude NSAID sensitivity. Hence, oral challenge with aspirin is used to confirm the diagnosis. The prevalence of AERD in adult asthma populations when oral aspirin challenge is used is around 9–20%.[57] Among adult asthmatics who also had nasal polyps and pansinusitis, when oral challenge was given, the prevalence of AERD increased to 34%.[58] About 66–97% of adult asthmatics who gave a history of aspirin/NSAID-induced respiratory reactions had positive oral challenges to aspirin. The ability to tolerate low-dose aspirin does not exclude the possibility of aspirin intolerance. This was shown in a study conducted among 163 patients with AERD. About seven patients who were taking low-dose aspirin (81 mg) were not having any symptoms. Following stoppage of aspirin for 10 days and rechallenge with aspirin, they developed typical reactions.[59]

DETECTION OF ASPIRIN SENSITIVITY

Currently, there are no acceptable, reproducible, practical in vitro tests, which will identify patients at the risk of developing AERD. The gold standard test is through aspirin challenge.[2] Though important mainly as a research tool, practically it is used before aspirin desensitization when patients require long-term treatment with NSAID or aspirin as in cardiovascular disease, rheumatological diseases, and AERD treatment.

ASPIRIN CHALLENGE

They can be inhaled or oral. Intranasal or intrabronchial (inhaled challenges) are performed in Europe using a liquid lysine acetylsalicylic acid derivative. Oral challenges are used in the United States.

Steps

1. Location
   Procedures are usually performed by a trained allergy specialist or a pulmonologist with expertise, facilities, and infrastructure for airway management and anaphylaxis.
2. Pre-procedure preparation
   Asthma should be reasonably controlled before performing the test because unstable asthma is associated with severe reactions. Suspected patients are asked to avoid antihistaminics for 1 week prior to the test. Drugs used for asthma control like oral/inhaled steroids with long-acting beta 2 agonists, intranasal steroids, theophyllines, and oral leukotriene inhibitors are continued. These drugs tend to reduce the severity of pulmonary manifestations, but retain most of the nasal and ocular signs, which will aid the clinician in diagnosis. However, anticholinergics, cromolyn, and short-acting inhaled beta 2 agonists should be discontinued 24 hours before challenge. For most AERD asthmatic patients, discontinuation of oral steroids increases bronchial irritability, and aspirin challenges cannot be accurately and safely performed. Leukotriene inhibitors will not affect the upper respiratory tract reactions, but attenuate the bronchospasm.[60]

   In patients with chronic idiopathic urticaria, discontinuing antihistamines prior to the oral challenge often results in urticarial flares. This may coincide with the drug challenge but may also be unrelated to the aspirin challenge. Patients with active urticaria if given aspirin challenge may have a higher prevalence of aspirin sensitivity. In such patients, antihistaminics should be tapered to the lowest effective dosage to help in identifying a reaction and minimizing flares. So, the recommendation is to stop antihistaminics before aspirin challenges in patients with AERD, but to continue them in those with urticaria.[61]
3. Procedure
   Start challenge if the baseline prebronchodilator FEV1 is equal to or more than 70% of best predicted or have an absolute FEV1 of >1.5 L whichever is greater. Challenges are given for 3 days, and first day is used for placebo. The first day of placebo challenges is done to ensure airway stability with vital signs and pulmonary function measured hourly. Days 2 and 3 are used for incremental aspirin dosage challenges. On the placebo day, the FEV1 values should vary by <10% from baseline values, and the FEV1 starting value on day 2 must be within 10% of the value on day 1. Oral aspirin is given in incremental doses every 3 hours and observed for manifestations. The usual starting dose is 30 mg, and doses are increased at intervals. If the historical reaction was severe, second dose is increased to 45 mg, and if the reaction was mild, dose used is 60 mg.

   Example of a protocol

	Aspirin dosage (mg)		
Time	Day 1	Day 2	Day 3
7 AM	Placebo	30	100–150
10 AM	Placebo	45–60	150–325
1 PM	Placebo	60–100	650

4. Criteria for positive reactions
   In AERD following ingestion of NSAIDs, reactions typically develop within 30 minutes to 3 hours. The reactions are dose dependent with small doses producing minimal nasal congestion and larger doses producing even severe bronchospasm. The classic reaction is rhinoconjunctivitis and bronchospasm with an FEV1 decline of >15%. If rhinoconjunctivitis alone occurs (upper respiratory), a decline in FEV1 of <15% is sufficient. If bronchospasm (lower respiratory) alone occurs, the FEV1 decline should be >20%. Other manifestations like laryngospasm, systemic manifestations like abdominal pain, flushing, urticaria, and rarely hypotension can occur. Most patients with AERD develop bronchoconstriction at low doses of 30–120 mg. Fatal reactions have rarely occurred following full NSAID doses.

   Once reactions occur, it is reversed immediately with symptomatic treatment, and subsequent challenges are postponed to the next day. If aspirin 650 mg is administered without reaction and patient is not taking more than 10 mg prednisolone per day or leukotriene modifier, the person does not have AERD. If clinical suspicion is high with a negative reaction, rechallenge with aspirin when patient is stable and without the use of oral steroid/leukotriene inhibitors should be done.

INHALED CHALLENGE

Aspirin lysine is used for the inhalation challenge. Bronchospasm occurs early by 30 minutes, which can be reversed with beta 2 agonists. Here the test can be completed in a single day and takes less than 5 hours.

INHALED VS. ORAL CHALLENGE

A study comparing inhaled and oral aspirin challenges found that, both routes accurately detected bronchospastic reactions. Urinary concentrations of leukotriene E4 (LTE4) were higher with oral challenge. Since inhaled aspirin is not directed toward the naso-ocular surfaces, the development of naso-ocular reactions is less with inhaled aspirin lysine. So, both these tests are equally specific for AERD, but oral aspirin challenge has a higher diagnostic sensitivity and mimicks the real-life situation. The disadvantage with oral challenges is the duration for testing, oral challenges requiring up to 3 hours from ingestion to reaction. So only three oral challenges can be conducted between 7 AM and 4 PM, whereas inhalation challenge requires only a half day.[62]

TESTS FOR ASPIRIN-INDUCED URTICARIA

There are no available in vitro tests to detect aspirin-induced urticaria. So oral aspirin challenge is required. Antihistaminics should be discontinued before doing the challenge. Most patients react to doses between 150 and 650 mg of aspirin, and a time delay of 2–4 hours is expected between ingestion and onset of hives. The starting dose is usually 150 mg, which is increased to 325 mg and then 650 mg. Sometimes a double-blind oral challenge incorporating the suspected provoking dose of aspirin and placebo doses may be needed to confirm specificity of the original challenge.

TREATMENT OF AERD

General Measures

Avoidance of aspirin and all cross-reacting NSAIDs prevents all reactions in patients with AERD and chronic idiopathic urticaria. Unless patients are known or suspected to have reacted to aspirin or NSAIDs, or have underlying nasal polyps, sinusitis, asthma, or chronic urticaria, it is unnecessary to advise them to avoid all NSAIDs. In patients with selective NSAID-induced urticaria, it is not necessary to avoid dissimilar NSAIDs. Because of the property of selectivity, there is no immunologic cross-reactivity between NSAIDs. Safe alternatives are those NSAIDs with very weak COX-1 activity, acetaminophen, and COX-2 selective inhibitors like the coxibs.

Management of asthma and allergic rhinitis should be as per standard guidelines. Abnormal leukotriene metabolism should be controlled with leukotriene modifying agents like leukotriene receptor antagonists (montelukast/zafirlukast) and leukotriene synthesis inhibitors (zileuton). Leukotriene-modifying drugs help in controlling the nasopulmonary manifestations as well as protecting from exacerbations due to accidental NSAID consumption. Multiple studies and randomized controlled trials have confirmed the efficacy of leukotriene-modifying agents in the control of AERD.[63,64]. A recent meta-analyses have shown that leukotriene receptor antagonists improve severity of symptoms and reduce eosinophil levels and polyp size compared to placebo.[65] The greatest symptom improvements were observed in headache, facial pain, sneezing, nasal pruritus, postnasal drip, and smell disturbance. They may provide additional benefit to inhaled steroids with regard to these symptoms, but not in overall disease severity. Usually patients are started on montelukast because of the ease of administration. If patients are not improving with montelukast, then zileuton may also be added or substituted. The combination therapy of montelukast and zileuton is based on the evidence that patients with AERD have elevated levels of cysteinyl leukotrienes and receptor numbers, as well as an upregulation of 5 lipoxygenase enzyme.[66] Zileuton is given four times daily and requires liver function test monitoring. A study conducted by Ta et al. has shown better symptom control with zileuton.[55]

If the patient develops an acute severe reaction following ingestion of aspirin, remember the rule of maintaining airway, breathing, and circulation. Bronchospasm can be controlled with beta 2 agonists. For laryngospasm, intramuscular epinephrine along with inhaled epinephrine is given. Nasal congestion and sinusitis can be relieved with topical decongestants like oxymetazoline and oral antihistaminic-decongestant combinations. Intravenous H1 antihistaminics like diphenhydramine and H2 blockers like ranitidine will control the systemic reactions. In case of anaphylaxis, intramuscular adrenaline 1 mL of 1/1,000 solution is injected intramuscular into the anterolateral aspect of thigh and repeated every 2–3 minutes as required. Facilities for intubation and mechanical ventilation must also be available.

Specific Treatment

In addition to the above measures, major goals in controlling AERD include preventing nasal polyp formation, treatment of secondary sinusitis, and anti-inflammatory therapy to both the upper and lower respiratory tracts. Treatment therefore includes high doses of topical steroids both nasal and inhaled, which reduces inflammation and nasal polyp formation. Some patients require, in addition, systemic steroids. Adequate control of sinus infections using antibiotics and oral steroid bursts may be needed to shrink nasal polyps and re-establish sinus drainage. Refractory nasal polyps on medical treatment require sinus surgery like functional endoscopic sinus surgery with polypectomy. Definitive treatment of aspirin allergy/AERD includes aspirin desensitization as mentioned below.

ASPIRIN DESENSITIZATION

Aspirin desensitization means eliminating reactions to aspirin by slowly and steadily increasing exposure to oral aspirin. This was first described by Widal in 1922.[67] The exact mechanism by which desensitization is effective is unknown. It is proposed that desensitization along with daily aspirin consumption reduces IL-4-induced expression of leukotrienes by blocking the transcription factor, signal transducer and activator of transcription 6 (STAT-6).[68,69]

All AERD patients can be desensitized to aspirin, but it is difficult in chronic urticaria. It reduces upper and lower airway symptoms in patients with AERD, with dramatic effects especially in the upper airway symptoms. But there are no data to show that aspirin is effective in asthmatics with nasal polyposis *without* aspirin intolerance.

The indications for aspirin desensitization in AERD include

1. Patients requiring very high doses of systemic steroids.
2. Recurrent nasal polyposis despite optimal and standard medical management after surgical resection.
3. Recurrent headaches not responding to conventional management and requiring intermittent bursts of NSAIDs.
4. Inflammatory conditions like arthritis, which requires daily NSAID usage.
5. Ischemic heart diseases/vascular diseases like Kawasaki syndrome, which require daily aspirin consumption.

Szczeklik and Stevenson described a strategy for desensitizing patients with AERD.[1] This protocol, known as "Scripps Clinic Protocol," involves reintroducing the dose of aspirin that initiated an aspirin reaction during the previous day. This process is continued slowly with escalation of doses till the patient can tolerate a dose of 650 mg without any reaction. Following the desensitization procedure, the desensitized state persists for 2–5 days with sensitivity returning after 7 days. So, a desensitized person can remain without aspirin for around 5 days maximum, beyond which sensitivity is restored. In addition, this procedure causes cross desensitization to other NSAIDs also. Following the desensitization procedure, the patient will have to take a dose of 325–650 mg aspirin twice daily to maintain desensitization. Patients with ischemic heart disease who take around 75 mg of aspirin as antiplatelet dose will remain tolerant to this dose, but they will not be able to tolerate larger doses.[70] Remember that an ability to tolerate low-dose aspirin does not exclude the possibility of NSAID intolerance/AERD. This was shown in a study conducted among 163 patients with AERD. About seven patients who were taking low-dose aspirin (81 mg) were not having any symptoms. Following stoppage of aspirin for 10 days and rechallenge with aspirin, they developed typical reactions.[59]

Some patients are unable to complete the desensitization procedure because of side effects like refractory nausea, diarrhea, abdominal pain, erythematous and pruritic rash, or rarely persistent respiratory symptoms. In most situations, an AERD patient with concomitant arthritis or coronary artery disease with a need for antiplatelet can be desensitized to aspirin and then take aspirin indefinitely, or the patient can be switched over to any other NSAID as long as the aspirin or NSAID is consumed daily. But daily aspirin rather than NSAID consumption has been found to reduce the upper and lower respiratory symptoms if it is AERD.

Aspirin Therapy in Cardiovascular Diseases

The prevalence of aspirin sensitivity in cardiovascular patients is not well known. Besides substitution with an alternative class of antiplatelet agents such as thienopyridines (clopidogrel), aspirin desensitization is an option for allergic patients who require long-term therapy for cardiovascular diseases. Schaefer and Gore reported a 45-year-old female patient with a history of asthma and allergic rhinitis and acetylsalicylic acid (ASA) sensitivity. This patient after developing a myocardial infarction was treated with coronary stenting and discharged with ticlodipine 250 mg twice-daily therapy. Later, she underwent the oral aspirin challenge test and desensitization in an outpatient setting and was able to take dual antiplatelets successfully.[71] Wong et al. desensitized 11 patients with a history of aspirin-induced urticaria/angioedema with a rapid desensitization protocol.[72] Nine out of the eleven patients tolerated the protocol and took aspirin without reactions for 1–24 months. The protocol is shown below.

Time (minutes)	Aspirin dose (mg)
0	0.1
15	0.3
30	10
45	30
60	40
85	81
110	162
135	325

This protocol has been found especially useful in unstable angina due to the rapid desensitization, but the initial dosages are difficult to obtain commercially. In patients with a positive aspirin challenge, the decision to continue aspirin should be based on a risk benefit approach. Those who require aspirin as primary prevention should avoid aspirin if they showed a positive challenge. Coronary artery disease patients who require aspirin as secondary prevention, those with vascular stents and those having recurrent ischemic events with single antiplatelets, would require a rapid desensitization protocol followed by daily aspirin therapy. Current recommendation from the American College of Cardiology and the American Heart Association regarding aspirin desensitization in cardiovascular patients is that, if true allergy is present, other antiplatelet agents such as dipyridamole, ticlopidine, or clopidogrel may be substituted.[73]

Newer Drugs for AERD

Biological therapies like monoclonal antibodies have been tried also with mixed results.

Omalizumab

The anti-IgE monoclonal antibody omalizumab is approved by the US Food and Drug Administration and recommended in GINA guidelines as step 5 treatment for inadequately controlled moderate-to-severe asthma. It could be considered for patients with concomitant chronic rhinosinusitis and nasal polyposis. Some isolated case reports have shown omalizumab to be effective in controlling asthma as well as reducing aspirin sensitivity.[74-76] In a study involving AERD patients, omalizumab was given to patients with chronic rhinosinustis with nasal polyposis and asthma, half of whom had AERD. Though omalizumab showed improved airway symptoms and quality of life compared to placebo, the effects were less pronounced in the AERD patients.[77]

Mepolizumab

The anti-IL-5 monoclonal antibody mepolizumab has been used in patients with severe asthma and eosinophilia. In a small randomized trial among patients with nasal polyposis refractory to conventional medical management, mepolizumab injections were found to reduce the polyps as assessed by polyp score. The exact role in AERD is yet to be studied.[78]

CONCLUSION

Aspirin, the prototype NSAID which is primarily a COX-1 inhibitor, induces both allergic and nonallergic reactions. Drug hypersensitivity reactions can be selective or cross-reactive, i.e., hypersensitivity reactions inducible by other NSAIDs also. The classical example of cross-reactive reactions is AERD. AERD is a syndrome complex of patients with chronic rhinosinusitis, nasal polyposis, asthma, and drug intolerance to aspirin. The typical patient develops acute upper and lower respiratory symptoms, 30 minutes to 3 hours, following consumption of an NSAID most commonly aspirin. AERD affects 5–20% of all patients with asthma. The mechanisms include an alteration in arachidonic acid metabolism with an imbalance of pro- and anti-inflammatory mediators. Further, aspirin-induced COX-1 inhibition and increased leukotriene production are believed to be responsible for the manifestations. A strong clinical suspicion should be kept in patients with chronic rhinosinusitis and history of recurrent nasal polypectomies with or without drug reactions. Though clinical history is suggestive, definite diagnosis requires an aspirin challenge test. Treatment includes management of upper and lower airway control with anti-inflammatory medicines and antileukotriene drugs. Avoidance of NSAID especially COX-1 inhibitors should also be done if AERD is present. Chronic rhinosinusitis with polyps refractory to medical management may require surgical management. Aspirin desensitization in an adequate resuscitation unit followed by daily aspirin will be helpful in selected AERD patients (as described earlier). The desensitization procedure will help AERD patients in controlling symptoms as well as tolerating different NSAIDs. Newer therapies like monoclonal antibodies have been tried, and results are promising.

REFERENCES

1. Szczeklik A, Stevenson DD. Aspirin induced asthma: Advances in pathogenesis and management. J Allergy Clin Immunol. 1999;104:5-13.
2. Park HS, Kowalski ML, Sanchez-Borges M. Hypersensitivity to aspirin and other nonsteroidal antiinflammatory drugs. In: Adkinson NF Jr, Bochner BS, Burks W, Busse WW, Holgate ST, Lemanske RF Jr, O'Hehir RE, editors. Middleton's allergy: principles and practice. 8th ed. Philadelphia (PA): Elsevier/Saunders; 2014. 1296.
3. Stevenson DD, Sanchez-Borges M, Szczeklik A. Classification of allergic and pseudoallergic reactions to drugs that inhibit cyclooxygenase enzymes. Ann Allergy Asthma Immunol. 2001;87:177-180.
4. Kowalski ML, Asero R, Bavbek S, et al. Classification and practical approach to the diagnosis and management of hypersensitivity to NSAID drugs. Allergy. 2013;68:1219-1232.
5. Stevenson DD, Kowalski ML. An epidemic of over diagnosing drug allergies. Allergy Asthma Proc. 2014;35:92-94.
6. Torres MJ, Barrionuevo E, Kowalski M, Blanca M. Hypersensitivity reactions to nonsteroidal anti-inflammatory drugs. Immunol Allergy Clin North Am. 2014;34:507-524, vii-viii.
7. Suresh KB, Sundeep SS. Aspirin and Asthma. Chest 2000;118:1470-1476.
8. Jenkins C, Costello J, Hodge L. Systematic review of prevalence of aspirin induced asthma and its implications for clinical practice. Br. Med J. 2004,328:434-436.
9. Spector SL, Wangaard CH, Farr RS. Aspirin and concomitant idiosyncrasies in adult asthmatic patients. J Allergy Clin Immunol. 1979;64:500-506.
10. Rachelefsky GS, Coulson A, Siegel SC, Stiehm ER. Aspirin intolerance in chronic childhood asthma detected by oral challenge. Pediatrics. 1975;56:443-448.
11. Kasper L, Sladek K, Duplaga M, et al. Prevalence of asthma with aspirin hypersensitivity in the adult population of Poland. Allergy. 2003;58(10):1064-1066.
12. Hedman J, Kaprio J, Poussa T, Nieminen MM. Prevalence of asthma, aspirin intolerance, nasal polyposis and chronic obstructive pulmonary disease in a population-based study. Int J Epidemiol. 1999;28(4):717-722.
13. Vally H, Taylor ML, Thompson PJ. The prevalence of aspirin-intolerant asthma in Australian asthmatic patients. Thorax. 2002;57:569-574.
14. Rajan JP, Wineinger NE, Stevenson DD, White AA. Prevalence of aspirin-exacerbated respiratory disease among asthmatic patients: A meta-analysis of the literature. J Allergy Clin Immunol. 2015;135(3):676-681.
15. Berges-Gimeno MP, Simon RA, Stevenson DD. The natural history and clinical characteristics of aspirin-exacerbated respiratory disease. Ann Allergy Asthma Immunol. 2002;89:474.
16. Szczeklik A, Nizankowska E, Duplaga M. Natural history of aspirin induced asthma: AIANE investigators. European network on Aspirin Induced asthma. Eur Respir J. 2000;16:432-436.
17. Stevenson D, Simon RA. Sensitivity to Aspirin and NSAID drugs. in Middleton EJ, Reed CE, Ellis EF, et al: Allergy: Principles and practise, 4th edn, Volume 2, St Louis 1993, Mosby. pp. 1747-1767.
18. Erdogan T, Karakaya G, Kalyoncu AF. Comorbid diseases in aspirin-exacerbated respiratory disease and asthma. Allergol Immunopathol. (Madr). 2014 accessed from doi:10.1016/j.aller.2014.07.008
19. Warren RP. Effect of Aspirin in chronic urticaria. Br J Dermatol. 1960;72:350-355.
20. Champion RR, Roberts SO, Carpenter RG. Urticaria and angioedema: A review of 554 patients. Br J Dermatol. 1969;81:588-595.
21. Mathison DA, Lumry WR, Stevenson DD. Aspirin in chronic urticaria and/or angioedema: Studies of sensitivity and desensitisation. J Allergy ClinImmunol. 1982;69:135.
22. Sanchez-Borges M, Capriles-Hulett A. Atopy is a risk factor for non-steroidal antiinflammatory drug sensitivity. Ann Allergy Asthma Immunol. 2000;84:101-106.
23. Sanchez-Borges M, Capriles-Hulett A, Caballero-Fonseca F. Cutaneous reactions to aspirin and nonsteroidal anti-inflammatory drugs. Clin Rev Allergy Immunol. 2003;24: 125-135.
24. Shore SA, Austen KF, Drazen JM. Lung biology in health and disease: Lung cell biology. In: Eicosanoids and the lung, L'Enfant C, Massaro D (Eds), Marcel Dekker, New York; 1989.
25. Laitinen LA, Laitinen A, Haahtela T, et al. Leukotriene E4 and granulocytic infiltration into asthmatic airways. Lancet. 1993;341:989.
26. Picado C, Fernandez-Morata JC, Juan M, et al. Cyclooxygenase-2 mRNA is downexpressed in nasal polyps from aspirin-sensitive asthmatics. Am J RespirCrit Care Med. 1999;160:291.
27. Pierzchalska M, Szabó Z, Sanak M, et al. Deficient prostaglandin E2 production by bronchial fibroblasts of asthmatic patients, with special reference to aspirin-induced asthma. J Allergy Clin Immunol. 2003;111:1041.
28. Sestini P, Armetti L, Gambaro G, et al. Inhaled PGE2 prevents aspirin-induced bronchoconstriction and urinary LTE4 excretion in aspirin-sensitive asthma. Am J Respir Crit Care Med. 1996;153:572.
29. Laidlaw TM, Cutler AJ, Kidder MS, et al. Prostaglandin E2 resistance in granulocytes from patients with aspirin-exacerbated respiratory disease. J Allergy Clin Immunol. 2014;133:1692.

30. Corrigan CJ, Napoli RL, Meng Q, et al. Reduced expression of the prostaglandin E2 receptor E-prostanoid 2 on bronchial mucosal leukocytes in patients with aspirin-sensitive asthma. J Allergy Clin Immunol. 2012;129:1636.
31. Bochenek G, Nagraba K, Nizankowska E, Szczeklik A. A controlled study of 9 alpha, 11 beta-PGF2 (a prostaglandin D2 metabolite) in plasma and urine of patients with bronchial asthma and healthy controls after aspirin challenge. J Allergy Clin Immunol. 2003;111:743.
32. Campo P, Ayuso P, Salas M, et al. Mediator release after nasal aspirin provocation supports different phenotypes in subjects with hypersensitivity reactions to NSAIDs. Allergy. 2013;68:1001.
33. Cahill KN, Bensko JC, Boyce JA, Laidlaw TM. Prostaglandin D_2: a dominant mediator of aspirin-exacerbated respiratory disease. J Allergy Clin Immunol. 2015;135:245.
34. Dahlén B. Treatment of aspirin-intolerant asthma with antileukotrienes. Am J Respir Crit Care Med. 2000;161: S137.
35. Laidlaw TM, Kidder MS, Bhattacharyya N, et al. Cysteinyl leukotriene overproduction in aspirin-exacerbated respiratory disease is driven by platelet-adherent leukocytes. Blood. 2012;119:3790.
36. Christie PE, Tagari P, Ford-Hutchinson AW. Urinary leukotriene E4 concentrations increase after aspirin challenge in aspirin sensitive asthmatic patients. Am Rev Respir Dis. 1991;143:1025-1029.
37. Smith CM, Hawksworth RJ, Thien FC. Urinary leukotriene E4 in bronchial asthma. Eur Respir J. 1992;5:693-699.
38. Knapp HR, Sladek K, Fitzgerald GA. Increased excretion of leukotriene E4 during aspirin-induced asthma. J Lab Clin Med. 1992;119:48.
39. Antczak A, Montuschi P, Kharitonov S, et al. Increased exhaled cysteinyl-leukotrienes and 8-isoprostane in aspirin-induced asthma. Am J Respir Crit Care Med. 2002;166:301.
40. Daffern P, Muilenburg D, Hugli TE, et al. Association of urinary leukotriene E4 excretion during aspirin challenges with severity of respiratory responses. J Allergy Clin Immunol. 1999;104:559-564.
41. Narayanankutty A, Reséndiz-Hernández JM, Falfán-Valencia R, Teran LM. Biochemical pathogenesis of aspirin exacerbated respiratory disease (AERD). Clin Bio Chem. 2013;46:566.
42. Sanak M, Levy BD, Clish CB. Aspirin tolerant asthmatics generate more Lipoxins than aspirin intolerant asthmatics. Eur Respir J. 2000;16:44-49.
43. Juergens UR, Christiansen SC, Stevenson DD, et al. Arachidonic acid metabolism in monocytes of aspirin sensitive asthmatic patients before and after oral aspirin challenge. J Allergy Clin Immunol. 1992;90:635-645.
44. Fischer AR, Rosenberg MA, Lilly CM, et al. Direct evidence for a role of the mast cell in the nasal response to aspirin in aspirin-sensitive asthma. J Allergy Clin Immunol. 1994;94:1046.
45. Yamashita T, Tsuyi H, Maeda N. Etiology of nasal polyps associated with aspirin sensitive asthma. Rhinology. 1989;8:15-24.
46. Cowburn AS, Sladek K, Soja J, et al. Overexpression of leukotriene C4 synthase in bronchial biopsies from patients with aspirin-intolerant asthma. J Clin Invest. 1998;101:834.
47. Maclouf JA, Murphy RC. Transcellular metabolism of neutrophil-derived leukotriene A4 by human platelets. A potential cellular source of leukotriene C4. J Biol Chem. 1988;263:174.
48. Nasser S, Christie PE, Pfister R, et al. Effect of endobronchial aspirin challenge on inflammatory cells in bronchial biopsy samples from aspirin-sensitive asthmatic subjects. Thorax. 1996;51:64.
49. Kowalski M, Grzegorczyk J, Pawliczak R. Decreased apoptosis in nasal polyps of patients with aspirin hypersensitivity. Allergy. 2002;57:493-500.
50. Laidlaw TM, Kidder MS, Bhattacharyya N, et al. Cysteinyl leukotriene overproduction in aspirin-exacerbated respiratory disease is driven by platelet-adherent leukocytes. Blood. 2012;119:3790.
51. Sousa AR, Parikh A, Scadding G, et al. Leukotriene-receptor expression on nasal mucosal inflammatory cells in aspirin-sensitive rhinosinusitis. N Engl J Med. 2002;347:1493.
52. Kowalski ML, Pawliczak R, Wozniak J, et al. Differential metabolism of arachidonic acid in nasal polyp epithelial cells cultured from aspirin-sensitive and aspirin-tolerant patients. Am J Respir Crit Care Med. 2000;161:391.
53. Samter M, Beers RF Jr. Intolerance to aspirin. Clinical studies and consideration of its pathogenesis. Ann Intern Med. 1968;68:975.
54. Szczeklik A, Stevenson DD. Aspirin-induced asthma: advances in pathogenesis, diagnosis, and management. J Allergy Clin Immunol. 2003;111:913-921.
55. Ta V, White AA. Survey-defined patient experiences with aspirin-exacerbated respiratory disease. J Allergy Clin Immunol Pract. 2015;3(5):711-718.
56. Cardet JC, White AA, Barrett NA, et al. Alcohol-induced respiratory symptoms are common in patients with aspirin exacerbated respiratory disease. J Allergy Clin Immunol Pract. 2014;2:208.
57. McDonald J, Mathison DA, Stevenson DD. Aspirin intolerance in asthma: detection by challenge. J Allergy Clin Immunol. 1972;50:198-207.
58. Weber RW, Hoffman M, Raine DA, et al. Incidence of bronchoconstriction due to aspirin, azo dyes, non azo dyes and preservatives in a population of perennial asthmatics. J Allergy Clin Immunol. 1979;64:32-37.
59. Lee-Sarwar K, Johns C, Laidlaw TM, Cahill KN. Tolerance of daily low-dose aspirin does not preclude aspirin-exacerbated respiratory disease. J Allergy Clin Immunol Pract. 2015;3:449.
60. Pleskow WW, Stevenson DD, Mathison DA, et al. Aspirin sensitive rhinosinusitis/asthma: spectrum of adverse reactions to Aspirin. J Allergy Clin Immunol. 1983;71:574-579.

61. Namazy JA, Simon RA. Sensitivity to nonsteroidal anti-inflammatory drugs. Ann Allergy Asthma Immunol. 2002;89:542-550.
62. Dahlen B, Zetterstrom O. Comparison of bronchial and per oral provocation with aspirin in aspirin sensitive asthmatics. Eur Respir J. 1990;3:527-534.
63. Dahlén SE, Malmström K, Nizankowska E, et al. Improvement of aspirin-intolerant asthma by montelukast, a leukotriene antagonist: a randomized, double-blind, placebo-controlled trial. Am J Respir Crit Care Med. 2002;165:9.
64. Lee DK, Haggart K, Robb FM, Lipworth BJ. Montelukast protects against nasal lysine-aspirin challenge in patients with aspirin-induced asthma. Eur Respir J. 2004;24:226.
65. Wentzel JL, Soler ZM, DeYoung K, et al. Leukotriene antagonists in nasal polyposis: a meta-analysis and systematic review. Am J Rhinol Allergy. 2013;27(6):482-489.
66. Dahlén B, Nizankowska E, Szczeklik A, et al. Benefits from adding the 5-lipoxygenase inhibitor zileuton to conventional therapy in aspirin-intolerant asthmatics. Am J Respir Crit Care Med. 1998;157:1187.
67. Widal MF, Abrami P, Lermeyez J. Anaphylaxis et Idiosyncrasie. Presse Med. 1992;30:189-192.
68. Steinke JW, Culp JA, Kropf E, Borish L. Modulation by aspirin of nuclear phospho-signal transducer and activator of transcription 6 expression: Possible role in therapeutic benefit associated with aspirin desensitization. J Allergy Clin Immunol. 2009;124:724.
69. Katial RK, Strand M, Prasertsuntarasai T, et al. The effect of aspirin desensitization on novel biomarkers in aspirin-exacerbated respiratory diseases. J Allergy Clin Immunol. 2010;126:738.
70. Pleskow WW, Stevenson DD, Mathison DA, et al. Aspirin desensitisation in aspirin sensitive asthmatic patients: clinical manifestations and characterisation of the refractory period. J Allergy Clin Immunol. 1982;69: 11-19.
71. Schaefer OP, Gore JM. Aspirin sensitivity: the role for aspirin challenge and desensitization in postmyocardial infarction patients. Cardiology. 1999;91:8-13.
72. Wong JT, Nagy CS, Krinzman SJ, et al. Rapid oral challenge-desensitization for patients with aspirin-related urticaria-angioedema. J Allergy Clin Immunol. 2000;105:997-1001.
73. Srinivasan R, Jeffrey AB, Vijay GK. Approach to "Aspirin Allergy" in cardiovascular patients. Circulation. 2004;110: e1-e4.
74. Aksu K, Kurt E. Aspirin tolerance following omalizumab therapy in a patient with aspirin-exacerbated respiratory disease. Allergol Immunopathol. 2013;41:208.
75. Bobolea I, Barranco P, Fiandor A, et al. Omalizumab: a potential new therapeutic approach for AERD. J Investig Allergol Clin Immunol. 2010;20:448.
76. Bergmann KC, Zuberbier T, Church MK. Omalizumab in the treatment of AERD. J Allergy Clin Immunol Pract. 2015;3:459.
77. Gevaert P, Calus L, Van Zele T, et al. Omalizumab is effective in allergic and nonallergic patients with nasal polyps and asthma. J Allergy Clin Immunol. 2013;131: 110.
78. Gevaert P, Van Bruaene N, Cattaert T, et al. Mepolizumab, a humanized anti-IL-5 monoclonal antibody, as a treatment option for severe nasal polyposis. J Allergy Clin Immunol. 2011;128:989.

CHAPTER 37

Aspirin-exacerbated Respiratory Disease

B Vidyasagar, BJ Arun

INTRODUCTION

Powder from the bark of white willow tree (*Salix alba*) used for pain relief was described as early as 460 BC by Hippocrates. "Salicylic acid" name was derived from Latin name of the tree *Salix*. In 1853, salicylic acid was neutralized by buffering with sodium salicylate and acetyl chloride creating acetylsalicylic acid (aspirin) by French chemist Gerhardt. It was abandoned until 1887[1] when Hoffmann Felix, a German chemist, rediscovered it in 1887, which he used to treat his father's arthritis. Since then, it has remained as the safest, least expensive, and most consumed analgesic.[2] Aspirin is being used for the prophylaxis of thromboembolic episodes as it possesses antiplatelet properties other than analgesic and antipyretic properties.[2] The association of aspirin with asthma was described by Widal et al. in 1922.[2] Brief historical perspective of aspirin and aspirin exacerbated asthma (AEA) is listed in Table 37.1.[1] The triad of asthma, aspirin sensitivity, and nasal polyps came to be known as 'Samter's triad' named after Samter and Beers who described the clinical entity in 1968.[3]

There exist many terminologies that link aspirin to asthma, such as aspirin intolerant asthma (AIA), AEA, aspirin-exacerbated respiratory diseases (AERD). However, in recent times, AERD is given more clinical relevance as earlier terms only emphasise on one component of the reaction. As described in earlier literature, AIA refers to onset of asthmatic symptom in a patient who never had respiratory symptom prior to taking aspirin and AEA refers to worsening symptoms of asthma on exposure to aspirin/ nonsteroidal anti-inflammatory drugs (NSAIDs) in a patient having pre-existing asthma.

AERD refers to clinical spectrum of asthma, chronic rhinosinusitis (CRS) with nasal polyposis, and acute upper and lower respiratory tract reactions to ingestion of aspirin

Table 37.1: Historical perspective of aspirin and aspirin-exacerbated asthma.

Date	*Person*	*Discovery*
460 BC	Hippocrates	Described properties of powders derived from bark of white willow tree (*Salix alba*)
1853	Gerhardt	Created ASA by acetylation of phenolic hydroxyl group of salicylic acid
1874	Kolbe	Synthesis of salicylic acid, used as a painkiller, although with severe GI side effects
1889	Hoffman	Rediscovered the medicinal properties of ASA without GI irritation; mass marketing by Bayer
1922	Abrami and Lemoyez	Reported a case of anaphylaxis to 100 mg ASA
1967	Samter and Beers	Reported the phenomena of ASA intolerance, nasal polyposis, asthma
1967	Vanselow	Bronchial asthma induced by indomethacin
1971	Sir John Vane	Identified mechanism of action of ASA as inhibition of cyclooxygenase pathway
1973	Lockey et al	Reported mechanism of the mode of inheritance of AEA as autosomal recessive
1980	Stevenson	Reported successful desensitization to ASA
1994	Szczeklik	Reported eicosanoids (cysteinyl leukotrienes) in pathogenesis of AEA

AEA, aspirin-exacerbated asthma; ASA, acetylsalicylic acid; GI, gastrointestinal.
Allergy, Asthma, and Clinical Immunology, Volume 4, Number 2, 2UUS.

(acetyl salicylic acid) and/or other cyclooxygenase-1 (COX-1) inhibiting drugs or NSAIDs. Symptoms of reaction to aspirin begin typically anywhere from 20 minutes to 3 hours after ingestion, presenting as nasal congestion and wheeze, and may continue to resolve over few hours of time.

PREVALENCE

Prevalence among general population is less than 5%[4,5] although some studies mention much higher rates.[6-8] A database study of around 13,000 randomly selected adults from Poland showed a prevalence of 0.6% among general population and 4.3% with known asthma diagnosis. But with nasal polyps, it ranged from 14% to 22%, and with chronic sinusitis, it ranged from 0.7% to 2.6%.[1] In steroid-dependent asthma, aspirin sensitivity may be as high as 20–40%.[6-8] In another study, 49% of 80 adults presenting to allergy and immunology clinic with CRS and nasal polyp reacted to aspirin challenge, while 36% reported sensitivity to NSAIDs.[9] The prevalence may be underdiagnosed as evidenced by European network of aspirin-induced asthma (AIANE) study, where 18% of participants were unaware of aspirin sensitivity[1] before undergoing unblinded aspirin provocation tests.

PATHOPHYSIOLOGY

Aspirin-related asthma typically occurs in the fourth decade in contrast to classic atopic asthma which occurs before the age of 20 years. Familial predisposition is rare as one study showed 2 out of 500 patients having positive family history. However, one study showed an increased expression of HLA-DQw2 in one group of such patients. Other studies have implicated the upregulation of the expression of leukotriene C4 (LTC4) synthase, which was found to be increased in the blood eosinophils of patients with AIA.[10]

The reactions to aspirin in suspected patients is not immunoglobulin (IgE) mediated hence classified as "pseudoallergic." These reactions are triggered by structurally different medication that can inhibit the COX-1 enzyme and evoke an abnormal biochemical response different from pharmacological action of NSAIDs. In contrast, IgE-mediated reaction occurs following antibody formation to a specific drug or haptenated drug. However, 30–70% of AERD patients are atopic[11,12] and a portion of these have high specific IgE levels to inhalant allergens.[13,14] Peripheral eosinophilia occurs in 50% of patients and is correlated with severity of nasal symptoms.[15-18]

The pathophysiology of AERD is not fully understood; dysregulation of arachidonic acid metabolism, particularly overproduction of leukotrienes, predominantly involved in bronchoconstriction and proinflammatory mechanisms is responsible. Arachidonic acid derived from membrane phospholipids of various cells undergoes metabolism via two different pathways resulting in lipid mediators (Flowcharts 37.1 and 37.2).

Metabolism of arachidonic acid through 5-lipoxygenase pathway produces leukotrienes (LTs), cysteinyl leukotrienes (cysLTs), LTC4, LTD4, and LTE4 which are bronchoconstrictors; induce increased mucus secretions, nasal mucosal swelling, and airway edema; and attract eosinophils.[19-21] LTB4 is another proinflammatory leukotriene having effects on neutrophils and monocytes.

Arachidonic acid metabolism through cyclooxygenase pathway (two isoforms: COX-1—cycloendoperoxidase H synthase and COX-2—prostaglandin synthase) yields prostaglandins and thromboxanes.[22]

Prostaglandin PGE which is a potent bronchodilator with anti-inflammatory property is decreased in polyp tissue and lower airway of AERD patients are reduced at baseline and fall further after aspirin challenge.[23-25] Levels of PGE2 also reduce after ingestion of other COX-1 inhibitors. The significant role of PGE2 in AERD patients is highlighted by a study in which PGE2 synthase 1 deficient mouse showed increasing airway resistance, cysLT production, and mast cell activation like in human AERD patients when challenged with lysine-aspirin,[26] and there was suppression of anti-IgE-induced cysLT production from activated mast cell cultures from AERD patients on exposure to PGE_2.[27,28]

In contrast, PGD_2 and its metabolites PGD_2S, which is a potent bronchoconstrictor, is increased in patients with AERD at baseline and further increased after aspirin challenge.[22,29,30] There appears to be a baseline dysregulation of arachidonic acid metabolism in patients with AERD, and increased production of inflammatory mediators and a decreased production of anti-inflammatory mediators compared to patients with asthma without AERD.[30-34] This dysregulation is accentuated by COX-1 inhibitors.

There is also an increase in the number of activated mast cells and eosinophils in the bronchial tree[35-37] of patients with AERD, bronchial mast cell being the primary source of leukotrienes (LTC4) in patients with AERD although eosinophils can also produce it in large amounts.[38]

Flowchart 37.1: Aspirin inhibits the COX pathway and consequently diverts arachidonic acid metabolites to the IX pathway. This also leads to a decrease in the levels of PGE_2, the anti-inflammatory PC. LTC_4 synthase overexpression further increases the number of cysteinyl LTs tilting the balance toward inflammation.

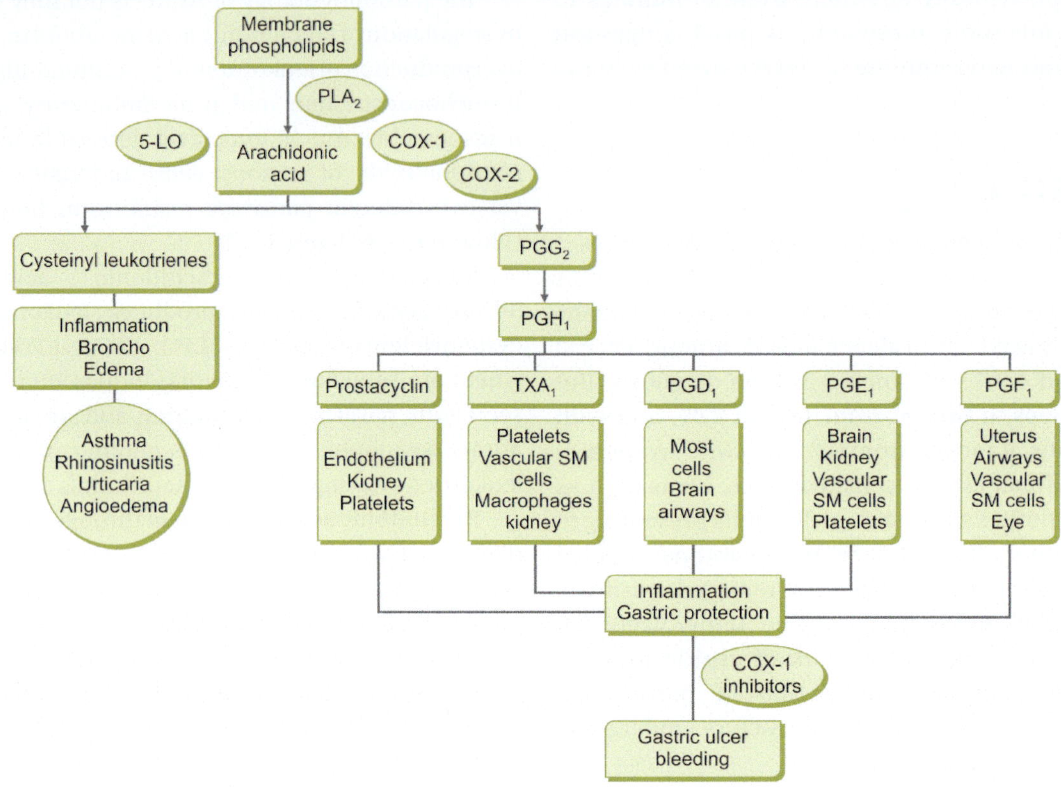

Flowchart 37.2: Enzymatic pathways of arachidonic acid metabolism.

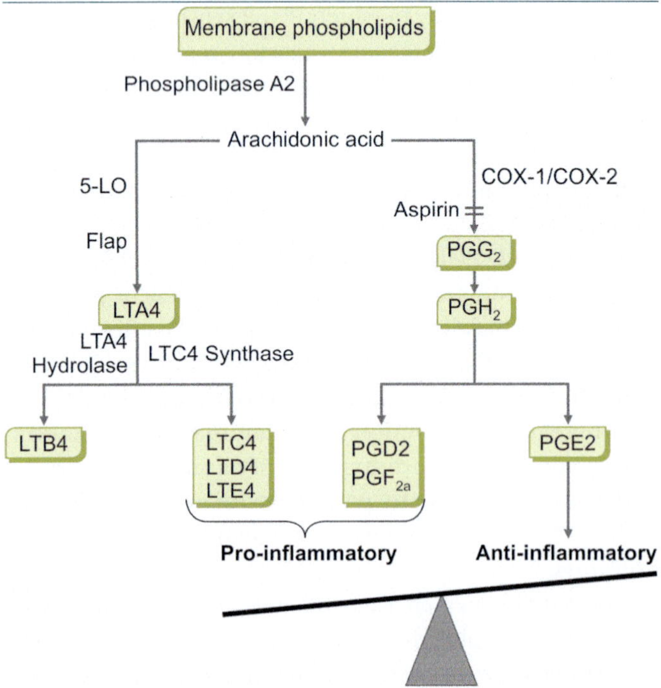

Source: From Sanchez-Borges M, Capriles-Hulett A, Caballero-Fonseca F. Cutaneous reactions to aspirin and nonsteroidal anti-inflammatory drugs. Clin Rev Allergy Immunol. 2003;24:125-135.

Although mast cells have been implicated in asthma pathology traditionally, there is also accumulating evidence of role of platelet in providing enzymes needed for LT production. The percentage of platelet–leukocyte aggregates correlated with a marker of systemic cysLT production and abnormal aggregation was demonstrated in peripheral blood and nasal polyps of patients with AERD.[39]

Blunting response or blocking effect on bronchoconstriction induced by aspirin on premedication with inhibitors of leukotriene synthesis or receptor antagonist further reinforces this pathophysiologic mechanism.[21,40-42]

CLINICAL PRESENTATION

Reactions to aspirin can take two distinct forms:

1. *Cutaneous*: Leading to urticaria and angioedema.
2. *Respiratory*: Resulting in rhinoconjunctivitis and bronchospasm.

The AERD represents chronic form of asthma and CRS with nasal polyposis and exacerbation of respiratory symptom on exposure to aspirin or other NSAIDs. It is usually diagnosed in adulthood, although children can be affected, and the three components develop serially over the period of years,[11,43] although some may progress to asthma rapidly from rhinosinusitis.

By the age of 30 years, most patients would have developed refractory rhinitis followed by chronic hypertrophic eosinophilic rhinosinusitis which may present as nasal polyposis, anosmia, nasal congestion, etc. Computed tomography of paranasal sinuses may show mucosal thickening, polyps, and sinusitis. As nasal symptoms worsen, patient starts to present with lower airway inflammatory signs as in asthma. AERD symptoms worsen in some patients over time even after avoiding NSAIDs.[4,6,44,45] However, nasal symptoms are more disturbing in many patients.

Symptoms of aspirin reaction are dose related, more severe reaction occurring at larger doses, typically starting 30 minutes after ingestion and may be slow to resolve.[46] Most sensitive patients react at 30–120 mg of aspirin when challenged with increasing doses, few require >325 mg.[46]

Typical reaction to aspirin consists of one or more of following.

- *Nasal and ocular symptoms*: Watery rhinorrhea, periorbitaledema, congestion, redness of eyes.
- *Respiratory symptoms*: Wheeze, dyspnea, cough, chest tightness, typically like in asthma.

Rare and severe symptoms include laryngospasm, abdominal cramps, hypotension, and flushing/erythema and may become difficult to distinguish from anaphylaxis.

DIAGNOSIS

A history of reaction to NSAID and presence of all three clinical entities such as asthma, nasal symptoms, and episodes of exacerbation of upper and lower airway symptoms would make diagnosis easy, but problem occurs when one is faced with a patient presenting with isolated nasal or lower respiratory symptoms. In such cases, a detailed history followed by clinical examination and then by aspirin challenge testing may be diagnostic.

Sometimes, there may be other concurrent asthma triggers in patients, such as lower respiratory infection, connective tissue diseases, and menstruation which by themselves can trigger asthma, NSAID in such cases may be incidental or coincidental used for symptom relief resulting in worsening asthma symptoms. When history is suggestive of reaction to an NSAID, details to be sought on similar reaction to other NSAIDs as the patient may be having drug-specific IgE-mediating response.

Aspirin challenge still remains the diagnostic test; however, this should be attempted in a setup having facilities and expertise required to handle any form of severe reaction that might occur during the procedure. Aspirin challenge is generally performed orally with increasing doses of aspirin, starting from low dose, such as 30–41.5 mg and advanced by doubling the dose every 3 hours. Patients undergoing such a test need to be treated with LT receptor antagonists as premedication reduces the respiratory symptoms dramatically but still ocular and nasal symptoms would be apparent in most patients. Antihistamines are avoided for a week as they tend to blunt nasal symptoms. Inhaled corticosteroids (or nasal) can be continued up to the procedure as they reduce the likelihood of a serious bronchoconstriction, but not all manifestations are suppressed to enable a diagnosis of aspirin sensitivity.

MANAGEMENT

Management of AERD is mainly about controlling chronic sinusitis asthma on its merits in addition to suppression of the consequences of abnormal leukotriene metabolism. There exist many national and international detailed guidelines on how to manage and monitor these clinical conditions. All NSAIDs and COX-1 inhibitors need to be avoided by these patients, and in special situations, aspirin desensitization can be done where patients are required to take NSAID therapy for definitive indications.

Leukotriene modifiers should be a part of management of patients with AERD. It not only prevents nasal and pulmonary symptoms but also protects patients from severe exacerbation due to accidental exposure to NSAIDs. 5-LO (5-lipoxygenase) inhibitors such as zileuton should be used twice on a daily basis with regular liver function monitoring. LTRAs (montelukast, zafirlukast) appear to be much safer and used once on a daily basis. Many studies demonstrated that respiratory symptoms improve significantly when LTRAs are added to pre-existing therapy.[30,47,48] Though combination of LTRA and zileuton are not studied, combination therapy may be beneficial to patients in whom disease control cannot be achieved adequately by either drugs.[49-51]

All NSAIDs should be avoided in patients with AERD; however, acetaminophen in lower doses and COX-2-selective inhibitors are well tolerated in most patients requiring alternatives for pain and inflammation. Up to 20% of AERD patients react to dose of 1,000 mg[52] of acetaminophen. Though AERD patient can be desensitized to aspirin, the mechanism which alters the response to NSAIDs is not completely understood. Some of the indications where aspirin desensitization is absolutely required may be recurrent nasal polyposis with resistant symptomatology with adequate or combined LTRA and zileuton treatment. Patients requiring NSAIDs for other inflammatory conditions such as arthritis and aspirin for antiplatelet effects in cardiovascular and cerebrovascular events.[53] However, patients who undergo desensitization are required to take aspirin on a daily basis to maintain desensitization status; but when the patient misses the daily dose, there exists a "refractory period" of not more than 5 days after which the patient becomes sensitive again.

SUMMARY AND CONCLUSION

- AERD includes patients with CRS, nasal polyposis, and asthma who have recurrent exacerbations of upper and lower respiratory tract symptoms following ingestion of aspirin or any other NSAID.
- It affects 5–20% of asthmatics, pathophysiology being dysregulation of arachidonic acid metabolism with selective inhibition of bronchodilator and anti-inflammatory mediators and increased channelization of arachidonic acid metabolism to bronchoconstrictors and proinflammatory mediators' production by COX-1 inhibitors.
- AERD is diagnosed clinically based on classical history and symptomatology on exposure to suspected drug; however, definitive diagnosis can only be made by aspirin challenge test.
- Apart from treating resulting clinical entities by available clinical guidelines, addition of leukotriene modifiers such as zileuton/LTRA is absolutely required in the management of AERD patients.
- In selected patients, aspirin desensitization followed by daily low-dose aspirin therapy is beneficial which also allows patient to tolerate intermittent NSAID therapy for other indications as long as desensitization state is maintained.

REFERENCES

1. Varghese M, Lockey RF. Aspirin-exacerbated asthma. Allergy Asthma Clin Immunol. 2008;4:75-83.
2. Babu KS, Salvi SS. Aspirin and asthma. Chest. 2000;118:1470.
3. Samter M, Beers RF Jr. Intolerance to aspirin. Clinical studies and consideration of its pathogenesis. Ann Intern Med. 1968;68:975.
4. Hedman J, Kaprio J, Poussa T, Nieminen MM. Prevalence of asthma, aspirin intolerance, nasal polyposis and chronic obstructive pulmonary disease in a population-based study. Int J Epidemiol. 1999;28:717.
5. Schiavino D, Nucera E, Milani A, et al. The aspirin disease. Thorax. 2000;55:S66.
6. Jenkins C, Costello J, Hodge L. Systematic review of prevalence of aspirin-induced asthma and its implications for clinical practice. BMJ. 2004;328:434.
7. Vally H, Taylor ML, Thompson PJ. The prevalence of aspirin intolerant asthma (AIA) in Australian asthmatic patients. Thorax. 2002;57:569.
8. Weber RW, Hoffman M, Raine DA Jr, Nelson HS. Incidence of bronchoconstriction due to aspirin, azo dyes, non-azo dyes, and preservatives in a population of perennial asthmatics. J Allergy Clin Immunol. 1979;64:32.
9. Nabavi M, Esmaeilzadeh H, Arshi S, et al. Aspirin hypersensitivity in patients with chronic rhinosinusitis and nasal polyposis: frequency and contributing factors. Am J Rhinol Allergy. 2014;28:239.
10. Gregory P Geba. Chapter 47: Aspirin- and exercise-induced asthma. Fishman's Pulmonary Diseases and Disorders. 4th ed. New York City: McGraw-Hill Education; Volume one, 2008: 799–814.
11. Fahrenholz JM. Natural history and clinical features of aspirin-exacerbated respiratory disease. Clin Rev Allergy Immunol. 2003;24:113.
12. Dursun AB, Woessner KA, Simon RA, et al. Predicting outcomes of oral aspirin challenges in patients with asthma, nasal polyps, and chronic sinusitis. Ann Allergy Asthma Immunol. 2008;100:420.
13. Shi J, Misso NL, Duffy DL, et al. Cyclooxygenase-1 gene polymorphisms in patients with different asthma phenotypes and atopy. Eur Respir J. 2005;26:249.
14. Barranco P, Bobolea I, Larco JI, et al. Diagnosis of aspirin-induced asthma combining the bronchial and the oral challenge tests: a pilot study. J Investig Allergol Clin Immunol. 2009;19:446.
15. Poznanovic SA, Kingdom TT. Total IgE levels and peripheral eosinophilia: correlation with mucosal disease based on computed tomographic imaging of the paranasal sinus. Arch Otolaryngol Head Neck Surg. 2007;133:701.
16. Fountain CR, Mudd PA, Ramakrishnan VR, et al. Characterization and treatment of patients with chronic rhinosinusitis and nasal polyps. Ann Allergy Asthma Immunol. 2013;111:337.
17. Newman LJ, Platts-Mills TA, Phillips CD, et al. Chronic sinusitis. Relationship of computed tomographic findings to allergy, asthma, and eosinophilia. JAMA. 1994;271:363.
18. Bryson JM, Tasca RA, Rowe-Jones JM. Local and systemic eosinophilia in patients undergoing endoscopic sinus surgery for chronic rhinosinusitis with and without polyposis. Clin Otolaryngol Allied Sci. 2003;28:55.
19. Shore SA, Austen KF, Drazen JM. Lung biology in health and disease: Lung cell biology. In: L'Enfant C, Massaro D, eds. Eicosanoids and the Lung. New York, NY: Marcel Dekker; 1989.

20. Laitinen LA, Laitinen A, Haahtela T, et al. Leukotriene E4 and granulocytic infiltration into asthmatic airways. Lancet. 1993;341:989.
21. Dahlén B. Treatment of aspirin-intolerant asthma with antileukotrienes. Am J Respir Crit Care Med. 2000;161:S137.
22. Narayanankutty A, Reséndiz-Hernández JM, Falfán-Valencia R, Teran LM. Biochemical pathogenesis of aspirin exacerbated respiratory disease (AERD). Clin Biochem. 2013;46:566.
23. Picado C, Fernandez-Morata JC, Juan M, et al. Cyclooxygenase-2 mRNA is downexpressed in nasal polyps from aspirin-sensitive asthmatics. Am J Respir Crit Care Med. 1999;160:291.
24. Kowalski ML, Pawliczak R, Wozniak J, et al. Differential metabolism of arachidonic acid in nasal polyp epithelial cells cultured from aspirin-sensitive and aspirin-tolerant patients. Am J Respir Crit Care Med. 2000;161:391.
25. Pierzchalska M, Szabó Z, Sanak M, et al. Deficient prostaglandin E2 production by bronchial fibroblasts of asthmatic patients, with special reference to aspirin-induced asthma. J Allergy Clin Immunol. 2003;111:1041.
26. Liu T, Laidlaw TM, Katz HR, Boyce JA. Prostaglandin E2 deficiency causes a phenotype of aspirin sensitivity that depends on platelets and cysteinyl leukotrienes. Proc Natl Acad Sci USA. 2013;110:16987.
27. Wang XS, Wu AY, Leung PS, Lau HY. PGE suppresses excessive anti-IgE-induced cysteinyl leucotrienes production in mast cells of patients with aspirin exacerbated respiratory disease. Allergy. 2007;62:620.
28. Bochenek G, Nagraba K, Nizankowska E, Szczeklik A. A controlled study of 9alpha,11beta-PGF2 (a prostaglandin D2 metabolite) in plasma and urine of patients with bronchial asthma and healthy controls after aspirin challenge. J Allergy Clin Immunol. 2003;111:743.
29. Campo P, Ayuso P, Salas M, et al. Mediator release after nasal aspirin provocation supports different phenotypes in subjects with hypersensitivity reactions to NSAIDs. Allergy. 2013;68:1001.
30. Antczak A, Montuschi P, Kharitonov S, et al. Increased exhaled cysteinyl-leukotrienes and 8-isoprostane in aspirin-induced asthma. Am J Respir Crit Care Med. 2002;166:301.
31. Knapp HR, Sladek K, Fitzgerald GA. Increased excretion of leukotriene E4 during aspirin-induced asthma. J Lab Clin Med. 1992;119:48.
32. Ferreri NR, Howland WC, Stevenson DD, Spiegelberg HL. Release of leukotrienes, prostaglandins, and histamine into nasal secretions of aspirin-sensitive asthmatics during reaction to aspirin. Am Rev Respir Dis. 1988;137:847.
33. Daffern PJ, Muilenburg D, Hugli TE, Stevenson DD. Association of urinary leukotriene E4 excretion during aspirin challenges with severity of respiratory responses. J Allergy Clin Immunol. 1999;104:559.
34. Lee TH, Woszczek G, Farooque SP. Leukotriene E4: perspective on the forgotten mediator. J Allergy Clin Immunol. 2009;124:417.
35. Cowburn AS, Sladek K, Soja J, et al. Overexpression of leukotriene C4 synthase in bronchial biopsies from patients with aspirin-intolerant asthma. J Clin Invest. 1998; 101:834.
36. Nasser S, Christie PE, Pfister R, et al. Effect of endobronchial aspirin challenge on inflammatory cells in bronchial biopsy samples from aspirin-sensitive asthmatic subjects. Thorax. 1996;51:64.
37. Fischer AR, Rosenberg MA, Lilly CM, et al. Direct evidence for a role of the mast cell in the nasal response to aspirin in aspirin-sensitive asthma. J Allergy Clin Immunol. 1994;94:1046.
38. Cai Y, Bjermer L, Halstensen TS. Bronchial mast cells are the dominating LTC4S-expressing cells in aspirin-tolerant asthma. Am J Respir Cell Mol Biol. 2003;29:683.
39. Laidlaw TM, Kidder MS, Bhattacharyya N, et al. Cysteinyl leukotriene overproduction in aspirin-exacerbated respiratory disease is driven by platelet-adherent leukocytes. Blood. 2012;119:3790.
40. Israel E, Fischer AR, Rosenberg MA, et al. The pivotal role of 5-lipoxygenase products in the reaction of aspirin-sensitive asthmatics to aspirin. Am Rev Respir Dis. 1993;148:1447.
41. Christie PE, Smith CM, Lee TH. The potent and selective sulfidopeptide leukotriene antagonist, SK&F 104353, inhibits aspirin-induced asthma. Am Rev Respir Dis. 1991;144:957.
42. Nasser SM, Bell GS, Foster S, et al. Effect of the 5-lipoxygenase inhibitor ZD2138 on aspirin-induced asthma. Thorax. 1994;49:749.
43. Szczeklik A, Nizankowska E, Duplaga M. Natural history of aspirin-induced asthma. AIANE Investigators. European Network on Aspirin-induced Asthma. Eur Respir J. 2000;16:432.
44. Berges-Gimeno MP, Simon RA, Stevenson DD. The natural history and clinical characteristics of aspirin-exacerbated respiratory disease. Ann Allergy Asthma Immunol. 2002;89:474.
45. Szczeklik A, Stevenson DD. Aspirin-induced asthma: advances in pathogenesis, diagnosis, and management. J Allergy Clin Immunol. 2003;111:913.
46. Hope AP, Woessner KA, Simon RA, Stevenson DD. Rational approach to aspirin dosing during oral challenges and desensitization of patients with aspirin-exacerbated respiratory disease. J Allergy Clin Immunol. 2009; 123:406.
47. Dahlén SE, Malmström K, Nizankowska E, et al. Improvement of aspirin-intolerant asthma by montelukast, a leukotriene antagonist: a randomized, double-blind, placebo-controlled trial. Am J Respir Crit Care Med. 2002;165:9.
48. Dahlén B, Nizankowska E, Szczeklik A, et al. Benefits from adding the 5-lipoxygenase inhibitor zileuton to conventional therapy in aspirin-intolerant asthmatics. Am J Respir Crit Care Med. 1998;157:1187.
49 White A, Ludington E, Mehra P, et al. Effect of leukotriene modifier drugs on the safety of oral aspirin challenges. Ann Allergy Asthma Immunol. 2006;97:688.

50. Lee RU, Stevenson DD. Aspirin-exacerbated respiratory disease: evaluation and management. Allergy Asthma Immunol Res. 2011;3:3.
51. Lee RU, White AA, Ding D, et al. Use of intranasal ketorolac and modified oral aspirin challenge for desensitization of aspirin-exacerbated respiratory disease. Ann Allergy Asthma Immunol. 2010;105:130.
52. Settipane RA, Schrank PJ, Simon RA, et al. Prevalence of cross-sensitivity with acetaminophen in aspirin-sensitive asthmatic subjects. J Allergy Clin Immunol. 1995;96:480.
53. Stevenson DD, Hankammer MA, Mathison DA, et al. Aspirin desensitization treatment of aspirin-sensitive patients with rhinosinusitis-asthma: long-term outcomes. J Allergy Clin Immunol. 1996; 98:751.

CHAPTER 38

Anticonvulsant Hypersensitivity Syndrome

Arun Raja V, Suneetha P, Alladi Mohan

INTRODUCTION

Conventional aromatic anticonvulsants are a common cause of drug allergy in hospitalized and general population.[1-3] Adverse drug reactions (ADRs) to anticonvulsant drugs result in treatment interruption, increase in morbidity, mortality, and impair quality of life in patients with epilepsy. ADRs are of two types. The more common Type A ADRs are dose dependent, predictable, and are usually reversible after discontinuation of the offending drugs. Type B ADRs are less common and occur unexpectedly in patients who are susceptible and are unrelated to the mechanism of action of the drug. Anticonvulsant hypersensitivity syndrome (AHS) is a Type B ADR with systemic manifestations that can be potentially fatal.

EPIDEMIOLOGY

True incidence of AHS is unknown because of its variable presentation and inaccurate reporting.

Global Scene

In 1950, Dilantin hypersensitivity syndrome was reported.[4] This syndrome was observed in patients several weeks after the starting of therapy with aromatic anticonvulsant drugs such as phenytoin as well as carbamazepine and phenobarbital. Shear and Spielberg[5] were the first to use the term AHS in 1988. AHS has been estimated to occur 1 in 1,000 to 1 in 10,000 exposures.[6] The risk of developing AHS within 60 days in new users of phenytoin or carbamazepine has been estimated to be 2.3–4.5/10,000 and 1–4.1/10,000, respectively.[7] Cross-sensitivity among aromatic AEDs is reported to range from 30% to 58%.[8,9] Cross-reactivity is more commonly seen in women and is especially evident between phenytoin and carbamazepine.[8,9]

Indian Scenario

Sparse data are available on this subject from India. In a study[10] from Jaipur (n = 33,000) in patients taking anticonvulsant drugs, incidence of cutaneous drug reactions was observed to be 558/33,000 (1.7%). AHS occurred in 60 patients; males outnumbered females (male:female = 4.5:1). Phenytoin was the most common drug (n = 39) followed by carbamazepine (n = 19). Cross-reactivity between phenytoin and carbamazepine was seen in three patients. Most of the patients recovered well; one patient died.[10]

RISK FACTORS

Several risk factors have been found to be associated with the occurrence of AHS and are summarized here.

Age

Metabolism of drugs is usually age dependent. Children younger than 12 years of age and adults older than 64 years have high risks for severe cutaneous adverse reactions with anticonvulsants.[11] Increased reactive metabolites in children result in increased susceptibility to hypersensitivity reactions as compared to adults. In elderly persons, discontinuation of anticonvulsant appears to be more frequent with the development of drug hypersensitivity. Lamotrigine-induced rashes are more common in children than in adults. The incidence of Stevens–Johnson syndrome in patients with lamotrigine is 10 times higher in children.[12]

Drug-related

A combination of valproate with lamotrigine increases the risk of lamotrigine-induced drug hypersensitivity reaction.[13] The prevalence of AHS reaction increased five times in patients with a history of anticonvulsant drug-induced eruption.[14] A multivariable analysis suggested that a history of rash with an anticonvulsant was the strongest predictor of lamotrigine-induced rash (odds ratio 3.62).[8]

Disease-related

Disorders such as systemic lupus erythematosus (SLE), family history of skin eruptions, and glucocorticoid treatment have been observed to be the risk factors for AHS.[15] Other potential risk factors include previous history of hypersensitivity to other anticonvulsant drugs, family history of AHS, traumatic brain injury, extremes of age, and presence of viral infections with human herpesvirus-6 (HHV-6), human herpesvirus-7 (HHV-7), cytomegalovirus, and Epstein–Barr virus.

Genetic Factors

Genetic markers are useful to predict individuals who are susceptible to develop AHS. A polymorphism in the promoter region of the tumor necrosis factor-alpha gene is also thought to be a predisposing factor for carbamazepine-induced AHS.[16] A strong association of human leukocyte antigen (HLA)-B*1502 with carbamazepine-induced severe cutaneous adverse reactions has been observed in Han Chinese patients.[17,18] This strong association was further confirmed by other extended cohorts of Han Chinese and other Asian populations (including Thai, Malaysian, and Indian groups). This association was not replicated in other populations, including Korean, Japanese, and Whites. HLA-A*3101 was reported to be associated with carbamazepine-induced hypersensitivity in European and North Asian carriers.[19] A potential protective role of HLA-B*0702 was suggested in patients with carbamazepine-induced severe cutaneous adverse reaction.[20]

PATHOGENESIS

The pathogenesis of AHS is multifactorial. The dosage of anticonvulsant used is not related to the onset or severity of AHS. Most of the AHS are Type IV (delayed) hypersensitivity reactions. Toxic metabolites of phenytoin, carbamazepine, and phenobarbital play a vital role in the development of AHS (Fig. 38.1).[1] During the metabolism of these drugs, reactive intermediates (such as arene oxides) are produced by cytochrome P450 oxidative metabolism. Detoxification is done by epoxide hydrolase; if deficient, these toxic metabolites bind to cellular macromolecules leading to cell death (necrosis or apoptosis) or initiate secondary immunological responses.[21] T cells regulate the immune response and release of cytokines resulting in cell death. Additional work has shown circulating immunoglobulin G antibodies (IgGs) in patients with AHS. These antibodies were directed against cytochrome P450 3A1.[22] It is possible that multiorgan involvement in AHS is a function of the expression of the antigen in different tissues.

The association between drug eruption and human herpes virus was first reported in a patient with phenobarbital-induced hypersensitivity syndrome.[23] Antibody titer of HHV-6 rose during the second to fourth week after the initiation of symptoms, and this episode of viral infection was related to the fulminant hemophagocytic syndrome.[23] Recently, reactivation of other types of herpes viruses was also discovered through different laboratory modalities. However, the mechanism for sequential viral reactivation and their pathogenetic roles in hypersensitivity drug reactions are still unclear. Antiviral CD8+ T cells possessing cross-reactivity to drugs play a central role in initiating this drug hypersensitivity reaction when the drugs and specific HLA alleles accidentally activate viral specific T cells.[24] Other theories

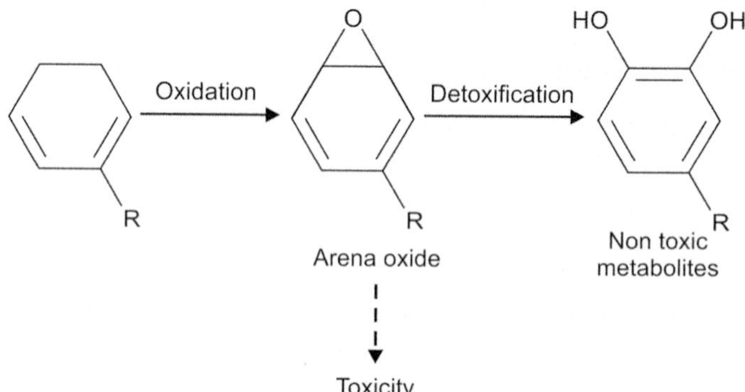

Fig. 38.1: Metabolic pathway for production of toxic metabolites of aromatic anticonvulsants (phenytoin, phenobarbitone, carbamazepine).

Source: Knowles et al. (1999).

that have been postulated include that AHS represents a form of graft-versus-host disease.[25]

The pathophysiology of lamotrigine-induced AHS is not known. Lamotrigine is extensively metabolized predominantly by N-glucuronidation. Only minor fractions of lamotrigine undergo phase I metabolism, resulting in the 2-N-oxide and the 2-N-methylated metabolites.[26] Whether one of the phase I products acts as a toxic metabolite is not known.

CLINICAL PRESENTATION

Anticonvulsant hypersensitivity syndrome has myriad of clinical manifestations ranging from cutaneous involvement to severe systemic organ system involvement. The condition develops frequently with initial symptoms starting 1–8 weeks after first exposure to the drug.[5] For phenytoin, the mean interval to onset is 17–21 days, and for carbamazepine, it is generally 21–28 days.[5] AHS syndrome occurs in previously sensitized individuals within 1 day of rechallenge. Fever and rash are usually followed by pharyngitis, lymphadenopathy, arthritis and general malaise. Fever is usually low grade but the temperature can be as high as 40°C. When present, atypical lymphocytosis occurs in the first week with a subsequent eosinophilia noted by second week.[5] Spectrum of clinical presentation of patients with AHS is given in Table 38.1.

Cutaneous Manifestations

A drug eruption occurs in approximately 90% of patients with AHS and can range from an exanthematous eruption to more serious SJS or toxic epidermal necrolysis (TEN).[27] The rash begins as a nonspecific morbilliform eruption

Table 38.1: Spectrum of clinical presentation in patients with AHS.

Organ system involved	*Severity*		
	Mild	Moderate	Severe (organ- or life-threatening)
Cutaneous	Exanthematous eruption	Urticarial eruption	SJS/TEN
Extracutaneous			
Hematological	Leukopenia	Agranulocytosis	Aplastic anemia, hypereosinophilia, hemophagocytic syndrome
Musculoskeletal	Elevated creatine kinase level	Myositis	Rhabdomyolysis
Renal	Hematuria	Nephritis	Acute kidney injury
Cardiovascular	Pericarditis	Myocarditis (hypersensitivity myocarditis and acute necrotizing eosinophilic myocarditis)	Congestive heart failure
Respiratory	Cough	Pneumonitis (acute interstitial pneumonitis, lymphocytic interstitial pneumonia), pleuritis	ARDS
Neurological			Meningitis, encephalitis
Endocrine	Sick euthyroid syndrome and thyroiditis, resulting in hyperthyroidism or hypothyroidism; syndrome of inappropriate antidiuretic hormone secretion		Thyrotoxicosis, fulminant type 1 diabetes mellitus
Gastrointestinal and hepatic	Mild elevations in liver function tests	Hepatitis, colitis	Fulminant hepatic failure, pancreatitis
Others	Pharyngitis, epididymitis, hypogammaglobulinemia		

AHS, anticonvulsant hypersensitivity syndrome; SJS, Stevens–Johnson syndrome; TEN, toxic epidermal necrolysis; ARDS, acute respiratory distress syndrome.
Adapted from Knowles et al. (1999).

progresses to a generalized form or even to erythroderma. Facial and acral edema with periorbital accentuation is pathognomonic (Figs. 38.2 and 38.3). Pustules, either follicular or nonfollicular, may also be evident. Initially, the upper trunk and face are affected with later involvement of the lower extremities. Blisters can form due to dermal edema.[27] As the rash resolves in the end-stage large sheet, desquamation are left behind. Atypical target lesions and pinhead-sized pustules may also be observed. Mucosal regions can be involved in such cases, the symptom is usually mild, and seen as cheilitis or erythematous pharynx rather than as extensive erosions seen in SJS/TEN.[28]

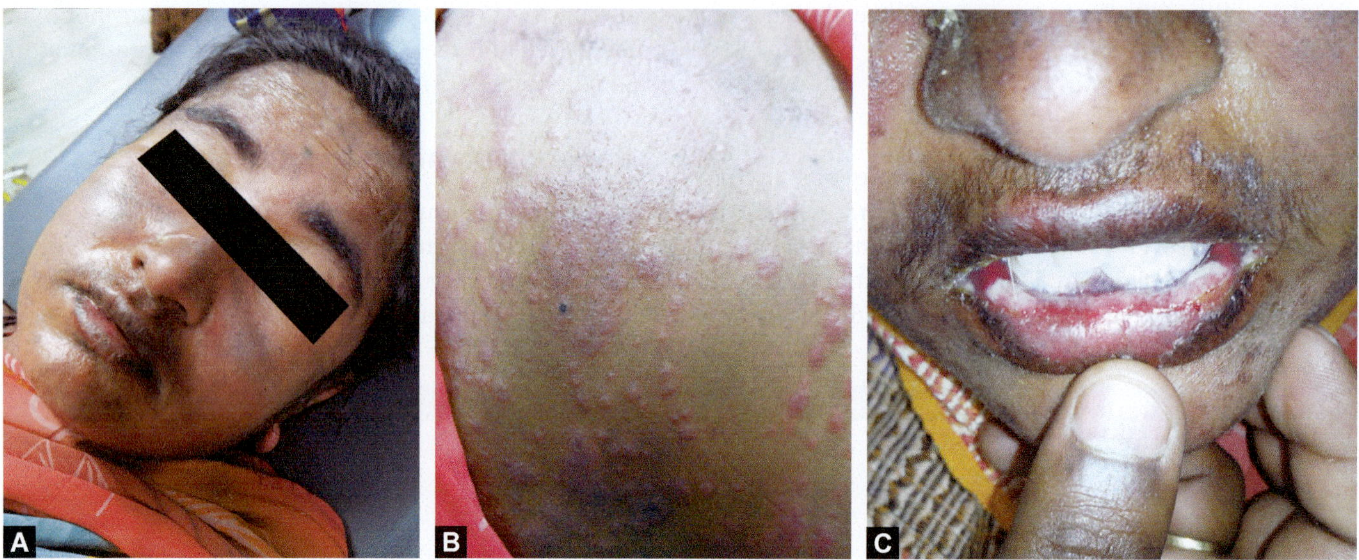

Figs. 38.2A to C: Clinical photograph of a patient with severe AHS due to phenytoin usage. (A) Facial edema with periorbital accentuation is evident; (B) The cutaneous eruption started as a macular erythema that evolved into a red, symmetrical, pruritic, confluent, papular rash; (C) Initially, the face and upper trunk were affected with later involvement of the lower extremities. Mucosal ulceration is also seen.

Courtesy: Dr B Vengamma, Senior Professor and Head, Department of Neurology, Sri Venkateswara Institute of Medical Sciences, Tirupati.

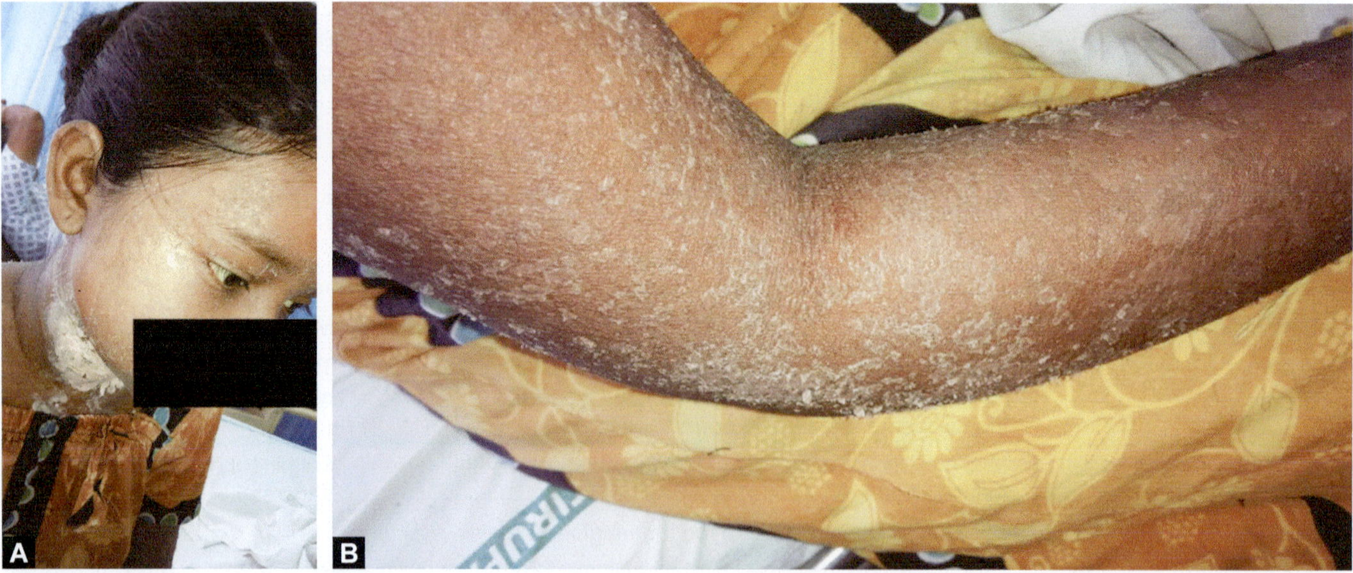

Figs. 38.3A and B: Clinical photograph of another patient with severe AHS due to phenytoin usage. (A) Jaundice is evident; (B) The cutaneous eruption started as a macular erythema initially in the face and upper trunk.

Courtesy: Dr B Vengamma, Senior Professor and Head, Department of Neurology, Sri Venkateswara Institute of Medical Sciences, Tirupati.

Extracutaneous Manifestations

Multiple organ involvement is another characteristic feature of AHS. Liver (50–87%) and kidneys (10–53%) are the most common organs involved.[29] Tender hepatomegaly with or without splenomegaly is seen. Liver involvement can range from mild elevation in liver enzymes to fulminant hepatic failure. The presence of icterus (Fig. 38.3A) is a poor prognostic sign. Severe hepatitis with jaundice increases the risk of mortality to 50%.[30] The degree of hepatitis is related to the interval between the onset of the syndrome and the discontinuation of the anticonvulsant. This emphasizes the importance of the prompt recognition of the syndrome and early discontinuation of offending drug. Recurrent elevation of liver enzymes, with or without relapsing fever and rash, may correlate with the reactivation of human herpes virus 6 (HHV-6).[31]

Renal involvement varies from a mild increase in serum creatinine to the development of end-stage renal disease. It usually presents as new-onset proteinuria, interstitial nephritis, rather than tubular necrosis, and it is the more common cause of acute renal failure in anticonvulsant hypersensitivity. Pulmonary involvement presents as nonproductive cough or shortness of breath, which may be complicated by acute interstitial pneumonitis, pleuritis, or adult respiratory distress syndrome.[32] Cardiac and muscular complications include myocarditis, rhabdomyolysis, and atrioventricular block.[33] Neurologic symptoms include headache, seizure, coma, or disturbed speech. Hippocampal involvement points to the diagnosis of limbic encephalitis, and syndrome of inappropriate secretion of antidiuretic hormone has been reported.[34] HHV-6 encephalitis associated with drug hypersensitivity syndrome has been described.[35] AHS syndrome may also result in acute pancreatitis, arthritis, or gastrointestinal bleeding. Other abnormalities include leukocytosis or leukopenia, thrombocytopenia, and hypogammaglobulinemia in the early stages.[36] Occurrence of pancytopenia is a marker of poor prognosis.[37] Hemophagocytic syndrome may also develop during the course of illness.[37] Thyroid involvement is also evident. The hyperthyroid phase of the illness, which develops during the acute phase of the reaction, may be missed by the clinician, because fever, tachycardia, and malaise appear to be part of the AHS. Within two months of onset of symptoms, hypothyroid may set in as part of an autoimmune thyroiditis.[38] Over the ensuing 12–18 months, resolution of the autoimmune thyroid disease associated with ACS occurs, allowing discontinuation of thyroid hormone replacement therapy.[38] Mortality in patients with AHS is 10% and is primarily associated with systemic organ involvement.[30]

DIAGNOSIS

Because of diverse clinical manifestations, diagnosis of AHS is a challenge. In a patient receiving anticonvulsant drug treatment, the diagnosis of AHS is suspected based on a characteristic clinical presentation. There is no single laboratory investigation to confirm the diagnosis, and several methods have been employed.

The lymphocyte toxicity assay (LTA) is a *drug* metabolite toxicity system in which murine hepatic microsomes are used as a source of cytochrome P450, which are incubated with the drug in question to generate reactive metabolites.[39] The optimal time to perform this test is 5–8 weeks after acute episode.[40] The lymphocyte transformation test (LTT) attempts to detect drug-specific T cells by measuring the proliferation of T cells. The LTT has a high specificity (85%), but has variable sensitivity.[41] The LTA and LTT are costly and hard to perform; currently, it is only being used in research centers.

Patch testing is used for diagnosing type IV or delayed type hypersensitivity reactions. A drug patch test is performed by applying a diluted drug in suitable media on the skin to detect inflammatory effects by drug-specific T cells. Overall, this method yields positive results in 51.5% patients; especially for carbamazepine, the positivity is more than 70%.[42] However, a systemic review[41] has shown that performing patch tests during or right after hypersensitivity episodes yielded low rates of positive results. The optimal time for performing this test is 2–6 months after the drug reaction.[41]

Drug provocation testing has occasionally been attempted in cases where the history is not typical and laboratory testing has been inconclusive or not available. However, the benefits of reaching a diagnosis of AHS must be carefully weighed against the risks of provoking the condition during drug provocation testing.

Histopathological examination of tissue biopsy specimens is sometimes carried out. Skin biopsy specimens from cutaneous lesions reveal a perivascular lymphocytic infiltrate in the papillary dermis, with eosinophils, atypical lymphocytes, and spongiosis. Histopathological examination of the affected lymph nodes may reveal either benign lymphoid hyperplasia or a pseudolymphoma pattern, which must be distinguished from lymphoma.

Diagnostic Criteria

There is still no universal consensus regarding the definition of AHS. The entity has been referred to with various names, such as Dilantin hypersensitivity syndrome, drug reaction with eosinophilia and systemic symptoms (DRESS) syndrome, drug-induced hypersensitivity (DIHS), among others. In 1996, Bocquet et al.[27] proposed the term DRESS syndrome to decrease the ambiguity of the denomination of hypersensitivity syndrome and to define this clinical entity more accurately. Subsequently, the European Registry of Severe Cutaneous Adverse Reaction (RegiSCAR)[43] and the Japanese Research Committee on Severe Cutaneous Adverse Reaction (J-SCAR)[44] have also defined diagnostic criteria for this condition. These diagnostic criteria are summarized in Box 38.1.[27,43,44]

DIFFERENTIAL DIAGNOSIS

The differential diagnosis for AHS includes other cutaneous drug reactions (e.g., SJS, TEN, fixed drug eruptions), acute infections (e.g., Epstein-Barr virus, hepatitis virus, influenza virus, *Streptococcus*), lymphoma or pseudolymphoma, collagen vascular diseases granulomatosis with polyangiitis (GPA; Wegener's granulomatosis), eosinophilic granulomatosis with polyangiitis (Churg-Strauss syndrome), polyarteritis nodosa, SLE, and serum sickness-like reaction.[28]

MANAGEMENT

In addition to clinical evaluation, laboratory investigations, such as complete blood count, liver function tests, urinalysis, serum creatinine, random blood glucose

BOX 38.1: Diagnostic criteria for AHS.

Diagnostic criteria proposed by Bocquet et al.[27] for the diagnosis of DRESS syndrome

i. Drug eruption
ii. Hematologic abnormalities (i.e., eosinophilia, eosinophil count >1.5 × 10^9/L) and the presence of atypical lymphocytes
iii. Systemic manifestations (i.e., lymphadenopathy, lymph node size >2 cm; hepatitis with transaminase levels twice the normal values; interstitial nephritis; pneumonitis, and carditis)

Presence of at least three criteria is required to establish the diagnosis

Diagnostic criteria proposed by European Registry of Severe Cutaneous Adverse Reaction study group:[43]

i. Acute rash
ii. The suspicion of a drug-related reaction
iii. Hospitalization
iv. Systemic features: (a) Fever (temperature >38.8°C); (b) Lymphadenopathy involving at least two sites; (c) Involvement of at least one internal organ (e.g., liver, kidney, heart, pancreas, or other organs); and (d) Hematologic abnormalities, including a lymphocyte count above or below the normal limits; an eosinophil count higher than laboratory limits; or a platelet count below laboratory limits

Presence of the first three criteria is essential and in addition presence of three of the four systemic features is required to establish the diagnosis. A final RegiSCAR score of less than 2 excludes AHS; a score of 2–3 indicates a possible diagnosis; a score of 4–5 suggests "probable" diagnosis; and a score greater than 5 is suggestive of a "definite" diagnosis.

Diagnostic criteria proposed by Japanese Research Committee on Severe Cutaneous Adverse Reaction (J-SCAR) group[44] for DIHS:

i. Maculopapular rash developing 3 weeks after beginning treatment with the causative drug
ii. Prolonged clinical symptoms after discontinuing the causative drug
iii. Fever (temperature >38.8°C)
iv. Hepatic abnormalities (ALT > 100 U/L) or other organ involvement
v. Leukocyte abnormalities (at least one of the following: leukocytosis [>11 × 10^9/L], atypical lymphocytes [>5%], or eosinophilia [>1.5 × 10^9/L])
vi. Lymphadenopathy
vii. HHV-6 reactivation

If all seven criteria are present, the patient is diagnosed to have with typical DIHS; if only criteria (i)–(v) are present, atypical DIHS is diagnosed

AHS, anticonvulsant hypersensitivity syndrome; DRESS, drug reaction with eosinophilia and systemic symptoms; DIHS, drug-induced hypersensitivity syndrome; ALT, alanine aminotransferase; HHV, human herpes virus.

baseline thyroid function tests, and other relevant tests must be done to look for internal organ involvement. Skin biopsy and excision biopsy of peripheral lymph node will be required to rule out other disorders which are close mimics.

Discontinuation of the anticonvulsant implicated as the causative agent following the development of a fever and rash is necessary to prevent progression of symptoms. Empirical use of antibiotics or anti-inflammatory medications should be avoided to prevent confusion between true deterioration due to newly administered drugs or paradoxical deterioration of clinical symptoms after withdrawal of causative drugs. In mild cases, use of topical corticosteroids and antihistamines may be beneficial. The risk of super-infection should always be kept in mind while using topical corticosteroid therapy.

Role of corticosteroids is controversial; if symptoms are severe, oral prednisolone is started at a dosage of 1–2 mg/kg/day.[45] This dosage should be slowly tapered over 6–8 weeks to avoid a flare-up of symptoms. Pulse therapy with high-dose methylprednisolone has been used when life-threatening clinical presentation with internal organ is involved.[46] Evidences from uncontrolled studies have shown that plasmapheresis,[47] immunosuppression, human intravenous immunoglobulin[48] may be efficacious in resistant cases. Benzodiazepines or one of the newer anticonvulsants (gabapentin, topiramate, vigabatrin) can be used for seizure control. Valproic acid is avoided in the acute phase because of the risk of developing hepatitis.

Cross-reactivity occurs with other aromatic anticonvulsants, so patients with AHS should avoid phenytoin, phenobarbital, and carbamazepine. The patient should obtain a "medical alert" stating a reaction to phenytoin, carbamazepine, and phenobarbital. Family counseling is a critical part of patient management because first degree relatives are at an increased risk.

LONG-TERM SEQUELAE

Autoimmune thyroid diseases and kidney failure requiring long-term hemodialysis were the most frequent sequelae for young patients and the elderly, respectively.[49] Variable autoimmune diseases were reported in the literature, and there were occasional reports of individual patients developing more than one particular disease, either simultaneously or sequentially.[50]

AHS due to Newer Anticonvulsants

Zonisamide is an anticonvulsant containing a sulfa moiety which has potential to trigger hypersensitivity reactions. The drug is generally a safe anticonvulsant with minimal adverse effects. Skin rash has been observed with zonisamide use in 1–2% of Japanese patients.[50] Maculopapular and purpuric eruptions have been noted in addition to mild oral mucosal involvement. There has been a recent report of a patient with clinical features of TEN attributable to zonisamide.[50] In this case, however, significant increases in HHV-6 IgG titers and detection of HHV-6 DNA in leukocytes were observed during the course of the illness, indicating that HHV-6 reactivation occurred.[50]

Lamotrigine, a new anticonvulsant, has also been implicated as the etiological cause of AHS.[51] Lamotrigine is an antiepileptic drug that inhibits the release of excitatory neurotransmitter glutamate or aspartate, acts on voltage-sensitive sodium channels, and stabilizes neuronal membranes. The drug is effective for multiple types of seizures. Lamotrigine has been recently reported to cause potentially life-threatening ADRs. The incidence of potentially life-threatening skin reactions occurs in 1 in 1,000 adults treated with lamotrigine and in 1 in 50–100 children.[52] The risk for exanthema is strongly associated with high initial serum levels and with a rapid increase in doses of lamotrigine. Slow introduction of the drug has been reported to reduce the incidence of rash.[52] In one study (n = 26), eosinophilia was noted in 19%, lymphadenopathy was reported in only 12% of the cases, and multiorgan involvement was reported in 46%; these rates are markedly lower than in AHS caused by other drugs.[51] In approximately 10% of patients, cutaneous eruption, usually severe, occurs typically within the first 4 weeks of treatment but has been reported to develop up to 6 months after lamotrigine initiation.[51] Cutaneous findings include a polymorphous eruption consisting of blanchable, erythematous, urticarial papules predominantly on the trunk, which spread to the face but spare the palms. Mucous membranes are rarely involved. Lymphadenopathy and hepatomegaly are commonly present. It has been reported that an adult patient developed transient diffuse alopecia and transverse onychodystrophy of all nails after resolution of lamotrigine drug hypersensitivity.[53]

CONCLUSION

Anticonvulsant hypersensitivity syndrome is characterized clinically by fever, rash, and internal organ involvement. Commonly used anticonvulsants such as phenytoin, phenobarbital, carbamazepine, and lamotrigine are among the most common etiological causes of AHS. The pathogenesis is unclear, but research supports the role of reactive metabolites in mediating toxicity. A possible genetic predisposition is being investigated. Patients developing symptoms suggestive of AHS need to be diagnosed early, and the offending drug should be discontinued immediately. Careful monitoring and supportive management can be lifesaving.

REFERENCES

1. Knowles SR, Shapiro LE, Shear NH. Anticonvulsant hypersensitivity syndrome: incidence, prevention and management. Drug Saf. 1999;21:489-501.
2. Thong BY, Tan TC. Epidemiology and risk factors for drug allergy. Br J Clin Pharmacol. 2011;71:684-700.
3. Ye YM, Thong BY, Park HS. Hypersensitivity to antiepileptic drugs. Immunol Allergy Clin North Am. 2014;34:633-43.
4. Chaiken BH, Goldberg BI, Segal JP. Dilantin sensitivity; report of a case of hepatitis with jaundice, pyrexia and exfoliative dermatitis. N Engl J Med. 1950;242:897-8.
5. Shear NH, Spielberg SP. Anticonvulsant hypersensitivity syndrome. In vitro assessment of risk. J Clin Invest. 1988;82:1826-32.
6. Gennis MA, Vemuri R, Burns EA, et al. Familial occurrence of hypersensitivity to phenytoin. Am J Med. 1991;91:631-4.
7. Tennis P, Stern RS. Risk of serious cutaneous disorders after initiation of use of phenytoin, carbamazepine, or sodium valproate: a record linkage study. Neurology. 1997;49: 542-6.
8. Arif H, Buchsbaum R, Weintraub D, et al. Comparison and predictors of rash associated with 15 antiepileptic drugs. Neurology. 2007;68:1701-9.
9. Alvestad S, Lydersen S, Brodtkorb E. Cross-reactivity pattern of rash from current aromatic antiepileptic drugs. Epilepsy Res. 2008;80:194-200.
10. Bhargava P. Anticonvulsant hypersensitivity syndrome study of 60 cases. Indian J Dermatol Venereol Leprol. 2001;67:317-9.
11. Chan HL, Stern RS, Arndt KA, et al. The incidence of erythema multiforme, Stevens-Johnson syndrome, and toxic epidermal necrolysis. A population-based study with particular reference to reactions caused by drugs among outpatients. Arch Dermatol. 1990;126:43-7.
12. Messenheimer JA, Giorgi L, Risner ME. The tolerability of lamotrigine in children. Drug Saf. 2000;22:303-12.
13. Messenheimer J, Mullens EL, Giorgi L, Young F. Safety review of adult clinical trial experience with lamotrigine. Drug Saf. 1998;18:281-96.
14. Hirsch LJ, Weintraub DB, Buchsbaum R, et al. Predictors of lamotrigine-associated rash. Epilepsia. 2006;47:318-22.
15. Pichler WJ. Delayed drug hypersensitivity reactions. Ann Intern Med. 2003;139:683-93.
16. Pirmohamed M, Lin K, Chadwick D, Park BK. TNF alpha promoter region gene polymorphisms in carbamazepine-hypersensitive patients. Neurology. 2001;56:890-6.
17. Chung WH, Hung SI, Hong HS, et al. Medical genetics: a marker for Stevens-Johnson syndrome. Nature. 2004;428:486.
18. Locharernkul C, Loplumlert J, Limotai C, et al. Carbamazepine and phenytoin-induced Stevens-Johnson syndrome is associated with HLA-B*1502 allele in Thai population. Epilepsia. 2008;49:2087-91.
19. Kim SH, Lee KW, Song WJ, et al. Adverse Drug Reaction Research Group in Korea. Carbamazepine-induced severe cutaneous adverse reactions and HLA genotypes in Koreans. Epilepsy Res. 2011;97:190-7.
20. Alfirevic A, Jorgensen AL, Williamson PR, et al. HLA-B locus in Caucasian patients with carbamazepine hypersensitivity. Pharmacogenomics. 2006;7:813-8.
21. Spielberg SP, Gordon GB, Blake DA, et al. Anticonvulsant toxicity in vitro: possible role of arene oxides. J Pharmacol Exp Ther. 1981;217:386-9.
22. Pirmohamed M, Kitteringham NR, Breckenridge AM, Park BK. Detection of an autoantibody directed against human liver microsomal protein in a patient with carbamazepine hypersensitivity. Br J Clin Pharmacol. 1992;33:183-6.
23. Descamps V, Bouscarat F, Laglenne S, et al. Human herpes virus 6 infection associated with anticonvulsant hypersensitivity syndrome and reactive haemophagocytic syndrome. Br J Dermatol. 1997;137:605-8.
24. Shiohara T, Kano Y, Takahashi R, et al. Drug-induced hypersensitivity syndrome: recent advances in the diagnosis, pathogenesis and management. Chem Immunol Allergy. 2012;97:122-38.
25. Gleichmann H. Studies on the mechanism of drug sensitization: T-cell-dependent popliteal lymph node reaction to diphenylhydantoin. Clin Immunol Immunopathol. 1981;18:203-11.
26. Rambeck B, Wolf P. Lamotrigine clinical pharmacokinetics. Clin Pharmacokinet. 1993;25:433-43.
27. Bocquet H, Bagot M, Roujeau JC. Drug-induced pseudolymphoma and drug hypersensitivity syndrome (Drug Rash with Eosinophilia and Systemic Symptoms: DRESS). Semin Cutan Med Surg. 1996;15:250-7.
28. Bachot N, Roujeau JC. Differential diagnosis of severe cutaneous drug eruptions. Am J Clin Dermatol. 2003;4:561-72.
29. Roujeau JC, Stern RS. Severe adverse cutaneous reactions to drugs. N Engl J Med. 1994;331:1272-85.
30. Morkunas AR, Miller MB. Anticonvulsant hypersensitivity syndrome. Crit Care Clin. 1997;13:727-39.
31. Tohyama M, Hashimoto K, Yasukawa M, et al. Association of human herpes virus 6 reactivation with the flaring and severity of drug-induced hypersensitivity syndrome. Br J Dermatol. 2007;157:934-40.
32. Kano Y, Ishida T, Hirahara K, Shiohara T. Visceral involvements and long-term sequelae in drug-induced hypersensitivity syndrome. Med Clin North Am. 2010;94:743-59.

33. Engel JN, Mellul VG, Goodman DB. Phenytoin hypersensitivity: a case of severe acute rhabdomyolysis. Am J Med. 1986;81:928-30.
34. Sakuma K, Kano Y, Fukuhara M, Shiohara T. Syndrome of inappropriate secretion of antidiuretic hormone associated with limbic encephalitis in a patient with drug-induced hypersensitivity syndrome. Clin Exp Dermatol. 2008;33: 287-90.
35. Fujino Y, Nakajima M, Inoue H, et al. Human herpes virus 6 encephalitis associated with hypersensitivity syndrome. Ann Neurol. 2002;51:771-4.
36. Kano Y, Inaoka M, Shiohara T. Association between anticonvulsant hypersensitivity syndrome and human herpes virus 6 reactivation and hypogammaglobulinemia. Arch Dermatol. 2004;140:183-8.
37. Chen YC, Chiu HC, Chu CY. Drug reaction with eosinophilia and systemic symptoms: a retrospective study of 60 cases. Arch Dermatol. 2010;146:1373-9.
38. Gupta A, Eggo MC, Uetrecht JP, et al. Drug-induced hypothyroidism: the thyroid as a target organ in hypersensitivity reactions to anticonvulsants and sulfonamides. Clin Pharmacol Ther. 1992;51:56-67.
39. Spielberg SP. In vitro analysis of idiosyncratic drug reactions. Clin Biochem. 1986;19:142-4.
40. Kano Y, Hirahara K, Mitsuyama Y, et al. Utility of the lymphocyte transformation test in the diagnosis of drug sensitivity: dependence on its timing and the type of drug eruption. Allergy. 2007;62:1439-44.
41. Elzagallaai AA, Knowles SR, Rieder MJ, et al. In vitro testing for the diagnosis of anticonvulsant hypersensitivity syndrome: a systematic review. Mol Diagn Ther. 2009;13:313-30.
42. Santiago F, Gonçalo M, Vieira R, et al. Epicutaneous patch testing in drug hypersensitivity syndrome (DRESS). Contact Dermatitis. 2010;62:47-53.
43. Kardaun SH, Sidoroff A, Valeyrie-Allanore L, et al. Variability in the clinical pattern of cutaneous side-effects of drugs with systemic symptoms: does a DRESS syndrome really exist? Br J Dermatol. 2007;156:609-11.
44. Shiohara T, Iijima M, Ikezawa Z, Hashimoto K. The diagnosis of a DRESS syndrome has been sufficiently established on the basis of typical clinical features and viral reactivations. Br J Dermatol. 2007;156:1083-4.
45. Chopra S, Levell NJ, Cowley G, Gilkes JJ. Systemic corticosteroids in the phenytoin hypersensitivity syndrome. Br J Dermatol. 1996;134:1109-12.
46. Sheretz E, Jegasothy B, Lazarus G. Phenytoin hypersensitivity reaction presenting with toxic epidermal necrolysis and severe hepatitis. J Am Acad Dermatol. 1985;12:178-81.
47. Chaidemenos GC, Chrysomallis F, Sombolos K, et al. Plasmapheresis in toxic epidermal necrolysis. Int J Dermatol. 1997;36:218-21.
48. Viard I, Wehrli P, Bullani R, et al. Inhibition of toxic epidermal necrolysis by blockade of CD95 with human intravenous immunoglobulin. Science. 1998;282:490-3.
49. Aota N, Shiohara T. Viral connection between drug rashes and autoimmune diseases: how autoimmune responses are generated after resolution of drug rashes. Autoimmun Rev. 2009;8:488-94.
50. Teraki Y, Murota H, Izaki S. Toxic epidermal necrolysis due to zonisamide associated with reactivation of human herpes virus 6. Arch Dermatol. 2008;144:232-5.
51. Schlienger RG, Knowles SR, Shear NH. Lamotrigine-associated anticonvulsant hypersensitivity syndrome. Neurology. 1998;51:1172-5.
52. Parri N, Bernardini R, Pucci N, et al. Drug rash with eosinophilia and systemic symptoms induced by lamotrigine therapy. Int J Immunopathol Pharmacol. 2007;20:643-5.
53. Schaub N, Bircher AJ. Severe hypersensitivity syndrome to lamotrigine confirmed by lymphocyte stimulation in vitro. Allergy. 2000;55:191-3.

CHAPTER 39

Hymenoptera Sensitivity

Narmada Ashok, PK Vedanthan

INTRODUCTION

In recent decades, humans have more than ever been changing the world's ecosystem for their growing demands.[1] Hence, exposure to insect bites and presentation to medical facilities with their varied manifestations has become a common scenario.[2] The clinical presentations are varied from an innocuous bite to life-threatening anaphylactic reactions.

There are about 30 orders of insects. However, the following orders of insects are clinically relevant as they can produce varied clinical manifestations from mild reactions to severe anaphylaxis. Following are the clinically relevant insects and their phylogeny: Anoplura belonging to lice order; flies and mosquitoes belonging to Diptera order; beetles belonging to Cleoptera order; the bedbugs and kissing bugs belonging to Hemiptera order; the fleas of the Siphonaptera order; the butterfly and moths belonging to Lepidoptera order; and the most important Hymenoptera order comprising the fire ants, bees, hornets, and wasps.[3]

The Hymenoptera order is one of the commonest causes of serious, at times fatal insect bites.

EPIDEMIOLOGY

The prevalence of insect bites from varied studies in India ranges from 5.27%[2,4] among children less than 12 years in South India to 10.6% in Western India.[2] They have no age or gender preponderance.[3] In India, the data regarding the incidence of hymenoptera insect bites are lacking.

Stinging insect allergy is the overall cause for more than 10% of all cases of anaphylaxis reported worldwide.[6] They are one of the main causes of fatal anaphylaxis in the United States and the United Kingdom occurring outside the hospital. The incidence of systemic reaction is more common in adult population (2–3.5%) compared to children (0.4–0.8%).[5,6] Irrespective of the severity of reactions, the incidence of insect bites is more than a million, and the incidence of fire ant stings is around 9.3 million. Large local reactions (LLRs) are seen in 17–56% of these bites.

The risk of recurrence of a systemic reactions is around 60–79% in adults.

HYMENOPTERA PHYLOGENY

The Hymenoptera are the third largest order of insects comprising the sawflies, wasps, bees, and ants. Over 1,50,000 species are recognized with many more yet to be described.[7] Biodiversity of Hymenoptera insect shows various patterns in space and time due to difference in climatic conditions and interaction between species and geography.[8]

There are three families of the Hymenoptera order of insects that are predominantly responsible for venom allergy in humans and are most studied:

- Apidae: Honeybees and bumble bees
- Vespidae: Yellow jackets, hornets, and paper wasps
- Formicidae: Fire ants.[6]

Indian studies have revealed a predominance of Apidae in the Western India,[8] and Vespidae-carpenter bees, leaf cutter bees, and ants are more common in South India.[1]

Apidae Family

Honeybees are more common in Apidae family. They live in colonies, and each of these colonies comprises up to 65,000 bees. Feral honeybees build their nests inside hollow trees or logs and are comparatively less common than domestic bees. The domestic bees tend to live in human-made hives and are generally used for commercial purposes like honey production and pollination. Generally, the honeybees are docile insects and usually they sting only when their colonies are provoked. They leave a barbed stinger with an attached venom sac in the victim's skin when they sting. This results in evisceration of the bees and its death. The stings most commonly occur to people who walk barefoot in lawns or who handle flowering plants. Beekeepers because of their occupation are more prone to bee sting. African bees are very aggressive and usually deliver the same venom when they perceive a threat to their hives. They tend to swarm and sting in large numbers causing deaths to both cattle and humans.

Vespidae Family

Yellow jackets, hornets, and wasps are the stinging insects in the Vespidae family that are of medical importance. Vespids make nests of masticated wood containing layers of combs with many individual cells. The comb layers are arranged vertically and, except for wasp nests, are encased in an outer layer of paper. The stingers of the vespids are smooth, and they are capable of stinging repeatedly unlike honeybees. However, they usually do not leave their stingers behind.

Yellow jackets are the commonest reason for vespid stings in human. They usually build their nests, and the nests are either in ground or in human-made structures. They are notorious scavengers. They search for their food in picnic areas and around trash containers. They are very aggressive, and no provocation is needed unlike other insects. Their colony number is largest during late summer, and if food supplies are also limited they are usually aggressive.

There are a variety of hornets, the new world hornets which closely resemble yellow jackets, yellow hornets and white-faced hornets which are actually aerial yellow jackets. These hornets are also very aggressive usually near their nests which they build in hollow trees. They typically fly at night and are attracted to bright lights. The new world hornets are usually aggressive. Yellow hornets are larger and more fearsome in appearance but less aggressive. The population of these insects is gradually increasing, but they are still only minor stinging threats. Wasp colonies are relatively small, and wasps are less aggressive than yellow jackets and hornets. Wasps tend to build their nests near human habitation (e.g., under the eaves of houses, on porches, and below deck railings), and hence, they are more susceptible to sting humans.

Formicidae Family

Fire ants are the medically important members of the family Formicidae. There are two types of fire ants: native and imported. Both can cause severe allergic reactions. However, imported fire ants are more aggressive and can inflict more stings compared to native ones. They are more common in soil where they build large mounds and when threatened they attack in large numbers and sting their victims repeatedly. After about 24 hours of sting, the characteristic sterile pustule appears.[9] Imported fire ants sting at an average of 3 times before removal, and most of the stings are in the feet or legs.

Identification of the Insect

Identification of the insect responsible for the reaction can be very useful in establishing the diagnosis, prescribing treatment and educating patients in avoidance measures (Table 39.1).

Table 39.1: Characteristics of insects most commonly responsible for venom allergy in humans.

Common names	*Scientific names*	*Habitat*	*Appearance*	*Sting features*
Honeybee	Apis mellifera	Trees and farmed in hives		Barbed stinger often left behind
Bumble bees	Bombus apidae	In underground holes or directly on the ground		Sting lacks barbs so can sting repeatedly

(Contd...)

(Contd...)

Common names	*Scientific names*	*Habitat*	*Appearance*	*Sting features*
Carpenter bees	Xylocopa	In dead woods, bamboo		Sting while provoked
European hornet	Vespa crabro	Build large nests in trees and shrubs and often goes undetected		Larger venom sack and painful
Yellow jacket	Vespula	In trees, shrubs, or in protected places. Encountered during yardwork, farming, gardening		Aggressive, more likely to sting than wasps. Lancer like stinger with small barbs, occasionally left behind Can sting repeatedly
Paper wasps	Polistes	Nests are open, and cells are not covered with a cap. Increased likelihood in outdoor events where food and drink is served		Rarely sting mainly if the nest is threatened
Imported fire ants	Formicidae	Large colonies in the ground, typically build bounds		Multiple stings from multiple ants. Inject formic acid

HYMENOPTERA VENOMS

The venoms are aqueous solutions. They generally contain enzymes (e.g., phospholipase, hyaluronidase) proteins, peptides, and vasoactive amines (e.g., histamine, dopamine). The toxic properties are caused by all these components. The proteins of the venoms are severely allergic.[9] A knowledge about the venoms and their cross-reactivity is essential, as this can explain reactivity when there is no prior history of bites from the culprit insect.

There is usually cross-reactivity within subfamily and less commonly within a family. In Apidae family, cross-reactivity is seen between bumble bee and honeybee and not between sweat bee and honeybee. Among Vespidae family, yellow jackets, hornets, and aerial jackets cross-react extensively. But cross-reactivity is reduced between wasps and Polistinae.[5,10] The venom enzymes also share certain cross-reacting carbohydrate determinants that can cause nonspecific skin reactions. Certain species have unique antigenic determinants that may explain certain cases where venom immunotherapy has failed; for example, in wasp family, *Polistes dominulus* has unique antigens not included in commercial wasp venom extract that will lead to negative skin testing or failure of therapy.

The ant venoms are unique in that they have a complex bend of alkaloids with limited protein content not shared with other insects.[5] They are toxic to human epithelium. They cause a sterile pustule at the site of bite. They have hemolytic, cytotoxic, and antibacterial properties. They can also activate platelets, neutrophils, and alternate complement pathway. They have little cross-reactivity to other hymenoptera species and have cross-reactivity between the genes.[10]

Reactions to Hymenoptera Venom

The reactions to venom of hymenoptera are highly variable among individuals and are difficult to predict. They are usually classified as

1. Local reactions—small and large
2. Systemic reactions—IgE-mediated reactions: mild, moderate, and severe
3. Nonallergic reactions.[6,11]

Small Local Reactions

Most stings cause small local reactions of no medical consequences. They are usually 2–3 cm in diameter. These normal sting reactions are characterized by pain, itching, redness, and swelling at the site of sting that resolve within several hours and are caused by the pharmacological properties of the venom.

Large Local Reactions

The LLRs are those areas which are usually more than 10 cm of either erythema, edema, pruritus, or induration. They can increase up to 15–20 cm or can cause massive swelling of the limb extending over a major joint. They are usually minimal in the first few hours, peak by 24–48 hours, and then subside after 5–10 days. Usually the systemic involvement is around 4–10%, and the risk of anaphylaxis is minimal in people who have had an LLR before. However, the morbidity is high if it involves closed spaces like the limbs (compartment syndrome) or the bite is near the oropharyngeal airways.[12]

Systemic Reactions

The systemic reactions can vary from mild urticaria to severe life-threatening anaphylaxis. Usually they are caused due to IgE-mediated reactions, which causes mast cell degranulation and release of mediators. Multiple systems are involved in IgE-mediated reactions.

Sterile Pustule

A pustule filled with yellow fluid containing epithelial debris occurs in the first 6–24 hours. The pustule remains up to a week or sometimes erodes after 72 hours.[10]

System	*Symptom of venom allergy*
Cutaneous	Pruritus, urticaria, angioedema
Gastrointestinal	Vomiting, diarrhea, abdominal pain, and incontinence
Cardiovascular	Tachycardia, hypotension, isolated cardiovascular collapse can occur
Neurological	Light headedness, dizziness, altered vision, seizures, collapse
Respiratory	Rhinitis, shortness of breath, tight chest, wheeze, strider, laryngeal edema

Systemic reactions occur within minutes of sting. Usually if the symptoms occur sooner, the reactions are very severe. Cutaneous signs and symptoms occur in 95% of children with systemic reactions and 80% of adults. They may also be the sole manifestation in 60% of children and 15% of adults. Compared to adults, children usually have a benign course.[3,9] Potentially life-threatening reactions occur in 3% of adults and 0.4–0.8% of children.

Nonallergic Reactions

Nonallergic reactions are very severe and serious and can occur due to toxic properties. They are usually associated when a patient has mastocytosis or when a patient has got multiple simultaneous stings. These reactions are usually indistinguishable from IgE.

System	*Symptom of venom allergy*
Cutaneous	Necrosis
Renal	Interstitial nephritis, rhabdomyolysis
Hematological	Hemolysis, cytopenias, disseminated intravascular coagulation (DIVC), vasculitis
Neurological	Guillain–Barre syndrome, myasthenia gravis, encephalitis
Respiratory	Alveolar hemorrhage

PATHOGENESIS OF REACTIONS

The IgE-mediated symptoms are due to cross-linking of antibodies bound to mast cells and basophils with the release of vasoactive mediators.

The non-IgE reactions are thought to be immune complex mediated which causes complement activation by antigen-antibody complexes and ensuing inflammatory mediators by massive infiltration of neutrophils but yet to be proven.[6,9,11]

RISK FACTORS FOR SEVERE ALLERGIC REACTIONS

1. *Age*: Adults are more prone to severe reactions. About 0.3–7.5% of adults experience systemic reactions in their first bite, and 57–75% of the adults who have experienced anaphylaxis will have severe reactions when restung. Age is a powerful predictor of severe reactions and for an increase of 10 years of age the chance of death due to these reactions increases by 70%.[13,14] Children usually suffer less from systemic reaction: Only 0.3–0.8% of children who are stung are prone to systemic reactions and even in them 60% of reactions are mild. Mostly these reactions are restricted to skin and very rarely there is cardiorespiratory compromise in contrast to adults.[14,15]
2. *Recurrent exposures*: The incidence of systemic reactions among beekeepers is 14% and 43%. There is an increased chance of sensitization among them as they sustain many stings each year. About 45% of the beekeepers who were stung less than 25 times a year had a history of anaphylaxis. However, when they are stung repeatedly they also develop tolerance. Beekeepers who were stung more than 200 times a year had no incidence of systemic reactions.[13,14]
3. *Increased baseline tryptase levels/mastocytosis*: Increased baseline tryptase levels from 4.5 μg/L to an increase of 20 μg/L with or without cutaneous mastocytosis will increase the risk of anaphylaxis by a factor of 3.8.[13] Baseline tryptase levels is an independent risk factor for potentially, life-threatening allergic sting reactions.
4. *Males*: They have been found to have an increased risk for systemic reactions, and this is more due to the fact that they are exposed more frequently due to outdoor activities than females.[13]
5. *Antihypertensive medications*: Patients on angiotensin converting enzyme inhibitors independent of age are more prone to severe reactions probably due to kinin-angiotensin system. However, no studies have conclusively proven that other antihypertensive medications especially beta blockers are a risk factor.[13]
6. *Earlier systemic reaction*: A significant association between earlier systemic sting reaction and severity of a subsequent sting reaction in several studies probably due to a boosting effect has been reported.[13]
7. *Cardiac and respiratory disorders*: They are not risk factors per se to cause severe allergic reactions but can increase the severity of reactions as they compromise on the reserve of the patient. Autopsies done on people who have had a fatal reaction showed coexistent cardiorespiratory comorbidity in 50% of cases.[14]
8. *Severity of local reaction does not predict risk of systemic reaction*: Only 5–10% of patients who experience LLR have severe systemic reaction.[16]

Evaluation of a Patient with Hymenoptera Stings

Most of the patients who get bitten by insect stings have mild reactions and usually do not report. However, those patients who report to medical care and have had history of large local reactions or systemic reactions need thorough evaluation and management. A detailed history is very helpful as a first part in evaluation.

Factors that might be helpful in identification include the following:

1. Type of activity during the time of bite
2. Location and timing of the bite
3. Common type of insects in the area
4. Visual identification of the dead insect
5. Presence of stinger indicates bee sting
6. Presence of pustule indicates fire ant bites but usually after 24 hours
7. Occupation of the patient is essential as further management greatly depends on this
8. Hobbies like trekking, bird watching, beekeeping
9. Comorbid conditions and concomitant medications can increase the morbidity (3).

EVALUATION AND MANAGEMENT OF VENOM ALLERGY

Management of venom allergy requires initial diagnosis by detailed evaluation, followed by testing for venom-specific IgE and immunotherapy where appropriate. The algorithm described in the figure aids in evaluation of patients with hymenoptera stings.

ALGORITHM FOR EVALUATION OF PATIENTS WITH HYMENOPTERA STINGS

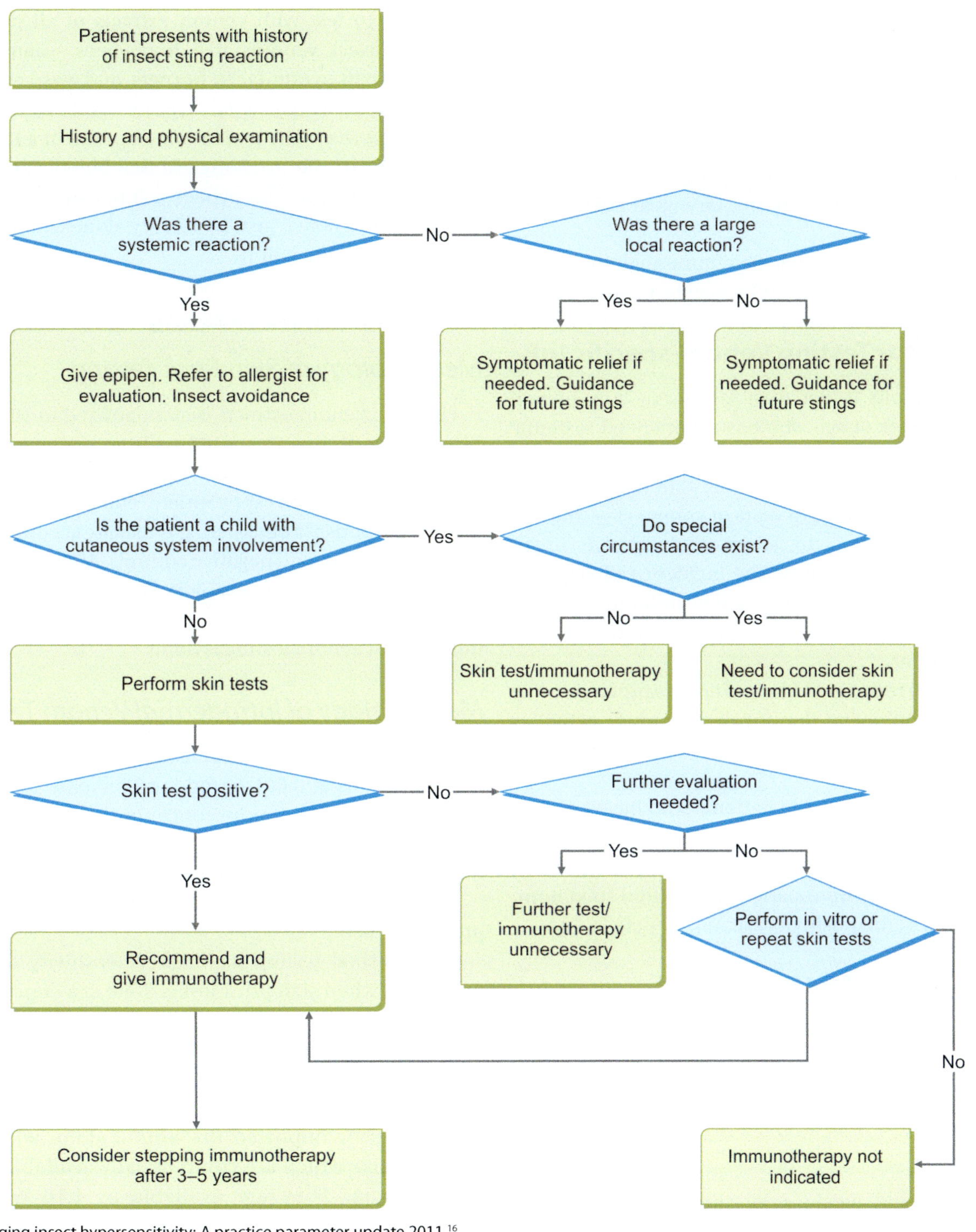

Source: Stinging insect hypersensitivity: A practice parameter update 2011.[16]

DIAGNOSIS OF VENOM ALLERGY

Patients who have had a systemic reaction to an insect sting should be referred for further evaluation.[5]

Diagnosis of Venom Allergy Requires

1. Strong history suggestive of systemic reaction to insect bite. The reactions may be mild limited to skin or severe causing bronchospasm, laryngeal edema, and hypotension.
2. Evidence of venom-specific immunoglobulin IgE either by doing a skin test or by in vitro IgE methods.

Indications for Testing Venom-specific IgE

Indication in adults (older than 16 years)—Any person older than 16 years of age who has experienced systemic reaction or anaphylaxis. Some countries do not do testing for adults who have cutaneous manifestation alone.

Indication in children (16 years or younger)—Children with systemic reaction to stings that involve organ other than the skin. However, the incidence of systemic reactions other than skin is very rare in children, and skin manifestations alone account for approximately 60% of all systemic reactions.

Patients with recurrent LLRs and are in a profession like beekeeping or hobbying that involves outdoor activities and who feel these LLRs significantly reduce the quality of life can be offered testing.

Testing is not indicated in patients who have no sting history but request testing as one or more family members have hymenoptera venom allergy. There is a 27–40% of people who have asymptomatic sensitization to venom, and the results of the positivity are not very clear.

Types of Testing Methods for IgE

1. Skin testing—Skin prick test or intradermal test
2. In vitro testing for IgE—radioallergosorbent test (RAST), ImmunoCAP, and Component-resolved diagnostics.

Skin Testing

Skin testing should be done by allergist/immunologist trained in this speciality.

Timing of Testing

It is ideal to wait for at least 4–6 weeks after the systemic reaction as antibody titres will be low during the first few weeks and hence can produce a false-negative test.

Choice of Venoms

It is ideal to test with venom extracts of all potentially relevant insect venoms like honeybees, yellow jacket, yellow hornets, white-faced hornets, and wasp even when the patient says a particular type of insect as the history can be imperfect. The patient may be sure of a honeybee, whereas the history may suggest that bite occurred while they were drinking. Honeybees will not sting unless until provoked and hence just the history alone cannot suggest which insect is the culprit.

Technique of Skin Testing

Methodology of Skin Prick Testing

Each of the venom extracts is standardized to 100 μg/mL. Most of the testing is started with a concentration of 1 μg/mL and increased to 100 μg/mL in 10-fold dilutions in fixed intervals in appropriate clinical settings till a positive response is obtained. It is usually accompanied by standard positive and negative controls. About 25% of them show positive reaction at a concentration of 100 μg/mL. Even at this concentration response is negative, then intradermal venom testing is done.

Methodology of Intradermal Venom Testing

The traditional approach is to begin with venom concentrations at 0.001 μg/mL and increase it in 10-fold dilutions till a maximum concentration of 1 μg/mL is reached. The testing is repeated at 20–30 minutes interval till a positive response is obtained.

The volume of the dilution used is 0.02–0.03 mL to produce a bleb.

Intradermal testing has higher sensitivity than skin prick even when skin prick test is done at a concentration of 100 μg/mL.[5,17] Hence, it is essential to do intradermal test even when the skin test is negative. The sensitivity of intradermal test is estimated to be about 90% or higher for 1 μg/mL concentration.

Testing for imported fire ants is done with whole body extracts which are commercially available though not in India. They are available as 1:10 w/v stock solutions. Skin prick testing is usually tested by diluting it to 1:100 w/v or 1:1,000 w/v. If negative intradermal testing is then performed. It is tested starting with 1:1,000,000 w/v and increased 10-fold until 1:500 to 1:1,000 w/v is reached.[5,10]

If the skin prick testing is negative but the history is very strongly suggestive of systemic reaction due to insect bites, it is necessary to proceed to testing for IgE by in vitro methods. About 5–10% of patients will have raised IgE levels with negative skin tests.

Serum Testing

Serum-Specific IgE by In vitro Methods

Indications for in vitro methods

1. When history is strongly suggestive of insect bite systemic reaction, but skin test is negative
2. Patients who cannot be tested for skin testing due to dermographism or skin diseases
3. Patients who are on drugs that can render skin test unreactive like tricyclic antidepressants
4. There is a discrepancy between the skin test results and the history

Methods used: In vitro RAST and a variety of methods like ImmunoCAP solid-phase assay and component-resolved diagnostics can be applied with the latest techniques giving more sensitive results. The venom-specific IgE is tested after a specific interval, and in the initial days the specific IgE may be low. A serum level of >0.35 kU/L is considered as positive result. It should be used as an adjunct to skin tests as both sensitivity and specificity are low compared to intradermal skin tests.

Component-resolved diagnosis (CRD) testing is being increasingly used in West in patients with dual sensitization to bee and wasp venom to know the culprit insect.

Cross-sensitivity: One of the main problems in interpreting the results is cross-sensitivity to venoms other than the culprit insects which can cause multiple sensitizations and increased IgE titres. Venom enzymes also share cross-reacting carbohydrate epitopes, for example, between honeybees and yellow jacket hornets that may also induce these multiple positive test results of unknown clinical significance. This can be found by RAST inhibition test where the test is modified with the inclusion of an initial incubation phase. In this phase, the patients' serum is incubated with venom from both the species separately or with carbohydrate epitopes. CRD is also a very useful tool in such situations.5,17

Serum tryptase levels: An elevated serum tryptase levels and mastocytosis are risk factors for severe reactions. Usually levels of about 20 μg/L is considered positive. Baseline tryptase levels (levels >11.4 μg/L) should be checked in all patients who develop a systemic reaction.[5] This is a marker to predict severe systemic reactions like anaphylaxis.

Serum total IgE: Not very useful.

In general, no single test can predict the severity of subsequent systemic reactions The combination of history with skin tests/in vitro tests can help to detect up to 95% of cases. Rest of the 5% of patients will require other advance modalities like basophil activation tests.

MANAGEMENT OF VENOM ALLERGY

The management depends on the severity of the reaction although avoidance advice is universal.

Avoidance

1. Infestations need to be removed using professional exterminators to eradicate infestations in the surroundings.
2. Suitable clothing like clothes with long sleeves and closed toed shoes should be worn.
3. Insect repellent creams can be used.
4. Avoiding bright-colored clothes that attract the insects, but there are studies which have refuted this point as they feel the insects are more attracted to ultraviolet patterns which the humans cannot be perceived by humans.[18]
5. Perfumes can help in avoidance when stepping outside; however, care needs to be taken regarding the type of cosmetic fragrances including alcohols and esters that may elicit defensive reactions by these insects.[18]
6. Generally, walk along the trails most frequented by all and avoid tall grasses when being adventurous.
7. Use of tightly covered food and waste receptacles; frequent cleaning of food residues; and frequent removal of wastes, fallen fruits, or animal feces are very effective to minimize local source of attraction.[18]
8. Generally, the attacks of insects come when they are accidentally stepped on or by taking the insects into the mouth along with food or drink, or striking with bare hands. This can be avoided by high vigilance while drinking or eating, by drinking using straws fitted to a tightly lidded cups, and avoiding directly drinking from cans or bottles, always checking the container before consuming while in open areas, and avoiding hitting the insects with bare hands even if they seem very small.[18]

9. When considering hobbies like gardening and beekeeping a prior history of bite or sensitization should be considered.
10. Stinger if present in the skin should be pulled out carefully and quickly as the presence of stinger will lead to injection of more venom in the body.
11. Imported fire ants can be avoided only by using lace-up shoes, thick socks, and pants.
12. Fire ants need to be exterminated, and insecticides are not very useful.[10]

TREATMENT

Acute Reactions

Local Reactions

1. Ice cold packs
2. Oral antihistamines—Cetrizine has quicker onset of action but any antihistamines can be used
3. Analgesics—Ibuprofen or naproxen can bring down the pain
4. Topical steroids: 0.5% or 1% (if ≥ 2 years of age) hydrocortisone may produce some decrease in itch and inflammation. The application can be done 1–2 times in a day for about a week
5. If infected, antibiotics are required.

Systemic Reactions

Mild—oral antihistamine when itching is the predominant symptom

Moderate and severe systemic reactions—are to be managed similarly

Airway obstruction/hypotension gives aqueous epinephrine intramuscularly and immediate emergency care and treatment with observation for 4 hours or longer.

Aqueous epinephrine should be given by intramuscular injections immediately. Usually the outer thigh is preferred as it results in higher and maximum plasma concentrations. The antigen source should be removed, and if possible, a tourniquet is placed above the bite site.

The doses can be repeated up to a maximum of 2–3 depending on the response. If there is a need to give repeated doses, then we need to consider epinephrine infusion. Coexistent hypotension needs to be treated with 20 mL/kg of normal saline rushed through a wide bore needle.

Dosage—0.3–0.5 mg of 1:1,000 dilution for adults and children more than 12 years and 0.01 mg/kg for children.

Special precautions—patients on beta blockers can be resistant to epinephrine. They will require fluids and glucagon to reverse anaphylaxis.

Prevention

Epinephrine autoinjectors should be given for emergency use and referral to an allergist or immunologist for the prevention of insect stings. Epipen is available as two strengths—Epipen 0.3 mg and Epipen junior 0.15 mg for children below 25 kg (Fig. 39.1).

Indications for Referral to an Allergist–Immunologist

1. Patients developing systemic reaction to insect stings or who has developed anaphylaxis for insect sting.
2. LLRs are usually referred to get informed discussion about the relative risk of future reaction and about the need for doing diagnostic testing and treatment. This helps to avoid unnecessary impairment of quality of life and unnecessary treatment.
3. History of generalized urticarial rashes after insect sting.
4. Patients having positive ST or ImmunoCap for insect venoms for discussion of results.
5. Patients who have coexisting condition that might complicate the treatment of anaphylaxis.

Venom Immunotherapy (VIT)

It is the only specific treatment available for currently reducing systemic reactions to future stings. It should be used in patients with specific IgE to respective venom and has a history of systemic reaction or anaphylaxis. Immunotherapy

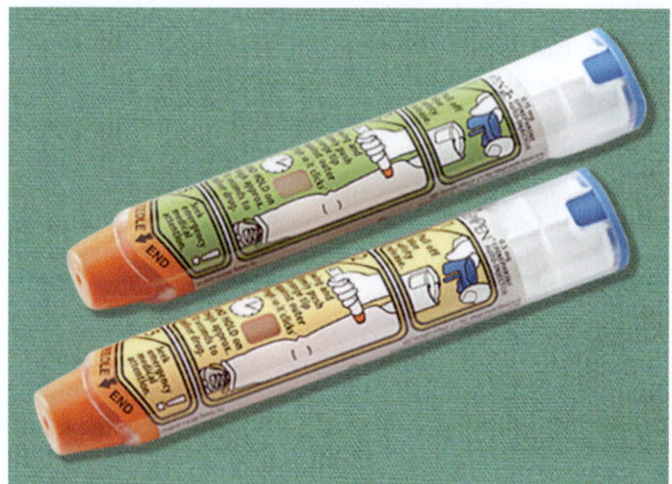

Fig. 39.1: Epinephrine autoinjectors (Epipen 0.3 mg and Epipen Junior 0.15 mg).

greatly reduces the risk of systemic reactions. It has an efficacy of 95–97%. The goal of immunotherapy is to reduce life-threatening reactions and will also alleviate anxiety for the patients. It improves the quality of life by allowing the patients to participate in outdoor activities.[19]

Indications for Venom Immunotherapy

Hymenoptera venom immunotherapy is the sole therapy that can produce immunomodulatory effects for patients who have had a systemic reaction to hymenoptera bites and reduces the chances of future stings.

1. Any adult above the age of 16 years who has a history of anaphylactic or systemic reactions and a positive skin test or elevated IgE levels by in vitro methods is a candidate for immunotherapy.
2. Children below 16 years who have had a systemic reaction other than skin manifestation has a future recurrent risk of 30% and hence needs to be started on immunotherapy.
3. Adults who have had *frequent* LLRs and also *have frequent hymenoptera* exposure like beekeepers, and *quality of life is sufficiently reduced* by these reactions can be considered for VIT.
4. Immunotherapy should be firmly advocated to adults with elevated baseline tryptase levels who had a systemic reaction even if mild.[5,19]

Immunotherapy Dosing Schedule

Up-dosing schedule is usually given weekly once or twice every week during the build-up phase which lasts for 12 weeks, and once a maintenance dose is reached, the dosage between injections is increased between doses to 4 weeks in case of inhalant allergens and 8 weeks in venom immunotherapy.

There are accelerated schedules like cluster schedule where the build-up phase is for 7 weeks, rush schedule where the build-up phase is for 3–4 days, and ultra-rush schedule where the build-up phase is just 1–2 days.

But in accelerated schedule the risk of both local and systemic reactions is greatly increased. Premedication needs to be given, and the time of observation should also be prolonged.[20]

A maintenance dosage of 100 μg (300 μg for mixed vespid) once monthly is the therapeutic goal.

The patients who have fire ant sensitivity are treated in the same way as the other hymenoptera species. Whole body extract with a monthly maintenance dose of 0.5 mL of 1:100 w/v extract is recommended for 3–5 years.[5]

Efficacy

Venom immunotherapy is very effective in preventing systemic reactions in patients who had prior reactions with insect sting. Effectiveness is highest for mixed vespid venoms. It is up to about 98% with a maintenance dose of 300 μg. Honeybee stings have a higher rate of recurrent anaphylactic reactions; however, honeybee venom immunotherapy is only 71% effective in controlling anaphylaxis. Few patients who have systemic reactions repeatedly usually have only milder reactions to future stings.[9,19]

Immunotherapy Failure

Venom immunotherapy at an accepted maintenance dosage is very effective but does not protect all patients. Failure should prompt defects in recognition of the culprit insect. If the insect is the same then increasing the dose to 200 μg might provide protection.

Documentation

Prior to initiating allergen immunotherapy, inform patients about the clinic's immunotherapy procedures, including the mandatory 30-minute wait time. Asthmatic patients in particular should be reminded not to discontinue their maintenance asthma medications without their physician's permission and to defer immunotherapy if their asthma is not well controlled. Review potential adverse reactions, including both local and systemic reactions. Informed consent needs to be signed prior to receiving their first injection. If the clinic's protocol requires carrying an epinephrine autoinjector, give a prescription to the patient with a reminder to carry it each time when he or she comes in for an allergy injection.[20]

Contraindications to VIT

1. Active immunologic diseases (e.g., immune complex diseases, active rheumatoid arthritis)
2. Active cancer within the last 5 years
3. Uncontrolled asthma, severe asthma—need to withhold injections if the peak flow reading is <70%
4. Chronic heart/lung disease (if unstable)
5. Treatment with beta blockers (relative contra-indication)
6. Pregnancy—If possible, discontinue VIT in pregnancy. If there is an increased risk for future stings, immunotherapy can be continued in the maintenance phase at which the treatment is tolerated. However, it should not be initiated in pregnancy.[6]

Consider Stopping VIT after 3–5 Years

Guidelines for stopping immunotherapy is slowly evolving. The criteria for discontinuing in serum-specific IgE to very low levels or negative skin response after starting immunotherapy. However, it has been noted that in spite of persistence of positive skin test response in 90% of patients, they may not develop systemic reactions even if immunotherapy is stopped after 3–5 years and hence can be discontinued after this period. Studies have reported a complete protection in 80–91% of patients 3 years after stopping immunotherapy.[21]

Hence, a decision about the duration of immunotherapy should be made individually after a discussion between the patient and the physician. Consideration should be given to lifestyle, occupation, coexistent disease, and severity of skin reactions. Fire ants immunotherapy does not have specific recommendations.[5,16]

Patients who have honeybee allergy, who had severe pretreatment reaction or who had systemic reaction during treatment, or who have received treatment for less than 5 years can develop recurrence after stopping immunotherapy. Patients who have significant cardiovascular or pulmonary disease, who require higher venom doses, or who have had mast cell disorders may require immunotherapy indefinitely.[9,21]

Those patients where immunotherapy is stopped should be counseled to carry an autoinjector epinephrine as recurrence may occur in 10% of them. Should they have serious reactions after a bite they need to immediately report to the allergy specialist.[21]

ABBREVIATIONS

CRD Component-resolved diagnostics
LLR Large local reaction
RAST Radioallergosorbent test
ST Skin testing
USA United States of America
UK United Kingdom

REFERENCES

1. Anita Kannagi V, Sivakumar V, S Santhi, et al. Hymnopteran diversity in a deciduous forest from South India. Int J Biodivers Conserv. October 2013;5:666-70.
2. Singh S, Mann BK. Insect bite reactions. Indian J Dermatol Venerol Leprol. 2013;79:151-64.
3. Kar S, Dongre A, Krishan A, et al. Epidemiological study of insect bite reactions from Central India. Indian J Dermatol. 2013;58:337-41
4. Karthikeyan K, Thappa DM, Jeevankumar B. Pattern of Pediatric dermatoses in a referral Center in South India. Indian Pediatrics. 2004;41:373-7.
5. Tankersley MS, Ledford D. Stinging insect allergy: state of the art 2015. J Allergy Clin Immunol Pract. 2015;3: 315-22.
6. Richard AG, Krishna MT. Insect venom allergy. In: Vedhanthan PK, Nelson H, Agashe SN, Mahesh PA, Katial R, ed. Textbook of Allergy for Clinicians. 2013: 256-67.
7. Hymenoptera - Wikipedia, the free encyclopaedia.htm
8. Rajkumari P, Sharmah D, Rahman A, Patgiri P. Diversity and distribution pattern of Hymenopteran insects in Jorhat District, Assam, India. Int J Sci Res. 2014;3: 1938-42.
9. Paschall VL. Allergy and Immunology, Hymenoptera venom allergy. www.clevelandclinicmeded.com/medical pubs/diseasemanagement/allergy/hymenoptera-venom-allergy/
10. deShazo RD, Williams DF, Goodard J, et al. Stings of imported fire ants: clinical manifestations, diagnosis and treatment. https://www.uptodate.com/contents/stings-of-imported-fire-ants-clinical-manifestations-diagnosis-and-treatment
11. Dutta TK, Mukta V. Indian guidelines and protocols: bee sting. Toxicology. New Delhi: Jaypee Brother Medical Publishers; 2013:Chapter 92:417-20. www.apiindia.org/medicine_update_2013/chapter92.pdf
12. Golden DBK. Large local reactions to insect stings. J Allergy Clin Immunol Pract. 2015;:331-3.
13. Rueff F, Pryzybila B, Beatrice M, et al. Predictors of severe systemic anaphylactic reactions in patients with Hymenoptera venom allergy: importance of baseline serum tryptase—a study of the European Academy of Allergology and Clinical Immunology Interest Group on Insect Venom Hypersensitivity. J Allergy Clin Immunol. 2009;124:1047-54. http://www.jacionline.org/article/S0091-6749(09)01269-X/fulltext
14. Bilo MB, Rueff F, Mosbech H, Bonifazi F. Diagnosis of hymenoptera venom. EAACI position paper. doi:xx.xxxx/eaacinet2005.xxxx
15. Quercia O, Incorvaia C, Marseglia GL, et al. Prevalence and incidence of reactions to insect stings in children: a reappraisal. Minerva Pediatr. 2014;66:257-60.
16. David BK, Golden, JM, Nicklas R. Stinging insect hypersensitivity: a practice parameter update 2011. J Allergy Clin Immunol. 2011;127:852-4.

17. Tracy JM, Golden DB, Feldweg AM. Diagnosis of hymenoptera venom allergy. February 2018. https://www.uptodate.com/contents/diagnosis-of-hymenoptera-venom-allergy/print?csi=465915a5-ce69-4790-a710-f931ab6cb547&source=contentShare#H15
18. Greene A, Breisch NL. Avoidance of bee and wasp stings: an entomological perspective. Curr Opin Allergy Clin Immunol. 2005;5:337-41.
19. Graft DF. Hymenoptera venom immunotherapy: efficacy, indications and mechanism of action. 2015. https://www.uptodate.com
20. Mehta V. Common Office Procedures. Milwaukee, WI: AAAAI Practice Management Resource Guide. 2014:1-29.
21. Muller UR, Ring J, When can immunotherapy for Insect sting allergy be stopped? J Allergy Clin Immunol Pract. 2014;3:324-8.

CHAPTER 40

Radiocontrast Allergy

Richa Gupta

INTRODUCTION

Radiocontrast allergy is the manifestation of allergic reaction either immediate or delayed-type hypersensitivity to the intravenous dye or radiocontrast media (RCM) used for X-ray-based imaging techniques such as radiography and computed tomography (CT).

RADIOCONTRAST MEDIA

Radiocontrast media are the drugs used to enhance the visibility of internal structures viz. vessels, tissues, organs, and urinary tracts during the various radiographic procedures, such as angiography, venography, urography, myelography, Endoscopic retrograde cholangiopancreatography (ERCP), and computed tomography. RCM are usually safe, and side effects are generally mild and self-limited.

Types of RCM

There are two basic types of contrast media[1] used for most radiologic studies:

1. Ionic high-osmolality contrast media.
2. Nonionic low-osmolality contrast media.

Both agents contain iodine, are derivatives of tri-iodobenzoic acid, and are administered intravenously (Table 40.1).

Table 40.1: Types of contrast agents.

High osmolality, ionic	*Low osmolality, nonionic*
• Diatrizoate sodium (Hypaque) • Iothalamate meglumine (Conray)	• Iodixanol (Visipaque) • Gadodiamide (Omniscan) • Gadoteridol (ProHance) • Iopamidol (Isovue) • Iopromide (Ultravist) • Ioversol (Optiray)

The nonionic contrast agents are more widely used as they have much better safety profile compared with the ionic agents, but are much expensive.

RISK FACTORS

There are certain conditions and patients are at increased risk for developing adverse reactions to contrast medium (Box 40.1).

The patients who have past history of anaphylaxis to the contrast agent are at high risk of developing similar reaction on re-exposure. Hence, history of previous such event should be meticulously included and reported to the radiographer. Similarly, patients with asthma[2] or history of other atopic diathesis have double the risk of developing adverse reactions compared to the general population, even if their asthma is under control. Certain preexisting medical conditions like cardiac or renal diseases also pose a risk for developing contrast reactions.

Diabetic patients on metformin are at high risk of developing severe lactic acidosis following IV administration of contrast media.[3] Hence, it is recommended to stop metformin at the time of procedure or before and

BOX 40.1: Conditions associated with increased risk for RCM allergy.

- History of reactions to contrast media
- Asthma
- Atopic status—history of food/medication allergy, hay fever
- Pre-existing medical conditions—heart, kidney, or thyroid disease
- Patients on beta blockers, metformin
- Elderly
- Females

for at least 48 hours post-contrast administration. The medication should be restarted only after renal functions have returned to normal.

Advance age and nephrotoxic drugs are risk factors for developing contrast media-induced renal failure.

Pregnant females should not receive contrast agents and should restore to alternate ways of imaging in case required.

CLINICAL MANIFESTATION

Two types of adverse events can occur with the administration of radiocontrast agent intravenously:

- Chemotaxic reaction.
- Hypersensitivity or allergic reactions.

Chemotaxic Reaction

Chemotaxic or physiologic reactions are related to the chemical properties of the agent and are dose and rate of infusion dependent. These reactions may include the following:

1. Vasovagal
2. Seizures
3. Arrhythmias
4. Organ toxicity especially renal (contrast-induced nephropathy or CIN) and thyroid (hypo or hyperthyroid).

Hypersensitivity or Allergic Reactions

Hypersensitivity reactions to radiocontrast are mainly idiosyncratic and largely independent of dose and rate of infusion. These reactions can be immediate or delayed. Hypersensitivity reactions to contrast media include both IgE and non-IgE-mediated anaphylaxis, with activation of mast cells, coagulation, kinin, and complement mechanisms; inhibition of enzymes; and platelet aggregation.[4]

Immediate Hypersensitivity Reaction

It occurs within 1 hour, usually within 5 minutes of radiocontrast administration. The incidence of immediate reactions to nonionic contrast media ranges from 0.01% to 0.04% (severe) to 3% (mild).[5] Mortality rate is less than 1 per 100,000 patients.[4]

Mild Hypersensitivity Reactions

- Immediate skin rashes
- Flushing or urticaria pruritus
- Rhinorrhea
- Nausea and/or vomiting
- Diaphoresis
- Coughing and dizziness.

Moderate Hypersensitivity Reactions

- Persistent vomiting
- Diffuse urticaria
- Headache
- Mild bronchospasm
- Abnormal heart rhythms.

Severe Hypersensitivity Reactions

- Coronary artery spasm
- Life-threatening cardiac arrhythmias (i.e., ventricular tachycardia)
- Overt bronchospasm
- Laryngeal edema, angioedema
- Cardiac failure and loss of consciousness
- Pulmonary edema
- Seizures, syncope.

Delayed Hypersensitivity Reaction

Delayed hypersensitivity reactions usually occur hours to weeks post-administration of radiocontrast medium. These reactions are usually self-limiting and cutaneous in the form of rash, erythema, urticarial, or angioedema. They may be at times accompanied by fever, nausea, vomiting, and dizziness. The reported incidence varies from 1% to 23%.

The pathophysiology of delayed cutaneous reactions is speculative but likely represents a spectrum of T-cell-mediated delayed hypersensitivity.[6]

Anaphylactic Reaction

Anaphylactic reactions are serious and potentially life-threatening reactions associated with the administration of contrast material. Anaphylactic reactions can occur within few minutes of administration of contrast and are not dose dependent. The clinical picture may vary from acute bronchospasm to profound hypotension and severe urticaria.

These reactions are not considered as "true" allergic reactions, because they can also occur in patients without prior exposure to contrast agent. The etiology of these anaphylactic reactions is not clear and IgE antibodies, associated with allergic reactions, have not been demonstrated in most patients with anaphylactic reactions.[7]

MANAGEMENT

General Principles

1. Identify potentially high-risk patients by careful clinical history and medications.
2. Past history of any reaction to radiocontrast agent—if so, the nature of reaction should be determined.
3. In patients who have had a previous allergic-type reaction to contrast media, premedication may be helpful.
   - Premedication protocol: Administer 50 mg of prednisone orally 13, 7, and 1 hour (s) before injection of the contrast medium, and 50 mg of diphenhydramine intravenously, intramuscularly, or orally 7 and 1 hour (s) before injection.[8,9]
4. Consider alternative imaging techniques.
5. Risks and benefits should be judged and discussed in length with the patient.

Treatment of Adverse Reaction

Mild to Moderate Reactions

Do not require any specific treatment as these reactions usually resolve spontaneously. In other cases, observation and/or symptomatic/general supportive care is sufficient in the management of these reactions.

Severe Reactions/Anaphylaxis

The anaphylactic reactions associated with radiocontrast allergy are managed as any other anaphylaxis. Principles of cardiac life support should be followed by securing patients airways and stabilizing cardiac functions—the key element in the management of anaphylactic reaction. Epinephrine is the mainstay of treatment of anaphylaxis. There is no contraindication per se for epinephrine in the settings of anaphylaxis. Epinephrine should be administered immediately (0.5 mg intramuscularly followed by every 5–10 minutes depending on the response). Oxygen and IV fluids should be given as early as possible as a part of treatment protocol. Antihistamines are second line of treatment for anaphylaxis and are usually given after initial resuscitation. Though corticosteroids have no immediate effect on anaphylaxis,[10] they should be administered to prevent a potential late-phase reaction (biphasic anaphylaxis) and also for patients with underlying airway disease. Other symptomatic and supportive treatments should also be instituted once patient is stabilized.

Delayed Reactions

Symptoms of delayed reactions usually do not require any specific treatment other than only supportive management, as these are mild and resolve spontaneously.

Allergy to RCM is not uncommon, and mild reactions may be seen in patients undergoing imaging with contrast. Awareness about the various risk factors and thorough prescreening of the patients allows for early recognition and treatment of these reactions. Further, use of low-molecular, nonionic agents in smaller amounts decreases the relative risk of severe reactions to RCM.

REFERENCES

1. Saljoughian M. Intravenous radiocontrast media: a review of allergic reactions. US Pharm. 2012;37:HS-14-6.
2. Maddox TG. Adverse reactions to contrast material: recognition, prevention, and treatment. Am Family Phys. 2002;66:1229-35s.
3. McCartney MM, Gilbert FJ, Murchison LE, et al. Metformin and contrast media—a dangerous combination? Clin Radiol. 1999;54:29-33.
4. Thomson KR, Varma DK. Safe use of radiographic contrast media. Aust Prescriber. 2010;s33:19-22.
5. Namasivayam S, Kalra M, Toress W, Small WC. Adverse reactions to intravenous iodinated contrast media: a primer for radiologists. Emerg Radiol. 2006;12:210-5.
6. Loh S, Bagheri S, Katzberg RW, et al. Delayed adverse reaction to contrast-enhanced CT: a prospective single-center study comparison to control group without enhancement. Radiology. 2010;255:764-71.
7. Carr DH, Walker AC. Contrast media reactions: experimental evidence against the allergy theory. Br J Radiol. 1984;57:469-73.
8. Greenberger PA, Patterson R. The prevention of immediate generalized reactions to radiocontrast media in high-risk patients. J Allergy Clin Immunol. 1991;87:867-72.
9. American College of Radiology. Manual on Contrast Media. 6th ed. Reston VA: The College; 2008. www.acr .org /Secondary Main Menu Categories /quality safety / contrast manual.aspx. Accessed June 8, 2009.
10. Choo KJ, Simons E, Sheikh A. Glucocorticoids for the treatment of anaphylaxis: Cochrane systematic review. Allergy. 2010;65:1205-11.

CHAPTER 41

Allergic Reactions to Anesthetics

PS Shankar

INTRODUCTION

During the anesthetic procedures and postoperative period, different drugs belonging to different pharmacological groups are administered to make the whole operative procedure safe. Anesthetic is an agent that produces anesthesia by causing paralysis of sensory nerve endings or nerve fibers at the site of application.

HYPERSENSITIVITY REACTIONS

Life-threatening hypersensitivity reactions may occur during surgery and anesthesia. The reactions during anesthesia differ according to a particular geographic area and range between 1 in every 6,000 to 1 in every 10,000 procedures. It includes both regional and general anesthesias.[1,2] There is no such system to document such episodes in India. Majority of mild reactions are not documented and ignored. Fortunately, serious allergic reactions to anesthetic medications are rare. Allergic episodes may be noted from factors other than the anesthetic agents such as antibiotics, blood preparations, neuromuscular blocking agents, heparin, protamine sulfate, colloids, polypeptides, and natural rubber latex.[3]

The allergic reactions are unpredictable and are considered as a part of adverse drug reaction (ADR). ADR is an unpredictable, unintended reaction to standard dose or overdose of a given agent. Commonly the reactions are usually dose dependent, and they are related to the pharmacological properties of a drug and/or its metabolites. Uncommonly, the reactions may be related to hypersensitivity and allergic responses. Such reactions are not dependent on specific pharmacology and are usually not dose dependent.[4] The allergic reactions should be recognized by the anesthetist, anesthesiologist, or nurse anesthetist. Allergic reactions develop within several minutes following the exposure to a triggering factor. The event can be severe and life-threatening if the reaction makes its onset quickly and rapidly.

ANESTHETICS

Anesthetics are categorized as general, spinal, epidural, and regional (local, topical) anesthetic agents. They may be given as general, inhalational, infiltrative, or local forms.

Local Anesthetics

Local anesthetic (LA) is a drug that causes reversible local anesthesia. It provides a local analgesic effect by blocking nerve conduction in the region where it is applied. It acts by altering the permeability of nerve cells to sodium ions. LAs are in use since 1884 when cocaine was discovered. Later, less-toxic and less-additive substances such as stovaine and procaine were introduced in 1903–1904. After half a century, several synthetic agents such as lidocaine, bupivacaine, and prilocaine were introduced as LA agents.

Classification

The LAs are classified into two groups:

1. Aminoamide (articaine, bupivacaine, etidocaine, lidocaine, lignocaine, meprivacaine, prilocaine).
2. Aminoester (benzocaine, cocaine, procaine, cyclomethycaine, piperocaine, propoxycaine, benzocaine, novocaine, tetracaine).

LA Solutions

The LA solutions used for injection consist of the following materials:

1. LA agent
2. Vehicle (water)

3. Preservatives (methyl paraben, bisulfate used to stabilize vasoconstriction)
4. Buffer.

Administration

The LAs may be administered by different methods:[5]

- Topical (surface anesthesia by application of LA spray solution or cream to the skin, or infiltrative anesthesia by injection of LA into the tissue to be anesthetized),
- Field block (subcutaneous injection of anesthetic in area that borders the field to be anesthetized),
- Peripheral nerve block (injection of anesthetic near a peripheral nerve innervating an area),
- Plexus block (injection of anesthetic in the vicinity of a nerve plexus),
- Epidural (injection of anesthetic into the epidural space with an effect on a spinal root),
- Spinal anesthesia (injection of anesthetic into the cerebrospinal fluid usually at the lumbar spine with effect on the spinal roots and part of the spinal cord), and
- Regional anesthesia (injection of anesthetic intravenously).

Allergic Reactions

LAs may be associated with adverse reactions in the form of allergy, tissue neurotoxicity, and systemic toxicity. Allergy and hypersensitivity reactions though an infrequent occurrence, they remain a major cause of concern for anesthesiologists. The reactions may take form of bronchospasm, urticarial, or angioneurotic edema.[6] Allergic reactions may be of two different types: (1) allergic contact dermatitis and delayed swelling at the site of administration, and (2) rarely urticaria and anaphylaxis. Ester-linked anesthetics are prone to produce allergic reactions which may necessitate the use of an amide preparation. True sensitivity reactions to amide-linked agents are extremely rare. Most esters are metabolized locally to pseudocholinesterase, while amides are metabolized in the liver.

Occurrence of allergic reactions is rare. They are mostly noted with esters due to sensitivity to their metabolite, paraminobenzoic acid (PABA). PABA is liberated by the hydrolysis of the amino ester. LA is likely to be the cause of allergic reaction. Cross-reactivity to an amino-amide drug has not been shown with allergy to an amino ester. Hence, amides are often used as an alternative in patients who exhibited allergy to esters. The amide class can be used with safety in patients who give a history of true allergy to an amino-ester LA. In general, a patient known to be allergic to one ester anesthetic is likely to be allergic to all ester anesthetics.

Nonallergic Reactions

Nonallergic reactions may resemble allergy in their manifestations. There may be a need to establish a diagnosis of allergy by using skin tests and provocative challenge tests. Some allergic manifestations may occur from preservative added to LAs (paraben). Though skin testing is available, they are rarely used. This is because the anesthesiologist obtains the history of suffering from an allergic reaction. If testing is performed, the amino-ester compounds have a high incidence of skin reactivity.[7] Skin testing may produce suspicious reactions that must be differentiated from true allergy. Most patients who are tested may show a reaction that may not be truly allergic. Such reactions may be related to an anxiety state or adrenaline used. Most of these patients describe some symptoms which they had experienced on an earlier occasion following administration of LA. Such reactions are usually due to systemic absorption of adrenaline and the condition has to be distinguished from true allergy.

Anaphylactic Reactions

Anaphylactic reactions are the most severe form of immune-mediated reactions. Such reactions are encountered following re-exposure to specific antigens and release of proinflammatory mediators. Such severe reactions may be noted following use of muscle relaxants during intraoperative period. Latex may induce such an anaphylactic reaction.

General Anesthetics

Anaphylactic reactions may be encountered during the use of general anesthetics, such as thiopentone, and rarely ketamine.[8] The manifestations present in a similar way as seen in LAs. However, it differs in three significant ways:

1. The patient may feel light-headedness and breathlessness while anesthetic is being administered.
2. During anesthesia, many drugs are administered simultaneously, and it is difficult to pinpoint which drug has caused the reaction.
3. During anesthesia, many other causes may be responsible for fall in blood pressure or airway obstruction.

During a general anesthesia, many drugs are administered. Many of them have a very low incidence of allergy. Thus, it becomes difficult to establish the diagnosis of anaphylaxis. Further when the patient is unconscious due to the influence of general anesthesia, it becomes difficult to determine the occurrence of an allergic reaction. The symptoms can only be recognized if they have a dramatic onset.

MANIFESTATIONS

Generally the symptoms are noted in the skin, particularly in regions rich in mast cells such as face, neck, anterior chest, and become generalized quickly.[9] Occasionally, the symptoms may be referred to cardiovascular, respiratory, and even alimentary tract. The individual may present with severe breathlessness, or nausea and vomiting. There is tachycardia and fall in blood pressure. The symptoms are very dramatic. Severe allergic reactions are referred to as anaphylaxis. During anaphylaxis the patient exhibits difficulty in breathing, puffiness of face, and a reddish skin rash. There is tachycardia and fall in blood pressure (Table 41.1).

The adverse reactions including allergic reactions are likely to occur at any stage of anesthesia. The events of most of the manifestations are noted within the first minutes following the intravenous medication administered.[10] The signs and symptoms are characteristic of immediate allergic reaction occurring through immunoglobulin (Ig)E. There can be delayed cell-mediated response (type IV) in the form of contact dermatitis.

DIAGNOSIS

The diagnosis is based on the clinical manifestations, the time of their onset and involvement of the body systems, and anesthetics or other agents used. Subsequently, investigations such as tests may be undertaken to determine allergen to allow its future avoidance. Skin testing may be useful in identifying cross-reactive substances and to select appropriate therapeutic alternatives. Such tests may be undertaken many days after the initial reaction to enable the immune system to react itself. It must be noted that the skin testing is not a foolproof technique as it can give false-positive and false-negative results.

Table 41.1: Allergic reactions.

Skin	Erythema, urticaria, pruritus, angioneurotic edema
Nose	Rhinitis
Eye	Conjunctivitis
Respiratory system	Breathlessness, wheeze
Alimentary tract	Nausea, vomiting, abdominal pain, diarrhea
Cardiovascular system	Tachycardia, hypotension, circulatory shock

TREATMENT

Successful immediate treatment requires prompt recognition of the condition. Adrenaline (epinephrine) has to be administered without losing time. Corticosteroids and antihistaminic agents may be used to provide relief. However, they have limited benefit during an acute situation. In severe anaphylactic reactions, the airway must be kept clear and there may be a need to insert an endotracheal tube. Oxygen has to be a administered. Intravenous fluids are to be given to keep the blood pressure at a normal level.

PRECAUTIONS

It is necessary to document the adverse drug reactions including allergic reactions in the anesthesia records and provide the patient with the information in the card giving description of the drug-related reactions. Precautions have to be taken in future not to administer similar agent in future.

The agent responsible for allergic episode has to be avoided in future. Skin testing is helpful to identify the agent and to determine appropriate therapeutic alternatives in future.

REFERENCES

1. Axon AD, Hunter JM. Anaphylaxis and anaesthesia—all clear now? Br J Anaesth. 2004;93:501-5.
2. Birnbaum J, Porri F, Pradal D, et al. Allergy during anaesthesia. Clin Exp Allergy. 1994;24:916-24.
3. Hepner F, Castalls MC. Anaphylaxis during the perioperative period. Anesth Analg. 2003;97:1381-95.
4. Michalska-Krzanowska G. Anaphylactic reactions during anaesthesia and the perioperative period. Anaesthesiol Intens Ther. 2012;44:104-11.
5. Eggleston ST, Lush LW. Understanding allergic reactions to local anesthetics. Ann Pharmacother. 1996;30:851-7.
6. Atkinson RS, Rushman GB, Lee AJ. A Synopsis of Anaesthesia, 9th ed. Bristol: Wright PSG; 1982: 656.

7. Incaudo G, Schatz M, Patterson R, et al. Administration of local anesthetic to patients with a history of prior adverse reactions. J Allergy Clin Immun. 1978;61:339-45.
8. Anderson JA. Allergic reactions to drugs and biologic agents. JAMA. 1992;268:2845-57.
9. Fisher MM, Baldo BA. The incidence and clinical features of anaphylactic reactions during anesthesia in Australia Ann Fr Anesth Reanim. 1993;12:97-104.
10. Fisher MM, Doig GS. Prevention of anaphylactic reactions to anaesthetic drugs. Drug Saf. 2004;27:393-410.

CHAPTER 42

Cow's Milk Protein Allergy

Major K Nagaraju

INTRODUCTION

Adverse reaction to cow's milk protein (CMP) in infants and children occurs due to nonimmunologic, physiological reasons such as lactose intolerance or due to an immune reaction to the milk proteins. Immune intolerance to CMP is referred to as CMP allergy (CMPA). Cow's milk allergy (CMA) usually affects children at a young age, increasing their vulnerability to malnutrition, impaired growth, and disrupted development of eating behavior. CMPA is hard to diagnose as it presents with a wide range of symptoms and clinical picture, because the clinical diagnostic criteria vary between clinics.[1] As a result, CMPA often goes undiagnosed in the primary care setting, causing much distress to infants and parents and, more importantly, retarding growth of infants. Hence, an accurate and early diagnosis of CMPA is urgently needed. Since 2008, the World Allergy Organization (WAO) has put efforts to overcome this challenge by forming a committee to set guidelines for physicians for the diagnosis and management of CMPA.

TYPES

There are two basic immune reactions that lead to CMPA, involving either immunoglobulin E (IgE)-mediated or cell-mediated mechanism.

IgE-mediated CMPA

The IgE-mediated response is more common in infants and children.[2] It is considered to be a phenotypic expression of atopy (Th2). The IgE response occurs earlier on in the atopic march and is followed by the development of other IgE-based allergic conditions such as atopic eczema, allergic rhinitis, and asthma.

Non-IgE-mediated CMPA

Certain patients develop T-helper 1-mediated immune response to CMP rather than a humoral response. These patients may present with symptoms distinct from those who suffer from IgE-mediated CMPA, such as gastrointestinal (GI) symptoms.

Diminished activity of regulatory T cells (Tregs) is implicated in both IgE- and cell-mediated CMPAs, as the upregulation of Treg responses was found to develop tolerance to CMP.

EPIDEMIOLOGY

The CMPA occurs in infants and in early childhood, usually disappearing in adulthood. Unlike other atopic allergies such as asthma and allergic rhinitis, data on CMPA are scanty and inaccurate; for example, the CMPA prevalence was perceived to be 1–17.5% as self-reported in preschool children,[2] which is an overestimate as several studies report it to be 2–7.5% in infancy.[3-6] However, comprehensive data on CMPA prevalence in India are lacking. According to a German multicenter study on allergies, the CMPA incidence in infants and children falls from 4% at 2 years to <1% at 10 years of age. Infants appear to be sensitized within a week of starting cow's milk diet.[3] A Danish study found 76% remission in IgE-mediated CMPA in children aged <3 years compared to 100% remission in children with non-IgE-mediated CMPA.[3] Other studies had similar findings. Acquisition of tolerance to cow's milk was associated with a fall in CMP-specific IgE in three studies.

Based on the various published studies from the European Union, it can be stated that the CMPA incidence in infants ranges from 1.5% (Finland), 2.22% (Denmark), 2.24% (the Netherlands), to 4.9% (Norway). Rona and colleagues performed a meta-analysis on the prevalence of allergy to cow's milk.

These data indicate that the CMPA prevalence is 0.5–2% in infants and children aged <5 years, 0.5% in children aged 5–16 years, and 0.5% in adults.[2] The prevalence of CMA is 0.21% in newborns and 0.35% in extremely premature babies (1,000 g), according to a recent Japanese multicenter trial.[7]

This is in agreement with the German multicenter study as incidence is <1% by 10 years of age. It is an interesting observation that infants exclusively breastfed show remarkably lower incidence of 0.5% compared to those fed formula milk or a mixed diet of breastfeeding and formula food.[4,6] Considering that the concentration of CMP, which is the sensitizing agent, is 100,000-fold lesser in breast milk than in cow's milk and derived formulas, this is not surprising.

IMMUNOPATHOGENESIS

Milk proteins reach the gut upon consumption, where they are processed at low pH by proteases. Upon absorption, CMPs enter the circulation and are measurable in micrograms per liter serum.[3] In infants, including those with CMPA, intact milk proteins are found in the circulation, possibly due to incomplete proteolysis and *increased gut permeability*.[1] Proteins are ingested by cells of the gut epithelium and enter the subepithelial layer of the intestine, where the antigens derived from the proteins are ingested, processed, and presented on the surface of the antigen-presenting cells (APCs).

The processed antigen exhibited by the APCs is recognized and bound by the T-cell receptors on T cells, which in turn activate B cells to produce antibodies against the antigen or activate Th1 cells that participate in cell-mediated immunity. Usually, either antibody- or cell-mediated allergic reaction occurs, but occasionally, a mixed pathology is noted. Activation of T and B cells occurs in the lymphoid follicles, followed by their migration via the lymphatic system to various organs. The activated cells then exert their activities in these organs with pathologic consequences that present as clinical symptoms of CMPA. It is believed that *downregulation of Treg* responses plays a role in modulating the immune response against the CMP antigens. Upregulation of the Treg activity promotes tolerance to these antigens. In addition, a Th1-skewed immune response as opposed to a Th2-skewed one promotes tolerance to CMP antigens.[8]

Factors governing disposition to develop CMPA include the individual's genetic makeup, the amount and frequency of consumption of sensitizing antigen(s), the biochemical nature/composition of the sensitizing antigen(s), and the rate of absorption of the sensitizing antigen(s) (Table 42.1).

As mentioned earlier, CMPA can be of two different types: IgE-mediated CMPA and IgE-independent, CMI-mediated CMPA. Clinically, the IgE-mediated CMPA presents early-onset allergy, whereas the non-IgE-mediated CMPA presents late-onset allergy due to differing underlying mechanisms.

The IgE-mediated immediate response is due to the binding of an antigen by specific IgE on mast cells and basophils, "bridging" the cells that are triggered to release histamine. This is considered a *Type I immunologic response*.[3,8] Some delayed symptoms result from non-IgE-mediated CMPA, due to complement fixation by antibodies (IgA or IgG) complexed to antigens (*Type III immunologic response*) or mediated by sensitized T lymphocytes that are stimulated by antigens to expand and release proinflammatory cytokines and lymphokines, recruiting proinflammatory cells such as mononuclear cells and neutrophils (*Type IV immunologic response*).[6,9]

The immaturity of the immune system, in general, along with the capacity for antigen processing by dendritic cells in the intestine, and the immunosuppressive characteristics of the immune cells of the Peyer's patches polarize the immune response to CMP toward either allergy or tolerance.

Two factors that promote tolerance to CMP are as follows:

1. *Gut microbiota* influences the immune function via modulation of APCs, Tregs, and T and B lymphocytes and helps to build tolerance.
2. Early and enhanced exposure to large amounts of soluble milk proteins (gradual increase of exposure to the dose of an allergen creates anergy—T and B cells recognize the antigens but fail to be active as they do not receive appropriate stimulatory signals).

Pathogen-associated molecular patterns on microorganisms are recognized by toll-like receptors that cause activation of Treg cells.[8] Treg involvement in tolerance has been substantiated by the finding that anaphylactic response increases in the absence or depletion of cells. Combined with the finding that specific gut bacteria protect against sensitization to food allergens, it is suggested that lack of exposure to microorganisms in early life results in lack of tolerance possibly due to T-cell deregulation and

Table 42.1: Allergens in cow's milk.[2]

Fraction of cow's milk	*Allergen (protein)*	*Prevalence*
Whey protein	α-lactalbumin (Bos d 4)	0–80%
	β-lactoglobulin (Bos d 5)	13–76%
	Bovine serum albumin (Bos d 6)	0–88%
	Bovine immunoglobulins (Bos d 7)	Not common
Casein (collectively called Bos d 8)	α 1	Sensitization 100%
	α 2	No data
	β	Sensitization −91.7%
	κ	

increased incidence of allergies. The bacteria, especially *Lactobacillus* and *Bifidobacterium*, modulate immunologic mechanisms. The probiotics reduce the inflammatory responses and help maintain the integrity of the gut lining.

Gut microbiota enhances the activity of dendritic cells that polarize the immune responses to Th1 and promote the secretion of gut IgA. The Th1 polarization has been shown to be not localized to the gut, but systemic in nature. In support of the role of probiotics in tolerance to cow's milk, a 2002 study found a significant decrease of bifidobacteria and lactobacilli in the guts and stools of infants with rectal bleeding that included those suffering from CMPA, while the remaining flora seemed similar to normal control subjects.[10]

The sensitizing antigens in CMP are highly resistant to denaturation by physical agents such as boiling, pasteurization, ultra-high temperature processing, and evaporation, which are the processes involved in the production of powdered infant formula. These antigens provoke allergic responses in spite of such extensive and vigorous processing. Moreover, the published studies report that milk sterilized at 121°C for 20 minutes provokes a stronger allergic response, suggesting that the antigenicity of the milk proteins is further increased.[11,12] Milk protein antigens from various domestic animal sources are related as *cross-reactivity* is observed among cow's, goat, sheep, and buffalo milk, and thus provoke the reaction in CMPA patients.[6]

CLINICAL FEATURES

There is not a single clinical feature/symptom pathognomonic of CMPA, and infants/children develop symptoms in at least two organs.[13] The rates of involvement of specific organs as reported in a Danish study are as follows: gastrointestinal (50–60%), skin (50–70%), and respiratory tract (20–30%).[3] The more recent symptom rates reported by the WAO are as follows: 32–60% (GI), 5–90% (skin), and 0.8–9% (anaphylaxis).[2]

SYMPTOMS OF IMMEDIATE CMPA

Published literature describes an immediate allergic reaction to as little as a single drop to a volume as high as 161 mL. Immediate reactions can be categorized as follows:[1,13]

- *Anaphylaxis*
  Milk and milk-dependent exercise (exercise following intake of milk) *induces anaphylaxis.* In one study, the incidence of anaphylaxis was reported to be 11–28%, with 11% being fatal outcome. A case has been reported in which the patient had life-threatening anaphylaxis upon inhaling dry milk powder; the allergen was lactose. In our experience in the clinic, we encountered two cases of intolerance to vapors from boiling cow's milk.
- *GI symptoms*
  Upper GI Symptoms
  - Oral allergy presents as lip swelling, oral pruritus, tongue swelling, and sensation of tightness in the throat.
  - Nausea and vomiting.
  - Colicky upper abdominal pain.

  Lower GI Symptoms
  - Lower abdominal pain.
  - Loose stools.
  - Occasional or persistent bloody stools. Blood was found in stools of newborn infants within 24 hours of feeding milk formula as a result of an immediate IgE-triggered allergic response.
- *Common cutaneous presentation*
  - Urticaria
  - Angioedema
  - Maculopapular rash
  - Flushing
  - Exacerbation of atopic dermatitis.
- *Respiratory symptoms*
  Respiratory involvement of an allergic reaction to CMP is not much common. Respiratory involvement in CMPA usually accompanies atopic dermatitis reaction to CMP. Some children suffering from CMPA develop

respiratory allergies later in life. Respiratory symptoms noted are as follows:

Upper Airway Symptoms
- Rhinorrhea
- Sneezing
- Nasal pruritus
- Nasal congestion.

Lower Airway Symptoms
- Dyspnea
- Chest tightness
- Wheezing.

SYMPTOMS OF LATE-ONSET CMPA

Late-onset CMPA symptoms present within a wide time window covering hours to days.[1,13] They present largely as GI symptoms, but cutaneous and respiratory symptoms are also seen; however, respiratory symptoms are rare.

1. *Cutaneous symptoms*
   a. Eczema/atopic dermatitis
   Eczema is frequently manifested in late-onset CMPA triggered by consuming cow's milk or inhaling vapors. Thirty-three percent of atopic dermatitis cases are accompanied by CMPA, irrespective of whether it is IgE dependent or IgE independent.[2] Removal of cow's milk or related products from the patient diet decreases the eczema, and this effect is dependent on the age of the patient and/or the severity of the eczema.[2]
   b. Red umbilicus
   A localized red rash surrounding the umbilical and/ or periumbilical region has been noted in 36 children. Upon elimination of the diet, the erythema disappeared within the second week. On cow's milk challenge, it reappeared within 24 hours.[14]
2. *GI symptoms*
   Most of the GI symptoms of lactose intolerance, such as intestinal discomfort, bloating, nausea, and diarrhea, are also present in CMPA.[1] Therefore, often CMPA goes undiagnosed as the patient is thought to suffer from lactose intolerance. Unlike formula-fed infants, breastfed infants develop CMPA very rarely at a rate of about 0.5% with mild symptoms, as the allergens in CMP are present in breast milk at a 100,000-fold lower level.[2]

Late-onset CMPA presents as a variety of GI symptoms as follows:

Upper GI Symptoms
- Cricopharyngeal spasm
- GERD-like symptoms
- Allergic eosinophilic esophagitis (EOE)
- Pyloric stenosis.

According to the published studies, about 40% incidence of GERD has been observed in a large cohort suffering from late-onset CMPA, along with delay in gastric emptying due to dysrhythmia, especially in infants and children. *Pre-pyloric lobular mass* in a 7-week-old baby has been reported, which subsided once milk was excluded from the baby's diet.[15]

Allergic EOE is a condition in which eosinophils are found in the esophagus. Biopsy of esophagus revealing a count of >15 eosinophils at both ends of the esophagus at 40-fold magnification indicates allergic EOE (Fig. 42.1). Allergic EOE incidence has increased in recent years. It is characterized by abdominal and chest pain, dysphagia, and food impaction that cannot be reversed with anti-reflux treatment.

Lower GI Symptoms
- CMP-induced enterocolitis syndrome
- CMP-induced enteropathy or gastroenteritis
- Proctocolitis
- Constipation
- Perianal dermatitis
- Irritable bowel syndrome
- Food protein-induced enterocolitis syndrome (FPIES).

Poddar et al. studied GI pathology in children with suspected CMPA by sigmoidoscopy.[16] They observed that 82% children suffered from aphthous ulcers and 92% children were positive upon rectal biopsy. Exclusion of milk from the children's diet resulted in disappearance of the pathology and improvement in their health, confirming

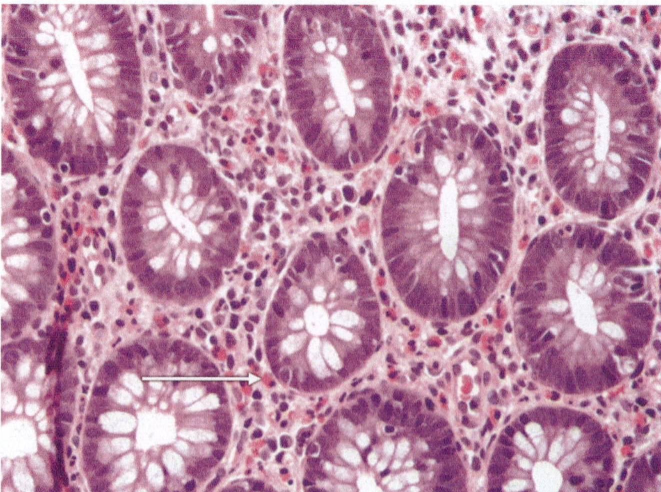

Fig. 42.1: Biopsy specimens of CMA showing >120 eosinophils/HPF in the lamina propria.

that they had suffered from CMPA. All children reacted positively to milk challenge within 6 months, clinching the author's finding that the GI pathology they observed was indeed due to CMPA.[16]

Enteropathy and *proctocolitis* due to CMPA are rare. Enteropathy causes vomiting, failure to thrive, and diarrhea. Sometimes, it is accompanied by blood in the feces and hypoproteinemia, which can be reversed by diet low in CMP allergen. According to a meta-analysis involving 314 patients, and literature from 1966 to 2013, allergic or eosinophilic proctocolitis occurs mainly in <6-month-old infants, mostly males, due to CMPA, with eosinophil infiltration of rectal mucosa.[17] Proctocolitis related to CMPA presents with *rectal bleeding*, accompanied by blood in stools, and a wide range of symptoms such as vomiting, diarrhea, and abdominal cramps. This condition can occur in breastfeeding infants and does not hamper the infants' health and growth. It is easily corrected by excluding cow's milk from the mother's diet. A Finnish study found that rectal bleeding in infants stopped upon elimination of cow's milk.[10] However, in this randomized study of 40 infants with rectal bleeding, where milk elimination was randomly assigned, only 18% patients turned out to suffer from CMPA.

Hence, the authors stress the use of the milk challenge test, while recommending a milk elimination test to prevent erroneous positive CMPA conclusion based merely on milk elimination. Most of the patients developed atopic eczema along with rectal bleeding; both symptoms subsided upon milk elimination and reappeared on milk challenge. Erythema of mucosal lining, eosinophil infiltration of lamina propria, and aphthous ulceration were seen by colonoscopy, indicating acute inflammation of the colon. All seven infants continued to suffer from CMPA at 1 year of age, when the study was stopped. Five of the seven children were also allergic to other foods (Fig. 42.2).[10]

Due to a variety of symptoms including bloody stools that are also caused by other disorders, CMPA can go undiagnosed. Apart from the classic tests such as milk challenge, gray-scale ultrasound and color Doppler imaging of the GI tract have been employed in a retrospective study of infants of 1–6 months with CMPA.[18] Twelve out of thirteen infants showed *thickening* (≥3 mm) and *enhanced vascularization* (five or more vessels in 2 cm^2 areas) of the GI wall, particularly in the colon. Reversals of these gut abnormalities were seen in repeat scan after 4 weeks on a cow's milk exclusion diet. Histopathology and colonoscopy correlated with the Doppler imaging; hence, this noninvasive technique holds promise for easier diagnosis of allergic colitis.[18]

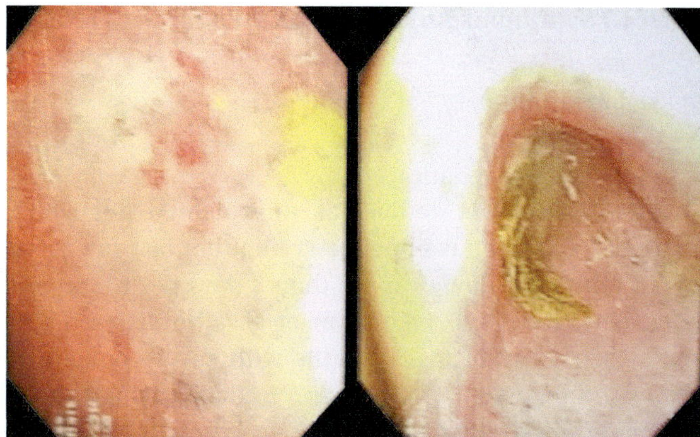

Fig. 42.2: Colonoscopy pictures of CMA showing aphthous ulcers with loss of vascularity.

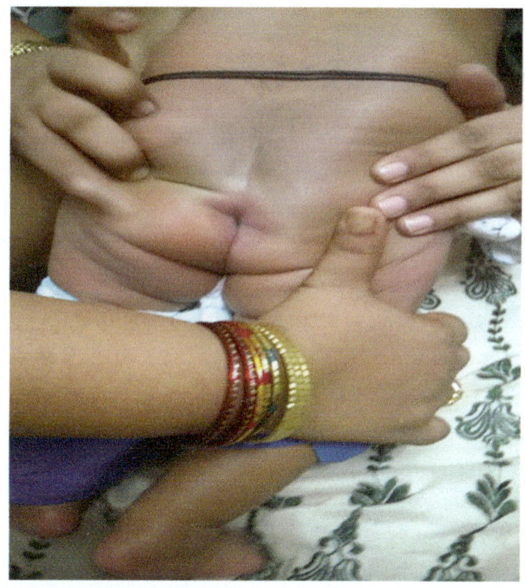

Fig. 42.3: Perianal excoriation due to CMPA.

Cow's milk-derived proteins are a major cause of inducing FPIES, which occurs within 1–3 hours after milk consumption. Usually, FPIES develops on first exposure to cow's milk and is characterized by symptoms of diarrhea, vomiting, and failure to thrive. In case of young infants, acute metabolic acidosis and perianal excoriation are also seen, which is confirmed by the presence of α-1-antitrypsin in the feces. Hypoproteinemia and anemia are often consequences of FPIES. Biopsy is characterized by massive influx of inflammatory cells in the lamina propria and enhanced infiltration of the crypts with eosinophils. Removal of milk from diet, along with introduction of hydrolyzed formulas, improves health in 80% of children with CMPA. Amino acid formulas (AAFs) are especially useful for treating stunted growth, with a 15–20% response (Fig. 42.3).[2]

Other GI Symptoms Attributed to CMPA

- Failure to thrive
- Malabsorption
- Infantile colic
- Frequent regurgitation.

Infantile colic is defined as unexplained persistent bouts of irritability, wailing, or crying that last for more than 3 hours per day, or more than 3 days per week and for at least 3 weeks.[2] Jakobsson et al. administered the hydrolyzed formula to 15 infants with severe colic and demonstrated a 60–70% reduction in daily crying time.[19] But caution should be exercised in generalizing these results to all infants with colic. Hydrolyzed formulas or a milk-free diet corrected this disorder according to some reports, indicating that infantile colic results from CMPA.[2,20,21]

Heiner's Syndrome

Infants/children with CMPA present a rare form of *pulmonary hemosiderosis* called Heiner's syndrome, characterized by repeat pulmonary infiltrates. Symptoms include tachypnea, chronic cough, rales, recurrent fever, wheezing, and failure to thrive. The patient sera contain antibodies that react with proteins from cow's milk. The disorder is corrected by excluding cow's milk from diet.

The CMPA can present with segmental enteritis,[22] segmental colitis,[23] recurrent necrotizing enterocolitis,[24] and Hirschsprung's disease-mimicking symptoms[25] in neonates.

Arunachalam and Mathai reported a neonate who presented with recurrent attacks of segmental enteritis due to CMPA and the last episode presented with signs of peritonitis. The child dramatically improved after elimination of cow's milk from his or her diet.[22]

Besides the more prominent symptoms, there are instances of recurrent abdominal pain and neurological syndromes such as Attention deficit hyperactivity disorder (ADHD) associated with CMPA reported in the literature.[2]

DIAGNOSIS

As already mentioned, late-onset CMPA often goes undiagnosed due to the similarity of symptoms induced by lactose intolerance.[1] Epidemiology of CMPA is not well studied in children and adults; therefore, accurate and systematic diagnostic methods have not been developed.

History

For the clinical assessment of CMPA, both *clinical symptoms* and *family history* are important.[5] The course of development of symptoms and tracking of the history of the condition are extremely important. Accurate information is needed on the introduction date of cow's milk into patient's diet, the duration of diet containing cow's milk, the amount of milk consumed, the frequency of its consumption, the method of milk preparation, and the sequence of events/symptoms observed upon milk consumption. An important indicator of CMPA is the resolution of the disorder after withdrawal of cow's milk from diet and resumption of the symptoms on reintroduction of cow's milk. Subjective analysis of symptoms using *milk symptom diaries* can aid the diagnosis.

Allergen Elimination Test

For diagnosing CMPA, cow's milk is eliminated from the patient's diet for a period and then reintroduced. If symptoms disappear on withdrawal and reappear on exposure to cow's milk, the test is positive. The allergen elimination and reintroduction test is particularly useful for late-onset CMPA as it is not IgE mediated.

Skin Prick Test

For IgE-mediated, early-onset, or immediate-onset CMPA, a useful confirmatory test is a simple skin prick with cow's milk, which results in induration around the prick area. If the induration is >7 mm, the likelihood of a positive milk elimination/challenge test is 90%.[26] In our clinic, we routinely perform the skin prick test when we suspect CMPA. First, a commercially available cow's milk formula is used. If the test is not conclusive, we repeat with fresh cow's milk, as the latter provokes a much stronger reaction with a more pronounced induration. The likelihood of a positive prick test correlating with a positive outcome for the milk challenge test is 58.8% with commercially available milk formula and is 91.7% with fresh milk.[27]

Immunologic Tests

High-specific serum IgE titers correlate with positive milk challenge tests.[26,28] Hence, detection of milk antigen-specific IgE is an important diagnostic measure. The radioallergosorbent test (RAST) was used to measure milk protein reactive antibodies in patient sera. In recent years, the ImmunoCAP assay has replaced RAST for IgE detection and quantification, which correlates well with the skin prick test.

The ImmunoCAP is a very popular and widely used immunologic test, as it has very high sensitivity (cutoff of 0.01 IU/l). Measurement of serum IgE levels is especially useful for diagnosis in very young infants, patients with atopic dermatitis, and patients suspected to suffer from IgE-mediated milk allergy.

Atopic Patch Test

This test is useful for detecting *non-IgE-mediated CMPA* leading to delayed hypersensitivity reaction. However, it is very difficult to do the atopic patch test in infants and young children, and nowadays, it is not generally practiced.

Milk Challenge Tests

As described earlier, the traditional allergen elimination/challenge test for CMPA consists of elimination of cow's milk from the patient's diet, provocation with the cow's milk, and re-elimination of cow's milk. Initially, when a patient presents with symptoms suspected to result from CMPA, It refers to symptoms will be mild or moderate. However, following the withdrawal of the allergen and the re-exposure to cow's milk, the patient often develops severe or anaphylaxis reaction, which could be life-threatening and need immediate medical attention.

We do the challenge tests only in the clinical setting with provision for efficient intervention and resuscitation. In case of patients with mild to moderate reactions to cow's milk, especially young children, an open milk challenge is often sufficient for accurate diagnosis. The American Academy of Allergy, Asthma and Immunology (AAAAI) has set guidelines for challenges tests.

Indications for Milk Challenge Tests (AAAAI):

- First diagnosis on initial suspicion of CMPA
- During follow-up of CMPA
- Estimation of tolerance to cow's milk
- Patients with atopic dermatitis or allergic EOE
- Patients with multiple food allergies.

Challenge tests should be avoided and postponed as much as possible in severe atopic patients, as life-threatening reactions are very common among these patients. Our practice of performing the milk challenge test involves gradually increasing the amount of cow's milk administered from a single drop to maximum uptake possible, along with monitoring any cutaneous or respiratory symptoms, and stopping the dosing at once when a reaction is seen. At the first drop of milk, if a patient presents with symptom (s), milk is not dispensed. The child/infant is kept under observation in clinic for 2 hours and under parental observation at home for 2 days. If any reaction is seen, the child/infant is fed a milk-free diet for 9–12 months, until the next challenge test to detect the immune allergic status. If no reaction occurs up to a week after the challenge, the child/infant is fed formula milk. *Dietary advice* is given to all patients irrespective of whether they develop an allergy. We perform open milk challenge test as well as single-blind challenge for CMPA on a routine basis in our clinic.

For ideal interpretation of the test, a double-blind, placebo-controlled provocation is required. A Double-blind, Placebo-controlled Food Challenge (DBPCFC) consists of gradual feeding of milk or placebo on different days during the provocation phase of the milk challenge. The placebo consists of an amino acid mixture with the taste of milk.[2] DBPCFC requires careful and lengthy preparation.

Indications for DBPCFC:[2]

- Delayed reactions with chronically developing symptoms
- Mandatory for subjective symptoms
- After an uncertain open milk challenge.

Allergen Microassays

For allergen detection, microassays are required to be well designed and carefully executed. The allergen microassays are used for testing their accuracy in comparison with oral milk challenge test in patients with suspected IgE-associated CMPA. These assays are not recommended as part of routine diagnostic methodology.

TREATMENT

The standard treatment of CMPA is the *elimination of cow's milk* and all related products such as formula food from the diet.[2] Breastfeeding is recommended and must be continued.[1,2] If the child is under 2 years of age, and breastfeeding is not possible, a substitute formula must be prescribed. If the child is older, no substitute milk formula is required.

The substitute formulas recommended for infants and children under 2 years of age suffering from CMPA are as follows:

- Partially hydrolyzed formula (pHF)
- Extensively hydrolyzed formula (eHF)
- Soy formula
- Soy hydrolyzed formula
- Rice hydrolyzed formula
- Amino acid formula
- Chicken- or lamb-based formulas.

Guidelines for management of CMPA recommend eHF rather than pHF so as to prevent ingestion of intact milk proteins as they may be allergenic.[1,2]

Use of eHF must be supplemented with calcium intake. eHF is recommended for infants under 6 months who present with symptoms of immediate CMPA, anaphylaxis, food protein-induced proctocolitis and enterocolitis, and atopic eczema. In India, formulas unrelated to milk, which provide essential proteins for growth such as *chicken-based formula*, are available. *Soy milk*-based formulas can be given to infants above 6 months, but those below will react to soy milk proteins in around 30% of the cases of CMPA,[29] and later develop soy allergy. AAFs are a safe option, and they are nonallergenic.[30] They are the treatment of choice for highly sensitized infants with CMPA that present with anaphylaxis and FPIES that present with failure to thrive and EOE. Soy milk-derived formulas can be used as a substitute for infants above 6 months who suffer from immediate nonanaphylactic CMPA, atopic eczema, and food protein-induced enterocolitis and proctocolitis, provided there is no failure to thrive.

Milk from other domestic animals such as goats, ewes, and buffalos can induce acute allergic reactions in CMPA patients as these milks contain proteins that cross-react with CMPs and cannot be used.[31] Unlike these milks, camel and equine milks do not contain a chief aggravating allergen β-lactoglobulin. Camel milk can be given to children above 2 years, whereas equine milk is used as a substitute for children suffering from delayed onset CMPA.[2,31]

Oral/Sublingual Immunotherapy

Immunotherapy is a controlled dosing of very low quantities of allergen, which is increased gradually and eventually leads to tolerance to a particular antigen. There are two possible immune states that can be achieved through milk allergen immunotherapy: desensitization and tolerance.[32] Immunotherapy is effective in alleviating symptomatology and distress in CMPA.

Keet et al. conducted a randomized clinical trial study in 30 children with CMPA.[33] After randomization, all subjects received sublingual immunotherapy (SLIT) for 4 weeks. They were then randomized equally into three groups: (1) continued SLIT escalation to 7 mg daily, (2) shifted with oral immunotherapy (OIT) to 1,000 mg (OITB), or (3) shifted with OIT to 2,000 mg (OITA). All children who underwent study were challenged with 8 g of milk protein after 12 and 60 weeks of therapy. If the 60-week challenge was passed by subjects, therapy was stopped and challenges were repeated after 1 week and 6 weeks to assess for tolerance. After therapy, one (10%) in the SLIT group, six (60%) in the SLIT/OITB group, and eight (80%) in the SLIT/OITA group passed the 8 g oral food challenge(OFC). However, all subjects completed maintenance therapy; the food challenge threshold was increased.[33]

In our clinic, currently 28 children with CMPA are undergoing OIT/SLIT and have completed 1 year with significant improvement. Allergic reactions and symptoms have abated.

Alternative therapies have been suggested for CMPA, but we do not recommend these, as reliable data on the risk/benefit ratio are not available, and effectivity remains unknown due to the absence of reported clinical trials carried out as per recommendations for proper randomization, double blinding, and placebo control. Scattered reports are favorable but without systematic trial data to rely on.

These therapies include the following:

a. Probiotics
b. Polyunsaturated fatty acids
c. Chinese herbal medicines.

PROGNOSIS

A 1994 Danish study found IgE specific for CMPs in most of the infants that developed CMPA, suggesting that sensitization to CMP could be at the fetal stage in the uterus.[3]

In most cases, children acquire tolerance to cow's milk by the age of 2, or latest by 4 years of age. The Danish study found that 50% of the babies suffering from CMPA in a birth cohort developed tolerance after 1 year.

Other studies found that 50–70% children became tolerant to cow's milk by age 2 years, while newer studies noted that 80–90% children gain tolerance by age 3–4 years.[3] However, persistent CMPA is noted in children who develop multiple allergic responses including respiratory symptoms with a high risk for prolonged disease. Multiple food allergies were reported in 50% children with CMPA, and inhalant allergies were reported in 50–80% children before puberty in the 1994 Danish study.[3] High anti-CMP IgE levels are found in serum of patients who develop persistent CMPA, suggesting that IgE levels predict the development of persistent CMPA.[3,4] Higher IL-10, BLG-IgG4, and the BLG-IgG4/IgE ratio were observed in CMPA patients during the tolerance phase compared to the symptomatic phase.[34]

A prospective Danish study is worth describing in some detail as it tracked 1,749 newborns, born in 1985 for CMPA/intolerance (CMPA/I) development until 2002.[35] Controlled milk elimination and challenge at fixed intervals was carried out until the children develop tolerance. The natural course of allergic symptomatology was analyzed along with serum IgE measurement and skin prick test. It was observed that 2.2% (39/117) infants remained allergic to cow's milk at 1 year of age. The prognosis of recovery from CMPA was 56% at 1 year and 97% at 15 years of age. Children with IgE-mediated CMPA were at high risk for developing persistent CMPA with multiple allergies to different allergens such as food and inhalants, which were associated with development of food allergies, asthma, and rhinoconjunctivitis. The rate of sensitization was as high as 39% in symptomatics, whereas it was up to 12% in asymptomatics, based on specific IgE. Asthmatics at age 10 had the highest rate of sensitization at 53%. In infants, the dominating symptoms were wheezing (20%), atopic dermatitis (14%), and food allergy (7%) at 1.5 years of age. Asthma and rhinoconjunctivitis increased up to 9% each at 10 years of age. The overall analysis of these data was that the incidence of any atopic disease at 1.5 years of age was 20%, decreasing at 5 years to 14% and rising at 10 years to 25% in children with CMPA.[35] CMPA is accompanied by the atopic march.[36]

Factors indicative of persistence of CMPA are as follows:
- Severe symptoms at diagnosis
- Respiratory symptoms
- Multiple food allergies
- Larger skin prick induration with fresh milk than processed/formula milk
- Initial higher milk-specific antibody titers.
- Sensitization to α-1-casein, β-casein, and κ-casein.

POINTS TO REMEMBER

- Non-IgE-associated CMPA occurs at higher incidence than IgE-mediated CMPA.
- Milk challenge tests are the gold standard for the diagnosis of CMPA.
- Fifty percent of children acquire tolerance to cow's milk by 2 years of age.
- eHFs are the treatment of choice as recommended by the guidelines on CMPA.
- Soy milk may not be used as a milk substitute in CMPA, as 30% of patients with CMA are allergic to soy milk too.

REFERENCES

1. Ewing WM, Allen PJ. The diagnosis and management of cow milk protein intolerance in the primary care setting. Pediatr Nurs. 2005;31:486-93.
2. Fiocchi A, Brozek J, Schünemann H, et al. World Allergy Organization (WAO) Diagnosis and Rationale for Action against Cow's Milk Allergy (DRACMA) Guidelines. Pediatr Allergy Immunol. 2010;21:1-125.
3. Høst A. Cow's milk protein allergy and intolerance in infancy. Some clinical, epidemiological and immunological aspects. Pediatr Allergy Immunol. 1994;5:5-36.
4. Høst A. Frequency of cow's milk allergy in childhood. Ann Allergy Immunol. 2002;89:33-7.
5. Vandenplas Y, Brueton M, Dupont C, et al. Guidelines for the diagnosis and management of cow's milk protein allergy in infants. Arch Dis Child. 2007;92:902-8.
6. Herbert B. Approach to milk protein allergy in infants. Can Fam Physician. 2008;54:1258-64.
7. Miyazawa T, Itahashi K, Imai T. Management of neonatal cow's milk allergy in high-risk neonates. Pediatr Int. 2009;51:544-7.
8. Vitaliti G, Cimino C, Coco A, et al. The immunopathogenesis of cow's milk protein allergy (CMPA). Ital J Pediatr. 2012;38:35.
9. Høst A, Jacobsen HP, Halken S, Holmenlund D. The natural history of cow's milk protein allergy/intolerance. Eur J Clin Nutr. 1995;49:S13-8.
10. Arvola T, Ruuska T, Kera J, et al. Rectal bleeding in infancy: clinical, allergological, and microbiological examination. Pediatrics. 2006;117:e760-8.
11. Morin S, Bernard H, Przybylski-Nicaise L, et al. Allergenic and immunogenic potential of cow's milk β-lactoglobulin and caseins evidenced without adjuvant in germ-free mice. Mol Nutr Food Res. 2011;55:1700-7.
12. Tsabouri S, Douros K, Priftis KN. Cow's milk allergenicity. Endocr Metab Immune Disord—Drug Targets. 2014;14:16-26.
13. Hill DJ, Firer MA, Shelton MJ, et al. Manifestations of milk allergy in infancy: clinical and immunologic findings. J Pediatr. 1986;109:270-6.
14. Iacono G, Di Prima L, D'Amico D, et al. The "red umbilicus": a diagnostic sign of cow's milk protein intolerance. J Pediatr Gastroenterol Nutr. 2006;42:531-4.
15. Morinvill V, Bernard C, Forget S. Foveolar hyperplasia secondary to cow's milk protein hypersensitivity presenting with clinical features of pyloric stenosis. J Pediatr Surg. 2004;39:E29-31.

16. Poddar U, Yachha SK, Krishnani N, Srivastava A. Cow's milk protein allergy: an entity for recognition in developing countries. J Gastroenterol Hepatol. 2010;25:178-82.
17. Lozinsky AC, Morais MB. Eosinophilic colitis in infants. J Pediatr (Rio J). 2013;90:16-21.
18. Epifanio M, Spolidoro JV, Missima NG, et al. Cow's milk allergy: color Doppler ultrasound findings in infants with hematochezia. J Pediatr (Rio J). 2013;89:554-8.
19. Jakobsson I, Lothe L, Ley D, Borschel MW. Effectiveness of casein hydrolysate feedings in infants with colic. Acta Paediatr. 2000;89:18-21.
20. Jakobsson I, Lindberg T. Cow's milk proteins cause infantile colic in breast-fed infants: a double-blind crossover study. Pediatrics. 1983;71:268-71.
21. Vandenplas Y, Salvatore S, Hauser B. Symptoms, diagnosis and management of colicky infants with regurgitations. Int Semin Paediatr Gastroenterol Nutr. 2002;11:1-7.
22. Arunachalam P, Mathai J. Neonatal segmental enteritis due to cow's milk allergy. J Indian Assoc Pediatr Surg. 2013;18:149-51.
23. Swischuk LE, Hayden CK Jr. Barium enema findings (? segmental colitis) in four neonates with bloody diarrhea—possible cow's milk allergy. Pediatr Radiol. 1985;15:34-7.
24. Srinivasan P, Brandler M, D'Souza A, et al. Allergic enterocolitis presenting as recurrent necrotizing enterocolitis in preterm neonates. J Perinatol. 2010;30:431-3.
25. Kawai M, Kubota A, Ida S, et al. Cow's milk allergy presenting Hirschsprung's disease-mimicking symptoms. Pediatr Surg Int. 2005;21:850-2.
26. Celik-Bilgili S, Mehl A, Verstege A, et al. The predictive value of specific immunoglobulin E levels in serum for the outcome of oral food challenges. Clin Exp Allergy. 2005;35:268-73.
27. Rance F, Juchet A, Bremont F, et al. Correlations between skin prick tests with commercial extracts and fresh foods, specific IgE and food challenges. Allergy. 1997;52:1031-5.
28. Vanto T, Juntunen-Backman K, Kalimo K, et al. The patch test, skin prick test, and serum milk-specific IgE as diagnostic tools in cows' milk allergy in infants. Allergy. 1999;54:837-2.
29. Klemola T, Vanto T, Juntunen-Backman K, et al. Allergy to soy formula and to extensively hydrolyzed whey formula in infants with cow's milk allergy: a prospective, randomized study with a follow-up to the age of 2 years. J Pediatr. 2002;140:219-24.
30. Sicherer SH, Noone SA, Koerner CB, et al. Hypoallergenicity and efficacy of an amino acid-based formula in children with cow's milk and multiple food hypersensitivities. J Pediatr. 2001;138:688-93.
31. Restani P, Gaiaschi A, Plebani A, et al. Cross-reactivity between milk proteins from different animal species. Clin Exp Allergy. 1999;29:997-1004.
32. Le UH, Burks AW. Oral and sublingual immunotherapy for food allergy. World Allergy Organ J. 2014;7:35.
33. Keet CA, Frischmeyer-Guerrerio PA, Thyagarajan A, et al. The safety and efficacy of sublingual and oral immunotherapy for milk allergy. J Allergy Clin Immunol. 2012;129:448-55.
34. Sommanus S, Kerddonfak S, Kamchaisatian W, et al. Cow's milk protein allergy: immunological response in children with cow's milk protein tolerance. Asian Pac J Allergy Immunol. 2014;32:171-7.
35. Høst A, Halken S, Jacobsen HP, et al. Clinical course of cow's milk protein allergy/intolerance and atopic diseases in childhood. Pediatr Allergy Immunol. 2002;13:23-8.
36. Høst A, Husby S, Hansen LG, et al. Bovine β-lactoglobulin in human milk from atopic and non-atopic mothers. Relationship to maternal intake of homogenized and unhomogenized milk. Clin Exp Allergy. 1990;20:383-7.

CHAPTER 43

Pregnancy and Allergy

Kiran Vishnu Narayan

INTRODUCTION

Allergic diseases can affect pregnancy by altering its smooth course, and pregnancy in turn can affect the natural course of allergic disorders. Though allergic rhinitis and asthma are common during pregnancy, they need to be managed optimally for ensuring the welfare of the mother and the baby. Commonly used diagnostic tests like skin prick test and provocation tests should be avoided during pregnancy. The principles of managing allergic diseases are followed similarly in pregnancy, except that immunotherapy should not be initiated when pregnant. A number of drugs that can be safely used for the management of allergy in normal conditions may have to be handpicked considering their risk–benefit ratio in pregnancy. In this chapter, we shall review the allergic diseases in pregnancy and discuss the management issues.

EPIDEMIOLOGY AND DIAGNOSIS

In general, around 20% of pregnancies are affected by allergies.[1,2] There is lack of data on the prevalence of allergic diseases from India. So, a comparison of global prevalence data is not possible. The most common allergic diseases include allergic rhinitis, rhinoconjunctivitis, asthma, urticaria, food allergy, and angioedema. A detailed medical history and knowing the differential diagnoses would help in treatment. Avoidance of the suspected allergens with the improvement of symptoms helps in pointing out the possible allergen. In suspected food allergy, a food diary would be extremely rewarding. Serological diagnostic tests should be preferred over skin prick tests, intradermal test, and food challenge tests as there is a minute but definite risk of anaphylaxis development, and these tests affect immunological responses related to pregnancy. Anaphylaxis during pregnancy may be detrimental for both the mother and the fetus.[3]

CLINICAL SITUATIONS

Rhinitis in Pregnancy

Commonly seen entities include pregnancy rhinitis, allergic rhinitis, rhinosinusitis, and drug-induced rhinitis.

Pregnancy Rhinitis

Nasal symptoms are common in pregnancy and are believed to be mainly due to the influence of hormones like placental growth hormone and estrogen. It is reported in 18–42% of pregnancies.[4] They produce both direct and indirect effects on the vascularity and mucus secretion of glands. There are significant physiological changes seen during pregnancy in the upper airway. Mucosal changes like hyperemia, edema, plasma leakage into the stroma, gland hyperactivity, and increased mucopolysaccharide deposition are seen. Nasal congestion occurs in the early first trimester, peaks late in pregnancy, and disappears within 8 hours of delivery.[5,6]

Rhinitis of pregnancy is defined as the nasal congestion present during the last 6 or more weeks of pregnancy, not due to an upper respiratory infection or allergic cause and disappearing completely within 2 weeks of delivery.[5] Complaints are persistent nasal congestion and watery discharge. As implied in the definition, nonhormonal factors responsible for rhinitis such as smoking, allergy, infections, and drug-induced causes should be excluded.

Management

Since it is a physiological condition, it does not require therapy usually. In patients with significant symptoms, nonpharmacological measures are advised. These include avoidance of allergens, irritants, and nasal lavages with saline. They poorly respond to pharmacological measures and can be tried. Intranasal steroids that are effective in nonpregnant individuals are not beneficial. The safe steroid in pregnancy is budesonide, which is not available in nasal spray preparations in India. Anticholinergics and nasal decongestants may also be tried. Decongestants, if used, should be given only for a short duration of 3 days or less as further use may result in drug-induced worsening or rhinitis medicamentosa.

Course

Rhinitis of pregnancy does not directly affect the outcome of pregnancy but can contribute to complications. The nasal congestion and resultant nasal obstruction causes the patient to have snoring and mouth breathing. The maxillary sinuses are a rich source of nitric oxide, which is a potent pulmonary arterial vasodilator, and the reduced concentrations may result in snoring-related complications including sleep-disordered breathing.[7] In addition, the neck circumference and Mallampati score also increase in pregnancy, which may also contribute to snoring and sleep-disordered breathing.[8] The above factors in combination may increase the risk of gestational hypertension, preeclampsia, and intrauterine growth retardation, although this association has not been confirmed.[9,10] They may also aggravate coexisting asthma or predispose to bacterial rhinosinusitis due to stasis.

Allergic Rhinitis and Rhinoconjunctivitis

They usually present before pregnancy or may manifest for the first time during pregnancy. The clinical manifestations are the same as in nonpregnant patients. Pre-existing rhinitis, as in asthma, may worsen, improve, or remain as such during pregnancy.[11] Common features include sneezing, rhinorrhea, watering of eyes, and nasoocular irritation. The triggering agents include house dust, dust mite, pollen, dander, and molds. Diagnosis can be made from the typical clinical picture especially in atopics or with a positive family history. The intracutaneous skin prick test can be used to diagnose specific allergens but extreme caution must be taken as some patients are sensitive even to the minute concentration of the antigen. So it is preferred to do in vitro tests like allergen-specific IgE or RAST (radioallergosorbent test).

Management of Allergic Rhinitis during Pregnancy: General Principles

Identifying and avoiding the allergy source is the best management for allergic diseases in pregnancy. Often the antigen is not identifiable or there are multiple allergens that are difficult to avoid. Avoiding triggers like dander, house dust, tobacco smoke, and irritating pollutants must also be done. Sleeping with the head end elevated may also give relief of nasal symptoms and in addition improve the functional residual capacity in pregnancy when compared to supine.[12,13]

In addition, irrigating the nasal cavities with saline helps in improving symptoms in allergic rhinitis.[14] The saline solution can be brought commercially or prepared at home by using pickling salt without preservatives, baking soda, and boiled and cooled water/distilled water. A mixture of three teaspoons of salt with one teaspoon of baking soda is put in a clean dry airtight container. Add one teaspoon of this mixture to around 240 mL of clean water. Tap water may be irritating to the nasal cavities, may contain environmental mycobacteria and parasites like *Naegleria fowleri*. The saline along with baking soda is used to neutralize the pH. The dilution may be increased if the mixture causes stinging. An initial burning sensation is anticipated, but it decreases over time with continuous use. A commercial nasal bulb or a pediatric dropper can be used to instill the saline into the upper nostril with head down and tilted to a side. This causes the saline to wash out through the other nostril. The plunger is directed toward the occiput rather than toward the frontal sinus. Breathing is done normally through the mouth. The saline rinsing should not be done if there is evidence of purulent nasal discharge or if there is severe nasal block. With no side effects of the drug, they pose minimal risk if properly performed. Caution should be taken to avoid contamination of the water used and the device used for instillation. Application can be done daily or intermittently whenever symptomatic. A randomized trial in pregnant women showed saline irrigation to be beneficial in allergic rhinitis.[15,16] Regular physical exercise leads to nasal vasoconstriction and in addition, nasal breathing exercises like yogic *pranayama* will also help.[17]

Drugs should generally be avoided in the first trimester but the risks of poor disease control and harm to the mother and fetus must also be thought of. Oral steroids can be used for short duration, but there exists a risk of cleft palate, pre-eclampsia, gestational diabetes, low birth weight, and preterm delivery.[18] Though there have been numerous case control studies on the side effects of steroids on cleft lip, most of these studies did not mention how long it was used or the exact dose used.[19-21] No statistically significant increased risk of steroids on the oral cleft lip or the palate was observed in a large nationwide cohort study on 832,636 live births in Denmark during a 12-year study period.[22] There are also no Cochrane meta-analyses available on this topic. So, oral steroids with their remarkable anti-inflammatory action can be used considering the risk-benefit ratio with the lowest dose needed and for the shortest duration possible. Intranasal steroids are applied topically for allergic rhinitis and no differences in safety or efficacy exist between the different agents available.

Other Drugs

Antihistaminics

In allergic diseases, the oral agents commonly prescribed include the first- and the second-generation antihistaminics. Fortunately, safety data available for these agents are reassuring.[23,24] The first-generation drugs like chlorpheniramine and diphenhydramine are considered safe during the first trimester. Chlorpheniramine is dosed at 4 mg every 4–6 hours. The maximum dosing per day should not cross 24 mg. Hydroxyzine should be used cautiously in the first trimester because of conflicting animal data reports. The second-generation agents like loratadine and cetirizine are preferred because they are less sedating and have lesser cholinergic side effects. Cetirizine at a dosage of 10 mg once daily and loratadine at a dosage of 10 mg once daily are safe in pregnancy.[25-27] Other second-generation antihistamines commonly used like levocetirizine, though categorized as group B, has not been extensively studied in humans. Fexofenadine is a group C drug and is better avoided during pregnancy. Inhaled antihistaminics are better avoided as human studies are not available regarding these drugs.

Decongestants

These drugs are widely used as over-the-counter medications. They cause vasoconstriction of the nasal mucosa and are useful in nasal congestion and stuffiness as well as rhinorrhea. All these can be controlled with inhaled steroids, which are considered safer. Available as oral as well as nasal preparations, they should be used with caution in both the pregnant and the nonpregnant population. The commonly available preparations are phenylephrine and pseudoephedrine.

Phenylephrine available at dosages of 10–40 mg in commercial preparations does not produce nasal vasoconstriction as pseudoephedrine in equivalent dosages. In addition, phenylephrine has caused eye and ear malformations and clubfoot. Pseudoephedrine has been associated with hemifacial microsomia, gastroschisis, limb reduction defects, and small intestinal atresia.[28] These drugs are to be avoided in the first trimester until definite safety data are available. Pseudoephedrine can be used in the second and third trimesters in women without hypertension. It is usually available in combination with antihistaminics at a dosage of 60–120 mg. In the second and third trimesters, these drugs are the choice if there is no hypertension. A Swedish study prospectively examined the pregnancy outcomes of 2,474 women who had reported use of oral decongestants in early pregnancy and 1,774 women who used these medications in later pregnancy. No teratogenic effects were detected in either group.[29] If oral decongestants are to be used, avoid phenylephrine because of uncertain efficacy and questionable safety. They also have a strong alpha-adrenergic action and hence will cause uteroplacental insufficiency because the uterine blood vessels selectively exhibit alpha-adrenergic receptors.[30,31]

Intranasal decongestants can be used for brief periods (a maximum of 3 days) for an immediate temporary relief of refractory nasal congestion. The data on intranasal decongestants are again conflicting with some human studies showing no teratogenicity and one study showing malformations.[28,32] In addition, patients have to be warned of not prolonging the use for more than the prescribed duration because of the risk of rhinitis medicamentosa.

Drug-induced Rhinitis: "Rhinitis Medicamentosa"

Decongestant nasal sprays are available as over-the-counter medicines. When these nasal sprays especially oxymetazoline are stopped after a prolonged application period, rebound nasal congestion occurs. The patient takes a higher dosage to get relief and after the medicine effect wanes, congestion reappears. This causes a cycle of congestion and increasing medication dosage to get relief. It usually occurs in patients with chronic rhinosinusitis, where they try every available medicine to get relief. This can be prevented by limiting the decongestant nasal sprays to less than 3 days. Treatment involves stopping the decongestants and simultaneously treating with intranasal steroids.

Immunotherapy

It should not be started during pregnancy as it may produce a systemic reaction and anaphylaxis.[33] If the patient was already on immunotherapy, it may be continued safely without increasing the dosage. Continuing immunotherapy at the same dose or at a lower dosage has shown to improve symptoms in the mother and reduce allergic sensitization in the child.[34] At any time during the treatment, if a patient develops a systemic reaction it is strongly advisable to stop the immunotherapy. These principles are the same for all forms of immunotherapy including sublingual. The above principles are based on two studies in 171 women receiving immunotherapy. The studies did not show an increase in toxemia, abortions, congenital malformations, perinatal deaths, or prematurity in the treatment groups compared to a control pregnant allergic group who were not given immunotherapy or to the general population.[35,36]

If the patient was on the build-up phase or had just recently started immunotherapy, it is advisable to stop the treatment if she becomes pregnant. This is because the benefits of immunotherapy take time to develop and it has no therapeutic efficacy.[37] But a prospective study from India by Shaikh et al. has shown that sublingual immunotherapy is safe in pregnancy even when it is initiated during pregnancy. This was based on his study on 155 pregnant patients who were on sublingual immunotherapy with either house dust mites or a mixture of five allergens. Twenty-four patients were initiated on sublingual immunotherapy while being pregnant. All patients including controls were given allergen avoidance measures. When compared to controls and the general population, the immunotherapy patients had lesser complications on follow-ups.[38]

Uncontrolled rhinitis may also aggravate the asthma and also predispose to sinusitis as mentioned earlier. Studies have shown that there is a relation between course and symptoms of rhinitis and asthma in pregnancy. A study done on 568 pregnant women by Kircher et al. showed that in those women whose asthma was controlled, rhinitis symptoms also improved. This also suggests and reiterates that rhinitis managed optimally during pregnancy improves the coexisting asthma also.[39]

Laryngopathia Gravidarum

This is an extremely rare disease usually occurring in multigravidae. It is a noninfectious laryngitis, which mimics laryngeal angioedema. It is believed to be due to the effect of hormones on the laryngeal mucosa because it disappears after delivery. There are two types, an acute variety occurring just before parturition and a chronic one occurring in early pregnancy. Clinical features include hoarseness of voice, odynophagia, progressive shortness of breath, cough, and cervical lymphadenopathy. Management includes maintaining a patent airway and sometimes requires artificial airways. The disease is self-limiting and both acute and chronic forms spontaneously improve after delivery.

Allergic Skin Disease

Anaphylaxis

Anaphylaxis is a life-threatening condition that must always be considered in undiagnosed hypotension. Anticipate anaphylaxis especially in patients with pre-existing severe allergic reactions to food and drugs. The fetus is protected from anaphylaxis because the placenta does not allow transmission of allergen-specific IgE. But hypotension and hypoxia developing with maternal anaphylaxis may be detrimental to the fetus. The management of anaphylaxis is essentially the same as in nonpregnant females. The primary step is to avoid pre-existing known allergens. If anaphylaxis occurs, immediate attention to maintaining an adequate circulation using isotonic fluids, maintaining an adequate airway, and oxygenation (SpO_2 above 95%) are mandatory. Positioning the patient in the left-lateral position with elevation of lower limbs will relieve the abdominal pressure of the uterus on the inferior vena cava and improve venous return. The drug of choice is adrenaline injection; 0.3–0.5 mL of 1:1,000 solution is injected intramuscularly into the anterolateral aspect of the thigh. Sometimes even intravenous injection may be needed in spite of reducing uteroplacental flow.[3]

Urticaria

Urticaria occurring for the first time in pregnancy is rare, but it tends to recur in subsequent pregnancies. It is believed to be due to an allergic sensitization to endogenous hormones. The pattern, appearance, and management are the same as in the general population.[40] A special type of urticaria is seen in pregnant ladies called pregnancy urticaria or pruritic urticarial papules and plaques of pregnancy (PUPPP). It is now known as polymorphic eruptions of pregnancy (PEP). This form is seen usually in primi mothers during the last trimester and is discussed later.

Atopic Eruption of Pregnancy

This is the most common pregnancy dermatoses, occurring in more than 50% of the patients. This is an eczematous or papular eruption occurring in early pregnancy in patients with an atopic background. They also tend to recur in subsequent pregnancies. Atopic eruption of pregnancy (AEP) is a conglomeration of conditions that include eczema, prurigo, and pruritic folliculitis of pregnancy. All these have shared clinical features and occur in patients with a personal or a family history of atopy. Most of these patients will also have a history of atopic dermatitis during infancy and childhood. It is believed to be due to an immunological shift with pregnancy-related enhancement of Th2 cytokines and suppression of Th1 cytokines.[41]

Eczema: It usually is a primary manifestation of atopic skin disease or in a minority maybe due to exacerbation of a previously controlled atopic dermatitis. Commonly involving the face, neck, and flexural areas as in classical atopic dermatitis, they are intensely itchy patches or papules.

Prurigo of pregnancy: These are red excoriated papules or nodules on the extensor surface of limbs and trunks.

Pruritic folliculitis of pregnancy: It looks like steroid-induced acne and contrary to its name is only mildly pruritic. A follicular papulopustular eruption, it initially appears on the abdomen and then it spreads throughout the body.

Differential Diagnosis of Eruptions

Other pregnancy-induced skin lesions that mimic AEP include allergic contact dermatitis, Pityriasis rosea, drug eruptions, PEP, and intrahepatic cholestasis.[42]

Polymorphic eruptions in pregnancy were previously known as PUPPP. They present with extremely pruritic red papules (unlike pruritic folliculitis of pregnancy) within the abdominal striae and then proceed to the extremities, chest, and back. It may sometimes be localized only to the abdominal striae and spare the periumbilical area. The face, palms, and soles are characteristically spared. Benign and self-limiting, they are usually seen in primiparous women and start in the last trimester or immediately after delivery. Treatment is with low to moderate potency topical steroids and oral antihistaminics. Caution is advised with high-potency steroids because of the risk of low birth weight.

Intrahepatic cholestasis of pregnancy presents only with excoriation marks and no typical skin lesions. It characteristically presents with severe pruritus mainly in the palms and soles and is due to elevated bile acids. It is associated with an increased incidence of stillbirths, preterm labor, intrauterine death, and neonatal fetal distress. So identifying this condition in pregnant patients with severe pruritus is important.[43]

Management of AEP

If the atopic eruptions are present before pregnancy, they should be well controlled before conception so that minimal medicines can be used. A preconception planning and spacing after stopping drugs is needed if the women are already on methotrexate or PUVA therapy.

Postpartum AEP-management is essentially the same like nonpregnant females. Avoiding triggers, adequate hydration, and emollients are to be used. Oral antihistaminics can control itching. Low to moderate potency topical steroids like 0.5–2.5% hydrocortisone are safe during pregnancy.[44,45] It is better to avoid topical tacrolimus as data on these agents are minimal.

DRUG SAFETY IN PREGNANCY

In pregnancy, drugs have to be prescribed considering the risk–benefit principle, i.e., risk of poor control of disease and progression balanced against the side effect and teratogenicity of the drug. Fortunately, only a few drugs have been documented to be harmful in humans.[46] Considering ethical issues, it is impossible to start any new drug in pregnancy and do a randomized study. Drugs used in pregnancy are divided into five groups (A, B, C, D, X), which are based on studies conducted in animals, humans, and on the risk–benefit ratio of drugs (Table 43.1).

The FDA modified the old classification of drugs (1979) used in pregnancy in 2015. It has been described as the *Pregnancy and Lactation Labelling Final Rule (PLLR)* and is based on information from studies on animal and humans of known drug side effects and dosage adjustments during pregnancy and postpartum. The complete list is not yet published. So till it is made available, the drugs should be prescribed as per the old classification.[47] As per the 1979 classification, none of the currently available allergy drugs belong to Category A.[48] Most of the drugs belong to either B or C. If drug prescription is required, it would be ethical to choose a Category B drug over C, if equally effective options are present. The safe B drugs in pregnancy would include cetirizine, levocetirizine, loratadine, chlorpheniramine, inhaled budesonide, and omalizumab. Whenever possible, it is preferable to give topical preparations like inhaled medicines in favor of systemic drugs to increase drug concentration at the site of action and thereby reducing systemic side effects.

Table 43.1: FDA-1979 safety classification of drugs in pregnancy.[49]

Category	*Description*
A	Adequate and well-controlled studies have failed to demonstrate a risk to the fetus in the first trimester of pregnancy (and there is no evidence of risk in later trimesters).
B	Animal reproduction studies have failed to demonstrate a risk to the fetus, and there are no adequate and well-controlled studies in pregnant women.
C	Animal reproduction studies have shown an adverse effect on the fetus and there are no adequate and well-controlled studies in humans, but potential benefits may warrant use of the drug in pregnant women despite potential risks.
D	There is positive evidence of human fetal risk based on adverse reaction data from investigational or marketing experience or studies in humans, but potential benefits may warrant use of the drug in pregnant women despite potential risks.
X (teratogenic)	Studies in animals or humans have demonstrated fetal abnormalities, and/or there is positive evidence of human fetal risk based on adverse reaction data from investigational or marketing experience, and the risks involved in use of the drug in pregnant women clearly outweigh potential benefits.

CONCLUSION

Allergic diseases are seen in about 20% of pregnancies and can be pre-existing, aggravated during pregnancy or developing first during pregnancy. Special precautions must be taken by the pregnant mother to avoid smoking and alcoholism because smoke exposure in utero increases the risk of developing childhood rhinitis, asthma, and eczema.[50] Alcohol consumption has shown to increase the serum IgE levels in cord blood and predispose to childhood atopic dermatitis.[50,51] In addition, observational studies have shown that high intake of oily fish rich in ω-3 PUFA during pregnancy is beneficial in reducing the incidence of childhood allergy.[52] Avoiding foods that have a tendency to produce allergy has not shown to reduce the risk of sensitization in the child. Nutritious foods like milk, eggs, and nuts should be continued to avoid malnourishment of the mother and baby.[1,53] The allergic conditions include allergic rhinitis, rhinoconjunctivitis, asthma, urticaria, food allergy, and angioedema. Avoidance of allergens and antihistaminics safe in pregnancy should control allergic rhinitis and dermatitis. In patients who are already on immunotherapy, it would be advisable to continue the same if there was definite improvement. Current consensus is to avoid initiating immunotherapy during pregnancy but some Indian studies are encouraging. This article gives an overview about the common allergic conditions expected during gestation and their management.

REFERENCES

1. Pali-Schöll I, Namazy J, Jensen-Jarolim E. Allergic diseases and asthma in pregnancy. World Allergy Organization, Allergic Diseases Resource Center, Updated 2016. http://www.worldallergy.org/professional/allergic_diseases_center/allergy_in_pregnancy/. Accessed November 30, 2017.
2. Bousquet J, Schunemann HJ, Samolinski B, et al. Allergic rhinitis and its impact on asthma (ARIA): achievements in 10 years and future needs. J Allergy Clin Immunol. 2012;130:1049-62.
3. Simons FE, Schatz M. Anaphylaxis during pregnancy. J Allergy Clin Immunol. 2012;130:597-606.
4. Bende M, Gredmark T. Nasal stuffiness during pregnancy. Laryngoscope. 1999;109:1108-10.
5. Ellegård EK. Pregnancy rhinitis. Immunol Allergy Clin North Am. 2006;26:119.
6. Toppozada H, Michaels L, Toppozada M, et al. The human respiratory nasal mucosa in pregnancy. An electron microscopic and histochemical study. J Laryngol Otol. 1982;96:613-26.
7. Lundberg JO, Weitzberg E. Nasal nitric oxide in man. Thorax. 1999;54:947-52.
8. Izci B, Vennelle M, Liston WA. Sleep disordered breathing and upper airway size in pregnancy and postpartum. Eur Respir J. 2006;27:321-7.
9. Franklin KA, Holmgren PA, Jönsson F, et al. Snoring, pregnancy-induced hypertension, and growth retardation of the fetus. Chest. 2000;117:137-41.
10. Ayrım A, Keskin EA, Ozol D, et al. Influence of self-reported snoring and witnessed sleep apnea on gestational hypertension and fetal outcome in pregnancy. Arch Gynecol Obstet. 2011;283:195-9.
11. Schatz M, Zeiger RS. Diagnosis and management of rhinitis during pregnancy. Allergy Proc. 1988;9:545-54.

12. Stroud RH, Wright ST, Calhoun KH. Nocturnal nasal congestion and nasal resistance. Laryngoscope. 1999; 109:1450-3.
13. Norregaard O, Schultz P, Ostergaard A. Lung function and postural changes during pregnancy. Respir Med. 1989;83:467-70.
14. Tomooka LT, Murphy C, Davidson TM. Clinical study and literature review of nasal irrigation. Laryngoscope. 2000;110:1189-93.
15. Rabago D, Zgierska A. Saline nasal irrigation for upper respiratory conditions. Am Fam Physician. 2009;80:1117-9.
16. Garavello W, Somigliana E, Acaia B, et al. Nasal lavage in pregnant women with seasonal allergic rhinitis: a randomized study. Int Arch Allergy Immunol. 2010; 151:37.
17. Schatz M, Zeiger RS, Falkoff R, et al. Asthma and allergic diseases during pregnancy. In: Adkinson NF, Bochner BS, Burks AW, et al. eds. Middleton's Allergy: Principles and Practice, 7th ed. Mosby, St. Louis; 2014:951.
18. Carmichael SL, Shaw GM, Ma C, et al. Maternal corticosteroid use and orofacial clefts. Am J Obstet Gynecol. 2007;197:585-7.
19. Czeizel AE, Rockenbauer M. Population-based case-control study of teratogenic potential of corticosteroids. Teratology. 1997;56:335-40.
20. Pradat P, Robert-Gnansia E, Di Tanna GL, et al. First trimester exposure to corticosteroids and oral clefts. Birth Defects Res sA Clin Mol Teratol. 2003;67:968-70.
21. Rodríguez-Pinilla E, Martinez-Frias ML. Corticosteroids during pregnancy and oral clefts: a case-control study. Teratology. 1998;58:2-5.
22. Hviid A, Molgaard-Nielsen D. Corticosteroid use during pregnancy and risk of orofacial clefts. CMAJ. 2011;183: 796-804.
23. Schatz M, Petitti D. Antihistamines and pregnancy. Ann Allergy Asthma Immunol. 1997;78:157.
24. Gilbert C, Mazzotta P, Loebstein R, Koren G. Fetal safety of drugs used in the treatment of allergic rhinitis: a critical review. Drug Saf. 2005;28:707.
25. Diav-Citrin O, Shechtman S, Aharonovich A, et al. Pregnancy outcome after gestational exposure to loratadine or antihistamines: a prospective controlled cohort study. J Allergy Clin Immunol. 2003;111:1239.
26. Moretti ME, Caprara D, Coutinho CJ, et al. Fetal safety of loratadine use in the first trimester of pregnancy: a multicenter study. J Allergy Clin Immunol. 2003;111:479.
27. Källén B. Use of antihistamine drugs in early pregnancy and delivery outcome. J Matern Fetal Neonatal Med. 2002;11:146.
28. Yau WP, Mitchell AA, Lin KJ, et al. Use of decongestants during pregnancy and the risk of birth defects. Am J Epidemiol. 2013;178:198.
29. Källén BA, Olausson PO. Use of oral decongestants during pregnancy and delivery outcome. Am J Obstet Gynecol. 2006;194:480.
30. Smith NT, Corbascio AN. The use and misuse of pressor agents. Anesthesiology. 1970;33:58.
31. Rayburn WF, Anderson JC, Smith CV, et al. Uterine and fetal Doppler flow changes from a single dose of a long-acting intranasal decongestant. Obstet Gynecol. 1990;76:180.
32. Heinonen OP, Slone D, Shapiro S. Birth Defects and Drugs in Pregnancy, PSG Publishing, Littleton, MA, 1977.
33. Oykhman P, Kim HL, Ellis AK. Allergen immunotherapy in pregnancy. Allergy Asthma Clin Immunol. 2015;11:31.
34. Lieberman J. Should we encourage allergen immunotherapy during pregnancy? Exp Rev Clin Immunol. 2014;10: 317-9.
35. Shaikh WA. A retrospective study on the safety of immunotherapy in pregnancy. Clin Exp Allergy. 1993;23:857.
36. Metzger WJ, Turner E, Patterson R. The safety of immunotherapy during pregnancy. J Allergy Clin Immunol. 1978;61:268.
37. Cox L, Nelson H, Lockey R, et al. Allergen immunotherapy: a practice parameter third update. J Allergy Clin Immunol. 2011;127:S1-55.
38. Shaikh WA, Shaikh SW. A prospective study on the safety of sublingual immunotherapy in pregnancy. Allergy. 2012;67:741-3.
39. Kircher S, Schatz M, Long L. Variables affecting asthma course during pregnancy. Ann Allergy Asthma Immunol. 2002;89;463-6.
40. Champion RH, Roberts SO, Carpenter RG, Roger JH. Urticaria and angio-oedema. A review of 554 patients. Br J Dermatol. 1969;81:588.
41. Ambros-Rudolph CM, Müllegger RR, Vaughan-Jones SA, et al. The specific dermatoses of pregnancy revisited and reclassified: results of a retrospective two-center study on 505 pregnant patients. J Am Acad Dermatol. 2006;54:395-404.
42. Ambros-Rudolph CM. Disorders of pregnancy. In: Burgdorf WHC, Plewig G, Wolff HH, Landthaler M, eds. Braun-Falco's Dermatology. 3rd ed. Heidelberg: Springer Medizin Verlag; 2009:1160-9.
43. Hillman SC, Stokes-Lampard H, Kilby MD, Intrahepatic cholestasis of pregnancy. BMJ. 2016;353:i1236.
44. Chi CC, Kirtschig G, Aberer W, et al. Evidence-based (S3) guideline on topical corticosteroids in pregnancy. Br J Dermatol. 2011;165:943-52.
45. Chi CC, Wang SH, Kirtschig G. Safety of topical corticosteroids in pregnancy. JAMA Dermatol. 2016;152:934-5.
46. Scialli A, Lone A. Pregnancy effects of specific medications used to treat asthma and immunological diseases. In: Schatz M, Zeiger RS, Claman HN, eds. Asthma and Immunological Diseases in Pregnancy and Early Infancy. New York, NY: Marcel Dekker; 1998.
47. Dinatale M, Sahin L, Johnson T, et al. Medication use during pregnancy and lactation: introducing the pregnancy and lactation rule. Pediatr Allergy, Immunol Pulmonol. 2017;30:132-4.
48. Food and Drug Administration. Content and format of labeling for human prescription drug and biological products: requirements for pregnancy and lactation labeling. Fed Regist. 2014;79:72064-72103. Available at: www.gpo.gov/fdsys/pkg/FR-2014-12-04/pdf/2014-28241.pdf.

49. Noakes PS, Holt PG, Prescott SL. Maternal smoking in pregnancy alters neonatal cytokine responses. Allergy. 2003;58:1053-8.
50. Gonzalez-Quintela A, Vidal C, Gude F. Alcohol-induced alterations in serum immunoglobulin E (IgE) levels in human subjects. Front Biosci. 2002;7:e234-44.
51. Carson CG. Risk factors for developing atopic dermatitis. Dan Med J. 2013;60:B4687.
52. Kremmyda LS, Vlachava M, Noakes PS, et al. Atopy risk in infants and children in relation to early exposure to fish, oily fish, or long-chain omega-3 fatty acids: a systematic review. Clin Rev Allergy Immunol. 2011;41: 36-66.
53. Kramer MS, Kakuma R. Maternal dietary antigen avoidance during pregnancy or lactation, or both, for preventing or treating atopic disease in the child. Evidence-based Child Health. 2014;9:447-83.

CHAPTER 44

Allergy March

PA Mahesh, Amrutha D Holla

INTRODUCTION

There is an increase in the prevalence of atopic and allergic diseases throughout the world, especially in the developed countries, where on average approximately 20% of the general population suffer from one or the other allergic manifestations.[1] It was observed that many children suffered from skin allergies [atopic dermatitis (AD)] initially and then progressed to develop allergic rhinitis (AR) and asthma. In many such cases with asthma, AR preceded asthma. This concept to describe the progression was coined as 'atopic march'.[1,2] Atopy is defined as the propensity of an individual to develop IgE antibodies (sensitization) to various environmental triggers and is key for the development of dermatitis, rhinitis, and asthma.[3] There is a large body of evidence supporting the concept of atopic march including both mouse models and human cross-sectional and longitudinal studies.[1,4-10]

COMPONENTS OF THE 'ALLERGY MARCH'

The key components of the Allergy March include AD that generally starts in early childhood and is subsequently followed by food allergy. Frequently, food allergy can coexist with AD. This is followed in the next few years by AR and then with asthma. It is important to note that though atopic march is a frequent occurrence, the exact sequence mentioned earlier may not be followed. AD can be followed by asthma without the development of symptoms of food allergy or AR. The first symptom could be AR, which then can lead to asthma without there being skin manifestations (AD) or food allergy. Also, it has been shown that subjects may develop asthma first and then develop AD. It is important to note that the atopic march can occur at any age and not just in childhood.[11]

ATOPIC DERMATITIS AND THE 'ALLERGY MARCH'

Some of the studies on atopic march have used the term 'eczema' for these atopic skin manifestations, leading to some confusion regarding the terminology. The terms eczema and AD mean the same atopic skin manifestations and have been used interchangeably.[1] AD has been used in the USA, and the term atopic eczema is used in Europe.[12] AD is an important risk factor for asthma and has been demonstrated in longitudinal studies. Children with AD and specific IgE antibodies to environmental allergens by the age of 2–4 years have a higher risk of progression to AR and asthma when compared to children with AD without any sensitization to environmental allergens.[1,13,14] Severity of AD has a bearing on the risk for developing asthma. Seventy percent of patients with severe AD develop asthma, whereas 20–30% of subjects with mild AD develop asthma and 8% of subjects without AD in the general population will develop asthma.[1] AD starts very early in life. Eighty-five percent of the children who develop AD do so before 5 years of age, and 45% develop the condition before they are 6 months old.[15] *These studies favored the concept of atopic march.*

ATOPIC DERMATITIS AND ONSET OF ALLERGIC RHINITIS AND ASTHMA

Many studies have confirmed the association of AD with the development of AR and asthma. The pediatric studies included both birth cohort studies and AD cohort studies. There were cross-sectional studies and stronger, prospective longitudinal studies. The strongest design to study the atopic march would be a prospective longitudinal study preferably lasting over a decade of follow-up.

The birth cohort studies demonstrated a risk of developing asthma in children with AD of 2.14 compared to children who did not have AD.[1] The German Multicenter Atopy Study, which was a birth cohort study, evaluated 1,314 newborn children for atopic disease and followed up them until 7 years of age.[16] In more than 40% of the children in this study, the AD resolved within the first 3 years. Early wheeze and the presence of atopic sensitization were associated with asthma in the school age of these children and not AD. *This was a negative study for the atopic march, as the authors did not observe an increased risk of AD with the onset of asthma at school age.* Another birth cohort study, the Tucson's Children's Respiratory Study, observed that AD was indeed a risk factor for the development of future asthma and was an independent risk factor. The study included 1,246 newborn babies and followed up for 22 years. For the final analysis, 849 children were available. *This study favored the concept of the atopic march for childhood asthma, but not for the onset of asthma in adulthood.*[17]

In a cross-sectional study of 2,270 children with physician diagnosed AD, evaluated for additional allergic manifestations using the ISAAC questionnaire, it was observed that 66% of the children with AD developed AR or asthma or both within 3 years of age. The presence of additional allergic diseases was significantly associated with poorer AD control.[10] *This study favored the concept of atopic march.*

The Tasmanian Longitudinal Health Study observed that childhood AD was associated with an increased risk of asthma throughout childhood and adult life, and that the atopic march is likely not limited just in childhood, but persists into adulthood as well.[18] In the Melbourne Atopic Cohort Study (MACS), AD in the first 2 years of life increased the risk of asthma at age 6–7 years.[19] This association was stronger in boys than in girls. In a cohort of 94 children with AD with an onset in infancy followed up until 7 years of age, it was observed that though AD resolves in a good number of children, 43% of the children developed asthma and 45% developed AR subsequently.[20] Severe disease at study inclusion was associated with higher prevalence of food-specific IgE on follow-up. Early onset of AD was associated with higher risk of sensitization to inhalant allergens. Early onset of food allergies was associated with an increased risk of AR and sensitization to both food and aeroallergens. The Prevention of Allergy among Children in Trondheim (PACT) study in the general population observed that AD before the age of 2 years was associated with an increased risk of asthma at age 6.[21] The Swedish Dampness in Buildings and Health (DBH) study also confirmed the association between AD and the subsequent development of AR and asthma.[22] Children with an earlier onset of AD, more severe AD, and persistent AD had higher risk than other children. Carlsten observed that the atopic march is confined to children with early onset AD.[23] It was also one of the few studies to show the association of AD with the development of food allergy. *All these studies favored the concept of atopic march.*

FOOD ALLERGY AND THE ONSET OF ALLERGIC RHINITIS AND ASTHMA

Food allergy also starts early in childhood and frequently co-exists with AD and is observed in about 35% of the children with AD.[24] It is an important trigger for worsening of AD. Food allergy in children independent of AD can progress to the development of AR and asthma. In a cohort of 118 children with cow's milk allergy at infancy, increased airway inflammation and bronchial hyper-responsiveness were observed at 8 years of age.[25] *This study favored the concept of Allergy March.* Further studies are necessary to confirm this association between food allergy and the onset of asthma, though food allergy itself is one of the factors associated with severe asthma. Since AD coexists with food allergy, longitudinal studies involving cases with food allergy alone, without AD, are necessary to quantify the risks of developing asthma in a patient who has developed food allergy.

ALLERGIC RHINITIS AND THE ONSET OF ASTHMA

Various studies, both epidemiological and immunological, have confirmed the association between AR and asthma. These two diseases share common risk factors as well as common pathophysiology. A Danish study by Pedersen observed that 40% of the patients with asthma had AR before the onset of asthma.[26] Of critical importance, this study noted that 75% of the subjects who developed asthma after the onset of AR did so within 2 years. A smaller proportion developed it later; 12% between 2 and 5 years and 5% from 6 to 10 years. A similar study in India by Mahesh PA observed that the highest risk of developing asthma was within the first 2 years after the onset of AR, and within 5 years, 90% of subjects with AR, who were 20 years or younger had developed asthma and 80% of subjects with AR, who were older than 20 years, had developed asthma.[27] Studies at Brown University in the USA with a follow-up for 23 years observed that AR often preceded asthma and was an important risk factor for the onset of asthma.[28,29] Some studies have demonstrated even higher prevalence of asthma in patients with AR. Leynaert[30] reported that 75% of the subjects with asthma had AR, and it is a risk factor for asthma and usually precedes asthma in most patients.

IDENTIFYING CHILDREN AT RISK FOR THE ATOPIC MARCH

Children who have already developed AD are obviously at a higher risk for developing atopic march. In addition, there are some other risk factors that predispose a child to develop allergies, which can progress. These include an elevated cord blood IgE at birth, the presence of specific IgE to foods, and aeroallergens, in early infancy, and positive skin prick tests to foods such as egg and aeroallergens such as house dust mites in the first year of life.[31]

MECHANISMS ASSOCIATED WITH THE ATOPIC MARCH

Though significant research has been conducted, the exact mechanisms of events related to the Allergy March are yet to be clearly elucidated.[1] The first event to occur is the AD. The key mechanisms underlying AD seem to be the defect in the epidermal barrier in the individual.[32] What are the reasons for defective epidermal barrier? Reduced lipids in the epidermis such as ceramide and sphingosine are important.[33] Dysfunctional filaggrin leading to poor keratinization causing defective cornified envelope of the epidermis is said to be one of the most important defects leading to AD.[34,35] The transepidermal water loss that is associated with these defects in the epidermis further contributes to AD and its severity.[36] The keratinocytes in subjects with AD show an abnormal response of inflammatory cytokines on environmental exposure to allergens and staphylococcal superantigens from the staph colonizing the skin of AD subjects.[37] These superantigens in addition can bind directly to the T-cell receptors leading to an abnormal Th-2 type cytokine responses, and these responses in the skin contribute to the development of similar responses in other organ systems such as the nose and the lungs. In addition, in such a milieu in the epidermis, easy access of the allergens deeper into the skin leads to interaction and antigen presentation and processing from the Langerhans cells with interaction with the T lymphocytes in the draining lymph nodes promoting Th-2 responses systemically.[35] The key links between AD and progression to AR and asthma is schematized in Figure 44.1.

Epidermal Differentiation Complex

The key proteins that make up the important structure of the outer layer of the epidermis are filaggrin (filament aggregating protein), loricrin, involucrin, small proline-rich proteins, and the S-100 calcium-binding proteins.[1] Deficient proteins hamper the adequacy of the epidermal barrier and predispose to AD. Filaggrin aggregates the keratin filaments and forms stratum corneum, which is important for water permeability and to block the entry of allergens into the skin.[12] The genetic mutations in chromosome 1q21 coding for filaggrin[38] are the most important that has shown strong associations not only with AD but also with the presence of AR and asthma. Two important loss-of-function mutations are observed in humans. These are R510X and 2282del4 variants.[39,40] The filaggrin protein is neither present in the upper nor lower respiratory tract, and mutations in *filaggrin* cannot affect the airway epithelial barrier.[41] Asthma and AR are present only in patients with *filaggrin* mutations who have AD, especially if the AD has developed before the age of 2 years. Therefore, it is suspected that the association of *filaggrin* mutations and AR and asthma is due to the increased risk of sensitization to allergens due to the defective skin epidermal barrier.[42,43] Thus, there is strong evidence from multiple studies regarding the causative role of filaggrin in AD and subsequent atopic march.[44] In addition to genetic mutations reducing the filaggrin protein levels, there are also acquired mechanisms for reduction in proteins belonging to the epidermal differentiation complex. Th2 cytokines such as Il-4 and Il-13 can reduce the secretion of filaggrin in the AD skin and sphingosylphosphorylcholine, a pro-inflammatory molecule reduces filaggrin production from keratinocytes.[45] Th2 cytokines also reduce the levels of two cornified envelope proteins, loricrin, and involucrin.

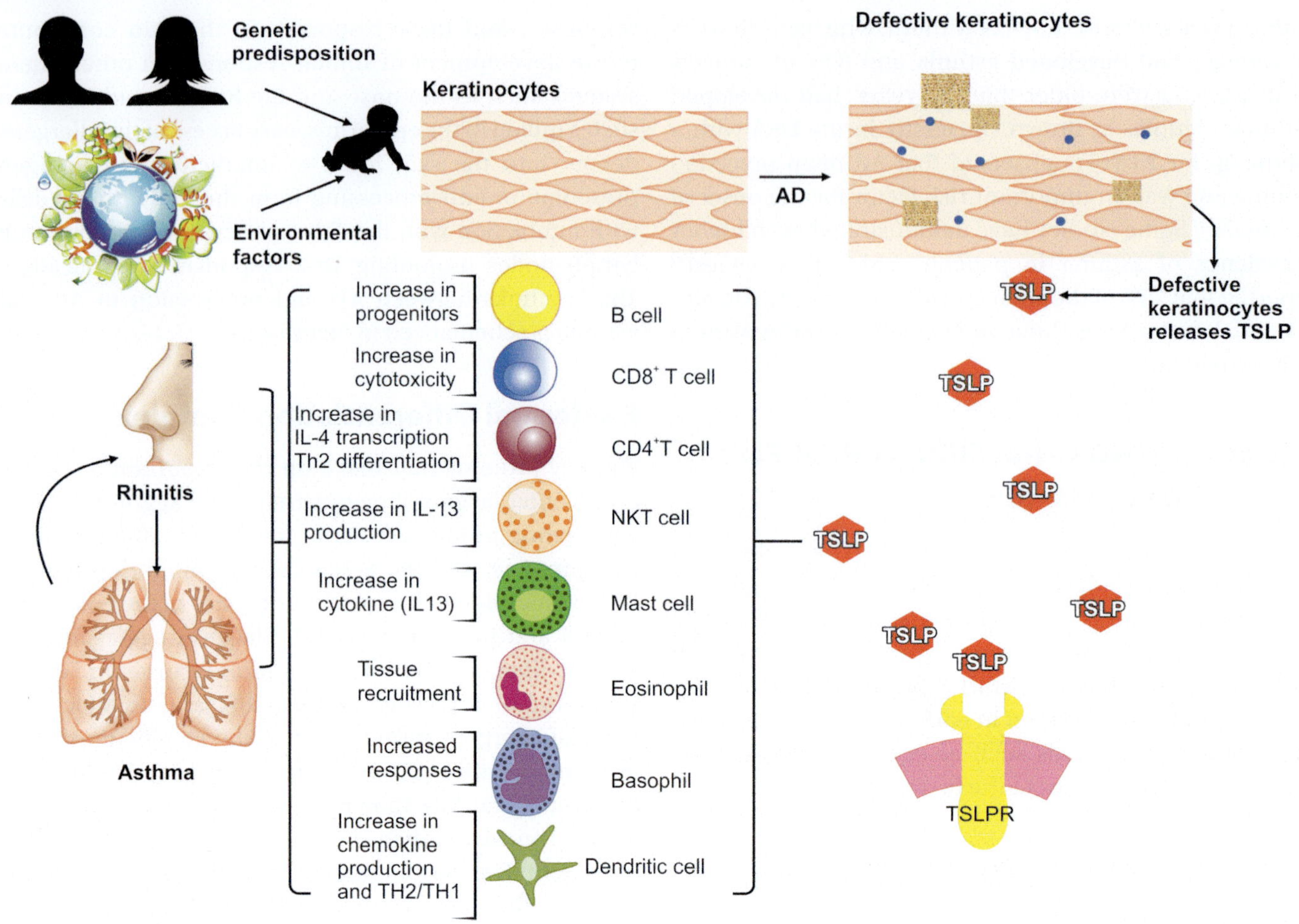

Fig. 44.1: Key mechanisms for progression of atopic dermatitis to allergic rhinitis and asthma.
Courtesy: Sangeetha Vishweswaraiah.

ANIMAL MODELS SUPPORTING THE ALLERGY MARCH

Studies in various animal models have confirmed that epidermal barrier dysfunction can be caused by repeated exposures of the antigens to the skin, which leads to AD-like picture and can further lead to systemic sensitization and symptoms similar to AR and asthma with lung inflammation and airway hyper-responsiveness.[1] The key pathways that are involved in the atopic march in the mouse models are thymic stromal lymphopoietin, IL-17, and filaggrin pathways. A mouse model with repeated exposure of inhalant allergens to the skin developed systemic Th2 responses leading to AR.[46] Repeated epicutaneous exposure of mouse skin to sensitizers like ovalbumin can lead to systemic sensitization to ovalbumin and bronchial hyper-responsiveness on methacholine challenge and asthma-like picture.[47] Stratum corneum is an important defense mechanism. Disruption of the stratum corneum and exposure to ovalbumin and a major food allergen like peanut leads to a strong Th2 cytokine response from the draining lymph nodes with a significant elevation of allergen-specific IgE.[48] Zheng et al. have demonstrated elevated levels of thymic stromal lymphopoietin (TSLP) released from keratinocytes of IL-13 transgenic mice that can explain the link of AD in the development of asthma. Deletion of TSLP prevents the atopic march from AD to asthma, confirming its relevance and role in the atopic march.[49] IL-17 is also likely to play a role in the atopic march. Ovalbumin-sensitized mice produced IL-17 on inhalational challenge by ovalbumin associated with bronchial hyper-responsiveness, and this effect could be reversed by blocking IL-17.[50] In mouse models with *filaggrin* mutations, impaired epidermal barriers are associated with inflammatory infiltrates in the skin secondary to local allergen exposure associated with priming of the cells involved in the allergic pathways, Th2 responses, and production of specific IgE.[51] The exact sequence of events from a disrupted epidermal barrier leading to AD and to the development of asthma is yet to be elucidated. Along with *filaggrin* mutations, there are other cofactors that have not yet been recognized for the development of AD since many subjects who have these same mutations do not develop AD.[1]

HOW CAN WE HALT THE ALLERGY MARCH?

It is important first to generate further evidence whether the Allergy March is indeed causal. If it is so, then planning interventions to arrest the progression of the disease from AD to AR and asthma would have important treatment implications. The two possible levels of interventions could be classified as primary and secondary prevention strategies.[11] Primary prevention is introduced to children before the onset of AD as well as other allergic diseases such as AR and asthma. Secondary prevention is introduced after the onset of AD but before the onset of AR and asthma to reduce its incidence. A summary of preventive strategies is listed in Box 44.1.

BOX 44.1: Strategies to prevent or halt the atopic march.

Primary Prevention

- Strengthening the skin barrier—emollients
- prebiotics, probiotics, and synbiotics
- Other interventions—modifying maternal diet, early introduction of allergenic foods

Secondary Prevention

- Pharmacotherapy
  - Antihistamines
  - Pimecrolimus
- Environmental modifiers
  - Pets
  - Daycare attendance
  - Maternal and infant diet
- Immunotherapy
  - SCIT
  - SLIT
  - SCIT with anti-IgE

Primary Prevention

Certain areas have shown promise. The key focus is on developing interventions to maintain the infant dermal barrier function. The hypothesis being if the sensitization occurs due to a defective cutaneous barrier, strengthening it would reduce sensitization and thus further clinical progression to AR and asthma.[11] Interventional studies are being conducted using standard emollients as well as ceramide-dominant emollients.[52,53] In this context, further research on the infant traditional management practices of using different oils in India needs further study regarding their efficacy in preventing AD. AD is much lower in the Indian population when compared to the Western world.

Clinical studies have evaluated the role of prebiotics, probiotics, and synbiotics.[54,55] Probiotics and live beneficial bacteria are shown to help regulate the immune system better, especially in children since all of them have a Th2 bias at birth, which matures to a Th1 predominant pathway later. Prebiotics are foods that contain ingredients usually fibers that favor the growth of the beneficial bacteria in the gut. Though some trials have shown promise, including the use of *Lactobacillus* in pregnant women, further details are being awaited to have a final say in the matter. In this context, the role of frequent consumption of fermented foods in the Indian dietary habits in protecting the individuals against the development of allergies needs to be further studied. Synbiotics are a combination of pre- and probiotics.

Other interventions that are currently being studied include modification of the infant and maternal diets including addition of certain fatty acids, timing of introduction of solids in the infant's diet, whether early introduction of allergenic foods such as peanuts would be beneficial in preventing the onset of allergic diseases. There is some evidence regarding the utility of vitamin D during pregnancy and infancy, but further research is needed to confirm its role in allergy prevention.[1,11]

Secondary Prevention

These interventions are given after the child has developed AD to prevent the development of AR and asthma or after the development of AR to prevent the development of asthma. They can be classified as pharmacological, environmental, and immunotherapeutic. Pharmacological interventions include use of antihistamines and calcineurin inhibitors, environmental modifiers include factors associated with the hygiene hypothesis, and immunotherapeutic interventions include either subcutaneous or sublingual immunotherapy.

Pharmacological Interventions

The role of antihistamines was evaluated in two longitudinal studies in the early treatment of the atopic child (ETAC)[56] and the early prevention of asthma in the atopic child (EPAAC).[57] There was some benefit in the prevention of asthma in children with AD in a subgroup of children sensitized to grass pollens and house dust mites, but strong evidence regarding its usefulness is lacking. In a study evaluating the time interval between developing asthma in subjects with AR, it was observed that regular use of antihistamines had a protective role in preventing asthma in subjects with AR.[27] The same study observed significant protection in subjects who ever used nasal steroids in univariate analysis, but not multivariate analysis. The role of regular use of nasal steroids in preventing asthma needs to be further evaluated. The Study of the Atopic March (SAM) evaluates the role of pimecrolimus in children with AD and results are awaited.[11] Another randomized trial used ketotifen in children of 1–36 months old for 1 year and observed there was some benefit in preventing asthma in children who used ketotifen.[58]

Environmental Modifiers

Pets and daycare attendance: The role of environmental modifiers has to be evaluated in further detail, and there is a need for randomized controlled interventional studies. Most of the evidence that is available thus far is by association studies that cannot be well controlled for the environmental modifier in question and rule out other confounders. The idea that environmental modifiers could be important came about by the observations that not all children with AD will go on to develop respiratory allergies. It was observed that children with AD who had cats at home and those who attended daycare had a lower incidence of asthma in a longitudinal study.[59] There are many contradicting studies on hygiene hypothesis, some attributing protection to animals such as dogs, and some studies observe that cats increase the risk but not dogs and these results need to be interpreted with caution. The question for the clinician and the parent having a child with AD is whether I keep a cat in the house and how much protection it would give my child in preventing the onset of asthma. A randomized control trial of allocating the children with AD to either receiving cat or a dog or none at all and followed up for 5 years may be able to answer this issue with some conviction. Without that study design even in longitudinal cohort studies, other confounding factors may not have been taken care of sufficiently. Though strong evidence is yet to emerge, it is prudent to avoid the exposure of the child to secondhand tobacco smoke, mosquito coils, and incense sticks, which increase the levels of many important air pollutants indoors.

Maternal and infant diet: There are some evidences to suggest that modification of the maternal diet with supplementation of omega-3 unsaturated fatty acids (from fish) and selenium during pregnancy can protect the infant from developing allergies, whereas there are other studies that show no effect.[31] Again it is controversial whether the child should avoid contact with known allergens or not including consumption of foods that are important allergens such as peanut. It is agreed that all infants should be breastfed, but it is controversial whether a feeding mother should avoid important food allergens such as peanut in her diet.

Immunotherapy

Immunotherapy is probably the only known treatment for allergy that can modify the natural course of the disease. It has been traditionally used as subcutaneous immunotherapy (SCIT) since more than a 100 years, after it was first introduced by Noon in 1911. SCIT has been shown to have a sustained resolution of allergic symptoms even after discontinuation of the SCIT for a prolonged period of time.[60] Recently, there is a lot of promise shown by sublingual immunotherapy (SLIT), which is ideally suited for children who are the most important candidates for interventions to halt the atopic march.[61] It would be very difficult for very young children to be able to go through SCIT involving regular injections for a period of 5 years. There are also studies that have used a combination of immunotherapy with anti-IgE therapy and have shown very good results in children with seasonal AR.[62]

REFERENCES

1. Zheng T, Yu J, Oh MH, Zhu Z. The atopic march: progression from atopic dermatitis to allergic rhinitis and asthma. Allergy Asthma Immunol Res. 2011;3:67-73.
2. Spergel JM, Paller AS. Atopic dermatitis and the atopic march. J Allergy Clin Immunol. 2003;112:S118-27.
3. Johansson SG, Bieber T, Dahl R, et al. Revised nomenclature for allergy for global use: Report of the Nomenclature Review Committee of the World Allergy Organization, October 2003. J Allergy Clin Immunol. 2004;113:832-6.

4. Zhu Z, Oh MH, Yu J, et al. The Role of TSLP in IL-13-induced atopic march. Sci Rep. 2011;1:23.
5. Ricci G, Patrizi A, Baldi E, et al. Long-term follow-up of atopic dermatitis: retrospective analysis of related risk factors and association with concomitant allergic diseases. J Am Acad Dermatol. 2006;55:765-71.
6. Martinez FD, Wright AL, Taussig LM, et al. Asthma and wheezing in the first six years of life. The Group Health Medical Associates. N Engl J Med. 1995;332:133-8.
7. Kulig M, Bergmann R, Klettke U, et al. Natural course of sensitization to food and inhalant allergens during the first 6 years of life. J Allergy Clin Immunol. 1999;103:1173-9.
8. Ohshima Y, Yamada A, Hiraoka M, et al. Early sensitization to house dust mite is a major risk factor for subsequent development of bronchial asthma in Japanese infants with atopic dermatitis: results of a 4-year followup study. Ann Allergy Asthma Immunol. 2002;89:265-70.
9. van der Hulst AE, Klip H, Brand PL. Risk of developing asthma in young children with atopic eczema: a systematic review. J Allergy Clin Immunol. 2007;120:565-9.
10. Kapoor R, Menon C, Hoffstad O, et al. The prevalence of atopic triad in children with physician-confirmed atopic dermatitis. J Am Acad Dermatol. 2008;58:68-73.
11. Dharmage SC, Lowe AJ, Matheson MC, et al. Atopic dermatitis and the atopic march revisited. Allergy. 2014;69:17-27.
12. Patrizi A, Pileri A, Bellini F, et al. Atopic dermatitis and the atopic march: what is new? J Allergy (Cairo). 2011;2011:279425.
13. Novembre E, Cianferoni A, Lombardi E, et al. Natural history of "intrinsic" atopic dermatitis. Allergy. 2001;56: 452-3.
14. Wuthrich B, Schmid-Grendelmeier P. Natural course of AEDS. Allergy. 2002;57:267-8.
15. Kay J, Gawkrodger DJ, Mortimer MJ, Jaron AG. The prevalence of childhood atopic eczema in a general population. J Am Acad Dermatol. 1994;30:35-9.
16. Illi S, von Mutius E, Lau S, et al. The natural course of atopic dermatitis from birth to age 7 years and the association with asthma. J Allergy Clin Immunol. 2004;113:925-31.
17. Stern DA, Morgan WJ, Halonen M, et al. Wheezing and bronchial hyper-responsiveness in early childhood as predictors of newly diagnosed asthma in early adulthood: a longitudinal birth-cohort study. Lancet. 2008;372: 1058-64.
18. Burgess JA, Dharmage SC, Byrnes GB, et al. Childhood eczema and asthma incidence and persistence: a cohort study from childhood to middle age. J Allergy Clin Immunol. 2008;122:280-5.
19. Lowe AJ, Carlin JB, Bennett CM, et al. Do boys do the atopic march while girls dawdle? J Allergy Clin Immunol. 2008;121:1190-5.
20. Gustafsson D, Sjoberg O, Foucard T. Development of allergies and asthma in infants and young children with atopic dermatitis—a prospective follow-up to 7 years of age. Allergy. 2000;55:240-5.
21. Saunes M, Oien T, Dotterud CK, et al. Early eczema and the risk of childhood asthma: a prospective, population-based study. BMC Pediatr. 2012;12:168.
22. von Kobyletzki LB, Bornehag CG, Hasselgren M, et al. Eczema in early childhood is strongly associated with the development of asthma and rhinitis in a prospective cohort. BMC Dermatol. 2012;12:11.
23. Carlsten C, Dimich-Ward H, Ferguson A, et al. Atopic dermatitis in a high-risk cohort: natural history, associated allergic outcomes, and risk factors. Ann Allergy Asthma Immunol. 2013;110:24-8.
24. Eigenmann PA, Sicherer SH, Borkowski TA, et al. Prevalence of IgE-mediated food allergy among children with atopic dermatitis. Pediatrics. 1998;101:E8.
25. Malmberg LP, Saarinen KM, Pelkonen AS, et al. Cow's milk allergy as a predictor of bronchial hyperresponsiveness and airway inflammation at school age. Clin Exp Allergy. 2010;40:1491-7.
26. Pedersen PA, Weeke ER. Asthma and allergic rhinitis in the same patients. Allergy. 1983;38:25-9.
27. Mahesh PA, Vedanthan PK, Holla AD, et al. Time interval and the factors associated with the development of asthma in patients with allergic rhinitis. Lung. 2009;187:393-400.
28. Settipane RJ, Hagy GW, Settipane GA. Long-term risk factors for developing asthma and allergic rhinitis: a 23-year follow-up study of college students. Allergy Proc. 1994;15:21-5.
29. Greisner WA, 3rd, Settipane RJ, Settipane GA. Co-existence of asthma and allergic rhinitis: a 23-year follow-up study of college students. Allergy Asthma Proc. 1998;19:185-8.
30. Leynaert B, Neukirch C, Kony S, et al. Association between asthma and rhinitis according to atopic sensitization in a population-based study. J Allergy Clin Immunol. 2004;113:86-93.
31. Van Bever HP, Samuel ST, Lee BW. Halting the allergic march. World Allergy Organ J. 2008;1:57-62.
32. Cork MJ, Robinson DA, Vasilopoulos Y, et al. New perspectives on epidermal barrier dysfunction in atopic dermatitis: gene-environment interactions. J Allergy Clin Immunol. 2006;118:3-21; quiz 22-3.
33. Arikawa J, Ishibashi M, Kawashima M, et al. Decreased levels of sphingosine, a natural antimicrobial agent, may be associated with vulnerability of the stratum corneum from patients with atopic dermatitis to colonization by *Staphylococcus aureus*. J Invest Dermatol. 2002;119:433-9.
34. McGrath JA. Filaggrin and the great epidermal barrier grief. Australas J Dermatol. 2008;49:67-73; quiz 73-64.
35. McGrath JA, Uitto J. The filaggrin story: novel insights into skin-barrier function and disease. Trends Mol Med. 2008;14:20-7.
36. Gupta J, Grube E, Ericksen MB, et al. Intrinsically defective skin barrier function in children with atopic dermatitis correlates with disease severity. J Allergy Clin Immunol. 2008;121:725-30 e722.
37. Allakhverdi Z, Comeau MR, Jessup HK, et al. Thymic stromal lymphopoietin is released by human epithelial cells in response to microbes, trauma, or inflammation and potently activates mast cells. J Exp Med. 2007;204:253-8.

38. O'Regan GM, Sandilands A, McLean WH, Irvine AD. Filaggrin in atopic dermatitis. J Allergy Clin Immunol. 2009;124:R2-6.
39. Mischke D, Korge BP, Marenholz I, et al. Genes encoding structural proteins of epidermal cornification and S100 calcium-binding proteins form a gene complex ("epidermal differentiation complex") on human chromosome 1q21. J Invest Dermatol. 1996;106:989-92.
40. Stemmler S, Parwez Q, Petrasch-Parwez E, et al. Two common loss-of-function mutations within the *filaggrin* gene predispose for early onset of atopic dermatitis. J Invest Dermatol. 2007;127:722-4.
41. Ying S, Meng Q, Corrigan CJ, Lee TH. Lack of filaggrin expression in the human bronchial mucosa. J Allergy Clin Immunol. 2006;118:1386-8.
42. Weidinger S, Illig T, Baurecht H, et al. Loss-of-function variations within the *filaggrin* gene predispose for atopic dermatitis with allergic sensitizations. J Allergy Clin Immunol. 2006;118:214-9.
43. Weidinger S, Rodriguez E, Stahl C, et al. *Filaggrin* mutations strongly predispose to early-onset and extrinsic atopic dermatitis. J Invest Dermatol. 2007;127:724-6.
44. Marenholz I, Nickel R, Ruschendorf F, et al. *Filaggrin* loss-of-function mutations predispose to phenotypes involved in the atopic march. J Allergy Clin Immunol. 2006;118:866-71.
45. Choi H, Kim S, Kim HJ, et al. Sphingosylphosphorylcholine down regulates *filaggrin* gene transcription through NOX5-based NADPH oxidase and cyclooxygenase-2 in human keratinocytes. Biochem Pharmacol. 2010;80:95-103.
46. Akei HS, Brandt EB, Mishra A, et al. Epicutaneous aeroallergen exposure induces systemic Th2 immunity that predisposes to allergic nasal responses. J Allergy Clin Immunol. 2006;118:62-9.
47. Spergel JM, Mizoguchi E, Brewer JP, et al. Epicutaneous sensitization with protein antigen induces localized allergic dermatitis and hyperresponsiveness to methacholine after single exposure to aerosolized antigen in mice. J Clin Invest. 1998;101:1614-22.
48. Strid J, Hourihane J, Kimber I, et al. Disruption of the stratum corneum allows potent epicutaneous immunization with protein antigens resulting in a dominant systemic Th2 response. Eur J Immunol. 2004;34:2100-9.
49. Zheng T, Oh MH, Oh SY, et al. Transgenic expression of interleukin-13 in the skin induces a pruritic dermatitis and skin remodeling. J Invest Dermatol. 2009;129:742-51.
50. He R, Kim HY, Yoon J, et al. Exaggerated IL-17 response to epicutaneous sensitization mediates airway inflammation in the absence of IL-4 and IL-13. J Allergy Clin Immunol. 2009;124:761-70 e761.
51. Fallon PG, Sasaki T, Sandilands A, et al. A homozygous frameshift mutation in the mouse Flg gene facilitates enhanced percutaneous allergen priming. Nat Genet. 2009;41:602-8.
52. Lowe AJ, Tang ML, Dharmage SC, et al. A phase I study of daily treatment with a ceramide-dominant triple lipid mixture commencing in neonates. BMC Dermatol. 2012;12:3.
53. Simpson EL, Berry TM, Brown PA, Hanifin JM. A pilot study of emollient therapy for the primary prevention of atopic dermatitis. J Am Acad Dermatol. 2010;63:587-93.
54. Thomas DW, Greer FR. American Academy of Pediatrics Committee on Nutrition: American Academy of Pediatrics Section on Gastroenterology, Hepatology, and Nutrition. Probiotics and prebiotics in pediatrics. Pediatrics. 2010;126:1217-31.
55. del Giudice MM, Rocco A, Capristo C. Probiotics in the atopic march: highlights and new insights. Dig Liver Dis. 2006;38:S288-90.
56. Diepgen TL. Early Treatment of the atopic child study G. Long-term treatment with cetirizine of infants with atopic dermatitis: a multi-country, double-blind, randomized, placebo-controlled trial (the ETAC trial) over 18 months. Pediatr Allergy Immunol. 2002;13:278-86.
57. Simons FE. Early Prevention of Asthma in Atopic Children Study G. Safety of levocetirizine treatment in young atopic children: An 18-month study. Pediatr Allergy Immunol. 2007;18:535-42.
58. Iikura Y, Naspitz CK, Mikawa H, et al. Prevention of asthma by ketotifen in infants with atopic dermatitis. Ann Allergy. 1992;68:233-6.
59. Gaffin JM, Spergel JM, Boguniewicz M, et al. Effect of cat and daycare exposures on the risk of asthma in children with atopic dermatitis. Allergy Asthma Proc. 2012;33:282-8.
60. Cools M, Van Bever HP, Weyler JJ, Stevens WJ. Long-term effects of specific immunotherapy, administered during childhood, in asthmatic patients allergic to either house-dust mite or to both house dust mite and grass pollen. Allergy. 2000;55:69-73.
61. Pajno GB. Sublingual immunotherapy: the optimism and the issues. J Allergy Clin Immunol. 2007;119:796-801.
62. Kuehr J, Brauburger J, Zielen S, et al. Efficacy of combination treatment with anti-IgE plus specific immunotherapy in polysensitized children and adolescents with seasonal allergic rhinitis. J Allergy Clin Immunol. 2002;109:274-80.

CHAPTER 45

Allergy and Infection

Anura Weerasinghe

INTRODUCTION

Sensitization to allergens has long been recognized as the first step in the development of allergy. The spectrum of allergen varies from nonliving proteins to living microbes. In this chapter, the role of infection in the development and worsening of allergy is discussed.

IMMUNOPATHOGENESIS OF ALLERGY

Allergy has two distinct phases, namely, sensitization and effector phases. First exposure to an allergen results in sensitization and subsequent exposure to the same allergen liberates mediators of allergy (Fig. 45.1) and causes wide spectrum of allergic reactions.[1]

Type I hypersensitivity results in the pathological process leading to lower airway obstruction. Histamine is immediately released by mast cells on exposure to an allergen. Repeated exposure to mast cells results in inflammation of the lower airways through the action of number of mediators released from mast cells (e.g., Interleukin 1), eosinophils [e.g., major basic proteins (MBP)] and Th1 cells (IL-4 and IL-5). IL-4 acts on B cells and produces IgE by inducing class switching, and IL-5 attracts eosinophils to the site of inflammation.[2]

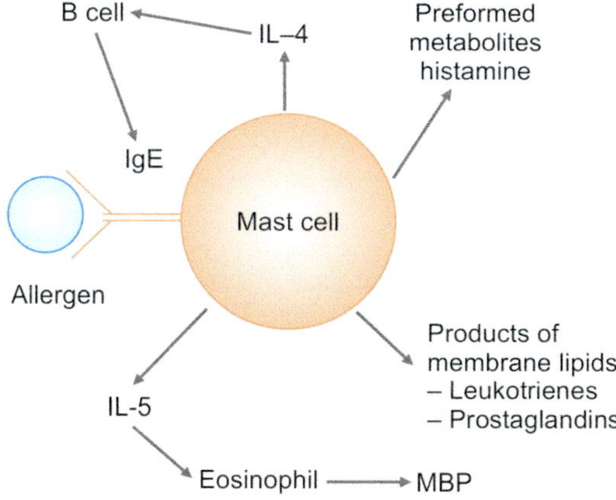

Fig. 45.1: Mediators of allergy.

CLINICAL MANIFESTATIONS OF ALLERGY

The clinical manifestations range from mild to severe (Box 45.1).

ROLE OF T CELLS IN ALLERGY

T lymphocytes are divided into two groups according to the cytokine profile. Th1 cells secrete IL-2 and INF-γ and Th2 cells secrete IL-4 and IL-5. Th2 cytokines are involved with allergy. Therefore, the infestations causing Th2 immune response result in allergy. In tropical pulmonary eosinophilia, mast cell stimulation and release of leukotriene is responsible for bronchospasm.

ASSOCIATION OF INFECTIONS WITH ALLERGY

Fungal, viral, helminthic, and some bacterial infections have found to be associated with allergy. Therefore, during evaluation of a patient with chronic allergy such as wheezing and urticaria, it is mandatory to look for those treatable associations (Box 45.2).

BOX 45.1: The spectrum of clinical manifestations.

- *Respiratory system*: Runny nose and wheezing
- *Cardiovascular*: Hypotension (anaphylactic shock)
- *Gastrointestinal system*: Abdominal pain
- *Skin*: Itching, erythema, hives (Urticaria), and subcutaneous swelling (angioedema)

BOX 45.2: Treatable associations of allergy.

- Filariasis[3]
- Toxocariasis[4]
- Aspergillosis[5]
- Worm infestations
- *Helicobacter pylori* infection

RESPIRATORY INFECTIONS

During infancy, a number of respiratory viruses have been implicated in the pathogenesis of the asthma.[6] In early life, respiratory syncytial virus (RSV) and parainfluenza virus cause bronchiolitis. A number of long-term prospective studies of children with documented RSV have shown that approximately 40% of these infants will continue to wheeze or have asthma in later childhood. Rhinovirus infections in early life are also emerging as risk factors for recurrent wheezing.[7] On the other hand, evidence also indicates that certain respiratory infections early in life, such as measles and RSV or repeated viral infections, can protect against the development of asthma. The "hygiene hypothesis" of asthma suggests that exposure to infections early in life influences the development of a child's immune system along a "nonallergic" pathway. Although the hygiene hypothesis continues to be investigated, this association may explain observed associations between large family size, later birth order, daycare attendance, and a reduced risk of asthma.[8] The influence of viral respiratory infections in the development of asthma may depend on an interaction with atopy.[9] The atopic state can influence the lower airway response to viral infections, and viral infections may then influence the development of allergic sensitization. The airway interactions that may occur when individuals are exposed simultaneously to both allergens and viruses are of interest but are not defined at present.

CONCLUSION

The relationship of infection and asthma is seen in both directions, in particular, protecting from the allergy and worsening the allergic condition. However, it is important to treat existing infection as it outweighs the risk of leaving it unattended.[10,11]

REFERENCES

1. Gunewardena M, Weerasinghe A, Herath J, Amarasena N. Myocardial infarction associated with eosinophilia: a variant of Kounis syndrome. BMJ. 2015;10:1136-46.
2. Chu HW, Martin RJ. Are eosinophils still important in asthma? Clin Exp Allergy. 2001;31:525-8.
3. Singh G, Ojha D. Chronic urticarial and filariasis. Dermatologia. 1968;136:173-5.
4. Ismail MA, Khalafallah O. *Toxocara canis* and chronic urticarial in Egyptian patients. J Egypt Soc Parasitol. 2005;35:833-40.
5. Hay RJ, Moore MK. Clinical features of superficial fungal infections. Br J Dermatol. 2006;110:677-83.
6. Swarbrick ET, Farrokhyar F, Irvine EJ. Inverse relation between the incidence of prototypical infectious diseases and the incidence of immune disorders from 1950 to 2000. N Engl J Med. 2002;347:911-20.
7. Illi S, von Mutius E, Lau S, et al. Early childhood infectious diseases and the development of asthma up to school age: a birth cohort study. BMJ. 2001;322:390-5.
8. Strachen DP. Allergic rhinitis is inversely linked to birth order and the size of the family. BMJ. 1989;299:1259-60.
9. Editorial. Farm life protects against atopy. BMJ. 2004;328:1211-12.
10. Weerasinghe A. Management of urticaria. Sri Lanka Prescriber. 2006;14:7-8.
11. Weerasinghe A. Management of allergic asthma. Sri Lanka Prescriber. 2015;22:5-8.

CHAPTER 46

Allergic Bronchopulmonary Aspergillosis

Rajendra Prasad , VK Jain, Nikhil Gupta

INTRODUCTION

Aspergillus is ubiquitous, occurring in mycelial form, which is thermotolerant and grows at 15–53°C, the optimum being 37–40°C and humid conditions. It is present in the environment, decaying vegetation, fallen leaves, mulch, water, saunas, basements, crawl spaces, bedding, some foodstuffs, and even in marijuana.

Pulmonary aspergillosis is a clinical spectrum of lung disease caused by the fungus *Aspergillus*. The classification of pulmonary aspergillosis includes saprophytic aspergillosis in the form of pulmonary aspergilloma, immune disease in the form of allergic bronchopulmonary aspergillosis (ABPA), IgE-mediated asthma, hypersensitivity pneumonitis, allergic *Aspergillus* sinusitis (AAS), and infectious disease in the form of invasive and semi-invasive pulmonary aspergillosis.[1] One of the latest studies also categorized aspergillosis-related respiratory disorders into upper and lower respiratory tract disorders.[2] ABPA is the most common disease among allergic bronchopulmonary mycoses. ABPA is a hypersensitivity immunological lung disorder caused by species of the dimorphic fungus *Aspergillus*, commonly *Aspergillus fumigatus* (about 95%) and rarely by *Aspergillus flavus*, *Aspergillus niger*, *Aspergillus oryzae*, *Aspergillus sydowii*, *Aspergillus terreus*, *Aspergillus glaucus*, *Aspergillus nidulans*, and *Aspergillus clavatus*. Other fungi like *Candida*, *Helminthosporium*, *Curvularia*, *Drechslera*, *Pseudallescheria boyii*, and *Fusarium vasinfectum* have also been found to cause an identical syndrome,[3] clinically manifesting as chronic asthma, recurrent pulmonary infiltrates, and bronchiectasis.[4-12,58] The condition has immunologic features of immediate hypersensitivity (type I), antigen-antibody complexes (type III), and eosinophil-rich inflammatory cell responses (type IVb), based on the revised Gell and Coombs classification of immunologic hypersensitivity.[13,14] The first case of ABPA was reported in England[15] in 1952 and in India[16] in 1971. Since then a number of cases have been reported from all over the world. Concomitant occurrence of ABPA and AAS is now being increasingly recognized, which is also called as "sinobronchial allergic mycosis" (SAM syndrome).[17] ABPA is commonly associated in patients with chronic bronchial asthma and cystic fibrosis but can also occur in nonasthmatics.[18] A new phenotype of asthma has been described recently, namely severe asthma with fungal sensitization (SAFS). SAFS can be conceptualized as a continuum of fungal sensitization, with asthma at one end and ABPA at the other end. It is diagnosed by the presence of severe asthma, fungal sensitization, and exclusion of ABPA.[19]

PREVALENCE

The ABPA has long been reported to be common in the UK, where it is the cause of 50–80% of the cases of the pulmonary eosinophilia.[10] The exact prevalence of ABPA is not known but contemporary estimates suggested that ABPA complicates 1–11% of all chronic cases of bronchial asthma.[20-28] Many case series of ABPA were reported from India.[29-32] A very recent study from India, however, found a higher prevalence of *Aspergillus* sensitization (39.5%) and ABPA (27%) in 564 patients with asthma.[33] Alok Nath et al. in their latest study on 350 patients found the prevalence of Aspergillus hypersensitivity (AH) and ABPA to be 35.1% and 21.7%, respectively.[34] The condition is being increasingly recognized, and the estimated prevalence rates in recent publications have been reported ranging from 5.9% to 20.5% for ABPA and 38–43% for AH.[35,36] Prevalence data from this part of the country are sparse.

IMMUNOPATHOLOGY

The ABPA patients are atopic with a history of chronic asthma. The basic underlying immunopathophysiologic process in ABPA is a hypersensitivity reaction to fungus in the bronchial tree. In susceptible individuals after inhalation of fungal spores in the bronchi, fungi germinate and form vegetative elements (hyphae). Local immunologic reactions and stagnation of tenacious sputum in bronchial airways favor the trapping of fungal spores and further colonization. Antigenic substance of the fungus stimulates formation of IgE, IgG, and IgA antibodies. ABPA is immunologically classified as it gives both type I (immediate) and type III (Arthus, antigen-antibody immune complex) hypersensitivity reactions. Type I reaction is IgE mediated and responsible for accumulation of eosinophils, bronchospasm, and edema leading to acute symptoms of diseases. Type III reaction results in polymorph aggregation, inflammation of bronchial and peribronchial tissues, and is responsible for the radiological features of ABPA. Recently, the possible role of type IV b[13,37] hypersensitivity reaction has also been observed in patients with ABPA and in the presence of parenchymal granuloma and mononuclear cell infiltration seen on histopathology. Long-standing involvement of the bronchial tree leads to bronchiectasis, fibrosis, lung contraction, and lobar shrinkage.[10]

CLINICAL PRESENTATION

Patients are usually atopic with a previous history of bronchial asthma. The onset is insidious with constitutional symptoms like anorexia, fatigue, weight loss, headache, generalized aches and pains, and low-grade fever. The frequency and severity of symptoms of underlying asthma are not fully controlled with usual anti-asthma therapy. It is characterized by repeated episodes of exacerbation with periods of remission, if untreated, may progress to fibrotic lung disease. It may occur at any age but usually occurs in the age group of 20–40 years. Patients with chronic fibrotic disease may present with cyanosis, cor pulmonale, and respiratory failure. However, symptoms have little or no relationship to the severity or chronicity of the disease, as one-third of the patients may be relatively asymptomatic in spite of extensive radiological shadows.[38]

Golden brown rubbery flecks or plugs in sputum are characteristic and have been reported in 5–54% of cases.[27] These plugs consist of fungal hyphae with eosinophils and mucous. Cough, breathlessness, and wheezing are the common symptoms seen in ABPA. Hemoptysis has been reported in 34–85% of cases, while pleuritic chest pain may be present in 50% of cases. In one of his studies, the author found that hemoptysis is found in 28.6% of patients.[39] Chronic cases of ABPA may rarely present with symptoms of bronchiectasis. Upon clinical examination of the chest, wheezing and diffuse crepitations are the common findings but tachypnea, cyanosis, features of cor pulmonale, and sometimes hypertrophic osteoarthropathy may be seen. The disease is often incorrectly diagnosed as tuberculosis, bronchiectasis, and bacterial pneumonia.[10] Almost half of the ABPA patients are initially misdiagnosed as pulmonary tuberculosis.[28]

DIAGNOSTIC APPROACH

The ABPA is suspected in any patient with asthma with lung shadows on chest skiagram and peripheral blood eosinophilia. All the features are not necessary to diagnose ABPA. The important diagnostic criteria are the presence of recurrent pulmonary infiltrates, peripheral blood eosinophilia, and a positive skin test to the *Aspergillus* antigen. Criteria for the diagnosis of SAFS include the history of poorly controlled asthma (>500 µg/day of fluticasone or the equivalent, near continuous oral corticosteroids for >6 months, or >2 oral steroid tapers per year), total serum IgE < 1,000 IU/mL, positive immediate skin test reactivity to *A. fumigatus*, elevated specific serum IgE to *A. fumigatus* or absence of serum precipitins (by gel diffusion) and elevated specific serum IgG to *A. fumigatus* and No radiographic evidence of bronchiectasis or infiltrates.[19]

Radiological Features

Chest X-ray

Radiological features in patients of ABPA may be transient (acute) or permanent (chronic). Transient shadows may clear with or without steroid therapy and are mainly due to pulmonary infiltrates and stagnation of secretions in damaged bronchi.[40,41] Transient shadows are perihilar infiltrates mimicking adenopathy, air fluid levels from dilated central bronchi filled with fluid and debris. Parenchymal abnormalities are more common and present in 80–90% of patients with ABPA as ill-defined homogeneous shadows without the evidence of loss of volume, which may be of 5–15 mm in size or more as massive/lobar in extent, may be unilateral or bilateral, more in upper lobes, resolve (fleeting/migratory shadows) often after expectoration of bronchial plugs but tends to recur in same/other places. Sometimes pulmonary shadows mimic carcinoma.

Fleeting shadows are characteristic of ABPA, the author in one of his studies found 66.7% of patients had fleeting shadows. Author described 'walking pneumonia' as a clue to the diagnosis of ABPA.[42] Bronchial abnormalities occur in 50–70% of episodes of acute ABPA consists of tramline, parallel lines, and ring shadows, which represents a normal or an abnormal bronchial wall. The impacted bronchus may appear as a full wine glass having an open upper end with a tapering lower end,[43] a gloved finger of 2–3 cm long and 5–8 mm wide, and inverted V, Y, or toothpaste shadows. Gloved-finger shadows are due to distally occluded bronchi filled with secretions. Tram lime shadows are the thickened walls of undilated bronchi, so the distance between lines is that of a normal bronchus, while parallel lines shadows represent walls of bronchiectatic bronchi, and the distance between walls is greater than normal. Permanent (chronic) changes reflect histological abnormalities secondary to repeated acute episodes of ABPA and are often associated with physiologic abnormalities. Rarely cavitations, local emphysema, pulmonary fibrosis or contracted upper lobe, honeycombing, collapse due to mucous impaction, and spontaneous pneumothorax[44] are recognized, even total collapse of lung has been reported.[45]

Computed Tomography

Conventional tomography has been shown to be more sensitive than the plain chest radiograph. Computerized tomography might be useful in the assessment of the extent of disease. HRCT is a sensitive noninvasive technique for the recognition of ABPA. Proximal bronchiectasis is due to the deposition of the immune complex in proximal airways. Bronchiectasis, centrilobular nodules, and mucoid impaction are the main features of ABPA.[46] Proximal bronchiectasis with ABPA may be seen in 40% of the patients[47] and characterized by a string of pearls and signet ring appearance as described by Webb et al.[48] Proximal bronchiectasis (in second-, third-, and fourth-order large bronchi) is an important diagnostic feature of ABPA with normal small bronchi and bronchioles.[49]

Radiological Classification of ABPA

The ABPA is classified into ABPA-S (mild), ABPA-CB (moderate), and ABPA-CB-ORF (other radiologic findings).[50] In ABPA-S all the diagnostic features of ABPA are present except the evidence of proximal bronchiectasis on HRCT. It is believed that patients with ABPA-S have milder clinical course and less severe immunological findings when compared to ABPA-CB. In ABPA-CB, all findings of ABPA including proximal bronchiectasis on HRCT present, however, in ABPA-CB-ORF all findings of ABPA and central bronchiectasis along with other radiological features such as pulmonary fibrosis, bleb, bullae, pneumothorax, parenchymal scarring, emphysematous change, multiple cyst, fibrocavitary lesions, aspergilloma, ground glass appearance, collapse, mediastinal lymph node, pleural effusion, and pleural thickening. Newly proposed radiological classification of ABPA based on computed tomography chest findings categorizes ABPA as ABPA-S (serological ABPA), ABPA-B (ABPA with bronchiectasis), ABPA-HAM (ABPA with high attenuation mucus), and ABPA-CPF (ABPA with chronic pleuropulmonary fibrosis).[51]

Laboratory Investigations

- Peripheral blood eosinophilia (usually 1,000–3,000/m^3), leukocytosis, and raised ESR in acute episodes and sputum contain eosinophils in most of the cases.
- *Serological tests*: Increase in total IgE and specific IgE and IgG-precipitating antibodies (in 70%) against *A. fumigatus*.[52,53] Both total and specific IgE levels are high during the development of pulmonary infiltrates and decrease after remission. The total IgE levels are greater than 1,000 IU/mL, may be as high as 20,000 IU/mL in acute cases except in cases that are in remission or on steroids therapy.[54] Precipitating antibodies against *A. fumigatus* are present in most of cases of ABPA with pulmonary infiltrates and diminished after steroid therapy.[55]
- *Skin test*: Positive skin tests (types 1 and 3) are more reliable than precipitin tests. Immediate type 1 skin reaction is positive in most of the cases but also positive in 25% of asthmatics without ABPA. Late-onset (type 3) erythema and edema occur usually after 4–6 hours and reaches the peak within 8 hours and subsides by 24 hours due to the deposition of IgE, IgM, IgA, and complement components.
- *Sputum smear and culture for Aspergillus*: Nearly two-thirds of the patients of ABPA show positive smear and a culture for *Aspergillus*, and positive culture with *Aspergillus* species in sputum has been reported in 58% cases of ABPA.[10]

- Pulmonary function test is neither sensitive nor specific and does not help to define the extent of disease or exclude it, during remission patient may have normal lung function even in the presence of bronchiectasis. The status depends upon the stage at which they are performed. Acute and chronic pulmonary function changes in ABPA have been described. In acute episodes, obstructive changes are observed, while during irreversible stages with bronchiectasis and fibrosis, restrictive changes are found. In chronic cases, diffusion capacity is reduced.

Classical Diagnostic Criteria for ABPA

Major Criteria

The major criteria include bronchial asthma, radiological pulmonary infiltrates, immediate skin test positivity to *A. fumigatus* antigens, elevated total serum IgE, precipitating antibodies against *A. fumigatus* antigens, peripheral blood eosinophilia, elevated serum IgE and IgG against *A. fumigatus,* and central/proximal bronchiectasis with normal tapering of distal bronchi.[5]

Minor Criteria

The minor criteria include a history of expectorating golden brown plugs in sputum, positive sputum smear and culture for *Aspergillus* species, and late type III (Arthus) skin reactivity to *A. fumigatus.*

The presence of six of eight major criteria makes the diagnosis almost certain.

Latest criteria do not differentiate between major and minor, the eight diagnostic criteria laid down to detect ABPA suggested by Greenberger 1997[7] are as follows:

Asthma (mild or severe) or cystic fibrosis, immediate cutaneous reactivity to *Aspergillus* antigens, current or previous pulmonary infiltrates, elevated total IgE concentration (>l mg/L), precipitin antibodies to *A. fumigatus,* peripheral blood eosinophilia, elevated serum IgE and/or IgG-against *A. fumigatus,* and proximal bronchiectasis.

Staging of ABPA

Five stages of ABPA have been described according to Patterson et al. and are as follows:[7]

1. *Acute stage*: Symptomatic presenting with fever, sputum production, and symptoms of asthma. High level of serum IgE and eosinophilia, with radiological pulmonary infiltrates. Steroids are indicated to achieve remission.
2. *Remission stage*: Control of respiratory symptoms, radiological clearing, decline in IgE levels, and eosinophilia. Steroids are not required in this stage.
3. *Exacerbation stage*: Occurs when the patient presents with all features of acute stage or when there is a twofold rise in the total serum IgE levels. Radiological study shows appearance of new infiltrates. Management requires induction of remission with steroids. Maintenance steroids are not necessary.
4. *Steroid-dependent asthma*: Patient is symptomatic suffering from asthma and needs long-term steroids. Lab investigations present a rise in serum IgE. Radiology is variable.
5. *Fibrosis*: Dyspnea and other manifestations of fibrotic lung disease with irreversible obstructive and/or restrictive pulmonary functions are present, serum IgE level is variable. High-IgE levels may reflect continued activity. Radiological study shows pulmonary fibrosis. Management requires long-term steroid that may not reverse these changes completely. Cor pulmonale, respiratory failure, and death may occur.

TREATMENT

Oral corticosteroid remains the cornerstone for the treatment of ABPA.[56] The goal of therapy is to achieve symptom resolution, clearance of radiographic infiltrates, and establishment of a stable baseline serum level of total IgE. There are two dose schedules of oral glucocorticoid therapy, low dose and high dose. In low-dose oral glucocorticoid therapy, prednisolone 0.5 mg/kg/day is given for 2 weeks, then on alternate days for 6–8 weeks and then tapered 5–10 mg every 2 weeks, and then discontinued. In high-dose glucocorticoid therapy, prednisolone 0.75 mg/kg is given for 6 weeks, followed by 0.5 mg/kg for 6 weeks, and then tapered 5 mg every 6 weeks to continue for a total of at least 6–12 months. Higher dose and prolonged use of steroids are associated with better outcome.[57] During the acute episode, usual starting dose of prednisolone is 0.5 mg/kg daily for 2 weeks, then reduced to an alternate-day regime for 2–3 months, after that it should be tapered off in the next 2–3 months. Repeat chest X-ray in 1 month should demonstrate clearing of the infiltrates. The total serum IgE level also regresses along with the infiltrates. The failure of the total serum IgE level to decrease suggests continuation of active disease and requires additional corticosteroids.

Following successful infiltrate clearing, there is a reduction in total serum IgE and remission of the patient's symptoms. The total serum IgE level, chest X-ray, and absolute eosinophil count should then be followed at 6 to 8-week intervals regularly. The goal of glucocorticoid therapy is not normalization of total serum IgE but reduction in total serum IgE by 35–50% from baseline that defines remission by 6 weeks. Serial total serum IgE levels are important for follow-up care.[51] A sudden doubling of total serum IgE levels over baseline usually heralds activity of diseases. Such activity can be aborted or even prevented with increased dose of prednisone at the time when the elevated level of IgE is noted.

Patients who have remission of ABPA may discontinue prednisone. The remission may last for years or may be permanent. In patients with recurrent flares of ABPA or in those with severe persistent asthma, long-term corticosteroid therapy may be necessary to control their symptoms. Patients in the fibrotic stage of ABPA may have increased sputum volume as a result of infection. Measures such as postural drainage and antibiotics may be useful, but with deterioration, exercise tolerance decreases and oxygen therapy may be needed.

Optimization of baseline asthma therapy is essential. In addition, prophylactic measures should be instituted when indicated to prevent the adverse effects of long-term corticosteroid treatment such as osteoporosis. Thus, patients who will be taking prednisolone for more than 2–3 months should be considered for bone mineral density analysis to direct commencement of calcium/vitamin D supplementation with or without bisphosphonates.[58]

Role of Anti-fungal Drugs

Pooled analysis showed that itraconazole could significantly decrease IgE levels by >25% when compared to placebo, and showed reduction in steroid dose by ≥50%, increase in exercise tolerance by ≥25%, improvement of ≥25% in results of spirometry, resolution of pulmonary opacities, but failed to reach statistical significance, and did not cause significant improvement in lung function. Itraconazole modified the immunologic activation associated with ABPA and improved the clinical outcome at least over the period of 16 weeks. A decline in exacerbation rates was also seen. At present, itraconazole should be limited in cases, where oral steroids are contraindicated or refused by patients. In patients requiring high doses of oral steroid, itraconazole may allow reduction in steroid doses, but should not replace the need of steroid; the major concern being no long-term trials and adrenal suppression with itraconazole. Thus, long-term trials are required before firm recommendation can be made for the use of itraconazole in ABPA. In a recent randomized trial of itraconazole vs prednisolone in acute-stage ABPA, it was found that oral glucocorticoids were more effective than itraconazole monotherapy in producing treatment response in patients with acute-stage ABPA complicating asthma. However, time to first exacerbation and the number of subjects experiencing exacerbation were similar in both groups. An important concern with azole therapy is emerging risk of azole-resistant *Aspergillus* species.[59] The use of omalizumab in ABPA has been associated with improvement in symptoms, reduction in exacerbations and asthma hospitalizations, improvement in lung function, and reduction in dose of oral steroids.[51] Recently, voriconazole has also been tried in the treatment of ABPA.[56-63]

CONCLUSION

Presently, ABPA is one of the important emerging immunologically mediated respiratory diseases, commonly present in patients of asthma. It should be highly suspected in patients presenting with the history of asthma, peripheral blood eosinophilia, recurrent pneumonia, or transient (fleeting) pulmonary infiltrates mimicking pulmonary tuberculosis. In such suspected patients, detailed evaluations are needed to prove the diagnosis. Early diagnosis and proper treatment may alter the prognosis of the disease and further prevent end-stage lung fibrosis.

REFERENCES

1. Binder RE, Falling LJ, Pugatch RD, et al. Chronic necrotizing pulmonary aspergillosis: a discrete clinical entity. Medicine. 1982;61:109-24.
2. Shah A, Panjabi C. Allergic bronchopulmonary aspergillosis: a perplexing clinical entity. Allergy Asthma Immunol Res. 2016;8:282-97.
3. Greenberger FA, Patterson R. Diagnosis and management of allergic bronchopulmonary aspergillosis. Ann Allergy. 1986;56:444-8.
4. Greenberger PA. Allergic bronchopulmonary aspergillosis. J Allergy Clin Immunol. 2002;110:685-92.
5. Rosenberg M, Patterson R, Mintzer R, et al. Clinical and immunologic criteria for the diagnosis of allergic bronchopulmonary aspergillosis. Ann Intern Med. 1977;86:405-14.
6. Greenberger PA, Patterson R, Ghory A, et al. Late sequelae of allergic bronchopulmonary aspergillosis. J Allergy Clin Immunol. 1980;66:327-35.

7. Patterson R, Greenberger PA, Radin RC, Roberts M. Allergic bronchopulmonary aspergillosis: staging as an aid to management. Ann Intern Med. 1982;96:286-91.
8. Patterson R, Greenberger PA, Halwig JM, et al. Allergic bronchopulmonary aspergillosis: natural history and classification of early disease by serologic and roentgenographic studies. Arch Intern Med. 1986;146: 916-8.
9. Patterson R, Greenberger PA, Lee TM, et al. Prolonged evaluation of patients with corticosteroid-dependent asthma stage of allergic bronchopulmonary aspergillosis. J Allergy Clin Immunol. 1987;80:663-8.
10. Greenberger PA, Patterson R. Allergic bronchopulmonary aspergillosis and the evaluation of the patient with asthma. J Allergy Clin Immunol. 1988;81:646-50.
11. Greenberger PA, Miller TP, Roberts M, Smith LL. Allergic bronchopulmonary aspergillosis in patients with and without evidence of bronchiectasis. Ann Allergy. 1993;70:333-8.
12. Greenberger PA. Clinical aspects of allergic broncho-pulmonary aspergillosis. Front Biosci. 2003;8:S119-27.
13. Rajan TV. The Gell-Coombs classification of hypersensitivity reactions: a re-interpretation. Trends Immunol. 2003;24: 376-9.
14. Geha RS, Sampson HA, Askenase PW, et al. Allergy and hypersensitivity. In: Janeway CA, Travers P, Walport M, et al. eds. Immunobiology. New York, NY: Garland; 2001:517-56.
15. Hinson KFW, Moon AJ, Plummer NS. Bronchopulmonary aspergillosis—a review and report of eight new cases. Thorax. 1952;7:317-33.
16. Shah JR. Allergic bronchopulmonary aspergillosis. J Assoc Physicians India. 1971;19:835-41.
17. Vernarske DL, deShazo RD. Sinobronchial allergic mycosis. The SAM syndrome. Chest. 2002;121:1670-76.
18. Hoshino H, Tagaki S, Kon H, et al. Allergic bronchopulmonary aspergillosis due to *A. Niger* without bronchial asthma. Respiration. 1999;66:369-72.
19. Agarwal R. Severe asthma and fungal sensitization. Curr Allergy Asthma Rep. 2011;11:403-13.
20. Mc-Carthy DS, Pepys J. Allergic bronchopulmonary aspergillosis, clinical immunology and clinical features. Clin Allergy. 1971;1:261-86.
21. Handerson AH, English MP, Vecht RJ. Pulmonary aspergillosis: a survey of its occurrence in patients with chronic lung disease and a discussion of the significance of diagnostic tests. Thorax. 1968;23:513-18.
22. Schwartz HJ, Greenberger PA. The prevalence of allergic bronchopulmonary aspergillosis in patients with asthma. Determined by serologic and radiologic criteria in patients at risk. J Lab Clin Med. 1991;117:138-42.
23. Eaton T, Garrett J, Milne D, et al. Allergic bronchopulmonary aspergillosis in the asthma clinic: a prospective evaluation of CT in the diagnostic algorithm. Chest. 2000;118:66-72.
24. Adiseshan N, Simpou J, Gandevia B. The association of asthma with aspergillus and other fungi. Aust N Z J Med. 1971;1:385-91.
25. Donnelly SC, McLaughlin H, Bredin CP. Period prevalence of allergic bronchopulmonary mycosis in a regional hospital outpatient population in Ireland 1985-1988. Irish J Med Sci. 1991;160:288-90.
26. Al-Mobeireek AF, Gad El-Rab MO, Al-Hedaithy SSA, et al. Allergic bronchopulmonary mycosis in patients with asthma: period prevalence at a university hospital in Saudia Arabia. Respir Med. 2001:95:341-47.
27. Maurya V, Gugani HC, Sarma PU, et al. Sensitization to aspergillus antigens and occurrence of allergic bronchopulmonary aspergillosis in patients with asthma. Chest. 2005;127:1252-59.
28. Prasad R, Garg R, Sanjay, Dixit, R. A study on prevalence of allergic bronchopulmonary aspergillosis in patients of bronchial asthma. Internet J Pulm Med. 2008;9.
29. Khan ZU, Sandhu RS, Randhawa HS, et al. Allergic bronchopulmonary aspergillosis—a study of 46 cases with special reference to laboratory aspects. Scand J Respir Dis. 1976;57:73-87.
30. Chetty A, Bhargava S, Jain RK. Allergic bronchopulmonary aspergillosis in Indian children with bronchial asthma. Ann Allergy. 1985;54:46-9.
31. Shah A, Bhagat R, Panchal N, et al. Allergic broncho-pulmonary aspergillosis with middle lobe syndrome and allergic aspergillus sinusitis. Eur Respir J. 1993;6:917-8.
32. Behera D, Guieria R, Jindal SK, et al. Allergic broncho-pulmonary aspergillosis—a retrospective study of 35 cases. Indian J Chest Dis Allied Sci. 1994;36:173-9.
33. Agarwal R, Gupta D, Aggarwal AN, et al. Allergic bronchopulmonary aspergillosis: lessons from 126 patients attending a chest clinic in north India. Chest. 2006;130: 442-8.
34. Nath A, Khan A, Hashim Z, Patra JK. Prevalence of Aspergillus hypersensitivity and allergic bronchopulmonary aspergillosis in patients with bronchial asthma at a tertiary care center in North India. Lung India. 2017;34:150-4.
35. Agarwal R, Gupta D, Aggarwal AN, et al. Clinical significance of hyperattenuating mucoid impaction in allergic bronchopulmonary aspergillosis: an analysis of 155 patients. Chest. 2007;132:1183-90.
36. Attapattu MC. Allergic bronchopulmonary aspergillosis in a chronic asthmatic. Ceylon Med J. 1983;28:251-3.
37. Geha RS, Sampson HA, Askenase PW, et al. Allergy and hypersensitivity. In: Janeway CA, Travers P, Walport M, et al. eds. Immunobiology. New York, NY: Garland; 2001; 517-56.
38. Safirstein BH, D Souza MF, Simon G, et al. Five year follow-up of bronchopulmonary aspergillosis. Am Rev Respir Dis. 1973;108:450-59.
39. Prasad R, Garg R, Sanjay, Shukla AD. Allergic broncho-pulmonary aspergillosis: a review of 42 patients from a tertiary care center in India. Lung India. 2009;26:38-40s.
40. McCarthy DS, Simon G, Hargreave FE. The radiological appearances in allergic bronchopulmonary aspergillosis. Clin Radiol. 1970;21:366-75.
41. Goldberg B. Radiological appearance in pulmonary aspergillosis. Clin Radiol. 1962;13:106.
42. Prasad R, Garg R, Sanjay. Walking pneumonia in a patient of bronchial asthma: a clue to the diagnosis of allergic bronchopulmonary aspergillosis. Pulmon. 2007;9:120-3.

43. Menon MPS, Das AK. Allergic bronchopulmonary aspergillosis (Radiological aspect). Ind J Chest Dis. 1977; 19:157-69.
44. Rickettl AI, Greenberger PA, Glassroth J. Spontaneous pneumothorax in allergic bronchopulmonary aspergillosis. Arch Intern Med. 1984;144:151-2.
45. Ellis RH. Total collapse of the lung in aspergillosis. Thorax. 1965;20:118-23.
46. Ward S, Heyneman L, Lee MJ, et al. Accuracy of CT in the diagnosis of allergic bronchopulmonary aspergillosis in asthmatic patients. Am J Roentgenol. 1999;173:937-42.
47. Neeld D, Goodman LR, Gurney JW, et al. Computerized tomography in the evaluation of allergic bronchopulmonary aspergillosis. Am Rev Respir Dis. 1990;142:1200-5.
48. Webb WR, Muller NL, Naidich DP, ed. High-resolution CT of the Lung, 2nd ed. New York, NY: Lippincot-Raven Publishers; 1996: 234-41.
49. Scadding J. The bronchi in allergic aspergillosis. Scand J Respir Dis. 1967;48:372-77.
50. Kumar R. Mild, moderate, and severe forms of allergic bronchopulmonary aspergillosis: a clinical and serologic evaluation. Chest. 2003;124:890-2.
51. Agarwal R, Chakrabarti A, Shah A, et al. Allergic bronchopulmonary aspergillosis: review of literature and proposal of new diagnostic and classification criteria. Clin Exp Allergy. 2013;43:850-73.
52. Greenberger PA. Allergic bronchopulmonary aspergillosis and funguses. Clin Chest Med. 1988;9:599-608.
53. Wang JLF, Patterson R, Rosenberg M, et al. Serum IgE and IgG antibody activity against *Aspergillus fumigatus* as a diagnostic aid in allergic bronchopulmonary aspergillosis. Am Rev Respir Dis. 1978;117:917-27.
54. lmbeau SA, Nichols D, Flaherty D, et al. Relationships between prednisolone therapy, disease activity, and the total IgE level in allergic bronchopulmonary aspergillosis. J Allergy Clin lmmunol. 1978;62:91-5.
55. Malo J, Hawkins R, Pepys J. Studies in chronic allergic bronchopulmonary aspergillosis: 1. Clinical and physiological findings. Thorax. 1977;32:254-61.
56. Fink JN. Therapy of allergic bronchopulmonary aspergillosis. Indian J Chest Dis Allied Sci. 2000;42:221-4.
57. Agarwal R. Allergic bronchopulmonary aspergillosis. Chest. 2009;135;805-26.
58. American College of Rheumatology Task Force on osteoporosis Guidelines. Recommendations for the prevention and treatment of glucocorticoid-induced osteoporosis. Arthritis Rheum. 1996;39:1791-801.
59. Tucker RM, Haq Y, Denning DW, Stevens DA. Adverse events associated with itraconazole in 189 patients on chronic therapy. J Antimicrob Chemother. 1990;26:561-6.
60. Agarwal R, Dhooria S, Sehgal IS, et al. A randomised trial of itraconazole vs prednisolone in acute-stage allergic bronchopulmonary aspergillosis complicating asthma. Chest. 2018;153:656-64.
61. Mulliez P, Croxo C, Roy-Saint Georges F, et al. Allergic bronchopulmonary aspergillosis treated with voriconazole. Rev Mal Respir. 2006;23:93-4.
62. Bandres Gimeno R, Munoz Martinez MJ. Prolonged therapeutic response to voriconazole in a case of allergic bronchopulmonary aspergillosis. Arch Bronconeumol. 2007;43:49-51.
63. Erwin GE, Fitzgerald JE. Case report: allergic bronchopulmonary aspergillosis and allergic fungal sinusitis successfully treated with voriconazole. J Asthma. 2007;44:891-5.

CHAPTER 47

Allergic *Aspergillus* Sinusitis

Ashok Shah

INTRODUCTION

Allergic fungal diseases are mainly caused by three main phyla: (1) *Ascomycota,* (2) *Basidiomycota*, and (3) *Zygomycota*. The genus *Aspergillus* belongs to the *Ascomycota* phylum.[1] It is a universal mold, causing disease, both in the healthy and immunocompromised, with diverse clinical manifestations and pathology. Three main forms: allergic aspergillosis, invasive disease and saprophytic colonization have been well identified.[2] Most commonly acquired through the inhalational route, it lodges in the airways, both upper and lower, to cause an array of respiratory disorders (Box 47.1). Allergic bronchopulmonary aspergillosis (ABPA), predominantly occurring in asthmatics, was first described by Hinson and colleagues[3] in 1952. Allergic *Aspergillus* sinusitis (AAS) is a more recently described entity, and it is known for its clinicopathological similarity to ABPA. Indeed, several cases of concomitant ABPA and AAS have been described,[4-15] and the term sinobronchial allergic mycosis (SAM) syndrome[11] has been proposed as fungi other than *Aspergillus* have been implicated.

BOX 47.1: *Aspergillus*-related respiratory disorders.[1]

Allergic aspergillosis
IgE-mediated asthma
Allergic bronchopulmonary aspergillosis
Allergic *Aspergillus* sinusitis
Hypersensitivity pneumonitis
Saprophytic colonization
Aspergilloma
Invasive disease
Invasive disseminated aspergillosis
Chronic necrotizing pneumonia

Fungal diseases of the nose and sinuses can be invasive or noninvasive (Box 47.2).[16] In a descriptive epidemiological study from rural north India, the prevalence of chronic fungal rhinosinusitis was found to be 0.11%. Of the patients with chronic fungal rhinosinusitis, allergic fungal rhinosinusitis constituted more than half and *Aspergillus flavus* was the predominant (97.6%) fungus in all types of chronic fungal rhinosinusitis.[17] In another study from south India, fungal rhinosinusitis was diagnosed in 44% of patients with chronic rhinosinusitis with allergic form being the most common.[18]

Allergic fungal sinusitis (AFS) is now known as a distinct clinical entity, the central features being chronic rhinosinusitis and the presence of "allergic mucin": eosinophil-rich mucus with a peanut butter consistency observed during surgery.[19] Safirstein,[20] in 1976, described a case of ABPA with nasal polyposis and a history of passage of hard nasal plugs. Few years later, Millar and colleagues[21] described the first case of allergic aspergillosis of the maxillary sinuses. This condition subsequently came to be known as AAS.[22] When fungi other than *Aspergillus* are involved, it is known as AFS.[23]

Similarities to ABPA were noticed and a set of diagnostic criteria evolved. We have reported that one-fourth of the patients with perennial rhinitis had positive skin reactivity to *Aspergillus* antigens.[24] Since rhinitis

BOX 47.2: Fungal rhinosinusitis disorders.[15]

Noninvasive fungal rhinosinusitis disorders
Sinus mycetoma
Allergic fungal sinusitis
Invasive infectious diseases
Acute (fulminant) invasive fungal sinusitis
Chronic invasive fungal sinusitis
Granulomatous invasive fungal sinusitis

is an important predisposing factor for sinusitis, these patients could possibly be at a greater risk of developing AAS. Fungi other than *Aspergillus* such as *Alternaria, Curvularia, Bipolaris, Exserohilum, Drechslera,* and *Cladosporium* were implicated.[25-28] About 5-10% of patients with chronic rhinosinusitis are estimated to be suffering from AFS.[29-31]

CLINICAL FEATURES

It usually affects people of younger age group.[32] The presentation is generally subtle, and patients may give a history of rhinorrhea, sneezing, nasal blockage, passage of nasal plugs, and asthma. Nasal polyps and crusts can be found on physical examination, causing gradual obstruction of the ostia leading to accumulation of allergic mucin in the closed spaces of the sinuses. The expanding mass may cause facial dysmorphism, sometimes so slowly as to even escape being noticed until at a later stage. It can erode into the sinus walls to extend into the adjacent spaces such as the orbit, causing proptosis and sometimes even loss of vision.[33] A history of previous surgeries, often several in number, for recurrent sinusitis is common. Superimposed bacterial infection may lead to pain.[34] Some may complain of post-nasal drip or frontal headache. Patients with a history of asthma or those with chest symptoms should be carefully evaluated for ABPA.

In a recent study from India, it was found that allergic fungal rhinosinusitis was more aggressive in children with increased fungal load as compared to adults. Moreover, it was less responsive to treatment with higher recurrence rates in children.[35]

DIAGNOSTIC CRITERIA

A set of criteria is required to make a diagnosis of AAS. This includes radiological and histopathological features, as well as demonstration of fungal elements obtained from the sinus (Box 47.3).[36,37] Histopathological confirmation from the inspissated mucus is a sine qua non for the diagnosis of AAS, and "allergic mucin" is the characteristic nasal pathologic material. It comprises eosinophils, Charcot-Leyden crystals, cellular debris, and scattered fungal hyphae.[38] Diabetics and immunocompromised are excluded from the diagnosis and so are patients with invasive fungal disease. Other laboratory features, akin to those in ABPA, help with making a diagnosis and include elevated total IgE, fungal-specific IgE and IgG, cutaneous hypersensitivity to *Aspergillus* antigens. Precipitating antibodies to *Aspergillus* antigens and peripheral blood eosinophilia may also be seen.[38]

BOX 47.3: Diagnostic criteria for AAS.[31,32]

Sinusitis of one or more paranasal sinus on X-ray film

Necrosed amorphous tissue along with edematous polyps infiltrated with eosinophils on histopathological evaluation of material from the sinus

Demonstration of fungal elements in nasal discharge or in material obtained at the time of surgery by stain or culture

Absence of diabetes, previous or subsequent immunodeficiency disease, and treatment with immunosuppressive drugs

Absence of invasive fungal disease at the time of diagnosis or subsequently

Other Features

Peripheral blood eosinophilia

Type I and type III cutaneous hypersensitivity to *Aspergillus*

Precipitating antibodies to *Aspergillus* antigens

Elevated total as well as *Aspergillus*-specific IgE levels

Radiological Features

The demonstration of sinusitis on one or more paranasal sinuses on plain sinus roentgenograms is one of the diagnostic criteria for AAS. The most common manifestation is haziness of one or more sinuses. Often, multiple sinuses are opacified. Bilateral involvement has been observed in up to 83% of cases reported.[10,39] When sequential time-related studies were performed, progressive involvement of multiple sinuses was the rule.[30] Other manifestations include mucosal thickening and varying degrees of bony sclerosis and/or destruction. These findings are, however, nonspecific as they may also be seen in chronic sinusitis or malignancy of the paranasal sinuses.

However, CT of the paranasal sinuses has now emerged as the gold standard for evaluation of AFS. The characteristic feature is the presence of heterogeneous densities, signifying opacification of the sinuses, with serpiginous areas of increased attenuation on noncontrast scans (Fig. 47.1).[30,40] It is opined that metallic elements such as iron and manganese, and also salts of calcium in the allergic mucin cause such hyperdense areas.[40] The serpiginous pattern of the central area of high attenuation has also been described as "star-filled sky" or "ground glass" patterns.[41] The extent of disease is better visualized on CT, and the features evaluated include bony erosion and intracranial involvement. It is important to determine

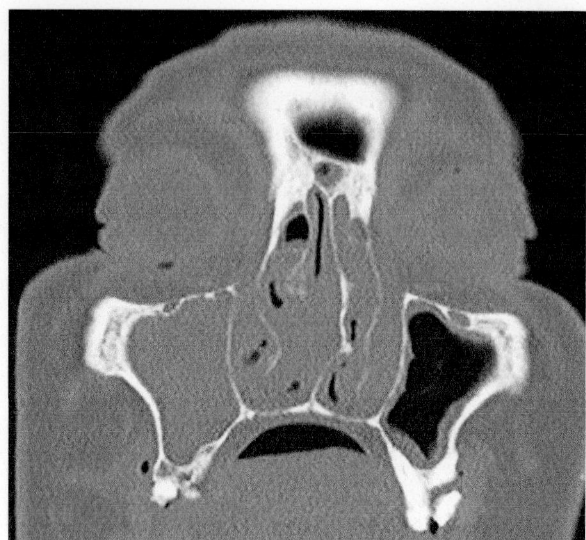

Fig. 47.1: Noncontrast computed tomography of the paranasal sinuses of a 35-year-old female with allergic *Aspergillus* sinusitis showing complete opacification of right maxillary, and posterior ethmoidal sinuses with intranasal polyps and erosion of inferior and middle turbinates.

these prior to definitive surgery. Limited bony destruction has been noted in up to 80% of patients with AFS, the exact mechanism of which is not clear.[30,42,43] This is either due to pressure necrosis causing reabsorption of the bone or bone-destroying enzymes produced by the fungus. Inflammatory mediators such as major basic protein produced by the allergic response could also be responsible.[29] This is in contrast to invasive fungal aspergillosis wherein bone destruction is evident.[16] Chronic disease of the sinuses with desiccated secretions often results in thickening and sclerosis of the adjacent sinus walls, while the presence of expansion and thinning of the sinus walls is suggestive of AFS.[40] CT also helps in distinguishing AFS from other forms of fungal sinusitis, which include acute (fulminant) invasive fungal sinusitis, chronic/indolent fungal sinusitis, and sinus mycetoma.[16,44,45] Sinus mycetoma appears as a focal round area of increased attenuation that is usually centered within a diseased maxillary sinus. Aggressive bone erosion with extension of disease into the adjacent soft tissues is a feature of acute invasive fungal sinusitis. Unlike AFS, sinus expansion and sinus wall modeling is uncommon in acute invasive fungal sinusitis.

Magnetic resonance imaging (MRI) is now thought to be more sensitive than CT in differentiating mycotic infections of the sinuses, but it is still not considered the primary diagnostic modality.[46] Hypointense central T1 signal, central T2 signal void, and increased peripheral T1/T2 enhancement have been demonstrated, in 10 patients of AFS, by Manning and colleagues[47] to be highly specific for AFS. A combination of CT and MRI findings provides a radiographic appearance highly specific for AFS.[47] Its utility as a noninvasive and alternative method for the diagnosis of AAS needs to be evaluated.

Chest X-ray should be done for all cases of AAS seeking evidence for involvement of the lower airways. CT scan of the chest should be done in all patients with chest symptoms or a history of asthma to rule out concomitant ABPA.

TREATMENT

Combined surgery and oral corticosteroids is required to control AFS. Surgery alone has seldom proved to be curative, and often patients have to undergo repeat procedures as recurrence is high.[10] However, it proves to be beneficial in providing drainage and aeration to the sinus mucosa, and also helps in reducing fungal load.

Based on the immunopathological similarity of AAS with ABPA, treatment patterns for the former have been formulated on existing medical therapies for the latter. Oral prednisolone, given for long durations, has met with considerable success in prolonging recurrence after sinus surgery.[48] The optimal duration of treatment is yet to be evaluated. Following the approach for ABPA, a safe option would be to start oral prednisone 0.5 mg/kg/day for 1–2 weeks, followed by alternate-day therapy for 6–8 weeks. It should then be tapered slowly over the next few months to a minimal dose necessary for maintenance of remission.

The adverse effects of long-term steroids are of immense concern. We recently assessed the feasibility of a biweekly prednisolone regimen in 26 patients with ABPA and found that this was as effective as alternate-day therapy in managing patients with ABPA and AAS.[49] Since oral prednisolone is often given repeatedly for long periods in these patients, a biweekly regimen would help in reducing the well-known adverse effects of long-term corticosteroid therapy.

Nasal sprays, by themselves, are not adequate to bring relief in symptoms. Antifungals, systemic and/or topical, do not seem to have a clear-cut benefit. It was presumed that antifungals, by reducing the fungal load, could reduce the antigenic stimulation and therefore the inflammatory response.[32] Their role in primary or adjunctive treatment needs to be evaluated.

REFERENCES

1. Rodrigues J, Caruthers C, Azmeh R, et al. The spectrum of allergic fungal diseases of the upper and lower airways. Expert Rev Clin Immunol. 2016;12:531-50.
2. Shah A. Allergic bronchopulmonary aspergillosis. Indian J Chest Dis Allied Sci. 1998;40:41-54.
3. Hinson KFW, Moon AJ, Plummer NS. Bronchopulmonary aspergillosis: a review and report of eight new cases. Thorax. 1952;7:317-33.
4. Sher TH, Schwartz HJ. Allergic *Aspergillus* sinusitis with concurrent allergic bronchopulmonary *Aspergillus*: report of a case. J Allergy Clin Immunol. 1988;81:844-6.
5. Shah A, Khan ZU, Chaturvedi S, et al. Concomitant allergic *Aspergillus* sinusitis and allergic bronchopulmonary aspergillosis associated with familial occurrence of allergic bronchopulmonary aspergillosis. Ann Allergy. 1990;64: 507-12.
6. Schwartz HJ, Witt WJ, Sher TH. Allergic bronchopulmonary aspergillosis and allergic aspergillus sinusitis: case report. Ann Allergy. 1992;69:447-8.
7. Shah A, Bhagat R, Panchal N, et al. Allergic broncho-pulmonary aspergillosis with middle lobe syndrome and allergic *Aspergillus* sinusitis. Eur Respir J. 1993;6:917-8.
8. Bhagat R, Shah A, Jaggi OP, Khan ZU. Concomitant allergic bronchopulmonary aspergillosis and allergic *Aspergillus* sinusitis with an operated aspergilloma. J Allergy Clin Immunol. 1993;91:1094-6.
9. Schwartz HJ. Allergic fungal sinusitis: experience in an ambulatory allergy practice. Ann Allergy Asthma Immunol. 1996;77:500-2.
10. Shah A, Panchal N, Agarwal AK. Concomitant allergic bronchopulmonary aspergillosis and allergic *Aspergillus* sinusitis: a review of an uncommon association. Clin Exp Allergy. 2001;31:1896-905.
11. Venarske DL, deShazo RD. Sinobronchial allergic mycosis: the SAM syndrome. Chest. 2002;121:1670-6.
12. Shah A, Panjabi C. Contemporaneous occurrence of allergic bronchopulmonary aspergillosis, allergic *Aspergillus* sinusitis and aspergilloma. Ann Allergy Asthma Immunol. 2006;96:874-8.
13. Erwin GE, Fitzgerald JE. Case report: allergic bronchopulmonary aspergillosis and allergic fungal sinusitis successfully treated with voriconazole. J Asthma. 2007;44:891-5.
14. Braun JJ, Pauli G, Schultz P, et al. Allergic fungal sinusitis associated with allergic bronchopulmonary aspergillosis: an uncommon sinobronchial allergic mycosis. Am J Rhinol. 2007;21:412-6.
15. Prasad R, Garg R, Dua R. Concomitant allergic bronchopulmonary aspergillosis and allergic *Aspergillus* sinusitis. Indian J Med Sci. 2007;61:532-4.
16. deShazo RD, Chapin K, Swain RE. Fungal sinusitis. N Engl J Med. 1997;337:254-9.
17. Chakrabarti A, Rudramurthy SM, Panda N, et al. Epidemiology of chronic fungal rhinosinusitis in rural India. Mycoses. 2015;58:294-302.
18. Krishnan KU, Agatha D, Selvi R. Fungal rhinosinusitis: a clinicomycological perspective. Indian J Med Microbiol. 2015;33:120-4.
19. Katzenstein AL, Sale SR, Greenberger PA. Pathologic findings in allergic aspergillus sinusitis: a newly recognized form of sinusitis. Am J Surg Pathol. 1983;7:439-43.
20. Safirstein BH. Allergic bronchopulmonary aspergillosis with obstruction of the upper respiratory tract. Chest. 1976;70:788-90.
21. Millar JW, Johnston A, Lamb D. Allergic aspergillosis of the maxillary sinuses (Abstract). Thorax. 1981;36:710.
22. Katzenstin A, Greenberger P, Sale S. Allergic aspergillus sinusitis: a newly recognized form of sinusitis. J Allergy Clin Immunol. 1983;72:89-93.
23. Robson J, Hogan P, Benn R, Gatenby PA. Allergic fungal sinusitis presenting as a paranasal sinus tumor. Aust N Z J Med. 1989;19:351-3.
24. Shah A, Sircar M. Sensitization to *Aspergillus* antigens in perennial rhinitis. Asian Pac J Allergy Immunol. 1991; 9:137-9.
25. Corey JP, Delsupehe KG, Ferguson BJ. Allergic fungal sinusitis: allergic, infectious, or both? Otolaryngol Head Neck Surg. 1995;113:110-9.
26. Manning SC, Schaefer SD, Close LG, Vuitch F. Culture-positive allergic fungal sinusitis. Arch Otolaryngol Head Neck Surg. 1991;117:174-8.
27. Bartynski JM, McCaffrey TV, Frigas E. Allergic fungal sinusitis secondary to dematiaceous fungi: *Curvularia lunata* and *Alternaria*. Otolaryngol Head Neck Surg. 1990;103:32-9.
28. Schubert MS. Goetz DW. Evaluation and treatment of allergic fungal sinusitis. I. Demographics and diagnosis. J Allergy Clin Immunol. 1998;102: 387-94.
29. Corey JP. Allergic fungal sinusitis. Otolaryngol Clin North Am. 1992;25:225-30.
30. Bent J, Kuhn F. Diagnosis of allergic fungal sinusitis. Otolaryngol Head Neck Surg. 1994;111:580-8.
31. Deshpande RB, Shaukla A, Kirtane MV. Allergic fungal sinusitis: incidence and clinical and pathological features of seven cases. J Assoc Physicians India. 1995;43:98-100.
32. Panjabi C, Shah A. Allergic *Aspergillus* sinusitis and its association with allergic bronchopulmonary aspergillosis. Asia Pac Allergy. 2011;1:130-7.
33. Marple BF, Gibbs SR, Newcomer MT, Mabry RL. Allergic fungal sinusitis-induced visual loss. Am J Rhinol. 1999;13: 191-5.
34. Marple BF. Allergic fungal sinusitis. Curr Opin Otolaryngol. 1999;7:383-7.
35. Patro SK, Verma RK, Panda NK, Chakrabarti A. Understanding paediatric allergic fungal sinusitis: is it more aggressive? Int J Pediatr Otorhinolaryngol. 2015;79: 1876-80.
36. deShazo RD, Swain RE. Diagnostic criteria for allergic fungal sinusitis. J Allergy Clin Immunol. 1995;96:24-35.
37. Shah A. (Editorial). Allergic bronchopulmonary and sinus aspergillosis: the co-occurrence. Chest (India). 2001;2: 234-5.

38. Shah A, Panjabi C. Allergic bronchopulmonary aspergillosis: a perplexing clinical entity. Allergy Asthma Immunol Res. 2016;8:282-97.
39. Waxman JE, Spector JG, Sale SR, Katzenstein AL. Allergic *Aspergillus* sinusitis: concepts in diagnosis and treatment of a new clinical entity. Laryngoscope. 1987;97:261-6.
40. Mukherji SK, Figueroa RE, Ginsberg LE, et al. Allergic fungal sinusitis: CT findings. Radiology. 1998;207:417-22.
41. Houser SM, Corey JP. Allergic fungal rhinosinusitis: pathophysiology, epidemiology and diagnosis. Otolaryngol Clinics North Am. 2000;33:399-408.
42. Manning SC, Vuitch F, Weinberg AG, Brown OE. Allergic aspergillosis: a newly recognized form of fungal sinusitis in the pediatric population. Laryngoscope 1989;99:681-5.
43. Cody DT, Neel HB, Ferreiro JA, Roberts GD. Allergic fungal sinusitis: the Mayo clinic experience. Laryngoscope. 1994;104:1074-9.
44. Goldstein MF, Atkins PC, Cogen FC, et al. Allergic *Aspergillus* sinusitis. J Allergy Clin Immunol. 1985;76: 515-24.
45. Morpeth JF, Rupp NT, Dolen WK, et al. Fungal sinusitis: an update. Ann Allergy Asthma Immunol. 1996;76:128-40.
46. Shah A. Allergic bronchopulmonary and sinus aspergillosis: the roentgenologic spectrum. Front Biosci. 2003;8:e138-46.
47. Manning SC, Merkel M, Kreisel K, et al. Computed tomographic and magnetic resonance diagnosis of allergic fungal sinusitis. Laryngoscope. 1997;107:170-6.
48. Schubert MS, Goetz DW. Evaluation and treatment of allergic fungal sinusitis. II: treatment and follow-up. J Allergy Clin Immunol. 1998;102:395-402.
49. Shah A, Panjabi C. Biweekly therapy with prednisolone is effective in the management of allergic bronchopulmonary aspergillosis [abstract]. Allergy Clin Immunol Int - J World Allergy Org. 2005;Suppl. 1:113.

CHAPTER 48

Pediatric Allergic Disorders and their Management

Shally Awasthi, Shambhavi Mishra

INTRODUCTION

Allergy represents the clinical expression of IgE-mediated allergic diseases that have a familial predisposition and that manifests in hyperresponsiveness in target organs, such as lung, skin, gastrointestinal tract, and nose. The increase in allergic diseases in recent times can be attributed to changes in environmental factors (tobacco and smoke exposure, air pollution, indoor and outdoor allergens, respiratory viruses, obesity, and perhaps a decline in certain infectious diseases). The "*hygiene hypothesis*," as originally formulated by Strachan in 1989, proposes that a cause of the recent rapid rise in atopic disorders could be a lower incidence of infection in early childhood, transmitted by unhygienic contact with older siblings. This is debatable, and several new theories have been proposed to explain the rise in allergic disorder. The "***old friends***" *hypothesis* was proposed by Graham Rook in 2003 as an alternative to or refinement of the hygiene hypothesis as an explanation for the rise in allergic disease. This states that besides exposure to microorganism, exposure to other organisms, such as intestinal helminths and others can result in allergy.[1]

COMPONENTS OF AN ALLERGIC RESPONSE

Allergens

These are mostly proteins but not all proteins are allergens.[2] Proteins that are allergenic must have B-cell epitopes, which facilitate binding to IgE and T-cell epitopes that induce type 2 T-lymphocyte response. In addition, the protein must be resistant to proteolysis. Subsequent exposure to the same protein will then lead to type I hypersensitivity. This requires the protein to have an adequate size so that it is large enough to bridge adjacent IgE antibody molecules on the surface of mast cells or basophils but it should not be too large as they have to pass through mucosal surfaces to reach the antigen presenting cells (APCs). Hence, most allergens lie within the range of 10–70 kDa MW. Some carbohydrates, too, can also induce allergic responses, such as biologics. Nonprotein structures can be rendered allergic by conjugation with a protein.

T cells

T-helper cells play a major role in allergic response. T-helper type 2 cells get stimulated and multiply in numbers. These are responsible for the secretion of cytokines IL-4, IL-5, IL-9, and IL-13, which in turn are responsible for IgE synthesis, eosinophilia, and mast cell activation.

T-helper type 1 cells: As a part of allergic immunological response, there is proliferation of T helper type 1 (Th1) also. They contribute to chronicity and the effector phase in allergic disease. Due to apoptosis of epithelial cells induced by Th1, eczematous lesions are formed in atopic dermatitis (AD) and in asthma, shedding of bronchial epithelium occurs. Th1 cells secrete IFN-γ, TNF-α, and Fas ligand.

Th17 and Th22 cells link the immune response to tissue inflammation with IL17 augmenting inflammation, while IL 22 plays a protective role.

T-regulatory (Treg) cells: They have the ability to suppress the effector T cells. Patients with mutation in gene translating for Treg cells develop severe immune dysregulation. Cytokines IL-10 and TGF-β are produced by them.

Antigen-presenting Cells

Dendritic cells, Langerhans cells, monocytes, and macrophages are the APCs that present the allergens to T cells and control the type of T-cell development. Among them, dendritic cells and Langerhans cells are responsible for the sensitization phase, and monocytes and macrophages are responsible for the elicitation phase of allergy.

IgE and Eosinophils

Receptor-bound IgE molecules are present on mast cells, basophils, dendritic cells, B cells, and platelets. Mast cells and basophils receptor cross-linking leads to anaphylaxis.

Eosinophils: Eosinophils are found both in peripheral blood and tissue. Their production and maturation is activated by IL-3, IL-5, and GM-CSF. Eosinophils participate in both innate and adaptive responses. They contain dense intracellular granules that are source of inflammatory proteins. They get recruited to local allergic tissue and cause inflammation.

Mast cells: They are distributed throughout the connective tissue, where they often lie adjacent to blood vessels and beneath the epithelial surfaces. They do not circulate in blood. They contain preformed granules containing mediators (histamine, serine proteases, and proteoglycans) and also membrane-derived lipid (cyclo-oxygenase and lipo-oxygenase products of arachidonic acid), cytokine, and chemokine mediators.

Mechanism of Allergic Response

Immune responses can be classified as follows:
- Early-phase response
- Late-phase response
- Chronic allergic disease.

Atopic March

The atopic march refers to the natural history of allergic diseases as they develop during infancy and childhood. Classically, the atopic march begins with AD and progresses to IgE-mediated food allergy (FA), asthma, and allergic rhinitis (AR)[3] (Fig. 48.1).

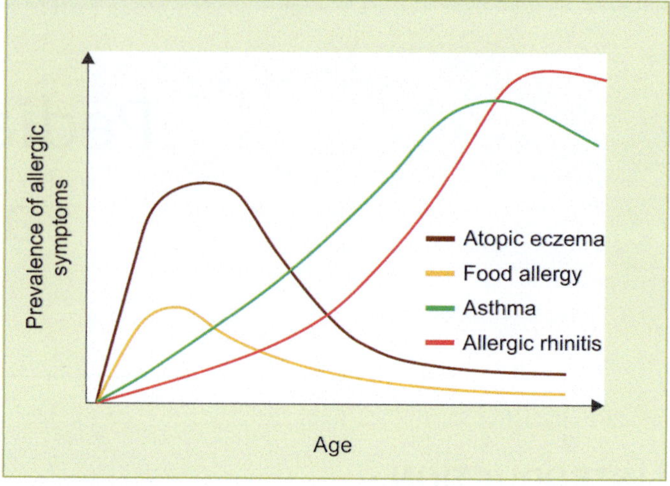

Fig. 48.1: Atopic march.
Source: Modified from Holgate S, Church MK eds. Allergy, London: Grower Medical Publishing. 1993.

Toward Diagnosis of Allergic Disorders

A complete and comprehensive history is an indispensable tool for diagnosis, especially in allergic disorders. The following points should be kept in mind while eliciting a history:
- There is high propensity of the presence of more than one allergic disorder, and hence all the symptoms must be described with their time and duration.
- A family history of allergy is common. The risk is 50%, when one parent is allergic, and 66% when both the parents are allergic.[4]
- The presence of temporal association with seasonal changes in the environment may indicate an allergic relation. It should be carefully enquired keeping in mind pollination and fungal spore dominance in air.
- The timing of symptoms or their recurrence can also be related to certain activities, such as dusting/lawn mowing/traveling/playing with pets/ingestion of certain foods.
- The symptoms can also be perennial or chronic in duration, when the indoor allergens are culprits, such as dust mites, animal dander, cockroaches, and fungi.
- The age of onset of symptoms is crucial. It helps identify potential allergens. For example, seasonal allergies develop over a long course of time after multiple cycles of sensitization.
- Equally essential is study of the environment of dwelling.

Physical Examination

General

The patient should be observed for characteristic behavior. Allergic salute, which is a horizontal crease over the bridge of the nose, is seen with AR due to persistent rubbing of the nose in upward direction. Allergic cluck is produced when tongue is placed against the palatal roof in an attempt to scratch it due to itchiness. Vigorous rubbing of eyes is observed in allergic conjunctivitis. The lips may reveal cheilitis due to drying of lips from continuous mouth breathing or repeated licking of the lips in an attempt to replenish moisture.

Systemic Examination

Respiratory: Observe the child for mouth breathing, sneezing, throat clearing, and rubbing of nose and eyes. Gastro-esophageal reflux (GER), coughing episodes, interference with feeding in infants their variation with position should be noted. Audible wheeze, tachypnea, presence of cyanosis, clubbing, and chest retractions can be present.

Local examination of the nose is crucial. In the nasal septum, turbinates, posterior pharynx, tonsils, adenoids, and nasal mucosa, the consistency of secretions must be noted. The frontal and maxillary sinuses should be palpated in older children. Ear examination to rule out otitis media is advisable.

Association of steroid side effects in chronic asthma patients may cause growth retardation, hypertension, and pulsus paradoxus, where there is a drop in systolic BP during inspiration of >10 mm Hg.

Skin: Eczematous changes in skin which in acute stage include red and itchy lesions, which later becomes dry, rough, and cracked. Blisters may accompany the acute stage that may weep. Dennie Morgan folds are infraorbital folds that are found in AD.

Ocular involvement: Excessive lacrimation, conjuctival injection, and chemosis may be noticed. The nature of discharge is ropy or stringy. Keratoconus may occur due to corneal trauma. Periorbital dermatitis is a result of rubbing of eyes. Cobblestoning of tarsal conjunctiva is present in vernal conjunctivitis.

Gastrointestinal: Poor weight gain and abdominal loss of fluids may result in dehydration in an acute episode, and GI loss of blood may cause pallor (anemia).

MANAGEMENT OF ALLERGIC DISORDERS

The overall plan can be divided as follows:

- Avoidance of allergen exposure
- Pharmacotherapy to control symptoms
- Immunotherapy.

Avoidance of Allergen Exposure

Identification of allergen requires a meticulous history taking, including elicitation of a temporal association between exposure and symptoms and, if possible, in vitro testing by skin pricks or blood test. Once identified, steps to reduce exposure are of foremost importance.

For dust mites, avoid using carpets or vacuum clean it weekly, encase pillow and mattress in allergen impermeable covers, and wash sheets and blankets weekly in hot water. Mites have been found to be killed by drowning rather than scalding and hence normal temperature soaking is all that is required.

Humidity should be not be allowed to rise above 50% as mites do not survive lower humidity. Attempts must be made to reduce objects that collect dust. Cyclonic vacuum cleaners have been found to be especially useful.[5]

Animal danders are best dealt with removal of the pet. If that is not possible, at least patient's bedroom should be kept pet free. Regular vacuuming is a must. High-efficiency particulate air filters (HEPA) can be used to reduce indoor airborne pet allergens. Pets need to be washed frequently. For example, Fel d1 produced by cat requires weekly cleaning of the pet. Cockroaches are a perennial allergen. Rat urine is source of allergy. Crevices in floor and walls must be sealed, food and water access removed, and regular extermination using baits or chemical treatment of infested areas is advisable.[5]

Molds grow in warm and humid conditions and are potent allergens. They can be kept in check by using dehumidifiers for reducing humidity to <50%. Any potential breeding place like water leaks, shower curtains, and contaminated carpets need to be cleaned or removed. Air conditioning and frequent handwashing must be observed strictly. Pollen exposure can also be dealt with similarly. Traveling in air-conditioned vehicle, avoiding lawn mowing, using masks when allergen cannot be avoided can be practiced.

Pharmacotherapy

This has been discussed in detail with respective disorders.

Immunotherapy

The use of allergen extracts for the treatment of allergic diseases was first published in the Lancet in 1911. It was discovered by Dr Leonard Noon, a British physician, and was done by subcutaneous route.[6] Allergen immunotherapy involves administering gradually increasing doses of allergens to a person with allergic disease for the purpose of reducing or eliminating the patient's adverse clinical response to subsequent natural exposure to those allergens. Earlier administered subcutaneously, now sublingual, oral, bronchial, and nasal therapies are available. Epicutaneous and intralymphatic therapies are under investigation. FDA has currently approved sublingual immunotherapy only.[7]

The disorders for which immunotherapy is currently used are AR, asthma, and insect venom hypersensitivity. The evidence for use of immunotherapy in other allergic disorders is lacking. A prerequisite for immunotherapy is finding evidence for sensitivity of patients to the particular allergen by a positive skin prick test or an in vitro test demonstrating an increased level of allergen-specific IgE. The same has to be verified by a history of allergic reaction in response to the allergen.

The therapy is not recommended for children <5 years of age because of increased risk of systemic reactions, difficulty in interpretation of an adverse event, and anaphylaxis management demanding expertise.[8] Cost consideration and compliance should be discussed before commencing therapy. Venom immunotherapy (VIT) is used in those that have the history of severe allergic reactions to animal sting, such as bee sting. VIT would gradually desensitize the patient and reduce response to animal bite/sting. In children <16 years of age, VIT is indicated for any systemic reaction, but not isolated skin reaction. In children >16 years of age, VIT is indicated for any systemic reaction as well as for even localized skin reaction.[7]

Contraindications

Autoimmune disorders, allergic bronchopulmonary aspergillosis, hypersensitivity pneumonitis, patients on β-blocker therapy, and ACE Inhibitor therapy, severe psychiatric disturbance, or any condition that impairs the ability to survive an allergic reaction. Pregnancy is a contraindication as well for initiation of therapy and if a pregnant adolescence is already on therapy then an increase in the dose of allergen, however, maintenance dose can be continued.[8]

Allergen Extracts

Allergen extracts need proper refrigeration. The practice of mixing numerous allergens into one mixture is unwise. Allergen extracts from cockroaches, dust mites, and molds should not be mixed with those from tree, grass, and weed pollens as the former contain proteases that may degrade other allergens.[7]

Adverse Effects

The most important concern with immunotherapy is its potential to cause severe or even fatal systemic reactions. This concern was so great that the practice of immunotherapy was virtually abandoned in the UK in the 1980s.[9] Risk factors identified include previous systemic reactions, a high degree of sensitivity, the use of newly prepared vaccines, administration error, administration during pollen season, hyperthyroidism, symptomatic asthma at the time of injection, and the concomitant use of β-blockers.[8]

Allergoids

The concept of allergoid was developed in the 1970s as an answer to the question of safety profile of immunotherapy. It is an allergen derivative for which the residual allergic reactogenicity relative to the natural allergen has been significantly reduced, while the original antigenic profile (both immunogenic and reactogenic) has been retained to a high degree and hence can be used at high doses .They have less reactive B-cell epitopes, which bind to IgE. They are prepared by using glutaraldehyde, formaldehyde for chemical modification of the allergen extracts, or by carbamylation. They have been found effective against house dust mites, grass pollen, and birch pollen. Compared to natural extracts which require 4–6 months of treatment for desensitization, allergoids updosing is completed in 4–8 weeks.[10]

Principles of Immunotherapy[7]

The dose of allergen extract is gradually increased until the dose of 4–12 μg of each allergen in the extract is reached.

- The dosing is initially done at a 5–10-day interval and in the case of hypersensitive patients, the schedule is more gradual. In about a 5–6-month time of weekly administration of doses, maintenance level is reached.
- A serious reaction to the previous dose warrants a dose reduction.
- When a fresh vial of allergen extract is being used, dose should be reduced by 25–75%, since potency is time dependent.
- Once the maintenance dosage level is reached, the inter-dosage interval is increased from several weeks to months.
- The patient should be observed for 30 min after the injection. A self-injectable epinephrine is advisable.
- The current recommendation for the course of immunotherapy is 3–5 years.

- No improvement after 1 year of immunotherapy is a reliable evidence for discontinuation of therapy.
- In VIT, it may need to be continued lifelong if an anaphylactic event following insect sting was present.
- In the case of relapse, resumption of therapy is expected to fetch positive results.

Rush immunotherapy: It refers to administration of multiple injections in a single day to reach maintenance dose more rapidly. The patients are pretreated with corticosteroids and antihistamines. Omalizumab administration may be considered in these patients.[9]

Sublingual immunotherapy (SLIT): SLIT is a treatment where allergen extracts are taken by mouth, held underneath the tongue for up to several minutes, and then spit out or swallowed.[9]

Oral Immunotherapy (OIT): This involves the daily ingestion of food to which the patient is allergic, which may be in pill or powder form, although generally it is given in powder form within food.[7]

Epicutaneous immunotherapy: A patch containing a regulated dose of allergen is being tried for FA.[9]

Local nasal immunotherapy: It is another modality that by far has been demonstrated to be useful only for AR and that too for short term.[9]

Prevention of Allergic Disorders

Prevention could be at various stages. Primary prevention entails stopping development of allergic disorders in the first place. Exclusive breastfeeding has since long been advocated to have a role in the prevention of atopic diseases. Some studies support use of fish oil supplements containing omega-3 fatty acids and use of probiotics as a preventive measure to be used in pregnant woman in the later half of the pregnancy to reduce risk of atopic eczema and FA in the offspring.[11] However, no substantial evidence regarding its efficacy is available as far as now.

ALLERGIC RHINITIS

The prevalence of self-reported allergic rhinitis (AR) has been estimated to be approximately 2–25% in children.[12] It is mostly commonly allergic rhinoconjuctivitis. It is an inflammatory disorder of the nasal mucosa marked by nasal congestion, rhinorrhea, and itching after accompanied by sneezing and conjunctival inflammation. Over 80% of patients with asthma have rhinitis, and 10–14% of patients with rhinitis have asthma.[13] Inhalant allergens are primarily responsible but food allergen can cause symptoms as well.

Allergic rhinitis and its impact on asthma (ARIA) classifies AR as intermittent or persistent, which is based on the duration of symptoms and severity of symptoms[14,15] (Flowchart 48.1).

- Intermittent - <4 days/week
- <4 consecutive weeks
- Persistent - >4 days/week
- >4 consecutive weeks

Clinical Manifestations

For the identification of allergen, synchrony of the occurrence of symptoms with environmental changes should be observed. Allergens cause itchiness of nose, eye, palates, or pharynx. Repeated rubbing of nose causes a transverse crease across the nose (allergic salute). Mouth breathing, nasal speech, and snoring may result. Secretions are clear or mucoid. Infraorbital cyanosis (allergic shiners) may be frequently observed. Allergic gape or continuous open-mouth breathing may cause high arched palate. Nasal examination shows edematous, boggy, and bluish mucus membranes.

Laboratory Findings

Eosinophilia can be demonstrated on nasal smears and total serum IgE may be elevated. However, both have low specificity and low sensitivity. Epicutaneous skin tests provide the best method for detection of allergen-specific IgE. Serum immunoassay for specific IgE to allergens can also be done. Alternatively the Phadia Immuno CAP assay RAST can be done.

Complications

Chronic sinusitis is the most common complication due to blockage of sinus ostea. It may or may not be associated with bacterial infection. Fungal allergens are often inciting agents. Asthma aggravation may be related to AR. Postnatal

Flowchart 48.1: Modified from ARIA classification of allergic rhinitis, 2008.

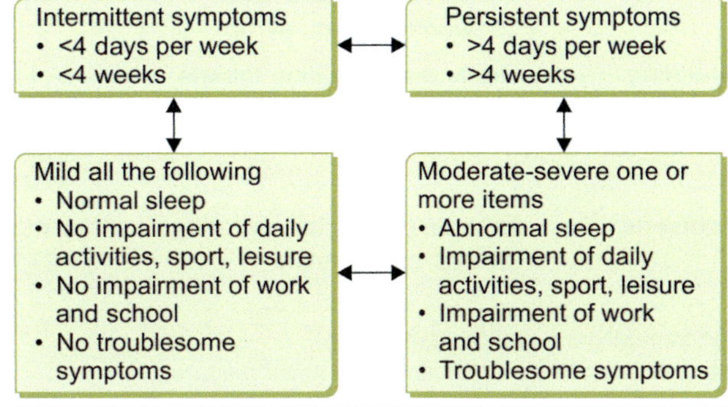

drip, Eustachian tube obstruction and middle ear effusion, hypertrophy of adenoids and tonsils, otitis media, and obstructive sleep apnea are some of the other complications.

Treatment

General Measures

Prevention of symptoms and symptomatic relief are two pillars of treatment. Knowledge of temporal variation of symptoms with season or occurrence of symptoms in association with indoor allergens may guide preventive measures that need to be taken to avoid allergen exposure as discussed before. Nasal saline irrigation gives relief in nasal rhinitis. For accompanying conjunctivitis, cold compression and lubrication are useful.

Pharmacotherapy

Evidence-based clinical practice guidelines, such as the ARIA guideline have recommendations for pharmacological management of AR.[12] These were developed based on studies that included exclusively adult patients. However, the suggestion is that careful extrapolation to the pediatric population can be attempted. One can assume that the relative effects of treatment of AR are likely similar among adults and children, but adverse effects might be more or less frequent.

Antihistamines

They are classified as first generation (relatively sedating) and second generation (relatively non-sedating). They are available for oral, nasal, and topical ophthalmic use (Table 48.1).

Corticosteroids

They constitute the most effective therapy for AR. Severely affected patients may be prescribed combinations with antihistamines (Table 48.2).

Mast Cell Stabilizers

Cromolyn sodium can be used as an intranasal spray 1-2 sprays QID. Its ophthalmic solution is available. Other ophthalmic solutions include lodoxamide 0.1%, 1-2 drops QID; nedocromil sodium 2% 1-2 drops BID, and pemirolast potassium 0.1%, 1-2 drops QID.

Table 48.1: Antihistamines for pediatric use with dosage and available formulations.

Drug	*Formulations*	*Dosage*
First-generation antihistamine		
Chlorpheniramine maleate	Tablets, syrups	2–5 years: 1 mg every 4–6 hours (maximum 6 mg/day) 6–11 years: 2 mg every 4–6 hours (maximum 12 mg/day) >12 years: 4 mg every 4–6 hours (maximum 24 mg/day)
Second-generation antihistamines		
Cetirizine	Syrup, chewable tablets, tablets, liquid-filled gels	6–12 months: 2.5 mg once daily; 12–23 months: initially 2.5 mg once daily, dosage may be increased to 2.5 mg twice daily; 2–5 years: 2.5 mg/day, may be increased to a maximum of 5 mg/day given either as a single dose or divided into two doses≥6 year: 5–10 mg/day as a single dose or divided into two doses.
Levocetirizine	Solution, tablets	6 months–5 years: maximum 1.25 mg once daily in the PM 6–11 years: maximum 2.5 mg once daily in the PM
Loratidine	Orally disintegrating tablets, tablets, liquid filled caps, chewable tablets, syrup	2–5 years: 5 mg once daily. >6 years: 10 mg once daily or 5 mg twice daily
Desloratidine	Orally disintegrating tablets, tablets, syrup	6–11 months: 1 mg once daily 12 months–5 years: 1.25 mg once daily 6–11 years: 2.5 mg once daily Adults and adolescents ≥12 years: 5 mg once daily
Fexofenadine	Tablets, orally disintegrating tablets, suspension	6 months–<2 years: 15 mg (2.5 mL) every 12 hours >2–11 years: 30 mg every 12 hours >12 years –adult: 60 mg every 12 hours; 180 mg once daily

Adapted from Milgrom and Sicherer (2016).
Azelastine is available as ophthalmic and nasal preparation.

Table 48.2: Corticosteroids with dosage and side effects.

Drug	*Dosing*	*Side effects*
Mometasone	(50 μg/spray) 2–12 years: 1 spray in each nostril qd >12 years: 2 sprays in each nostril qd	Burning and irritation of nasal mucosa, epistaxis growth monitoring for possible suppression
Fluticasone furoate	2–12 years: Initial dose: 1 spray (27.5 μg/spray) per nostril once daily (55 μg/day)	Burning and irritation of nasal mucosa, epistaxis Monitor growth
	Patients who do not show adequate response may use 2 sprays per nostril once daily (110 μg/day). Once symptoms are controlled, dosage may be reduced to 55 μg once daily ≥12 years and adolescents: Initial dose: 2 sprays (27.5 μg/spray) per nostril once daily (110 μg/day). Once symptoms are controlled, dosage may be reduced to 1 spray per nostril once daily Total daily dosage should not exceed two sprays in each nostril (110 μg)/day	
Beclomethasone	6–12 year: 1 spray in each nostril bid; may increase if needed to two sprays in each nostril bid >12 year: 1 or 2 sprays in each nostril bid	Burning and irritation of nasal mucosa, epistaxis Monitor growth
Budesonide	(32 μg/spray) 6–12 years: 2 sprays in each nostril qd >12 years: up to 4 sprays in each nostril qd (maximum dose)	Burning and irritation of nasal mucosa, epistaxis Monitor growth
Ciclesonide	(50 μg/spray) 2–12 years: 1–2 sprays in each nostril qd >12 years: 2 sprays in each nostril qd	Burning and irritation of nasal mucosa, epistaxis Monitor growth
Flunisolide	6–14 years: 1 spray each nostril Three times daily *or* two sprays in each nostril twice daily; not to exceed four sprays/day in each nostril ≥15 year: two sprays each nostril twice daily (morning and evening); may increase to two sprays three times daily; maximum dose: eight sprays/ day in each nostril (400 μg/day)	Burning and irritation of nasal mucosa, epistaxis Monitor growth
Triamcinolone	2–6 years; 1 spray in each nostril qd 6–12 year: 1–2 sprays in each nostril qd ≥12 years: two sprays in each nostril qd	Burning and irritation of nasal mucosa, epistaxis Monitor growth
Fluticasone propionate	(50 μg/spray) ≥4 years: 1–2 sprays in each nostril qd	Burning and irritation of nasal mucosa, epistaxis

Adapted from Milgrom and Sicherer (2016).

Decongestants and Vasoconstrictor Agents

Pseudoephedrine is an oral vasoconstrictor available in combinations with other agents. However, its use is not recommended in children less than 4 years of age due to side effects such as irritability and an increased risk of infant mortality. Intranasal decongestants should be used for less than 10 days and should not be repeated more than twice a month.[12] Oxymetazoline and phenylephrine are the examples of nasal decongestants. Oral formulations of phenylephrine in combination with antihistamines are available.

Other Agents

Leukotriene antagonists such as montelukast are approved for perennial AR in 6-month-old children.

Omalizumab: It is a humanized monoclonal antibody able to bind IgE. It is used subcutaneously.

Immunotherapy

In the case of failure of general measures to control rhinitis, due to persistent unavoidable exposure to allergen, immunotherapy should be considered.

Surgery

Turbinectomy, polypectomy, and functional endoscopic sinus surgery are sometimes indicated in AR, more so in chronic patients.

ATOPIC ECZEMA OR DERMATITIS

Atopic dermatitis (AD) is a chronically relapsing inflammatory skin disease. It presents in early childhood with onset prior to 5 years of age in approximately 90% of patients.[13] It also represents predisposition to develop AR and asthma in later childhood. This is termed as "the atopic march." AD has an underlying genetic cause as defective skin barrier due to mutation in protein filaggrin, which is essential for normal barrier function and exaggerated T-cell responses to environmental allergens and microbes.

The AD can be atopic or non-atopic dependent on IgE-mediated sensitization. Both forms are associated with eosinophilia. Acute and chronic AD have difference in cytokine expression as also in skin manifestations. Severely dry skin is a hallmark of AD. *Acute AD* skin lesions are in the form of papules, excoriation, and vesiculation. They are intensely pruritic and erythematous. S*ub-acute* presents with erythematous, excoriated, and scaly papules; and *chronic* with thickened skin with accentuated surface markings (lichenification) and fibrotic papules (Figs. 48.2A to C).

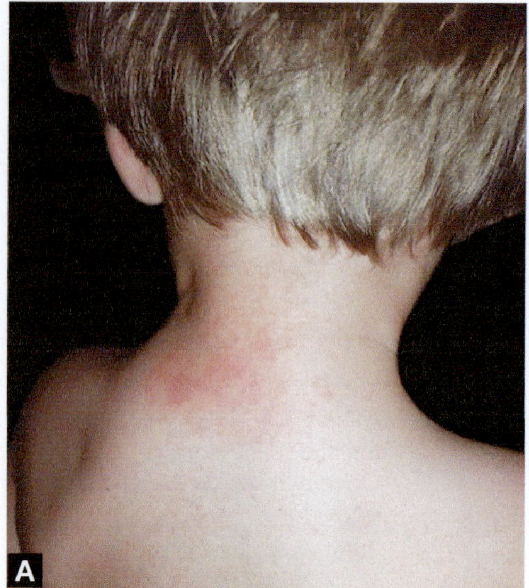

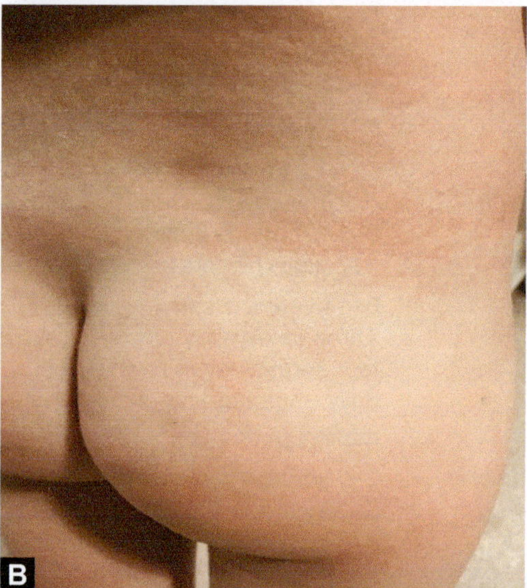

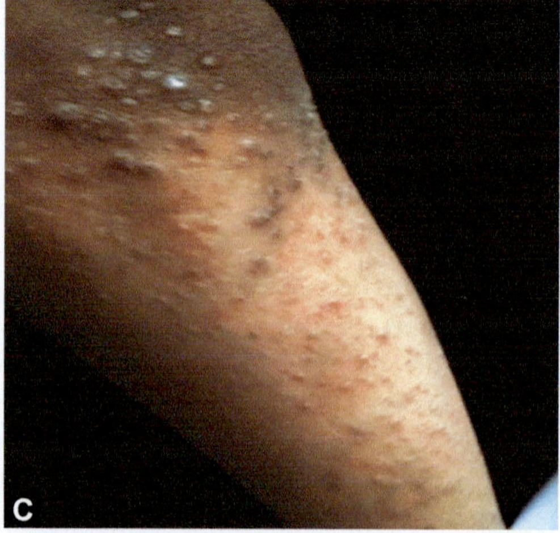

Figs. 48.2A to C: Atopic dermatitis.

Acute AD involves the face scalp and extensor surface of extremities. Diaper area is spared. Chronic has localization of rash to flexural folds of the extremities. AD often goes into remission as age advances.

Laboratory Investigations

There are no specific laboratory tests. However, it is possible to identify the allergen by measuring the specific IgE antibody or by skin prick testing.

Treatment

A multifaceted approach is required.

General Measures

Avoidance of irritants and/or specific allergen is a must. New clothing should be washed before use. Residual detergent in clothing maybe irritating, so use of liquid detergent is advised and extra care should be taken to rinse properly. Cotton/cotton blends for clothing should be preferred.

Hydration

Moisturizers are first-line therapy to ensure hydration. Lukewarm soaking bath for 15–20 minutes followed by application of an occlusive emollient to retain moisture can be taken. Therapeutic moisturizers/barrier creams penetration is aided by bath or hydration. Wet wrap therapy has been found to be highly soothing. It is used after emollient application wherein a wet dressing over the affected area is covered with a dry dressing.[16]

Pharmacotherapy

Topical Corticosteroids

Cornerstone of anti-inflammatory treatments is topical corticosteroids.[13,17] They reduce inflammation and pruritus in AD. Topical corticosteroids are divided into seven groups based on potency by vasoconstrictor assay. Use is guided by the distribution and severity of symptoms. Only low-potency corticosteroids should be used on face and intertriginous areas. Mid potency can be used for long periods. After a daily regime has been effective in control of symptoms, it is advisable to shift to a twice-weekly schedule to prevent relapse. Ointments have better occlusive properties, however in humid environments, creams are better. Solution should be used for scalp and hirsute areas. Corticosteroids can be discontinued when inflammation resolves but hydration must be continued. Side effects of topical corticosteroids include thickening of the skin, telangiectasias, bruising, hypopigm, acne, and striae. Systemic adverse effects include suppression of hypothalamic pituitary axis, more so in infants and young children.

Topical Calcineurin Inhibitors

These are immunomodulating agents that are indicated in cases where topical steroids are ineffective or in patients with face and neck dermatitis where treatment with low-potency steroids has not been effective. Pimecrolimus cream 1% is used to treat mild to moderate AD in children ≥2 years of age. Tacrolimus ointment 0.03% can be used in children 2–15 years of age and 0.1% for older patients, for moderate to severe AD. These drugs are used only for short-term and intermittent chronic treatment as they can cause cancer.

Tar Preparations

These are primarily used in shampoos. Side effects include irritability, folliculitis, and photosensitivity.

Antihistamines

These can be used as antipruritic agents. Sedating antihistamines are preferred due to their tranquilizing and anxiolytic effects.

Systemic Corticosteroids

They show a dramatic acute response followed frequently with severe rebound flair of AD after therapy termination. A short course of systemic corticosteroids is advisable to achieve control while continuing other therapies.

Cyclosporine

This immunosuppressive drug has been beneficial for severe refractory AD. Its side effects include renal impairment and hypertension.

Antimetabolites

These are immune suppressive agents. Examples are methotrexate and azathioprine, and mycophenolate mofetil (MMF) can be used. If MMF shows no response in 4–8 weeks, it should be stopped. Myelosuppression is a significant adverse effect of these drugs.

Phototherapy

Natural sunlight is beneficial but excessive use should be avoided as it can cause flare up. Narrowband UVB and psoralen followed by UVA is recommended. Ultraviolet A1 and Ultraviolet B modalities of treatment are available. Long-term use can cause cutaneous malignancies.

Experimental Stage Drugs

Interferon γ, Omalizumab, allergic immunotherapy, probiotics, and vitamin D supplementations are in experimental stage.

Recalcitrant Disease

Patients who are erythrodermic or appear toxic need hospitalization. It may induce marked clinical improvement due to removal of allergen and by ensuring compliance.

Complications

Exfoliative dermatitis is a known complication. It is associated with erythroderma, weeping, crusting, scaling, systemic toxicity, lymphadenopathy, and fever due to superinfection. Eyelid dermatitis and chronic blepharitis may cause corneal scarring. Atopic keratoconjunctivitis, keratoconus, and cataract may also result.

Prognosis

Resolution after age of 5 years is seen in 40–60%, however a study suggests 20% resolution and 65% reduction in severity. Lesions may relapse in adult life in previously treated adolescent cases.[17]

Prevention

Hypoallergenic hydrolyzed formula for infants with AD may help, as suggested by few studies. However, literature on this topic is inconsistent and insufficient. Probiotic and prebiotic use is also beneficial.[18] To avoid recurrences, it is essential to prevent inciting factors from actuation of an allergic response. Hence, irritants, such as humidity, chemicals, smoke, etc., should be avoided. Also, a concomitant infection must be readily treated as they are highly susceptible to microbial colonization. FA and aeroallergens can be triggering factors.

ADVERSE DRUG REACTIONS

The majority of adverse drug reactions are not immunologically mediated and maybe due to over dosage, pharmacological side effects, nonspecific release of pharmacologic effectors molecules, or drug interactions. The immunologically mediated reactions are unpredictable ones. They are dose independent and include idiosyncratic reactions, allergic (hypersensitivity) reactions, and pseudoallergic reactions, which are due to cross-reactive antigens.

Pathogenesis

The following are the four hypersensitivity reactions according to Gell and Coombs:[19]

- Type 1 reaction—immediate hypersensitivity reactions
- Type 2 reaction—cytotoxic antibody reactions
- Type 3 reaction—immune complex reactions
- Type 4 reaction—delayed-type hypersensitivity reactions.

Diagnosis

Diagnosis is largely based on finding a temporal association between a drug and an adverse reaction on the basis of medical history. Complete information about the dosage, route of administration, previous exposures, and dates of administration is important.

Use of skin testing is reliable to some extent in the case of penicillin. However, it cannot be said the same about other drugs, as exact immunogen is not known in every drug, as it could be its metabolites, or conjugated product with proteins. Moreover, some drugs cause non-specific irritant reactions. Hence, interpretation becomes difficult in such cases. A positive skin test to major or minor allergenic determinants of penicillin (major determinant is the moiety which could be derived or part of the parent drug molecule that shows allergenicity in a large population group and minor determinant leads to reaction in a small number of people) has a 60% positive predictive value for immediate hypersensitivity reaction to penicillin.[20]

Direct and indirect Coombs testing in drug-induced hemolytic anemias can be done. Specific serum IgE and IgM measurement and serum IgE immunoassay for identification of IgE to penicilloyl (a moiety that constitutes major allergenic determinant for penicillin molecule) are available. The degree of cross-reactivity of allergenic determinants formed from cephalosporins with IgE to other β lactum drugs is still unclear. The degree of clinical reaction is much lower than in vitro cross-reactivity. The presence of the same side chain as the penicillin increases chances of cross-reactivity. Carbapenems, another β lactam antibiotic, demonstrates a cross-reactivity on skin testing of approximately 1%. The degree is higher clinically. Aztreonam, having a monocyclic ring structure, can be safely administered to a penicillin allergic patient.[20]

Non-β Lactam Drugs

Sulfonamides: Maculopapular eruption with fever is the reaction that may occur after 7–12 days of therapy.[20]

Antiretroviral agents: These are reverse transcriptase inhibitors, protease inhibitors, and fusion inhibitors. Abacavir hypersensitivity reaction is life-threatening, dose independent, and is an absolute contraindication for any subsequent use.

Chemotherapeutic agents: Carboplatin, Paclitaxel, and Rituximab.

Biologics: Inliximab, Rituximab, and Abatacept.

Vaccines: Egg protein containing vaccines (MMR, MMRV, influenza, yellow fever, and rabies). Anesthetic agents: Local and general anesthesia.

Latex Allergy

Insulin: More to porcine and bovine than human insulin. The dose following the systemic reaction should be reduced to one-third and then successively increased to two to five units until desired control is reached.

Radio contrast media, narcotic analgesia, aspirin, and NSAIDS are some other agents that may induce an adverse drug reaction.

STEVENS–JOHNSON SYNDROME AND TOXIC EPIDERMAL NECROLYSIS

These are blistering mucocutaneous disorders induced by drugs. Epidermal detachment of less than 10% is suggestive of Stevens-Johnson syndrome or more than 30% detachment suggests toxic epidermal necrolysis. And 10–30% detachment suggests overlap of the two syndromes (Figs. 48.3A and B; Table 48.3).

Treatment

Withdrawal of the implicated drug is the foremost step. Alternative drug with no immunological cross-reactivity should be used. Management of anaphylactic reaction to an agent is done as described later in the chapter, with epinephrine, H_1 and H_2 receptor blocking agents, and systemic steroids and supportive care. Toxic epidermal necrolysis should be treated in a burn unit.

Corticosteroids are contraindicated because they can significantly increase the risk of infection. Antihistamines and corticosteroids for other reaction can be used.

INSECT ALLERGY

Allergic reactions to insects can vary from local cutaneous reactions to life-threatening anaphylaxis. Apart from insect stings, inhalation of particulate matter of insect origin can induce acute and chronic respiratory symptoms. The insect from order Hymenoptera are mostly involved in eliciting such responses. It includes honeybees, yellow jackets, yellow hornets, white-faced hornets, wasps, and fire ants.

Pathogenesis

The insect venom has numerous vasoactive substances, such as histamine; acetylcholine; kinins; enzymes, such

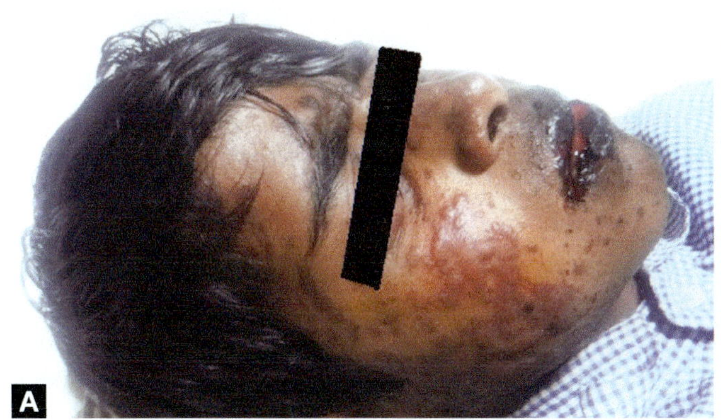

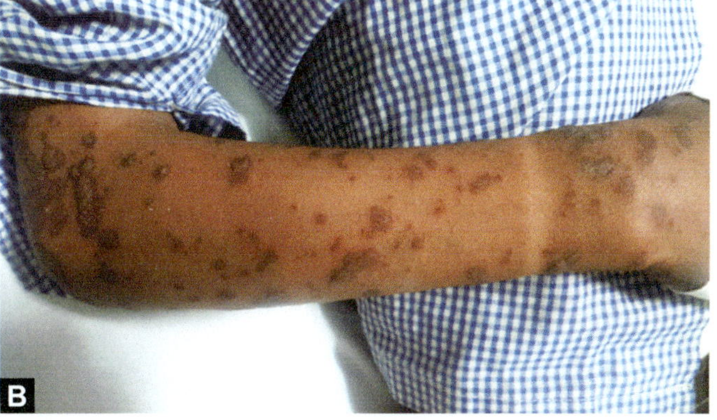

Figs. 48.3A and B: Stevens–Johnson syndrome.

Table 48.3: Adverse drug reaction syndromes.

Diagnosis	*Mucosal lesions*	*Skin lesions*	*Typical time to onset (weeks)*
Stevens–Johnson syndrome	Erosions at ≥2 sites	Purpuric macules and erosion on skin, mouth, and genitalia. Fever rhinorrhea and cough. ≤10% Detachment of epidermis is found	1–3 weeks onset time
Toxic epidermal necrolysis	≥2 sites	Similar lesions, however, detachment is ≥30%	1–3 weeks
Drug hypersensitivity syndrome or DRESS syndrome	Infrequent	Severe exanthematous rash, exfoliated dermatitis	1–6 weeks

Adapted from Boguniewicz et al. (2016).

as phospholipase and hyaluronidase; apamine; melutin; and formic acid. There is substantial cross-reactivity among vespid venoms. The localized responses are due to vasoactive or irritant materials and are not due to IgE-antibody-mediated allergic responses.[21]

Clinical Manifestations

Clinical manifestations range from local reactions or cutaneous reactions, such as urticaria and papulovesicular eruptions and angioedema to systemic reactions. These are laryngeal edema bronchospasms, hypotension, GI symptoms, fever, malaise, emesis, and nausea. Delayed systemic reactions occur 2 hours–3 weeks following the sting and include serum sickness, peripheral neuritis, vasculitis, nephritic syndrome, and encephalopathy. Inhalant allergy can be caused by insects and is similar to other inhalant allergens.

Laboratory Findings

Skin testing or in vitro testing is indicated for children with systemic reactions to confirm reactivity where VIT is being considered. Skin tests are usually accurate within 1 week of sting reaction. Skin tests are the most sensitive to detection of a venom allergy. If skin tests are negative, in vitro tests which include serum assay for venom-specific IgE, need to be used. In vitro tests howsoever have large numbers (20%) of false-positive and false-negative results. Hence, a negative in vitro test cannot be employed to reject venom sensitivity. If both come negative, skin test should be repeated, 4–6 weeks later. Chronic exposure to inhalant allergens needs high suspicion for diagnosis.[21]

Treatment

Treatment is similar to any other allergic phenomenon. Local cutaneous reactions should be dealt with cold compresses and topical medications to relieve itching. The use of a systemic antihistamine and oral analgesic is recommended. Self-injectable epinephrine in susceptible situation is advisable. Antibiotic application on sting site is not warranted. Open wounds due to scratching should be left open and topical antibiotics should be used. In the case of an anaphylactic reaction to the insect sting, the management is as per the discussion in the Anaphylaxis section.

Venom Immunotherapy

Hymenoptera venom is used mostly. It is indicated only if there is evidence of IgE sensitivity to venom documented by skin tests and/or specific serum IgE tests. The length of the therapy is individualized. Recommended duration of treatment is 3–5 years. Lifelong treatment is advisable for those with severe reaction and those with occupational exposures.

- *≤16 years*: Usually not indicated in the case of generalized cutaneous reaction as risk of further reaction is 10%. However, they may benefit in the case of a systemic reaction.
- *≥17 years*: In this age group, a generalized cutaneous reaction or systemic reaction or both warrant use of immunotherapy.
- Treatment should be carried for 3–5 years.[21]

Prevention

Bright-colored clothes and perfumes act as attractants and should be avoided. Patient preparedness in the case of an unavoidable exposure should be ensured. Self-injectable epinephrine, identification bracelet, and an action plan for allergic reaction management are essential.

FOOD ALLERGY

National Institute of Allergy and Infectious Diseases (NIAID) sponsored expert panel defines food allergy (FA) as an adverse health effect arising from a specific immune response that occurs reproducibly on exposure to a given food. An adverse reaction to a food can be food intolerance as well; however, these are physiologic responses which are by non-immune-mediated mechanisms.

FA can be IgE mediated or non-IgE mediated. Approximately 6–8% children get affected by IgE-mediated FA.[22]

Allergic reaction occurs with egg, milk, peanuts, tree nuts, wheat, and seafood mostly and was found to occur with rice (6.2%) followed by black gram (5.9%), lentil (5.5%), citrus fruits (5.3%), pea (3.8%), maize (3.8%), and banana (3.6%).[22] Genetically modified crops are also a concern as they contain transgene, which may be considered foreign by our body.

Pathogenesis

Food allergies are becoming increasingly common. It is deemed as one of the first steps in atopic march. As mentioned earlier, FA can be IgE mediated or non-IgE mediated and/or cell mediated. IgE mediated reactions occur within minutes to up to 2 hours after food ingestion. Non-IgE mediated can be delayed in onset for more than several hours to possibly days later.[23] IgE-mediated reaction causes release of mediators from mast cells, basophils, macrophages, and dendritic cells. In non-IgE-mediated reaction, allergen-specific T-cells secrete cytokines that cause chronic reactions.

Clinical Manifestations

Types of food allergy are manifested in Table 48.4.

Laboratory Findings

For the detection of FA, a number of tests are available. Skin prick testing which has a high negative productive value can be used in ruling out an allergen. Serum food-specific IgE can also be measured but has low specificity. The gold standard for diagnosis is double-blind, placebo-controlled food challenge. This can also be used for non-IgE-mediated FA. Elimination diets can also be tried followed by food challenges. The food needs to be eliminated for 10–14 days for IgE-mediated FA and up to 8 weeks for cell-mediated allergy.[24]

Table 48.4: Types of food allergy reactions.

IgE-mediated reaction	*Non-IgE-mediated reaction*	*Mixed reaction*
Skin: Urticaria (Fig. 48.4), angioedema, flushing GI: oral pruritus, nausea, abdominal pain, vomiting, diarrhea Respiratory: nasal congestion, rhinorrhea, nasal pruritus, sneezing, laryngeal edema, dyspnea, wheezing. Cardiovascular: Dysrhythmia, hypotension, loss of consciousness	Skin: Contact dermatitis, dermatitis herpetiformis (celiac disease) GI: food-protein-induced enterocolitis, proctocolitis, and enteropathy syndromes, celiac disease, eosinophilic eosophagitis. Respiratory: food-induced pulmonary hemosiderosis (Heiner syndrome)	GI: eosinophilic esophagitis/ gastroenteritis/ colitis Cutaneous: atopic dermatitis Respiratory: asthma

Adapted from Covar et al. (2016).

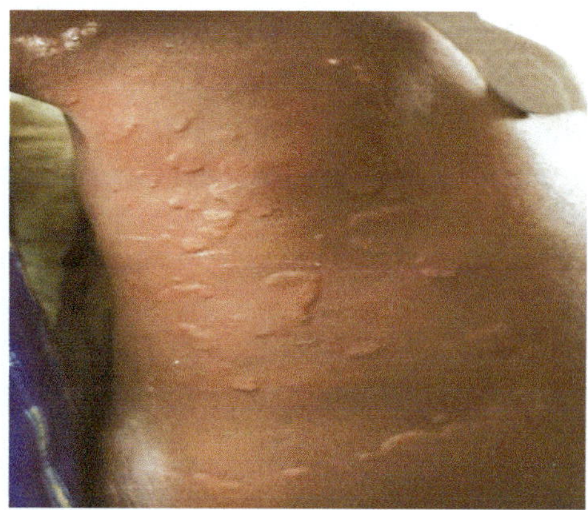

Fig. 48.4: Urticaria.

Treatment

The only validated treatment for FA is identification and elimination of foods. This however is difficult for the common foods with widespread use as ingredients in other processed foods. Hence, ingredients should be carefully checked for the presence of allergens in the case of atopic individuals.

The patient should carry an action plan in the case of accidental ingestion, and he should be provided with epinephrine autoinjector.

Immunotherapy

Oral, sublingual, and epicutaneous immunotherapy for IgE-mediated FA is still under evaluation. Anti-IgE combination with immunotherapy is more effective. Moreover, regular exposure to the tolerable amounts or forms of allergic food is helpful. Milk, egg, wheat, and soy allergy is mostly outgrown by adolescence but peanut or tree nut allergy continues. Egg in baked products and extensively heated milk is better tolerated and hence children diets can include these.

A number of guidelines are there, some of which are Clinical guideline 116 for FA in under 19 years and iMAP guidelines for milk protein allergy.[23, 25] Reintroduction of food to which the child is allergic is done in ladder pattern according to specific guidelines (milk ladder, egg ladder, wheat ladder, etc.) so as to slowly sensitize the baby for the development of tolerance.

Prevention

Introduction of allergic food after 6 months of exclusive breastfeeding may prevent development of allergy. However, one of the theories suggests that there is transcutaneous sensitization to food allergens in susceptible individuals, and sensitization occurs well before the introduction of food. Mother's diet should not be restricted during pregnancy or breastfeeding in atopic families. These practices lack in evidence-based approach.

OCULAR ALLERGIES

Ocular allergies are quite common due to the direct exposure of eyes to the environment and its high vascularity. The involvement is always bilateral. Occurrence is often linked with nasal allergic symptoms.

Pathogenesis

Conjunctiva is most commonly involved in ocular allergic disorders. Initially, an airborne allergen dissolves in tear film and binds to the IgE antibody. This initial sensitization process is not associated with an inflammatory response. Subsequent exposure to the allergen evokes an allergic reaction, which may be divided into an early phase and a late phase.[26,27]

Clinical Manifestations

Ocular allergies are classified into four types: [26]

- Allergic conjunctivitis/Hay fever conjunctivitis
- Vernal keratoconjunctivitis
- Atopic keratoconjunctivitis
- Giant papillary conjunctivitis.

Hay fever conjunctivitis/allergic conjunctivitis: It is a manifestation of type I or immediate hypersensitivity reaction mediated by IgE. It manifests as ocular itching, burning, chemosis or conjunctival swelling, and watery discharge. It can be seasonal or perennial. Perennial allergens are animal danders or dust mites. Perennial conjunctivitis is less severe than seasonal conjunctivitis.

Vernal keratoconjunctivitis (VKC): It is a chronic inflammatory process of the upper tarsal conjunctival surface. It is recurrent and potentially sight threatening. Patients generally have asthma or AD. Symptoms include itching, photophobia, foreign body sensation, and lacrimation. The absence of itching makes the diagnosis of VKC highly unlikely. The upper tarsal has giant papillae described as cobblestoning. Signs include a ropy stringy discharge, whitish spots in limbus (Trantas dots) and in conjunctiva (Horner points), and Dennie lines. Corneal involvement translates as grave prognosis.

Atopic keratoconjunctivitis: It is also a chronic inflammatory ocular disorder most commonly involving the lower tarsal conjunctiva. It presents a stronger association with asthma and AD. Presentation is similar to vernal keratoconjunctivitis. Cataract may occur. Eczema is more common and may involve periorbital skin and cheeks.

Giant papillary conjunctivitis: It involves chronic exposure to foreign bodies, such as contact lens.

Symptoms are similar to other conjunctivitis.

Contact allergy involves the eyelid mostly and at times the conjunctiva is a reaction to medication and contact lens solution and preservatives.

Diagnosis

Diagnosis is based on symptoms and signs. The presence of eosinophils in conjunctival scrapings aids in making the diagnosis, but their absence does not exclude it. Tear tryptase, a protease released primarily from activated mast cells, may serve as an objective parameter of disease activity.

Treatment

The primary goal is allergen avoidance. Cold compresses and regular lubrication may help provide relief. Pharmaceutical treatment includes oral or topical antihistamines, topical decongestants, mast cell stabilizers, and anti-inflammatory agents. Combination of these agents is better than either alone.

Combined use of antihistamine and a vasoconstrictor, such as pheniramine is more effective than either alone. Steroid sparing agents, such as topical tacrolimus and cyclosporine are also in use.

Allergy immunotherapy can be considered for both seasonal and perennial conjunctivitis (Table 48.5).

ANAPHYLAXIS

Anaphylaxis is a life-threatening allergic reaction to an allergen in a previously sensitized patient. It occurs when large quantities of inflammatory mediators

Table 48.5: Drugs for ocular allergies in pediatric patients.

Drug	*Dosing*	*Precautions*
Topical antihistamines		
Azelastine hydrochloride 0.05%	≥3 years: 1 gtt BID	Not to be used with contact lens
Emedastine difumarate 0.05%	≥3 years: 1 gtt BID	Not to be used with contact lens
Levocabastine 0.05%	≥12 years: 1 gtt BID-QID	Not to be used with contact lens
Mast-cell stabilizers		
Cromolyn sodium 4%	≥4 years: 1–2 gtt q4-6h	Not to be used with contact lens
Lodoxamide tromethamine 0.1%	≥2 years: 1–2 gtt QID	Not to be used with contact lens
Nedocromil sodium 2%	≥3 years: 1–2 gtt BID	Not to be used with contact lens
Perimolast potassium 0.1%	≥3 years: 1–2 gtt QID	Not to be used with contact lens
Multimodal medications		
Olopatadine hydrochloride 0.1% ,0.2%	≥3 years: 1 gtt BID (8 hour apart)	Not to be used with contact lens
Alcaftadine 0.25%	≥2 years: 1 gtt BID	Not to be used with contact lens
Bepotastine besilate 1.5%	≥2 years: 1 gtt BID	Not to be used with contact lens
Ketotifen fumarate 0.025%	≥3 years: 1 gtt BID	Not to be used with contact lens
Epinastine hydrochloride 0.05%	≥3 years: 1 gtt BID	Not to be used with contact lens
Nonsteroidal anti-inflammatories		
Ketorolac tromethamine 0.5%	≥3 years: 1 gtt QID	Not to be used with contact lens
Soft corticosteroids		
Fluorometholone 0.1%, 0.25%	≥2 years 1 gtt BID-QID initially (24–48 h)q4h	Increased intraocular pressure, viral infections, and cataract. Not to be used with contact lens

Adapted from Boguniewicz et al. (2016)

are rapidly released from mast cells and basophils. Anaphylactoid reactions mimic anaphylaxis but are not mediated by IgE antibodies. The term anaphylactoid has been termed outdated by World Allergy Organization (WAO) in their 2013 update.[28] They may be mediated through non-immune mast cell degranulating agents. However, WAO proposed the term "non-allergic anaphylaxis" for the same. The treatment guidelines are the same for both.

Clinical Manifestations

Anaphylaxis encompasses reactions leading to cutaneous, respiratory, cardiovascular, and gastrointestinal symptoms. The symptoms and signs vary depending on the organs affected. FA is the most common cause of anaphylaxis. Reaction to ingested allergen (food, medications) is delayed in onset (minutes to 2 hours) than from injected allergens. Diagnosis of anaphylaxis is difficult, mostly goes unnoticed in infants (Table 48.6).

Manifestations in Various Body Systems

General

Feeling of warmth, anxiety, impending doom, and fatigue.

Respiratory

- Nasal itching, rhinorrhea, congestion, sneezing
- Throat itching and tightness, stridor, hoarseness, dysphonia, dry staccato cough
- Lower airways: increased respiratory rate, shortness of breath, chest tightness, deep cough, wheezing/bronchospasm, decreased peak expiratory flow
- Cyanosis
- Respiratory arrest.

Skin, Subcutaneous Tissue, and Mucosa

- Itching, flushing, angioedema urticaria (hives), morbilliform rash, pilo erection

Table 48.6: Diagnosing anaphylaxis.[29]

Anaphylaxis is highly likely when any one of the following three criteria is fulfilled:
1. Acute onset of an illness (minutes to several hours) with involvement of the skin and/or mucosal tissue (e.g., generalized hives, pruritus or flushing, swollen lips/tongue/uvula)
And at least one of the following:
a Respiratory compromise (e.g., dyspnea, wheeze/bronchospasm, stridor, reduced peak PEF, hypoxemia)
b Reduced BP or associated symptoms of end-organ dysfunction (e.g., hypotonia [collapse], syncope, incontinence)
2. Two or more of the following that occur rapidly after exposure to a likely allergen for that patient (minutes to several hours):
a Involvement of the skin/mucosal tissue (e.g., generalized hives, itch/flush, swollen lips/tongue/uvula)
b Respiratory compromise (e.g., dyspnea, wheeze/ bronchospasm, stridor, reduced PEF, hypoxemia)
a Reduced BP or associated symptoms (e.g., hypotonia [collapse], syncope, incontinence)
b Persistent gastrointestinal symptoms (e.g., crampy abdominal pain, vomiting)
3. Reduced BP following exposure to known allergen for that patient (minutes to several hours):
a Infants and children: low systolic BP (age-specific) or >30% drop in systolic BP
b Adults: systolic BP <90 mm Hg or >30% drop from patient's baseline

Modified from Sampson et al. (2006).

- Periorbital itching, erythema and edema, conjuncitval erythema, tearing
- Itching of lips, tongue, palate, and external auditory canals; and swelling of lips, tongue, and uvula.

Gastrointestinal

Nausea, abdominal pain, vomiting, diarrhea, and dysphagia.

Cardiovascular System

- Chest pain
- Tachycardia, bradycardia (less common), other arrhythmias, palpitations
- Hypotension, feeling faint, urinary or fecal incontinence, shock
- Cardiac arrest.

Central Nervous System

Aura of impending doom, uneasiness (in infants and children, sudden behavioral change, e.g., irritability, cessation of play, clinging to parent); throbbing headache (pre-epinephrine), altered mental status, dizziness, confusion, tunnel vision.

Other

- Metallic taste in the mouth
- Cramps and bleeding due to uterine contractions in females.

Criteria for Anaphylactic Disease

The major anaphylaxis guidelines include the NIAID clinical criteria for diagnosis, a practical instrument for rapid identification of patients with a likely diagnosis of anaphylaxis.

Laboratory Findings

Serum IgE to specific antigens may be demonstrated but is not definite. Plasma histamine is unstable and cannot be used for diagnosis. Plasma tryptase may be helpful but has to be tested within 3 hours of the onset of reaction. However, tryptase levels are often normal in food-associated anaphylaxis. Serum creatinine kinase, ASOT, and LDH elevation is seen in myocardial infarction. ABG may show hypoxemia, hypercapnia, and acidosis.

Treatment

Anaphylaxis demands aggressive management. The initial management includes airway-breathing circulation management, which needs ensuring adequate airway with effective respiration, circulation, and perfusion (Flowchart 48.2).

The most important drugs include as shown in Table 48.7.

Flowchart 48.2: Algorithm for anaphylaxis management.

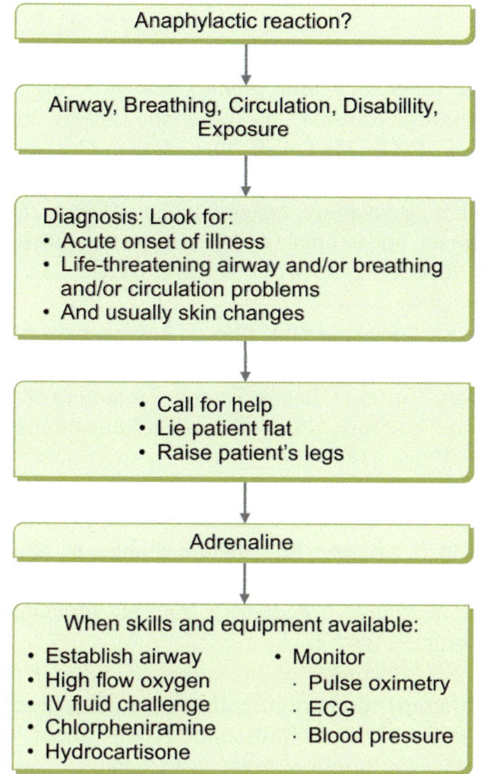

Adapted from Resus Council UK 2008.[30]

Table 48.7: Pharmacotherapy for anaphylaxis.

Drugs	*Dosing*	*Adverse reactions*
Epinephrine DRUG OF CHOICE	IM- 1:1000 dilution, 0.01 mg/kg up to 0.5 mg IM in lateral thigh ≥12 year 0.5 mg IM Can be repeated 2–3 times at 515 min interval. IV or intraosseous route 1:10,000 dilution, 0.01 ml/kg. For infusion :The dosing is 0.1–0.5 mcg/kg/min Endotracheal: 0.1 mg/kg q35 min; use 1:1000 concentration (0.1 mL/kg)	Tachycardia, anxiety, tremors, headache, nausea, hypertension
H_1 antihistamine antagonists		
Cetirizine	0.25 mg/kg up to 10 mg PO	Hypotension, tachycardia, somnolence
Diphenylhydramine	1.25 mg/kg up to 50 mg PO, IM, or IV	
H_2 antihistamine antagonists		
Ranitidine	1 mg/kg up to 50 mg IV Should be administered slowly	Headache, mental confusion
Cimetidine	4 mg/kg up to 200 mg IV Should be administered slowly	
Corticosteroids		
Methylprednisolone	Solu-Medrol (IV) 1–2 mg/kg up to 125 mg IV Depo-Medrol (IM) 1 mg/kg up to 80 mg IM	Hypertension, edema, nervousness
Prednisone	1 mg/kg up to 75 mg PO	
β agonist		
Nebulized albuterol	(0.83 mg/mL [3 mL]) via mask with O_2	Palpitation, nervousness, CNS stimulation, tachycardia
Volume expanders		
Crystalloids (normal saline or Ringer lactate)	30 mL/kg in first hour	
Colloids (hydroxyethyl starch)	10 mL/kg rapidly followed by slow infusion	
Post emergency management		
Antihistamine	Cetirizine (5–10 mg qd) or loratadine (5–10 mg qd) for 3 days	
Corticosteroids	Oral prednisone (1 mg/kg up to 75 mg) daily for 3 days	

Adapted from Sampson et al. (2016).

Supportive measures include supplemental oxygen, leg elevation for maintenance of blood pressure.

Refractoriness to epinephrine can be a difficult situation and can be dealt with glucagon or methylene blue use.

Anaphylactic reactions can be biphasic where symptoms occur after apparent resolution, mostly observed within 4 hours of first reaction.

Preventive Therapy\

- Confirmation of etiology on follow-up
- Avoidance of allergens
- Medical identification bracelet for allergy
- Epinephrine autoinjector and antihistamine availability
- Written plan for patient management
- Immunotherapy
- Patient education for recognizing early symptoms.

REFERENCES

1. Rook GAW, Brunet LR. Microbes, immunoregulation and the gut. Gut. 2005;54:317-20.
2. Akdis CA, Sicherer SH. Allergy and the immunologic basis of atopic disease. In: Kliegman, R, Stanton, B, St. Geme, JW, Schor, NF, Behrman, RE, eds. Nelson Textbook of Pediatrics, 20th ed. Philadelphia, PA: Elsevier;2016:1074-7.
3. Wahn U. The Allergic March. World Allergy Organization. September, 2015. http://www.worldallergy.org/education-and-programs/education/allergic-diseaseresource-center/professionals/the-allergic-march. Accessed June 3, 2018.
4. Kim JS, Bunyavanich S, Sicherer SH. Diagnosis of allergic disease. In: Kliegman R, Stanton B, St. Geme JW, Schor NF, Behrman RE, eds. Nelson Textbook of Pediatrics, 20th ed. Philadelphia, PA: Elsevier;2016:1078-82.
5. Portnoy JM, Kennedy K. Allergen Avoidance. World Allergy Avoidance. March, 2018. http://www.worldallergy.org/education-and-programs/education/allergic-diseaseresource-center/professionals/allergen-avoidance/. Accessed June 8, 2018.
6. Durham SR, Nelson H. Allergen immunotherapy: a centenary celebration. World Allergy Organ J. 2011 Jun; 4: 104-6. https://www.ncbi.nlm.nih.gov/pmc/articles/PMC3651049/. Accessed June 8, 2018.
7. Bunyavanich S, Kim JS, Sicherer SH. Principles of treatment of allergic disease. In: Kliegman R, Stanton B, St. Geme JW, Schor NF, Behrman RE, eds. Nelson Textbook of Pediatrics, 20th ed. Philadelphia, PA: Elsevier;2016:1087-8.
8. Gaur SN, Kumar R, Singh AB, et al. Guidelines for practice of allergen immunotherapy in India: 2017—An update. Indian J Allergy Asthma Immunol. 2017;31:3-33.
9. Wu AY-Y. Immunotherapy—Vaccines for allergic diseases. J Thoracic Dis. 2012;4:198-202.
10. Gaur SN. Allergoid preparations for allergen immunotherapy: A brief overview. Indian J Allergy Asthma Immunol. 2018; 32:1-3.
11. Garcia-Larsen V, Lerodiakonou D, Jarrold K, et al. Diet during pregnancy and infancy and risk of allergic or autoimmune disease: A systematic review and meta-analysis. PLOS Med. Feb 2018. https://doi.org/10.1371/journal.pmed.1002507. Accessed June 9, 2018.
12. Brożek JL, Bousquet J, Agache, I, et al. Allergic rhinitis and its impact on asthma (ARIA) guidelines—2016 revision. http://dx.doi.org/10.1016/j.jaci.2017.03.050. Accessed 29 march, 2018.
13. Covar RA, Fleischer DM, Cho C, Boguniewicz M. Allergic disorders. In: Hay Jr. WW, Levin MJ, Deterding RR, Abzug MJ, eds. Current Diagnosis and Treatment Paediatrics, 23rd ed. New York, NY: McGraw-Hill Education;2016:1131, 1135, 1136-9, 1147.
14. Bousquet J, Khaltaev N, Cruz AA, et al. Allergic rhinitis and its impact on asthma (ARIA) 2008. Allergy, 2008;63:8-160.
15. Milgrom H, Sicherer SH. Allergic rhinitis. In: Kliegman R, Stanton B, St. Geme JW, Schor NF, Behrman RE, eds. Nelson Textbook of Pediatrics, 20th ed. Philadelphia, PA: Elsevier;2016:1092-4.
16. Nicol NH, Boguniewicz M, Strand M, Klinnert MD. Wet wrap therapy in children with moderate to severe atopic dermatitis in a multidisciplinary treatment program. J Allergy Clin Immunol Pract. 2014;2:400-6.
17. Leung DYM, Sicherer SH. Atopic dermatitis (Atopic Eczema). In: Kliegman R, Stanton B, St. Geme JW, Schor NF, Behrman RE, eds. Nelson Textbook of Pediatrics, 20th ed. Philadelphia, PA: Elsevier;2016:1118-21.
18. Cabana MD. The role of hydrolyzed formula in allergy prevention. Ann Nutr Metab. 2017;70:38-45.
19. Coombs RRA. Gell PGH. In: Gell PGH, et al., eds. Clinical Aspects of Immunology. Oxford: Blackwells. 1975, 761-81.
20. Boguniewicz M, Cho CB, Sicherer SH. Adverse reactions to drugs. In: Kliegman R, Stanton B, St. Geme JW, Schor NF, Behrman RE, eds. Nelson Textbook of Pediatrics, 20th ed. Philadelphia, PA: Elsevier;2016:1145-9.
21. Wang J, Sicherer SH. Insect allergy. In: Kliegman R, Stanton B, St. Geme JW, Schor NF, Behrman RE, eds. Nelson Textbook of Pediatrics, 20th ed. Philadelphia, PA: Elsevier;2016:1122-4.
22. Gaur SN, Kumar R. Food allergy or food intolerance? Indian J Allergy Asthma Immunol. 2013;27:93-4.
23. Allergy UK. iMAP guidelines. 2017. https://www.allergyuk.org/healthprofessionals/mapguideline. Accessed June 9, 2018.
24. Nowak-We A, Sampson HA, Sicherer SH. Food allergy and adverse reactions to foods. In: Kliegman, R, Stanton, B, St. Geme, JW, Schor, NF, Behrman, RE, eds. Nelson Textbook of Pediatrics, 20th ed. Philadelphia, PA: Elsevier;2016:1143.

25. NHS UK. Food allergy in children and young people. 2011. https://www.nice.org.uk/guidance/cg116/resources/cg116-food-allergy-in-children-andyoung-people-full-guideline3. Accessed June 9, 2018.
26. Haq SM, Singh S, Song BJ, Trocme SD. Ocular allergic disorders. In: Duane's Ophthalmology. 2007. Philadelphia, PA: Lippincott Williams & Wilkins.
27. Boguniewicz M, Cho CB, Sicherer SH. Ocular allergies. In: Kliegman, R, Stanton, B, St. Geme, JW, Schor, NF, Behrman, RE, eds. Nelson Textbook of Pediatrics, 20th ed. Philadelphia, PA: Elsevier;2016:1125-6.
28. Lockey RF, Kemp SF, Lieberman PL, Sheikh A. Anaphylaxis. WAO White Book on Allergy: Update 2013.
29. Sampson HA, Muñoz-Furlong A, Campbell RL, et al. Second symposium on the definition and management of anaphylaxis: summary report—Second National Institute of Allergy and Infectious diseases/food allergy and anaphylaxis network symposium. J Allergy Clin Immunol. 2006;117:391-7.
30. Resuscitation Council (UK). Emergency treatment of anaphylactic reactions. Guidelines for healthcare providers. 2008. https://www.resus.org.uk/EasySiteWeb/GatewayLink.aspx?alId=824. Accessed June 9, 2018.

CHAPTER 49

Biomarkers in Allergy

Naveen K Bhatraju, Anurag Agrawal

INTRODUCTION

The prevalence of allergic diseases is on the rise, affecting millions of individuals worldwide and increasing the global health and economic burden. Available data suggests that about 30–40% of the world population is affected by one or more allergic conditions with increased prevalence of diseases in children and young adults. The rise in air pollution and global warming is predicted to further increase the burden of respiratory allergies. While avoidance of environmental allergen triggers is recommended as a preventive strategy, appropriate diagnosis is important for institution of targeted therapy and monitoring of allergic diseases. Measurement of a variety of biomarkers for the clinical assessment of allergic disorders is a routine practice in a clinical laboratory and some of these outcome measures are also utilized as surrogate markers for the evaluation of efficacy of targeted therapeutics in clinical trials. In this chapter, we provide a brief account of the various known and standardized biomarkers utilized in the aforementioned context and also highlight emerging biomarkers that may be utilized in the future for efficient diagnosis and design of personalized preventive or therapeutic strategies.

ALLERGY AND ALLERGIC DISEASES

The study of allergy and hypersensitivity is known as "allergology." The term allergy, from the Greek *allos* ("other") and *ergeon* ("work"), was introduced by Clemens von Priquet (1906) to describe the uncommitted biological response/altered reactivity of the immune system of an individual to a foreign agent (allergen) which may either result in immunity or allergic disease.[1] However, in recent times, clinical allergists use the term allergy, in a restricted sense, to describe the immunoglobulin E (IgE)/cell-mediated hypersensitivity reactions to the common environmental allergens (Box 49.1).

Allergic diseases include seasonal and perennial rhinitis, atopic dermatitis (AD)/eczema, atopic asthma, hypersensitive pneumonitis (alveolitis), conjunctivitis, urticaria and angioedema, mastocytosis, reactions to food and drugs, eosinophilic gastroenteropathies, allergic bronchopulmonary aspergillosis, and insect allergy. There has been a steady rise in the prevalence of the allergic diseases specifically allergic rhinitis (AR), atopic asthma, together with AD and food allergies in the last two decades.[2] The upsurge in the prevalence of these diseases is more apparent in middle and low-income countries with high incidence in children and young adults.[2,3] Allergic diseases during childhood have a severe negative impact on the quality of life of patients and their families. Moreover, a high degree of comorbidity has been observed among the allergic diseases. For instance, subjects with AD are more frequently presented with other atopic manifestations, such as AR, asthma, conjunctivitis, and food allergies, compared to patients without AD.[4,5] Therefore, an integrated approach for the diagnosis is essential for proper design of the therapeutic strategy. A wide array of biomarkers is being used in the clinical assessment of allergy, both in hospitals and research. Some biomarkers have also been shown to correlate with the disease severity and/or predict the disease risk and outcome of therapeutic response. These as well as diagnostic biomarkers would be discussed in the following sections. A brief explanation of what constitutes a biomarker is provided in Box 49.2.

BOX 49.1: Immunoglobulin E.

The early observation that allergic sensitization could be passively transferred to an otherwise normal individual, through blood transfusion, led to the hypothesis that serum-borne factors are responsible for the hypersensitivity reactions observed in subjects with allergic diseases. This was later substantiated by famous PK (Prausnitz–Küstner) test, which was a passive transfer of positive skin test, by Prausnitz and Küstner in 1921. Later in 1923, Coca and Cooke coined the term "atopy" to describe the inheritable immediate hypersensitivity reactions and attributed them to the serum-borne "bodies" which they called *reagins*. However, the actual discovery of the IgE was made after approximately five decades of these reports. Two research groups independently discovered a new class of immunoglobulins, with unique antigens and physicochemical properties, responsible for the reagin-mediated hypersensitivity. In 1968, WHO Immunoglobulin Reference Centre in Lausanne announced IgE as a new immunoglobulin class.

The IgE is a globular glycoprotein with a molecular weight of ~190,000 Da, containing four subunits. In adults, the IgE levels constitute about ~0.0005% of the total immunoglobulin levels in serum. IgE cannot cross the placental barrier in significant amounts and therefore the cord blood IgE levels remain low (<4.8 µg/L). The normal titers of these antibodies are found to vary in age-dependent manner with mean serum levels increasing up till 10–15 years of age and decrease thereafter through the eighth decade of life. The IgE levels in the serum of atopic individuals are greater than 800 µg/L by the age of 14 years and this abnormal increase has been found to be strongly associated with various atopic diseases such as AD, AR, and atopic asthma.

A first time exposure to an environmental allergen triggers the production of allergen-specific IgE in atopic individuals. Thus, secreted IgE binds to high-affinity Fcε receptors on mast cells and basophil cells, causing a sensitized state. Subsequent exposure to the same antigen results in the cross-linking of cell surface-bound IgE and an increase in intracellular calcium. The rise in intracellular calcium causes hypersensitivity reaction through release of preformed and newly synthesized mediators such as histamine, proteases, leukotrienes and prostaglandins.

While the role of IgE in allergy is well understood, the normal function of IgE is not yet clear. Defense against parasitic infections has been proposed to be the primary function of IgE. IgE has been suggested to have a gatekeeper function due to its ability to detect minute concentrations of foreign proteins entering the body and activate and recruit other parts of immune system. Several contradictory hypotheses have been proposed linking IgE and cancer. On one hand, it has been suggested that IgE-mediated enhancement in immune surveillance may be protective against cancer. On the other hand, increased levels of IgE have been suggested to be associated with increased cancer risk. But substantial evidence is awaited in support of either hypothesis.

BOX 49.2: Definition and types of biomarker.

Biomarker (shortened form of biological marker) can be defined as, "a characteristic that is objectively measured and evaluated as an indicator of normal biological processes, pathogenic processes, or pharmacologic responses to a therapeutic intervention." World Health Organization (WHO) in one of its reports stated that the true definition of biomarker includes "almost any measurement reflecting an interaction between a biological system and a potential hazard, which may be chemical, physical, or biological. The measured response may be functional and physiological, biochemical at the cellular level, or a molecular interaction." The characteristics of an ideal biomarker include ease of measure, reproducibility, accuracy, economic, ease of interpretation by clinician, and finally acceptable to the patient. If a biomarker is absent in the disease state, it is known as "negative biomarker." The biomarkers can be classified into three broad categories:

Type 0 biomarkers: These include measures that track disease progression and correlate with known clinical measures.

Type 1 biomarkers: These include measures that capture therapeutic efficacy of a drug.

Type 2 biomarkers: These are also called surrogate end points and include measures that could substitute for a clinical endpoint.

GENETIC BIOMARKERS

Genetic biomarkers are the earliest possible biomarkers and have evinced much interest in recent years. While it is generally accepted that the susceptibility to allergic diseases has a heritable component, it has been shown that complex interactions between genetic determinants and environmental risk factors shape the disease susceptibility, pathophysiology, and severity.[2,6-8]

The seminal report on linkage of chromosome 11q13 with atopy in 1989 was followed by over a thousand published studies reporting genetic associations of several other chromosomal regions, such as 1q23, 5q23, 2q12, 10q22.2, and 17q12, with various phenotypes of asthma and other allergic diseases.[6,7] Both hypothesis-driven approaches such as candidate gene approach and hypothesis independent approaches such as positional cloning by linkage and genome-wide association studies have provided significant insight into the genetic associations of various loci with atopy and atopic diseases.[7] The genes identified so far by these approaches could be classified into four groups:

1. *Environment-sensing genes*:
   Gene–environmental interactions have significantly furthered the understanding of pathophysiological mechanisms of allergic diseases. Single nucleotide polymorphisms (SNPs) in the genes encoding molecules involved in the interaction with environmental risk factors have been shown to directly modulate the effects of exposure and thus risk for developing allergic disease. Genes encoding the components, involved in interaction with levels of microbial exposure and other detoxifying enzymes that modulate the tobacco smoke or air pollution exposure-induced oxidant stress, are included in this group. For instance, polymorphisms in *CD14*, *toll-like receptor 2* (*TLR2*), and *toll-like receptor 4* (*TLR4*) genes, involved in lipopolysaccharide response, have been found to be associated with the risk for developing asthma, particularly in the presence of rural lifestyle.[2] SNP in the *glutathione-S-transferase* genes (*GSTM1*, *GSTM2*, *GSTM3*, *GSTM5*, *GSTT1*, and *GSTP1*) have also been shown to be associated with asthma susceptibility in subjects exposed to tobacco smoke and air pollution.[7]
2. *End-organ susceptibility genes*:
   Epithelium at the mucosal surfaces is the first to be exposed to the environmental allergens. Upon exposure, the epithelium of atopic subjects triggers an unusual inflammatory response through signaling to the immune system. The end-organ susceptibility genes are involved in the maintenance of epithelial barrier integrity at the mucosal surface and in signaling from epithelium to the immune system. These genes determine the clinical manifestation of the allergic disease but do not alter the susceptibility to allergy. For instance, polymorphisms in *filaggrin* (*FLG*) gene, which affect the dermal barrier function, have been found to be associated both with increased atopic sensitization and risk for AD. Similarly, subjects with certain genetic variants in *protocadherin-1* (*PCDH1*) gene, a member of a family of cell adhesion molecules, expressed in bronchial epithelium, have been identified to be susceptible to bronchial hyper-responsiveness.[7] Chitinases such as AMCase and YKL-40, that are considered to play a key role in modulation of allergic inflammation, have been demonstrated to be expressed at higher levels by epithelium and activated macrophages in asthmatics.[2,7]
3. *Immune response-regulating genes*:
   This group includes genes that regulate immune response and are associated with atopy, allergic sensitization, and allergic disease. For instance, genes that regulate Th1/Th2 differentiation and effector function such as *IL13*, *IL4RA*, *STAT6*, *TBX21* (encoding T-box transcription factor), *HLAG*, and *GATA3* are included in this group. Other genes such as *IRAKM* and *PHF11* that are suggested to influence the level of end-organ inflammation are also included in this group. Further, considerable overlap has been noticed between the genes included in this group and the susceptibility genes identified for other chronic inflammatory diseases such as ulcerative colitis and Crohn's disease.[2,7]
4. *Genes that regulate tissue response to chronic inflammation*:
   This group includes genes involved in determining the tissue response to chronic inflammation, such as airway wall remodeling and smooth muscle hyperexcitability during asthma and dermal remodeling during AD. For instance, *COL29A1*, a novel collagen encoding gene expressed in the skin has been linked to AD. Other genes such as *ADAM33*, expressed in both fibroblasts and smooth muscle, and *PDE4D*, expressed in smooth muscle and in inflammatory cells, are included in this group.[2,7]

Early Life Environment, Transgenerational Epigenetics, and Allergic Diseases

The dependence of onset of allergic diseases on the fetal immune and lung development is evident from a number of studies. It has been shown that phenotypic measures such as cord blood immune responses, airway function, and bronchial responsiveness in the neonatal period could predict subsequent development of allergic diseases.[7] Further, the available evidence from various genetic studies supports the role of early life developmental effects in allergic disease and suggests a possible interaction between atopy and lung development. For instance, polymorphism in *ADAM33* has been shown to be associated with early life lung function measures (specific airway resistance at age 3 years). Similarly, single nucleotide variants on the chromosome 17q21 have been shown to be associated with early onset of asthma (<4 years of age).[7] Accumulating evidence also suggests a role of epigenetic factors in allergic diseases.

The evidence for the importance of epigenetic factors in allergic diseases comes from both animal and human studies. Proxy markers for maternal nutrition such as altered birth weight, head circumference at birth, or both have been linked to increase in IgE levels and thus risk for allergic disease. Another study has shown a dose-dependent increase in the peripheral blood DNA methylation to an increase in environmental particulate exposure from traffic pollution. The concept of transgenerational epigenetic effects in allergic diseases has also received support from the observations such as increase in the risk of childhood asthma in grandchildren due to grandmaternal smoking. Enhanced airway inflammation after allergen challenge has also been observed in mice in utero exposed to supplementation with methyl donors. Although these studies suggest a significant role of epigenetic effects on the heritability of allergic diseases, future studies on large prospective birth cohorts, with information regarding the maternal environmental exposures during pregnancy, are required to establish the role of epigenetic factors in the heritability of allergic diseases.[2,7]

Clinical Utility of Allergic Disease Genetics

Although accumulating knowledge of allergic disease genetics has significantly furthered our understanding of disease pathogenesis, we are in no way near to utilizing this knowledge in clinical practice. This may in part be attributed to the poor predictive value of variation in any one gene. Further, differences in locally acting gene-environment interactions result in a range of disease subphenotypes requiring custom-designed treatment strategies. Increasing focus on understanding these gene-environment interactions would enable the clinicians to consider the genotypic risk factors, along with critical patient characterization, for better diagnosis and management of allergic diseases. For instance, it has been observed that *FLG* mutations, in infants with eczema and food allergen sensitivity, could predict the subsequent development of childhood asthma with 100% positive predictive value.[7] A significant progress has also been made toward identifying the genetic markers contributing to the severity of the disease ('modifier' genes) and those contributing to the interindividual differences in treatment responses (pharmacogenetics).

A number of clinical studies in patients with asthma have identified polymorphisms associated with the clinical response to bronchodilators, inhaled steroids, and leukotriene modifiers. For instance, R16G amino acid substitution altering the function and expression of *β_2-adrenoceptor* gene (*ADRB2*) has been found to be associated with differential therapeutic response to short and long-acting β agonists.[2,6,7] It has been shown that asthmatics homozygous for arginine (Arg/Arg16) in *ADRB2* has reduced peak expiratory flow (PEF) rate, in comparison to asthmatics homozygous for glycine (Gly/Gly16), in response to salmeterol (with or without concomitant corticosteroid treatment). However, considering the contradictory observations obtained in the subsequent studies, further work is required to fully evaluate the contribution of the *ADRB2* polymorphisms to the bronchodilator response. Similarly, another study based on candidate gene approach has identified *arg1* encoding *arginase 1* as a predictor of acute response to albuterol.[7] Interindividual differences in response to inhaled corticosteroids (ICSs) have also been linked to variations in a number of genes. For instance, genetic variance in genes encoding corticotropin-releasing hormone receptor 1 and stress-induced phosphoprotein 1 has been shown to be associated with improvements in forced expiratory volume (FEV_1) and magnitude of FEV_1, respectively. Similarly, polymorphisms in gene encoding T-box transcription factor (*TBX21*) have been associated with differential response to ICS in Asian population. In addition, variations in genes including *ORDML3*, cytochrome genes (*CYP3A4*, *3A5*, *3A7*), low-affinity IgE Fc receptor (*CD23* or *FcεR2*) have also been identified to be associated with response to ICS. Genetic variations in candidate genes of leukotriene pathway have also been shown to predict response to treatment with leukotriene modifiers such as montelukast and zileuton. For example, *polymorphisms in 5-lipoxygenase* (*ALOX5*) and *multidrug resistance protein 1* (*MRP1*) genes have been found to correlate with variations in FEV_1 response to montelukast and zileuton, and SNPs in the leukotriene C4 synthase (*LTC4S*) and leukotriene A4 hydrolase (*LTA4H*) have been found to contribute to the changes in exacerbation rates.

Although most of the association studies have reported genetic variations contributing to differential treatment response in asthma, a few studies have suggested genetic variations in genes involved in Th2 response as contributors to the disease severity and to the treatment response in chronic rhinosinusitis and AD.[6,7,9]

Although a number of genetic determinants have been discussed in this section, the applicability of these genetic determinants as biomarkers to identify responders and nonresponders to specific therapeutic strategies is limited. However, it is clear that there is a huge potential for pharmacogenetics to be harnessed for greater understanding of the complex allergic diseases en route to personalized medicine.

BIOMARKERS FOR DIAGNOSIS OF ALLERGIC DISEASES

Allergy diagnosis involves a thorough clinical history evaluation and physical examination, followed by a battery of primary and secondary confirmatory tests relevant to various aspects of allergic reaction. These include testing for allergen-specific IgE in vivo (skin testing) and in vitro (serological test), in vivo provocation challenge, testing for mast cell and basophil priming and for the presence of their mediators in serum/urine.[1,10]

Allergen-specific IgE

Once the allergic causality is identified, primary confirmatory tests may be performed to confirm allergen sensitization through detection of allergen-specific IgE in vivo (skin prick test [SPT]) and/or in vitro (serum specific IgE [ssIgE] testing).

In vivo skin tests are routinely used in the clinical practice to confirm the allergen sensitization and establish the allergic causality of the clinical symptoms. There are several reasons for widespread use of skin tests in clinical practice. Skin tests are easy to perform, minimally invasive, fast, reproducible (when performed correctly), and sensitive. Based on the method of allergen administration to the skin, there are two variants of skin tests: epicutaneous (skin prick/puncture, atopic patch test) and intracutaneous (intradermal injection test) skin tests. The negative and positive reactions are evaluated with reference to histamine (positive) control (1.8 or 10 mg/mL) or negative (diluent used to present the allergen) control. Depending on the scale used, +3- or +4-sized wheals are considered as positive. False-positive reactions can be observed due to several reasons such as bleeding and skin irritation caused by contamination of allergen extracts with naturally occurring histamine, cross-contamination of allergens (e.g., dust mite contamination of dog dander extracts), and dermatographism or active eczema. On the contrary, use of antihistamines or β-blockers may result in false-negative results. Further, variability of SPT results depends on various factors such as tester's skill, subject's skin responsiveness, quality of the allergen extract (concentration, purity, stability, and diluent vehicle used), device used for allergen application, and method used to measure and report the results.[11-13]

Although in vivo skin testing provides a highly sensitive, fast, and cost-effective measurement of allergen-specific IgE, the occasional risk of anaphylactic shock and death associated with it, along with other limitations discussed above, has prompted the development of a safe in vitro alternative. The measurement of serum-specific IgE (ssIgE) could be used to detect a wide range of allergens, overcoming the aforementioned risks and limitations but is less sensitive than skin testing. Three different autoanalyzers are presently available for ssIgE measurement: the immunoCAP by Phadia (UniCAP100, ImmunoCAP250), the immulite system from Siemens (Berlin, Germany), and the HYTEC-288 system from Hycor/Agilent technologies (Santa Clara, Calif). These three systems use non-isotopic antihuman IgE antibody and are to be calibrated by interpolation of response data from a heterologous total serum IgE calibration curve that has been referenced to WHO total serum IgE standard (11/234). The measured ssIgE is expressed in terms of kilo international units/liter (kIU/L) [1kIU/L = 2.4 IgE]. Conventionally the ssIgE levels greater than 0.35 kIU/L are considered to be positive, suggesting allergen sensitization. Although the performance of these three autoanalyzers is qualitatively similar, there exists a significant difference in the reported ssIgE levels among the three autoanalyzers and they cannot be used interchangeably.[10,14]

The development of microarray chip technology along with the progress made in the component-resolved diagnostics has revolutionized the allergy diagnosis by allowing the detection of multiple allergens in a single run using twenty microliters of serum. At present, the commercially available allergen chip, ImmunoCAP immunosorbent allergen chip (ISAC) or Immuno-solid-phase allergen chip (VBC Genomics-Phadia), has 103 allergens from 43 allergen sources spotted on the glass slides in triplicates.[15] A modified and advanced version of ISAC platform has been recently developed, MeDALL allergenchip.[16] This chip has 170 allergens spotted and allows monitoring of both IgE and IgG antibodies in the serum of allergic patient with high sensitivity and specificity. Point-of-care diagnostic platforms are available for sensitive detection of allergen-specific IgE in a drop of blood from finger prick (e.g., ImmunoCAP Rapid [Phadia], FastCheck System [Diagnostische Systeme & Technologien GmbH]).

A recent review comparing the performance characteristics of SPT and ssIgE in allergy diagnosis has shown that there is a considerable discordance between skin prick/puncture test and serum-specific IgE measurement and these tests cannot be used interchangeably.[17] They have also suggested that these two tests complement each other and have improved allergy diagnosis by decreasing the false-negative results. Further, it may also be important to note that a positive SPT or serological test merely implies allergen sensitization but not clinical allergy, i.e., a subject tested positive for the presence of specific IgE to a particular allergen may not always have an allergic reaction upon exposure to that particular allergen.[10,11] The clinical history links the positive result for allergen sensitization and allergic disease. In case of discordance between the clinical history and tests for the presence of allergen-specific IgE, in vivo provocation tests may be performed to judge the correctness of the observed discordance.

In Vivo Provocation Tests

In vivo provocation tests are secondary confirmatory tests performed in case of discrepancy between the clinical history and skin prick and/or serological tests. Provocation tests are performed to assess, both immediate and delayed, physiological changes induced by allergens at the organ level. Provocation tests are especially useful to assess the current reactivity of the patient to the allergens, to evaluate the strength of allergen sensitization, and also to exclude clinically silent sensitization. Provocation tests have also been recommended as endpoint measures for evaluation of AIT/VIT efficacy. The EMA guidelines suggest that these may be used as primary end points in early stage, proof-of-concept, and dose-ranging (phase-II) trials. Provocation challenges are to be performed by trained allergists in the presence of a doctor, at specialized centers with facilities to handle anaphylactic reactions. Different types of provocation tests including bronchial and nasal provocation tests, conjunctival provocation test, double-blind, placebo-controlled food challenge (DBPCFC) and drug provocation test are generally used for evaluation of clinical relevance of a variety of allergens. Please see Table 49.1 for the practical aspects of various provocation tests including indications, contraindications, and recommended washout periods. The detailed procedure and interpretation of these tests can be found elsewhere.[18] Although in vivo provocation tests are considered as a direct measure for establishing clinically relevant allergen sensitization, limited availability of facilities across the world for conducting provocation tests and associated anaphylactic risk restricts its use in routine diagnostics.

Basophil Activation Test

Basophil activation test is another diagnostic tool utilized as an indirect measure of allergen sensitization and is indicated in patients with positive clinical history, but test negative for skin test and/or serum-specific IgE. Basophil activation is measured by quantification of surface marker (CD63, CD203c) expression by flow cytometry or by measuring the levels of secreted mediators (histamine, leukotriene) after exposure to allergen in vitro. Details of basophil activation test are presented elsewhere.[19]

Potential Molecular Biomarkers in Allergy Diagnostics

The increase in understanding of molecular mechanisms underlying the pathophysiology of atopic diseases has allowed the discovery of many objective measures, which can provide complementary information to conventional disease markers and aid in monitoring the clinical course of the disease. Several such molecules have been identified by various groups and proposed as potential biomarkers.

Cytokines

The differential expression of cytokines such as interleukins (IL)-12, IL-18, and IL-31 has been found to be associated with various atopic manifestations. For instance, elevated local and/or serum levels of IL-31 has been shown to be associated with disease severity of various allergic diseases including AD, allergic contact dermatitis, mastocytosis, and AR.[20] In case of AD, elevated serum IL-31 levels have also been reported to be associated with subjective itch intensity. On the other hand, no correlation between IL-31 levels and pruritus was observed in AR patients, suggestive of alternative functions for IL-31.[20] Similarly, serum levels

Table 49.1: Practical aspects of in vivo provocation tests.

Provocation test	Indications	*Contraindications*	*Recommended washout periods*	*Response measures*	
				Clinical practice	*Research*
Nasal provocation test	• To resolve discrepancy between clinical history and SPT and ssIgE measurement • Confirmatory diagnostic procedure for occupational AR • To select an allergen for AIT in polysensitized patients • Secondary outcome measure for AIT in clinical trials	• Advanced nasal polyposis • Nasal surgery in the recent past (<3 months) • Respiratory tract infections in the past two weeks	• Pollen sensitization—1 month • Occupational allergy—1 week • Oral and topical antihistamines—>72 hours • Topical corticosteroids— >24 hours • Cromoglycate—>6 hours	Nasal and nonnasal symptom scores, visual analog scale, peak nasal inspiratory flow, anterior rhinoscopy	Inflammatory mediators and cytokines in nasal lavage, tears, or biopsy, nasal airway resistance, nasal NO, acoustic rhinometry
Bronchial provocation test	• To resolve discrepancy between clinical history and SPT and ssIgE measurement] • Diagnostic procedure for occupational asthma • To demonstrate late airway response • Proof-of-concept for efficacy of targeted therapies in clinical research	• Unstable asthma or unable to refrain medication for asthma during washout period • FEV_1 <70% of predicted or <2L or spirometry-induced bronchoconstriction • Active or recent respiratory tract infections (<4 weeks) • Frequent exacerbations or hospital admission for asthma in the past 1 year • Recent vaccination • use of systemic β-blockers • History of angina pectoris; myocardial infarction; compromised left ventricular function; cerebrovascular accident; arterial aneurysm; seizures; untreated hypertension; active hyperthyroidism; immunologic disorder; cancer, pregnancy, or lactation; severe drug allergy; or history of anaphylaxis	• Topical anti-inflammatory medication—>4 weeks • Systemic steroids—>8 weeks Antihistamines—>1 week • Bronchodilators—6–72 hours • Caffeine containing products—>8 hours • Should be performed outside allergen season	FEV_1	FEV_1

(Contd...)

(Contd...)

Provocation test	Indications	*Contraindications*	*Recommended washout periods*	*Response measures*	
				Clinical practice	*Research*
Conjunctival provocation test	• To identify clinically relevant allergens in polysensitized patients • To resolve discrepancy between clinical history and SPT and ssIgE measurement • Secondary outcome measure for AIT in clinical trials • Evaluation of novel topical drugs for ocular allergy	• Recent eye surgery (within 3–6 months) • History of retinal diseases or detachment	• Oral antihistamines and corticosteroids—2 weeks and topical — 2 days • Should be performed outside exposure periods	Total ocular signs and symptom scores, pruritus	Cellular and cytokine profiles in ocular secretions, conjunctival erythema, edema, eyelid edema, and ocular surface sensation
DBPCFC	• To resolve discrepancy between clinical history and SPT and ssIgE measurement • To demonstrate tolerance to suspected food allergens having cross-reactivity to other aeroallergens • To monitor response to AIT in clinical trials	• Exacerbated atopic diseases such as asthma, AD, urticarial, or AR • Unstable asthma, rhinitis, or AD • History of anaphylaxis	• Two weeks for the diet foods to be tested • Antihistamines for a period of five half-lives of the specific agent • Systemic steroids—7–14 days	Inspection of the skin, lung auscultation, abdominal auscultation, monitoring of blood pressure, heart rate, and oxygen saturation measurement, questionnaire for pruritus of mouth mucosa and/or skin, abdominal pain, and laryngeal symptoms	Facial thermography, exhaled NO
Drug provocation test	• Diagnosis of drug hypersensitivity (DHR) to NSAIDs, local anesthetics, β-lactams, non-β-lactam antibiotics, and other drugs for which safer tests are not standardized or inexistent • In cases where skin tests and ssIgE measurement results are inconclusive • Patients with prior severe DHR history • To demonstrate tolerance to specific drugs	• Severe life-threatening and/or uncontrollable DHR • Severe cutaneous reactions such as SJS, TEN, DRESS, vasculitis, and AGEP • Systemic reactions, hematologic responses, and any internal organ involvement • Severe concurrent illness or pregnancy	Test should be performed at least one month following the DHR	Anaphylactic reactions: Cutaneous and/or respiratory symptoms or alterations in vital signs (decrease in PEF rate, rhythm alteration, or hypotension)	Anaphylactic reactions

of IL-12 and IL-18 have been found to be higher in AD patients than in control subjects. Further, elevated serum IL-18 levels have been found to be significantly correlated with the severity of AD.[21]

Chemokines

Thymus and activation-regulated chemokine (TARC) or C–C chemokine ligand (CCL)17, a chemoattractant for type 2 helper (Th2) cells, has been proposed as a potential biomarker for monitoring disease severity of AD in clinical practice.[22] Elevated serum levels of TARC had been observed in both infantile and adult patients with AD.[23] Further, serum levels of TARC were found to be positively correlated with the severity scoring of AD (SCORAD) index.[22] In another study, it has been suggested that CCL17 may contribute to the acute exacerbation pathology in chronic hypersensitivity pneumonitis patients, through inducing accumulation of Th2 lymphocytes in lungs. They have also suggested high concentrations of serum TARC at the baseline to be a promising predictor of acute exacerbation in these subjects.[23] Other studies have revealed two other T-cell chemoattractant chemokines, macrophage-derived chemokine (MDC/CCL22), and cutaneous T-cell attracting chemokine (CTACK/CCL27) that are associated with disease severity in AD patients.[24] Of note, Nakazato et al. have found CCL27 to have the most significant correlation with the disease severity in infantile AD patients.[25]

Mast Cell Tryptase

Mast cell tryptase is a 134-kDa tetrameric serine esterase enzyme released from activated mast cells along with preformed histamine and newly synthesized leukotrienes. Two different types of mast cell tryptases—α-tryptase and β-tryptase which are indicators of mast cell number and mast cell activation, respectively—are measured in the sera of patients. High levels of baseline total serum tryptase levels (>20 ng/mL) in comparison to normal controls (1–10 ng/mL) are suggestive of systemic mastocytosis.[10,26] If the postmortem β-tryptase levels are greater than 10 ng/mL, anaphylaxis may be considered as a probable cause of death. However, it has been observed that significant high postmortem β-tryptase levels could be found even in the absence of anaphylaxis.[27] In case of patients with reported moderate or severe anaphylactic reactions to stings, measurement of baseline serum tryptase levels has been recommended due to its high predictive value.[28] In these patients, increased baseline serum tryptase levels have been shown to be associated with frequent and more severe anaphylactic reactions to stings, as well as greater failure rate with venom immunotherapy (VIT) and greater relapse rate after stopping VIT.[29]

Urinary Leukotrienes

Leukotriene B4 (LTB4) and cysteinyl leukotrienes (LTC4, LTD4, and LTE4) are important inflammatory mediators released from a variety of cells during an allergic reaction. Major sources of these mediators include mast cells, eosinophils, basophils, and macrophages. The secreted leukotrienes bring about bronchoconstriction, mucous metaplasia, and eosinophil chemotaxis through receptor-mediated mechanisms.[30] The concentration of leukotrienes could be measured in body fluids such as urine, plasma, and exhaled breath condensate. Elevated urinary LTE4 levels have been reported in patients with atopic asthma.[31] Raithel et al. demonstrated enhanced excretion of LTB4 and cysteinyl leukotrienes in urine of patients with indolent systemic mastocytosis and suggested that determination of urinary leukotrienes could be used for diagnosis and therapeutic monitoring of systemic mastocytosis.[32]

Fractional Exhaled Nitric oxide

Fractional exhaled nitric oxide (FENO) is a simple, noninvasive and reproducible biomarker of ongoing eosinophilic airway inflammation and has been recently recommended as a secondary outcome to evaluate the therapeutic efficacy and/or to characterize steroid responsive phenotypes in asthma clinical trials.[31] The FeNO levels have been shown to positively correlate with eosinophilic inflammation, with low (<25 ppb) and high (>50 ppb) FeNO levels indicating non-eosinophilic inflammation with poor corticosteroid response, and eosinophilic inflammation and corticosteroid responsiveness, respectively.[33] A recent study has suggested that FeNO could be a useful indicator of atopic phenotype among asthmatics.[34]

BIOMARKERS FOR EFFICACY OF ALLERGEN IMMUNOTHERAPY

The therapeutic strategies routinely used in clinical practice for resolution of allergic reactions include allergen avoidance, pharmacotherapy, and allergen immunotherapy (AIT). The individualized allergy management plan involves either of these or combinations of these therapeutic strategies based on careful consideration given to patient's preference, risk/benefit assessment of immunotherapy, and severity of the disease and response to previous treatment. Allergen avoidance, wherever feasible, is the primary prevention strategy best suited for high-risk children and is the most effective and economic treatment strategy for the allergic diseases.

Assessment of Indoor Allergen Levels

Indoor aeroallergen testing is achieved, in specialized laboratories, through evaluation of quantitatively extracted fine dust (<300 μm particle size) from air/surface dust samples collected with vacuum either from a general indoor environment or individual rooms. The soluble allergen extracts are assessed for the levels of indicator allergens, from a range of sources including dust mite, pet epidermal, rodent, cockroach and molds, by either monoclonal antibody (mAb)-based immunoenzymatic assays or multiplex bead-based assays. Der f 1 and 2 and Der p 1 and 2 allergens excreted in the fecal particles of dust mites (*D. farinae* and *D. pteronyssinus*), Fel d1 and Can f 1 allergens excreted by the sweat glands of cat and dog, Bla g 1 and 2 allergens released by the cockroach, Mus m 1 and Rat n 1 allergens excreted in the urine of mouse and rat, beyond certain threshold levels are considered as the "indicators" of allergen-laden indoor environments. The threshold levels for some of these allergens have been identified. The presence of detectable levels of cockroach, rat, and mouse allergens is considered to be an indicator of clinically relevant environment contamination. While greater than 2000 ng of Der p 1 allergen, Der f 1 allergen, or both in one gram of fine dust has been associated with increased risk of allergic symptoms in sensitized subjects, greater than 10,000 ng of these allergens per gram of fine dust have been associated with increased risk of sensitization.[10] Visible mold growth or musty odors indicate indoor mold contamination and specific testing is not essential in such cases. In the absence of any visible mold growth or characteristic odor, viable spore count is obtained, by culturing bulk dust samples either directly or preprocessed by gravity sampler or suction impactor, after 24, 48 and 72 hours. The levels of Alt a 1 and Asp f 1 allergens secreted by *Alternaria* and *Aspergillus* species, respectively, could be quantified by mAb-based immunoenzymatic assays. Environmental relative moldiness index test is an alternative PCR-based method for quantification of relative levels of 36 molds (26 molds associated with water damage and 10 molds not associated with water damage). The environmental relative moldiness index level of indoor environment has been found to be effective in predicting the development of respiratory illness (wheezing, rhinitis, or both) in asthmatic children.[10,13]

Outdoor allergen levels could also be measured by sampling airborne particles, using collection devices such as Rotorod sampler, Burkard Hirst trap, and Burkard spore watch, followed by microscopic assessment of number and types of pollen and mold spores per cubic meter of air sample. However, this data corresponds to the levels of aeroallergens of the previous 24 hours and therefore is of limited use to the public.

Allergen Skin Test Titration

Allergen skin test titration has been initially validated for research use and is used as a surrogate marker in many AIT clinical trials. The reduction in skin test titration has been found to be associated with effective immunotherapy, but at present, this measure is not considered to be practical for routine clinical use.[29,35]

Molecular Biomarkers for Evaluation of Immunotherapy

Growing knowledge of molecular mechanisms underlying the immunomodulatory effects of AIT has allowed the identification of several objective measures for evaluation of the efficacy of AIT or prediction of clinical responders to AIT. These measures have been found to be valuable secondary outcomes for the assessment of immunologic effects of AIT in clinical trials. Some of the measures include ssIgE /total IgE ratio (tIgE), allergen-specific IgG levels, cytokines such as interferon gamma (IFN-γ), interleukins (IL-5, IL-10, IL-12), nasal eosinophil cation protein, tryptase, transforming growth factor-β (TGFβ), and other inflammatory parameters.[29,36] Although their surrogacy for clinical endpoints is unproven, these objective measures can have additional value when used in clinical studies, particularly in early stage, proof-of-concept, and dose-ranging (phase-II) trials.

ssIgE/tIgE

The ratio of ssIgE/tIgE has been proposed as a potential predictor of AIT outcome based on a clinical study of timothy grass pollen immunotherapy. In this study, in vitro analysis of 279 monosensitized subjects receiving immunotherapy has revealed a significant correlation between ssIgE/tIgE ratio and clinical response (as measured by visual analog scores). Further, ssIgE/tIgE ratio has been shown to predict AIT clinical outcome with a sensitivity and specificity of 97.2% and 88.1%, respectively.[37] However, the results were not reproducible in another randomized, controlled, open-labeled, three parallel group study involving 48 asthmatic and rhinitis children sensitized to house dust mite receiving either immunotherapy or pharmacotherapy. The lack of reproducibility in this study may be partially attributed to small sample size. Further evaluation of ssIgE/tIgE ratios in large randomized double-blind, placebo-controlled studies is required before utilizing it as a biomarker for effective immunotherapy.

Cytokines

Long-term peripheral tolerance induction following immunotherapy is associated with immune deviation from a Th2 cell pattern (IL-4 and IL-5) of response to a more Th1(IFN-γ) and regulatory T (Treg)-cell pattern (IL-10 and TGFβ). In fact, induction and function of IL-10 and TGFβ producing $CD4^+CD25^+Foxp3^+$ Treg cells following AIT has been observed in several studies and is considered as an important mechanism of peripheral tolerance induction.[37-39] A time-dependent increase in IL-10 levels has been observed in a 12-month study of conventional grass pollen immunotherapy.[37] In this study they have also identified that a significant increase in IL-10 levels could be observed as early as 2–4 weeks during the buildup phase. The secreted IL-10 and TGFβ suppress the activity of allergen-specific Th2 cells and simultaneously stimulate B cells to undergo antibody isotype class switching, in favor of protective antibodies IgG_4 and IgA_2. Subcutaneous immunotherapy-induced inhibition of allergen-induced late cutaneous responses has been shown to positively correlate with increase in IL-12 (Th1 cell cytokine) mRNA expression in skin macrophages.[39,40] A simultaneous increase in IFN-γ and decrease in IL-4 has also been reported in this study. Together, these studies suggest that measuring interleukin patterns in immunotherapy clinical trials may help in objective assessment of efficacy of AIT.

Allergen-specific IgG_4 and IgA_2 Antibodies

IL-10 and TGFβ-induced antibody isotype class switching induces the production of IgG_4 and IgA_2. The secreted allergen-specific IgG_4 antibodies either directly disrupt the interaction between allergen and mast cell-bound IgE by directly competing for the same epitope or indirectly inhibiting the binding of IgE-allergen complexes to the low-affinity receptors on B-cells and thus inhibit the IgE-facilitated allergen presentation to T cells. The competitive inhibition of allergen binding to allergen-specific IgE could be measured in basophil histamine release assays and inhibition of IgE-facilitated allergen presentation could be assessed in facilitated allergen-binding (FAB) assays. Although elevated levels of IgG_4 is consistent with immunotherapy, many studies fail to find a correlation between elevated IgG_4 levels and effective immunotherapy.[37,39] A significant correlation with clinical efficacy has been reported for serum inhibitory activity measured by IgE-FAB assay.[41] However, the correlation is not sufficient to recommend the assay for evaluation of treatment response in clinical practice. Similar to IgG_4, IgA_2 is also a noninflammatory isotype which has been shown to increase after grass pollen immunotherapy. Induction of IgA_2 has been shown to promote IgG_4 production through an IL-10-mediated mechanism.[37]

CONCLUSION

The biomarkers presently being utilized in clinical trials and routine practice for the diagnosis, monitoring and management of allergic diseases suffer from one or more of the following shortcomings: (1) poor predictive value, (2) lack of reproducibility, (3) risk of adverse reactions, (4) time consuming, (5) costly/resource intensive, (6) invasive, and (7) require expertise and trained personnel. In addition, the symptoms of various allergic and nonallergic diseases overlap causing difficulties in diagnosis. Further, existence of endophenotypes with variable treatment response warrants better diagnostics for efficient management of allergic diseases. The application of microarray and proteomics for identification of molecule/s has certainly added new dimensions to the field of allergy biomarkers. For instance, glycoproteomics of plasma from patients with AD has revealed CD5L and apolipoprotein E (ApoE) as potential biomarkers.[42] Further, microRNA profiling studies have led to the identification of distinct profiles of microRNA associated with asthma and other allergic phenotypes.[6,43] In addition, novel noninvasive skin biomarkers such as skin autofluorescence and inflammatory cytokine profiles in skin washings have been shown to improve the diagnosis of psoriasis and AD.[44] However, the allergic diseases are considered to be complex involving interactions at multiple levels, and a system-level understanding of these interacting networks warrants better management of allergic diseases. Therefore, the need of the hour in the field of allergy biomarkers is the application of integrated systems approach combining the comprehensive data from genomics, proteomics, epigenomics, transcriptomics, and metabolomics with a goal of stratified/personalized medicine.

REFERENCES

1. Kay AB. Allergy and hypersensitivity: history and concepts-allergy and allergic diseases. In: Kay AB, Bousquet J, Holt PG, Kaplan AP, eds. Wiley-Blackwell Publishing, UK; 2008:3-22.
2. Pawankar R, Canonica GW, Holgate ST, et al. The WAO White Book on Allergy: Update 2013; 2013. http://www.worldallergy.org/definingthespecialty/white_book.php.
3. Pawankar R. Allergic diseases and asthma: a global public health concern and a call to action. World Allergy Organ J. 2014;7:1-3.
4. Böhme M, Lannerö E, Wickman M, et al. Atopic dermatitis and concomitant disease patterns in children up to two years of age. Acta Derm Venereol. 2002;82:98-103.
5. Suh, D, Sung J, Gause D, et al. Economic burden of atopic manifestations in patients. J Manage Care Pharm. 2007;13:778-89.
6. Ortiz RA, Barnes KC. Genetics of allergic diseases. Immunol Allergy Clin. NA 2015;35:19-44.
7. Holloway JW, Yang IA, Holgate ST. Genetics of allergic disease. J Allergy Clin Immunol. 2010;125:S81-94.
8. Vercelli D. Discovering susceptibility genes for asthma and allergy. Nat Rev Immunol. 2008;8:169-82.
9. Pawankar R, Canonica GW, Holgate ST, Lockey RF. White Book on Allergy; 2011. http://www.worldallergy.org/definingthespecialty/white_book.php.
10. Hamilton RG. Clinical laboratory assessment of immediate-type hypersensitivity. J Allergy Clin Immunol. 2010;125:S284-96.
11. Cox L, Williams B, Sicherer S, et al. Pearls and pitfalls of allergy diagnostic testing: report from the American College of Allergy, Asthma and Immunology/American Academy of Allergy, Asthma and Immunology Specific IgE Test Task Force. Ann Allergy Asthma Immunol. 2008;101:580-92.
12. Oppenheimer J, Nelson HS. Skin testing. Ann Allergy Asthma Immunol. 2006;96:S6-12.
13. Douglass JA, O'Hehir RE. Diagnosis, treatment and prevention of allergic disease: the basics. Med J Aust. 2006;185:228-33.
14. Wood RA, Segall N, Ahlstedt S, Williams PB. Accuracy of IgE antibody laboratory results. Ann Allergy Asthma Immunol. 2007;99:34-41.
15. Mari A, Alessandri C, Bernardi ML, et al. Microarrayed allergen molecules for the diagnosis of allergic diseases. Curr Allergy Asthma Rep. 2010;10:357-64.
16. Lupinek C, Wollmann E, Baar A, et al. Advances in allergen-microarray technology for diagnosis and monitoring of allergy: the MeDALL allergen-chip. Methods. 2014;66: 106-19.
17. De Vos G. Skin testing versus serum-specific IgE testing: which is better for diagnosing aeroallergen sensitization and predicting clinical allergy? Curr Allergy Asthma Rep. 2014;14:430-7.
18. Agache I, Bilò M, Braunstahl GJ, et al. In vivo diagnosis of allergic diseases—allergen provocation tests. Allergy. 2015;70:355-65.
19. Kleine-tebbe J, Erdmann S, Knol F, et al. Diagnostic tests based on human basophils: potentials, pitfalls and perspectives. Int Arch Allergy Immunol. 2006;141:79-90.
20. Rabenhorst A, Hartmann K. Interleukin-31: a novel diagnostic marker of allergic diseases. Curr Allergy Asthma Rep. 2014;14:1-7.
21. Aral M, Arican O, Gul M, et al. The relationship between serum levels of total IgE, IL-18, IL-12, IFN-γ and disease severity in children with atopic dermatitis. Mediators Inflamm. 2006;2006:1-4.
22. Landheer J, Kishida M, Kuroiwa R, et al. Utility of serum thymus and activation-regulated chemokine as a biomarker for monitoring of atopic dermatitis severity. J Am Acad Dermatol. 2014;71:1160-6.
23. Miyazaki Y, Unoura K, Tateishi T, et al. Higher serum CCL17 may be a promising predictor of acute exacerbations in chronic hypersensitivity pneumonitis. Respir Res. 2013;14:57.
24. Jahnz-Rozyk K, Targowski T, Paluchowska E, et al. Serum thymus and activation-regulated chemokine, macrophage-derived chemokine and eotaxin as markers of severity of atopic dermatitis. Allergy Eur J Allergy Clin Immunol. 2005;60:685-8.
25. Nakazato J, Kishida M, Kuroiwa R, et al. Serum levels of Th2 chemokines, CCL17, CCL22, and CCL27, were the important markers of severity in infantile atopic dermatitis. Pediatr Allergy Immunol. 2008;19:605-13.
26. Akin C, Valent P. Diagnostic criteria and classification of mastocytosis in 2014. Immunol Allergy Clin NA. 2014;34:207-18.
27. Randall B, Butts J, Halsey JF. Elevated postmortem tryptase in the absence of anaphylaxis. J Forensic Sci. 1995;40:208-11.
28. Golden DBK, Demain J, Freeman T, et al. Stinging insect hypersensitivity: a practice parameter update 2011. J Allergy Clin Immunol. 2011;127:852-4.e23.
29. Cox L, Nelson H, Lockey R, et al. Allergen immunotherapy: a practice parameter third update. J Allergy Clin Immunol. 2010;127:S1-55.
30. Niimi A. Cough, asthma, and cysteinyl-leukotrienes. Pulm Pharmacol Ther. 2013;26:514-9.
31. Szefler SJ, Wenzel S, Brown R, et al. Asthma outcomes: Biomarkers. J Allergy Clin Immunol. 2012;129:S9-23.
32. Raithel M, Zopf Y, Kimpel S, et al. The measurement of leukotrienes in urine as diagnostic option in systemic mastocytosis. J Physiol Pharmacol. 2011;62:469-72.
33. Dweik R, Boggs P, Erzurum S, Irvin C. et al. An official ATS clinical practice guideline: interpretation of exhaled nitric

oxide levels (FENO) for clinical applications. Am J Respir Crit Care Med. 2011;184:602-15.
34. Romero KM, Robinson CL, Baumann LM, et al. and PURA Study Investigators. Role of exhaled nitric oxide as a predictor of atopy. Respir Res. 2013;14:48.
35. Makatsori M, Pfaar O, Calderon MA. Allergen immunotherapy: clinical outcomes assessment. J Allergy Clin Immunol Pract. 2014;42:123-9.
36. Pfaar O, Kleine-Tebbe J, Hörmann K, Klimek L. Allergen-specific immunotherapy: which outcome measures are useful in monitoring clinical trials? Immunol Allergy Clin North Am. 2011;31:289-309.
37. Shamji MH, James LK, Durham SR. Serum Immunologic markers for monitoring allergen-specific immunotherapy. Immunol. Allergy Clin North Am. 2011;31:311-23.
38. Akdis M, Akdis CA. Mechanisms of allergen-specific immunotherapy. J Allergy Clin Immunol. 2007;119:780-9.
39. Viswanathan RK, Busse WW. Allergen immunotherapy in allergic respiratory diseases: from mechanisms to meta-analyses. Chest. 2012;141:1303-14.
40. Maggi E. T cell responses induced by allergen-specific immunotherapy. Clin Exp Immunol. 2010;161:10-8.
41. Till S. Mechanisms of immunotherapy and surrogate markers. Allergy Eur J Allergy Clin. Immunol. 2011;66:25-7.
42. Kim WK, Hwang HR, Kim DH, et al. Glycoproteomic analysis of plasma from patients with atopic dermatitis: CD5L and ApoE as potential biomarkers. Exp Mol Med. 2008;40:677-85.
43. Sinha A, Yadav AK, Chakraborty S, et al. Exosome-enclosed microRNAs in exhaled breath hold potential for biomarker discovery in patients with pulmonary diseases. J Allergy Clin Immunol. 2013;132:219-22.
44. Portugal-Cohen M, Horev L, Ruffer C, et al. Non-invasive skin biomarkers quantification of psoriasis and atopic dermatitis: cytokines, antioxidants and psoriatic skin auto-fluorescence. Biomed Pharmacother. 2012;66:293-9.

SUGGESTED READING

1. Fleming TR, Powers JH. Biomarkers and surrogate endpoints in clinical trials. Stat Med. 2012;31:2973-84.
2. Johansson SGO. The history of IgE: From discovery to 2010. Curr. Allergy Asthma Rep. 2011;11:173-7.
3. Kewal KJ. The Handbook of Biomarkers. (Humana Press, 2010).
4. Lassere MN, et al. Definitions and validation criteria for biomarkers and surrogate endpoints: Development and testing of a quantitative hierarchical levels of evidence schema. J Rheumatol. 2007;34:607-15.
5. Strimbu K, Tavel JA. What are Biomarkers? Curr Opin HIV AIDS. 2011;5:463-6.

CHAPTER 50

In Vitro Testing for Specific IgE

Major K Nagaraju, N Karthik

INTRODUCTION

Diagnosis of human allergic diseases (type I hypersensitivity reaction) is mainly through a detailed clinical history and the physical examination. The degree of suspicion for the diagnosis of allergic diseases increases with positive temporal association with allergen exposure. First identified in 1967 as reagin antibody, the role of immunoglobulin E (IgE) in allergy has been evaluated extensively.[1] Demonstration of allergen-specific IgE in algorithmic evaluation of allergic diseases is done either as in vivo tests such as skin prick test or as in vitro tests. In vitro tests measure the amount of circulating IgE antibody in the blood. The presence of specific IgE is not definitive of allergic diseases and fails to differentiate between sensitization and disease state. Allergen-specific IgE antibody is a marker of allergic sensitization. Along with this test, clinical history, and physical examination, we can strongly predict an allergic disorder. It is a diagnostic challenge for the clinician to differentiate clinically relevant allergen components within the allergen from the nonrelevant one. This chapter will provide an overview of types and methods of commonly available in vitro allergy testing and its role in the evaluation of allergic diseases with a look into the future prospects.

CHARACTERISTICS OF IDEAL IgE TEST

The tests for the detection of total or specific IgE should ideally:[2]

- Be highly accurate
- Be highly sensitive and specific
- Be reproducible
- Be standardized
- Have a good quality control
- Be easy to use
- Be automated (reduces human errors)
- Test a wide variety of allergens
- Be free of cross-reactivity
- Be affordable.

METHODS

Radioallergosorbent Test

Radioallergosorbent test (RAST) was the first method used for the identification of allergen-specific IgE. This method used radioactive labels for the identification of antigen–antibody complexes.

Immunoassay

Immunoassay is the most commonly used method for in-hospital testing and in laboratories. This method is based on the interaction between antigen and antigen-specific antibodies, which is identified using enzyme (enzyme immunoassay) or fluorescence-labeled markers (fluorescence enzyme immunoassay).[3]

PRINCIPLE OF ALLERGEN-SPECIFIC IGE IMMUNOASSAY

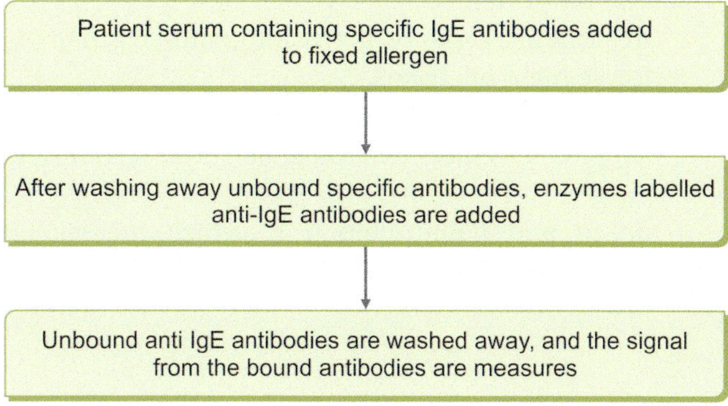

Indications for IgE Testing

- Allergic rhinitis[4]
- Allergic asthma
- Suspected food allergies
- Atopic dermatitis (AD)
- Insect bite allergies
- Drug allergies (IgE-mediated).

Why In Vitro Testing Needed?

Although skin testing for allergy diagnosis is the preferred method due to its immediate results, there are certain situations where in vitro testing has a significant role.[4]
These include the following:

- Extensive eczema of the skin making it unsuitable for doing allergy skin testing
- Patients on antihistamines and unable to stop the same
- Dermographism
- Immediately following an anaphylaxis
- Risk of anaphylaxis with minute amounts of allergen
- Older patients with cardiovascular disease or on beta-blockers or ACE inhibitors
- Practitioners not trained in allergy skin testing
- In younger infants.

CLASSIFICATION OF SPECIFIC IgE ANTIBODY IMMUNOASSAYS

- *Qualitative assays*
  The most diffuse and typical illustration is the multiallergen screening test in which different antigen specialities are present in a single reagent. No calibration curve is needed for this method. It indicates either positive or negative based on preassailed positive threshold.[5-8]
- *Semiquantitative assays*
  The variations in the positive signal detected are commonly presented: [5]
  - in terms of a series of increasing grades (e.g., I to IV, low to high) or classes.
  - in arbitrary units (U/mL) determined relative to a supplier-specific, heterologous dose-responsive curve.
  - or an end point dilution to which the signal becomes negative (e.g., titer).[5,9]
- *Quantitative assay*
  A quantitative assay provides an accurate and reproducible estimation of concentration of IgE and fulfills the analytical criteria for quantification.[5,8]

TYPES OF IMMUNOASSAYS

Nowadays, we are using two types of immunoassays for the measurement of specific IgE, which are based on the use of[8]

- Solid-phase immunoassays
- Liquid-phase immunoassays (the fluid-phase allergen is bound to the solid phase only after the allergen has complexed with the fluid-phase IgE antibody).

Solid-phase immunoassays make use of allergens bound to some forms of matrix or substrate, such as (allergosorbent or immunosorbent)[8]

- Insoluble dextran
- Cellulose
- Filter paper disc (RAST)
- Minicolumns (CAP)
- Thread (CLA)
- Microcrystalline particles
- Nitrocellulose (dot blot)
- Polystyrene tube (fast)
- Microtiter well-activated silica chip [immune solid-phase allergy chip (ISAC)].

Liquid-phase immunoassays are performed with solutions of antigens and antibodies. Biotin-labeled allergens (ADVIA Centaur) in the ligand (biotin) is covalently attached to a backbone (soluble polymer and amino acid copolymer) to which the allergen molecules are also attached (Immulite 2000).[8]

FACTORS INFLUENCING THE ACCURACY OF IN VITRO IgE TESTING

- Types of method used
- Methods of standardization
- Quality control
- Quality of reagents and buffers used
- Education, training, and experience of the technical staff
- Laboratory quality control practices.

Although several in vitro diagnostic products are introduced in the market, only few products are currently available and few have withdrawn their products from the market. More popular products are ImmunoCap (ThermoFisher, previously Phadia), Immulite (Siemens), and Hytec-288 (Hycor), which have the largest share in the global market and are also available in India. These methods are not interchangeable. They differ in allergen quantity, quantification of specific IgE, and cutoff points.[2,10-14]

TECHNIQUES COMMONLY AVAILABLE IN INDIA—WHICH ONE TO CHOOSE?

Reports given by the different laboratories are not uniform, and also, they will not mention what type of the method they used. The physicians ordering the test must mention which type of the method they wants to test for their patient in the request form. Several bogus tests are carried out by so many nonstandardized laboratories, especially in India, and it is the responsibility of the physicians to see whether the test is done properly and the results are good. All systems are calibrated using WHO 75/502 International human serum IgE reference preparation and are automated.[2,15] The analysis of different literatures shows that ImmunoCAP system is the most popular among the physicians partly due to its pioneer status in allergy diagnostics and partly due to its continuous innovation:[2,7]

- Clinicians must check which method the test was done before interpreting the results.
- Nowadays, radioimmunoassay is no more used as radiation is the concern.

POINTS TO REMEMBER WHILE ORDERING AND INTERPRETING THE RESULTS

- The presence of IgE indicates sensitization, which does not necessarily imply allergic disease. It may be genuine sensitization or may be cross-reactivity.
- Knowledge and experience of the clinician is very important.
- Correct method should be recommended while ordering the test.
- Negative test does not mean no allergy.
- Clinical history, environment, living conditions, and local aerobiological data guide the physicians to select the number of allergens to be tested.
- Large panel of tests should not be recommended.
- Correct interpretation of test results is guided by a clinical history and the physical examination (Table 50.1).

Table 50.1: Grading of immunoCAP results.

Range (KUA/L)	*Grade*	*Description*
0.1–0.35		Detectable, low
0.36–0.69	1	Low
0.70–3.49	2	Moderate
3.50–17.40	3	High
17.50–49.0	4	Very high
50.0–99.0	5	Very high
>100	6	Very high

MERITS OF IN VITRO SPECIFIC IgE TESTING

- Needs a very small amount of blood sample for results
- Good for screening purposes
- Useful when antihistamines cannot be withheld
- Useful in AD and other skin diseases where the skin is involved at the site
- Useful in dermographism
- Useful in food allergies, whether child outgrown with that food or not?[15]
- Safe in patients with history of anaphylaxis
- It is a general practitioner domain.
- As a part of workup in allergic bronchopulmonary aspergillosis (ABPA)
- It is useful in very young children, where the skin prick test is difficult to do.
- Total IgE will not interfere with the results, especially when we use immunoCap method.
- Useful in people who afraid of needle pricks
- Severely or poorly controlled asthmatics
- Highly uncooperative patients.

LIMITATIONS OF IN VITRO SPECIFIC IgE TESTING

- Expensive method
- Need costly equipment. Investment will be heavy.
- Requires regular maintenance and calibration of the equipment
- Not able to visualize the reaction by the patient/parent.
- Need to obtain blood samples.
- It takes some time to get the test results: we will get test results within 15-20 minutes in skin prick test.

WHEN TO REPEAT IN VITRO SPECIFIC IgE TESTS?

- To check whether food allergies have been outgrown and to find out whether allergen avoidance is necessary.[15]
- To check for increasing or decreasing specific IgE antibodies titers and to emphasize allergen avoidance measures.
- To look for newer allergen sensitization.
- To know the possible improvement or worsening of the allergic status.
- To check whether the patient has developed tolerance to a particular food allergen.
- By repeating the IgE-specific antibodies, the need for food challenges will be reduced.

Apart from these three techniques (ImmunoCAP, Immulite, and Hytec288), several newer variety of tests are available. The drawback remains the lack of correlation between these different tests:

- *EUROIMMUN*, a new entrant that provides in vitro test systems for the determination of specific IgE antibodies in patient sera with "CCD band" as an additional indicator for the clinical relevance of specific IgE results. *In the EUROLINE test system, membrane strips with 20 different allergens are used, allowing a detailed patient allergy profile to be obtained with a single test.* Moreover, the specific antibodies are determined semiquantitatively by comparing the intensities using "Euroline Scan System".[16]
- In a similar fashion, Omega Diagnostics have brought out "*Allergodip*" *dipsticks*. This is based on the principle of immunoassay for the determination of specific IgE without any laboratory equipment.[16]
- The latest development is the emergence of "*POC Panels*" named "*FAST CHECK POC*" from a German company. The product is available in Europe, but not yet available in India. It promises to revolutionize the allergy diagnostics by shifting the action directly at the physician's desk rather than referring to laboratory. Consequently, the results can be interpreted within 20 minutes, clinically correlated, and affordable.[16]
- All the aforementioned tests are not accepted by the physicians mainly due to the lack of standardization and the false-negative results.

COMPONENT-RESOLVED DIAGNOSIS

Specific IgE tests for allergic diseases only detect sensitization to whole allergen extracts, and we do not know to which molecule the patient is allergic. Component-resolved diagnosis (CRD) can distinguish sensitization to the clinically relevant allergic components from the clinically irrelevant allergic components. CRD will detect the IgE-specific components that are potentially dangerous such as lipid-transfer proteins or are less dangerous such as polcalcins and profilins. Food allergies in aeroallergen-sensitized patients are an excellent example where it is relevant to distinguish between cross-reacting allergens of low clinical significance and those with a high risk for systemic reactions.[13,17]

Advantages

- We can predict or assess the risk of clinical reaction.[13,17]
- It helps to differentiate between genuine sensitization and cross-reactivity.
- It identifies an appropriate antigen for targeting in allergen immunotherapy in polysensitized individuals.

MULTIPLEX SYSTEM (SEMIQUANTITATIVE)

ISAC is a multiplex system that enables the measurement of IgE antibodies to a fixed panel of 112 components from 51 allergen sources in a single step, using only 30 μL of serum or plasma. Microarray-based ISAC testing has a high sensitivity and specificity and showed a strong correlation with the in vitro IgE and skin prick test with extracts, specifically for respiratory allergens. The ISAC test will be able to identify cross-reactions between pollen and food-related sensitizations.[13,18]

Allergy explorer (ALEX) is a newly developed macroarray containing both extracted "whole" allergens and molecular components. This method allows the acquisition of an IgE profile comprising 282 reagents (157 allergen extracts and 125 components), resulting in the widest screening of potential allergens available.[4,13]

Multiplex system (ISAC/ALEX) is useful in the followings:

- Identifying the real sensitization profile of multisensitized patients.
- Revealing potential risk for severe food-related reactions.
- Identifying the IgE antibody profile in patients with unsatisfactory response to treatment.
- Ruling out allergy, when the patients present with allergic symptoms.
- Identifying the causative agent of allergen causing anaphylaxis.

CELL-BASED TECHNOLOGIES

Cell-based technologies are extensively used as an alternative to the measurement of allergen-specific IgE antibody. In this technology, the human basophil will be activated by the allergen. These assays are expensive and time-consuming and also require a special technical skill.[5]

TOTAL IgE MEASUREMENT

Total IgE measurement indicates the total amount of circulating IgE in human serum or plasma. IgE antibodies appear as a result of sensitization to allergens in patients suffering from asthma, rhinitis, AD, or food allergies. However, total IgE also increased in other conditions such as worm infestations, multiple myeloma, ABPA, and allergic fungal sinusitis.[19] Physicians must eliminate these causes by a clinical history and the physical examination before labeling as IgE-mediated disorder.[7]

Most laboratories report IgE concentrations in IU or ng per mL (1 IU = 2.4 ng IgE). Approximately one half of patients with allergic disease have serum IgE levels in the normal range. When a high value of IgE is chosen to distinguish allergic from nonallergic individuals, the specificity of the test is often greater than 90%, but the sensitivity is lesser than 30–50%. Lowering the threshold level increases the sensitivity but decreases the specificity. Serum IgE concentration is mostly age dependent. Very low levels of IgE are found in the cord serum with a progressive increase observed up to the age of 15 years and then with a decline from the second through the eighth decades of life.[9]

CLINICAL USE OF TOTAL IgE IN ALLERGIC DISEASES

- Total IgE measurement aids in the clinical diagnosis of IgE-mediated allergic disorders. In younger persons, high IgE levels strongly predict the probability of sensitization that may be useful to decide whether further investigation is warranted.
- Total IgE measurement provides a good indication of sensitization caused by high allergen exposure without atopy in a suspected occupational allergy.
- Total serum IgE levels are highest in AD, whereas patients with allergic asthma generally have higher levels than those with allergic rhinitis.

SUMMARY

- Diagnosis of IgE-mediated diseases is mainly made by a detailed clinical history and thorough the physical examination.
- ImmunoCAP technique is the gold standard in in vitro diagnosis of IgE-mediated disorders.
- Radioimmunoassay technique is no more used in the diagnosis of IgE-mediated disorders.
- When interpreting the in vitro test results, physicians must see which technique was used for the diagnosis of IgE-mediated allergies.
- CRD is very useful test to differentiate between genuine sensitivity from cross-reactivity.
- ISAC/ALEX is very useful in polysensitized patients.
- Total IgE levels will aid in the clinical diagnosis of IgE-mediated allergic disorders, especially in young children.

REFERENCES

1. Ishizaka K, Ishizaka T, Lee EH. Physiochemical properties of reaginic antibody. II. Characteristic properties of reaginic antibody different from human gamma-A-isohemagglutinin and gamma-D-globulin. J Allergy. 1966;37:336-49.
2. Goikoetxea MJ, Sanz ML, García BE, et al. Recommendations for the use of in vitro methods to detect specific immunoglobulin E: are they comparable? J Investig Allergol Clin Immunol. 2013;23:448-54.
3. Yalow RS, Berson SA. Immunoassay of endogenous plasma insulin in man. J Clin Invest. 1960;39:1157.
4. Heffler E, Puggioni F, Peveri S, et al. Extended IgE profile based on an allergen macroarray: a novel tool for precision medicine in allergy diagnosis. World Allergy Organ J. 2018;11:7.
5. Hamilton RG, Franklin Adkinson N. In vitro assays for the diagnosis of IgE-mediated disorders. J Allergy Clin Immunol. 2004;114:213-25.
6. Wood RA, Segall N, Ahlstedt S, Williams PB. Accuracy of IgE antibody laboratory results. Ann Allergy Asthma Immunol. 2007;99:34-41.
7. Kerkhof M, Dubois AE, Postma DS, et al. Role and interpretation of total serum IgE measurements in the diagnosis of allergic airway disease in adults. Allergy. 2003;58:905-11.
8. Johansson SGO, Yman L. In vitro assays for immunoglobulin E. Clin Rev Allergy. 1988;6:93-139.
9. Martins TB, Bandhauer ME, Bunker AM, et al. New childhood and adult reference intervals for total IgE. J Allergy Clin Immunol. 2014;133:589-91.
10. Sánchez-Borges M, Ivancevich JC, Rodríguez Pérez N, Ansotegui I. Evidence based approaches to diagnosis and management. In: Pawankar R, Canonica GW, Holgate ST, Lockey RF, Blaiss MS, ed. WAO White Book on Allergy: An Update; 2013:109-13.
11. Host A, Andrae S, Charkin S, et al. Allergy testing in children: why, who, when and how? Allergy. 2003;58:559-69.
12. Alessandri C, Zennaro D, Zaffiro A, Mari A. Molecular allergology approach to allergic disease in the paediatric age. Ital J Pediatr. 2009;35:1-12.
13. Sastre J. Molecular diagnosis in allergy. Clin Exp Allergy. 2010;40:1442-60.

14. Sicherer SH, Wood RA; American Academy of Pediatrics Section on Allergy And Immunology. Allergy testing in childhood: using allergen-specific IgE tests. Pediatrics. 2012;129:193-7.
15. Yunginger J, Ahlstedt S, Eggleston P, et al. Quantitative IgE antibody assays in allergic diseases. J Allergy Clin Immunol. 2000;105:1077-84.
16. Nagaraju K. Diagnosis of allergic diseases. In: Nagaraju K, ed. Manual of Paediatric Allergy. New Delhi: Jaypee Brothers Medical Publishers (P) Ltd; 2013:17-28.
17. Luengo O, Cardona V. Component resolved diagnosis: when should it be used? Clin Trans Allergy. 2014;4:28.
18. Jensen-Jarolim E, Jensen AN, Canonica GW. Debates in allergy medicine: molecular allergy diagnosis with ISAC will replace screenings by skin prick test in the future. World Allergy Organ J. 2017. 10. 10.1186/s40413-017-0162-3.
19. Chiriac AM, Bousquet J, Demoly P. Principles of allergy diagnosis. In: O'Hehir RE, Holgate ST, Sheikh A eds. Middleton's Allergy Essentials. Edinburgh: Elsevier; 2017:117-31.

CHAPTER 51

Diet and Allergy

Surya Kant

INTRODUCTION

"Allergy" is defined by American Academy of Allergy Asthma and Immunology as a chronic condition involving an abnormal reaction to an ordinarily harmless substance called an allergen.[1] Allergens can be divided into four categories:

- inhalants/aeroallergens (such as dust mite, mold, animal dander, tree weed, and grass pollen)
- ingestants (food and food additives, drugs)
- injectants (insect bites, stings, and some medications)
- contactants (cosmetics, heavy metals, solvents, glues, latex).

HISTORICAL ASPECTS OF DIET ASSOCIATED WITH SYMPTOMS OF ALLERGY AND ASTHMA

Hippocrates stated "Cheese does not harm all men alike; some can eat their fill of it without the slightest hurt, may, those it agrees with are wonderfully strengthened thereby. Others come off badly."

The term "allergy" was first defined by Austrian pediatrician Clemens von Pirquet [1874–1929] as "any form of altered biological reactivity" dates back to 1906; reactions to food were nothing new.[2]

Skin testing for allergy, which von Pirquet, Isaac Chandler Walker, and John Freeman developed during the 1900s and 1910s, brought laboratory experimentation into clinical practice. Suspecting an allergy to crabgrass pollen, for example, an allergist would inject crabgrass extract under the skin. If the surrounding area erupted in a wheal, the diagnosis was confirmed. Although skin testing provided a relatively reliable, although somewhat unconventional, procedure for detecting most allergens, its accuracy in cases of food allergy had begun to be questioned by the 1930s.[3] In contrast, later food allergists, such as Theron Randolph (1906–1995), would downplay the need to confirm immune system involvement in the diagnosis of allergy. The preferred test that emerged was the elimination diet, designed by Albert Rowe during the late 1920s. Patients prescribed that elimination diets would consume a bland, hypoallergenic diet and then ingest suspect foods to see whether a reaction followed. Foods were suspected of causing everything from asthma and eczema to migraine and psychiatric symptoms, and few foods were off the list of potential culprits. A survey by Virginia allergist Warren Vaughan (1893–1944) listed dozens of foods known to cause allergy and suggested that 60% of Americans were allergic to one food or another.[4]

DIET PROVOCATIVE OF SYMPTOMS OF ALLERGY AND ASTHMA

Although more than 170 foods have been identified as triggers of food allergy, those causing most of the significant allergic reactions include peanut, tree nuts, fish, shellfish, milk, egg, wheat, soy, and seeds.[5-8] Food allergy (to foods other than shellfish and fruits/vegetables) is more common in children than in adults.[9-12] The eight foods identified by the law are as follows:

- Mammalian milk (cow's and goat's milk): All milk products such as lassi or buttermilk, cheese, evaporated and condensed milk, ice cream, and yoghurt are allergic products.
- Eggs: All foods made from eggs, such as French toast, cakes, cookies, pancakes, home-made bread, and even egg-based vaccines should be avoided.
- Fish (bass, flounder, cod).
- Crustaceans shellfish (crab, lobster, shrimp).
- Soybean: Soya milk and other foods that contain soya should be avoided.

- *Wheat*: A person suffering from arthritis should not be given wheat—it can be replaced with rice, jowar, or nachni. This means that the allergic person should not be given foods made with cornstarch, semolina or suji, all-purpose or white flour. So upma, suji lapsi, suji kheer or toast, cakes, cookies, biscuits, and white sauce should be avoided.
- Tree nuts (almond, walnuts, pecans).
- *Peanuts*: All foods with peanuts should be avoided.

However, people who are allergic to peanuts can often eat tree nuts such as walnuts, cashew, hazel, almonds, or pecans, since they are from separate plant families. These eight foods and any ingredients that contain protein derived from one or more of them are designated as major food allergens by Food Allergen Labeling and Consumer Protection Act, 2004.[13]

PROTECTIVE DIET FOR ALLERGY AND ASTHMA

Their diet needs to be balanced for vitamins and minerals so that no extrasupplements are needed by the body, but the degree of severity increases the requirement. As the regular pattern of a healthy and wholesome breakfast, nutritious lunch, and light dinner is very important to be followed, the effect of medication on diet (drug and diet interaction) should be regularly monitored so that they may not trigger off any other serious side effects. However, diet is a complex combination of foods from various groups and nutrients, and some nutrients are highly correlated. It would be challenging to separate the effect of a single nutrient or food group from that of others in free-living populations.[14] Previous studies on the relationship of diet and nutrition with asthma have focused on either individual nutrients[15,16] (e.g., long-chain polyunsaturated fatty acids, vitamin D, and antioxidants) or individual food groups[17,18] (e.g., fruit, vegetables, and fish).

- Vitamin C appears to be the most abundant antioxidant in the extracellular fluid that lines the lung. It is a water-soluble vitamin that contributes to antioxidant activity through several mechanisms, including scavenging oxygen free radicals and suppressing macrophage secretion of superoxide anions. Epidemiologic studies have reported a protective effect of this vitamin on lung function.[19] Supplementation with vitamin C has been shown to decrease the severity and frequency of asthma.[20]
- Vitamin E comprises several fat-soluble components with distinct antioxidant properties.[21] Vitamin E effects have been studied, and there is evidence of beneficial effects of vitamin E on asthma.[22] High vitamin E intake is associated with reduced asthma incidence.[21]
- Getting enough vitamin D may help reduce the number of asthma attacks in children aged 6–15, according to the Vitamin D Council.[23] Sources of vitamin D include salmon, milk, fortified milk, fortified orange juice, and eggs.
- A study in the Journal of Allergy and Clinical Immunology[24] found that women with asthma who consumed higher levels of beta carotene, a form of vitamin A, had a better quality of life. Good sources of beta carotene are carrots, cantaloupe, sweet potatoes, leafy greens, broccoli, and spinach. Vitamin A has a protective effect on asthma. Vitamin A derivatives of retinol influence the development, maintenance, differentiation, and regeneration of lung epithelial cells and may play a central role in the development of airway disease.[25]
- Dietary fatty acids have an important role in asthma.[26-28] Fish oil may alleviate certain inflammatory respiratory diseases, preserve normal airway resistance, and modulate allergic sensitization.[29] There is also some evidence that the balance of the unsaturated fatty acids in diet may act directly to influence gene expression. Sources of omega-3 fatty acids are fish oil, fish, shellfish, and leafy vegetables. Sources of omega-6 fatty acids are vegetable fats such as margarine and processed foods.
- An apple a day may keep asthma away. According to a research review in *Nutrition Journal*,[30] apples were associated with a lower risk of asthma and an increased lung function.
- A survey published in the *European Respiratory Journal*[31] found that bananas might decrease wheezing due to asthma in children. This may be due to the fruit's antioxidant and potassium contents, which may improve the lung function.
- Breast milk is the best food for infants that must be exclusive diet for babies up to 1 year. Nature has provided it even the chemicals protecting allergy in the future for growing child. Researchers at Boston Children's Hospital and Harvard Medical School in the United States found that breastfeeding can promote tolerance to the foods that most often cause allergies.[32]

- A study in the *American Journal of Epidemiology*[33] found that children aged 11–19 who had low magnesium levels also had low lung flow and volume. Kids can improve their magnesium levels by eating magnesium-rich foods, such as spinach, pumpkin seeds, chard, dark chocolate, and salmon.

The role of food allergy in asthma is well recognized but is poorly quantified. The food items play a major role as food allergens on the basis of perception in asthmatic individuals. Some suspected food items are significantly associated with the demographic profile of asthmatic individuals.[34]

VARIOUS MANIFESTATIONS OF FOOD ALLERGY

Various manifestations of food allergy are listed in Table 51.1.

If patient is experiencing a severe allergic reaction to food that involves more than one body system [e.g., skin and respiratory tract and/or gastrointestinal (GI) tract], it is called anaphylaxis. Angioedema is a common symptom in patients with anaphylaxis.[35-37]

Table 51.1: Various food allergy manifestations.

Affected part of the body	*Immediate symptoms*	*Delayed symptoms*
Skin	Redness, itching, hives, measles like red bumps, swelling beneath the skin	Same as immediate symptoms plus rash similar to eczema and flushing
Eyes	Itching, tearing, redness, and swelling around eyes	Same as immediate symptoms
Upper respiratory	Nasal congestion, itching, running nose, sneezing, swelling of voice box, hoarseness, dry cough	–
Lower respiratory	Cough, chest tightness, shortness of breath, wheezing, visible signs of shortness of breath	Cough, shortness of breath, and wheezing
Gastrointestinal (GI) (oral)	Swelling of lips, tongue, or palate, itching in the mouth	–
GI (lower)	Nausea, colicky abdominal pain, reflex, vomiting, diarrhea	Same as immediate symptoms plus bloody stool irritability and food refusal with weight loss (young children)
Cardiovascular	Rapid heartbeat (occasionally slow heartbeat in anaphylaxis), low blood pressure, dizziness, fainting loss of consciousness	–
Others	Uterine contractions	–

TREATMENT

It is not supposed to use allergen-specific immunotherapy or immunotherapy with cross-reactive allergens to treat food allergy involving IgE. The safety of immunotherapy is uncertain. Early studies of allergen-specific immunotherapy have had promising results, but the therapeutic effect and the duration of benefit have not been proven. If a patient develops anaphylaxis, then an intramuscular injection of epinephrine should be initiated. After epinephrine has been given, the patient may be placed in a reclining position to help restore normal blood flow.[38] A healthcare professional may also give the patient any of the following secondary treatments:

- Medications to help the patient breathe
- Antihistamines to relieve itching and hives
- Corticosteroids to prevent pain, swelling, and redness
- Medications to help restore normal blood pressure and maintain a normal heart rate
- Supplemental oxygen therapy
- Intravenous fluids.

Epinephrine should be given immediately to treat anaphylaxis. Delays in giving epinephrine to patients can result in a rapid decline and death within 30–60 minutes. Epinephrine acts immediately, but it may be necessary to give repeat doses. The allergenic food should be removed from the mouth or skin. If an auto-injector is available, epinephrine will be injected into the thigh muscle.

PREVENTION

The main method of managing is by avoiding those foods causing allergy for that particular individual. Egg-based vaccinations such as influenza, MMR, and rabies should be avoided in patients suffering from egg allergy. Education is an essential part of management for all asthma patients. Education should not, however, be limited to providing knowledge, but ideally should be aimed at altering behavior. This will help patients participate in self-management plans and better control of their asthma.[39]

REFERENCES

1. National Asthma Education and Prevention Program. Expert Panel Report 3(EPR-3): guidelines for the Diagnosis and Management of Asthma Summary Report 2007. J Allergy Clin Immunol. 2011;127:145-52.
2. Von Pirquet C. Allergie. Munch Med Wochenschr 1906;30:1457-8.
3. Feinberg S. Allergy in General Practice. London, UK: Kimpton; 1934.
4. Vaughan WT. Minor allergy: its distribution, clinical aspects, and significance. J Allergy. 1935;5:184-96.
5. Sicherer SH, Munoz-Furlong A, Godbold JH, Sampson HA. US prevalence of self-reported peanut, tree nut, and sesame allergy: 11-year follow-up. J Allergy Clin Immunol. 2010;125:1322-6.
6. Gupta RS, Springston EE, Warrier MR, et al. The prevalence, severity, and distribution of childhood food allergy in the United States. Pediatrics. 2011;128:e9-17.
7. Ben-Shoshan M, Harrington DW, Soller L, et al. A population-based study on peanut, tree nut, fish, shellfish, and sesame allergy prevalence in Canada. J Allergy Clin Immunol. 2010;125:1327-35.
8. Osborne NJ, Koplin JJ, Martin PE, et al. Prevalence of challenge-proven IgE-mediated food allergy using population-based sampling and predetermined challenge criteria in infants. J Allergy Clin Immunol. 2011;127:668-76.
9. Rona RJ, Keil T, Summers C, et al. The prevalence of food allergy: a meta-analysis. J Allergy Clin Immunol. 2007;120:638-46.
10. Zuidmeer L, Goldhahn K, Rona RJ, et al. The prevalence of plant food allergies: a systematic review. J Allergy Clin Immunol. 2008;121:1210-8.
11. Luccioli S, Ross M, Labiner-Wolfe J, Fein SB. Maternally reported food allergies and other food-related health problems in infants: characteristics and associated factors. Pediatrics. 2008;122:S105-2.
12. Canadian Government: The Food and Drugs Act, Part 2 Food and Drugs Regulations, Part B Foods, Division 21 Foods for special dietary uses, Regulation B.24.018. http://www.hc-sc.gc.ca/fn-an/alt_formats/hpfb-dgpsa/pdf/legislation/e_d-text-2.pdf. Accessed December, 2005.
13. Bakolis I, Hooper R, Thompson RL, Shaheen SO. Dietary patterns and adult asthma: population-based case-control study. Allergy. 2010;65:606-15.
14. Jain P, Kant S, Mishra R, et al. Reported adverse food reactions overestimate true food allergy in asthmatics. Indian J Appl Pure Biol. 2012;27:257-65.
15. Hooper R, Heinrich J, Omenaas E, et al. Dietary patterns and risk of asthma: results from three countries in European Community Respiratory Health Survey-II. Br J Nutr. 2010;103:1354-65.
16. Kant S, Jain P, Gupta B. Diet and asthma. J Physiol. 2007;8:27-30.
17. Shaheen SO, Jameson KA, Syddall HE, et al. The relationship of dietary patterns with adult lung function and COPD. Eur Respir J. 2010;36:277-84.
18. Schwartz J, Weiss ST. Relationship between dietary vitamin C intake and pulmonary function in the First National Health and Nutrition examination survey (NHANES I). Am J Clin Nutr. 1994;59:110-4.
19. Gilliland FD, Berhane KT, Li YF, et al. Children's lung function and antioxidant vitamin, fruit, juice and vegetable intake. Am J Epidemiol. 2003;158:576-84.
20. Greenough A, Shaheen SO, Shennan A, et al. Respiratory outcomes in early childhood following antenatal vitamin C and E supplementation. Thorax. 2010;65:998-1003.
21. Litonjua AA. Fat-soluble vitamins and atopic disease: what is the evidence? Proc Nutr Soc. 2012;71:67-74.
22. Hoskins A, Roberts JL 2nd, Milne G, et al. Natural-source d-alpha-tocopheryl acetate inhibits oxidant stress and modulates atopic asthma in humans in vivo. Allergy. 2012;67:676-82.
23. Gupta A, Bush A, Hawrylowicz C, Saglani S. Vitamin D and asthma in children. Paediatr Respir Rev. 2012;13:236-43; quiz 243.
24. Mora JR, Iwata M, von Andrian UH. Vitamin effects on the immune system: vitamins A and D take centre stage. Nat Rev Immunol. 2008;8:685-98.
25. Katsoulis K, Kontakiotis T, Leonardopoulos I, et al. Serum total antioxidant status in severe exacerbation of asthma: correlation with the severity of the disease. J Asthma. 2003;40:847-54.
26. Wendell SG, Baffi C, Holguin F. Fatty acids, inflammation, and asthma. J Allergy Clin Immunol. 2014;133:1255-64.
27. Raj D, Kabra SK, Lodha R. Childhood obesity and risk of allergy or asthma. Immunol Allergy Clin North Am. 2014;34:753-65.
28. Papoutsakis C, Chondronikola M, Antonogeorgos G, et al. Associations between central obesity and asthma in children and adolescents: a case-control study. J Asthma. 2014;52:128-34.
29. Boyer J, Liu RH. Apple phytochemicals and its health benefits. Nutr J. 2004;3:5.

30. Okoko BJ, Burney PG, Newson RB, et al. Childhood asthma and fruit consumption. Eur Respir J. 2007;29: 1161-8.
31. Ohsaki A, Venturelli N, Buccigrosso TM, et al. Breast milk found to protect against food allergy. J Exp Med. 2017.
32. Gilliland FD, Berhane KT, Li YF, et al. Dietary magnesium, potassium, sodium, and children's lung function. Am J Epidemiol. 2002:155;125-31.
33. Caubet JC, Eigenmann PA. Allergic triggers in atopic dermatitis. Immunol Allergy Clin North Am. 2010;30: 289-307.
34. Jain P, Kant S, Mishra R. Perception of dietary food items as food allergens in asthmatics individuals in north Indian population. J Am Coll Nutr. 2011;30:274-83.
35. Leung DY. Our evolving understanding of the functional role of filaggrin in atopic dermatitis. J Allergy Clin Immunol. 2009;124:494-5.
36. van den Oord RA, Sheikh A. Filaggrin gene defects and risk of developing allergic sensitisation and allergic disorders: systematic review and meta-analysis. BMJ. 2009;339:b2433.
37. Warshaw EM, Belsito DV, DeLeo VA, et al. North American Contact Dermatitis Group patch-test results, 2003-2004 study period. Dermatitis. 2008;19:129-36.
38. Agnihotri S, Kant S, Mishra SK, Tripathi PM. Prevalence of asthma and its treatments: a resource. Dynamics Human Health. 2015;2.
39. Sodhi R, Prasad R, Kushwaha R, et al. A study to know the knowledge, attitude, and practices of patients of bronchial asthma. Int J Med Public Health. 2013;3:159-62.

CHAPTER 52

Need of Allergy as a Medical Specialty

Rajendra Prasad

Clemens von Pirquet of Vienna first coined the term allergy in 1906[1] to describe a special state of exceptional sensitivity of the body to certain foreign substances. Since then, though other fields of immunology were rapidly developing, the discipline of allergy remained underdeveloped till the discovery of serum factors responsible for allergy, i.e., IgE immunoglobulin, in 1967 by a Japanese couple.[2]

Until the early 1960s, a wrong notion prevailed that the malady of allergy is confined only to the temperate regions of the world.[3,4] Hence, researches in tropical and semitropical countries like India were not given due importance. However, subsequent studies established conclusively that the prevalence of allergic disorders was as high as in the Western countries, and it is now known that approximately 20–30% of our population suffers from one or other allergic disorders.[5-9] Although exact epidemiological studies have not been carried out in India, we can assume that about 250–300 million people must be suffering from one or the other allergic disorders, and these diseases will further increase with increased industrialization and urbanization. Bronchial asthma and rhinitis are the most common diseases seen in allergy clinics. Other diseases coming to allergic clinic are urticaria, dermatitis, and conjunctivitis. It is also known that not all such diseases are allergic but an allergic etiology can be demonstrated only in some of them. Thus, it is evident that allergy is a multidisciplinary subject, and such types of patients go to different specialists, such as general physician, chest physician, ENT surgeon, dermatologist, ophthalmologist, and so on. As allergy is a multidisciplinary subject, it needs cooperation from clinicians of diverse clinical disciplines such as general medicine, chest medicine, otorhinolaryngology, dermatology, gastroenterology, ophthalmology, and pediatric and other scientists like botanists, zoologists, aerobiologists, biochemists, and mycologists.

Teaching and training facilities available for specialty of allergy in most medical colleges of India are far from satisfactory. It is, therefore, no wonder that most of the doctors tend to attribute allergy what they do not understand or cannot diagnose or treat properly; similarly among educated laymen, it is fashion to suffer from allergy. They would often call it allergy when it is not allergy and when it is allergy, they would often not be aware of it. To face with these problems, the Government of India established the Department of Allergy in the VP Chest Institute, Delhi, in 1960. The CSIR Centre for Biochemicals was established in 1966 and started preparing antigens for allergy testing and immunotherapy. Indian workers in the field of allergy and applied immunology from different specialties organized together and formed an association named Indian College of Allergy and Applied Immunology (ICAI). The first allergy clinic was established in 1960 at the VP Chest Institute, Delhi, then in Jaipur and Lucknow. Training workshops in allergy and immunotherapy are being carried out twice in a year for 20–25 physicians under the joint auspices of CSIR Centre for Biochemicals Later CSIR Institute of Genomics and Integrative Biology (IGIB) and VP Chest Institute, Delhi, from 1975 and few workshops were also conducted by KG's Medical College, Lucknow. With the result of the abovementioned training in our country, there have been more than 600–700 allergy clinics, some in medical colleges and mostly in private sectors. Most of the allergy specialists running these allergy clinics are trained for 1–2 weeks in training workshops, and such type of training appears to be grossly inadequate. Young enthusiasts after such training often misused the allergy testing and immunotherapy and put immunotherapy into disrepute and made it controversial.

So better training is required for doctors who want to establish allergic clinics for service to the patients suffering from allergic diseases, and this can be made possible by adopting the following measures:

1. Better teaching of allergic diseases at undergraduate and postgraduate levels in all medical colleges.
2. Establishment of a few more dedicated Centers of Excellence in Allergy in medical colleges on the pattern of VP Chest Institute, which can serve as training centers for medical and paramedical workers who want to take up allergy speciality as their future career. These centers may also play a leading role in the field of research in such subjects.
3. Postgraduate medical degrees and diplomas in allergy and applied immunology may be started for which even Medical Council of India has already recommended.

REFERENCES

1. Von Pirquet, C. Allergic. Munch Med Wochenschr. 1906;30.
2. Ishizaka K, Ishizaka T. Identification of IgE antibodies as a carrier of reaginic activity. J Immunol. 1967;99:1187-98.
3. Holgate ST. Allergic disorders—science, medicine and the future. BMJ. 2000;320:231-4.
4. Beasley R, Keil U, von Mutius E, Pearce N. Worldwide variation in prevalence of symptoms of asthma, allergic rhinoconjunctivitis, and atopic eczema: ISAAC. Lancet. 1998;351:1225-32.
5. Anonymous. All India Coordinated Project on Aeroallergens and Human Health Report. Ministry of Environment and Forests, New Delhi; 2000.
6. Chhabra SK, Gupta CK, Chhabra P, Rajpal S. Prevalence of bronchial asthma in school children in Delhi. J Asthma. 1998;35:291-6.
7. Prasad R, Kumar R. Allergy situation in India: What is being done? Indian J Chest Dis Allied Sci. 2013;55:7-8.
8. Jindal SK, Aggarwal AN, Gupta D, et al. Indian study on epidemiology of asthma, respiratory symptoms and chronic bronchitis in adults (INSEARCH). Int J Tuberc Lung Dis. 2012;16:1270-7.
9. Kumar R, Kumari D, Srivastava P, et al. Identification of IgE-mediated food allergy and allergens in older children and adults with asthma and allergic rhinitis. Indian J Chest Dis Allied Sci. 2010;52:217-24.

CHAPTER 53

Allergen Avoidance in Naso-bronchial allergy

VK Jain, Shubhra Jain, Girish Jain

Allergy and allergic diseases have most common ailment in clinical practice and affect millions of people globally with economic lost. In the present era of modernization and industrialization, the majority of people spend more than 2/3 time of the whole day in indoor environments both at workplace and at home having common biological source of allergens especially house dust mite (HDM), insects, and fungal domestic animals in addition to nonallergenic irritants such as environmental tobacco smoke (ETS), NO_2, and ozone. The basic treatment is based on the avoidance of allergens/irritants, pharmacotherapy, allergen-specific immunotherapy, and patient education. The real challenge facing by practicing physicians is to create a low allergic environment in patients both indoor and outdoor environment effectively.[1]

HISTORICAL BACKGROUND

In 16th century, the first evidence of allergen avoidance in the treatment of allergic disorders is used when the Italian physician G. Cardano advised to Archbishop of St. Andrew, Scotland, to avoid his featherbedding, and he responded miraculously of asthma symptoms.[1] Leopold in 1925 treated asthma by environmental manipulation by keeping the patients of allergic disorders/asthma in a dust-free room.[2] In 1927, in Netherlands, Leeuwen kept patients in dust-free climate chamber rather than their homes and observed significant improvement.[3]

Allergens are antigens causing allergy mostly having proteins, occasionally carbohydrates reacting with IgE and IgG antibodies. In rare instances, low-molecular weight chemicals, i.e., isocyanates anhydrides acting as haptens also referred to as allergens for IgE antibodies.[4] Allergen avoidance is the foremost step applicable in all the three levels of prevention: primary, secondary, and tertiary for allergy and allergic diseases.[4-7] Allergen avoidance is important in both outdoor and indoor environments. The efficacy of specific control interventions may help to reduce allergy sensitization and relief of symptoms of respiratory diseases. Evidence supporting the efficacy of various approaches is still weak and a subject of controversy. However, specific airborne allergen control is still widely recommended as a holistic approach to prevent the immunological sensitization, development of allergic diseases, and reduce the severity of allergic respiratory symptoms. Before recommending the allergen avoidance in general one should know the specific allergen causing disease in a patient by performing skin prick test and immunoassay (ELISA/RAST) test (Fig. 53.1).[4]

NATURE OF ENVIRONMENTAL AEROALLERGENS

Allergenic proteins are present in component parts of biologic organisms (pollens and mold spores) and in the excretions of furred animals, mites, and insects.[25,26] They become airborne on particles of varying sizes that are characteristic of the source. Particles carrying HDM and cockroach allergens are relatively large (30 μm) and settle quickly, and their exposure is largely confined to fabrics in bedding or carpets.[26,27] Animal allergens are found on small buoyant particles (1–20 μm) that remain airborne and are widely distributed indoors.[28,29] Pollen and mold spores range from 6 to 150 μm, but they are buoyant and can be found in indoor and outdoor air samples.[26,30]

Thus, outdoor and indoor environments contain a complex mixture of particles carrying a variety of allergenic proteins. Their assays in the environment make it possible to estimate individual environmental allergen exposure and to assess the effectiveness of environmental allergen avoidance programs.

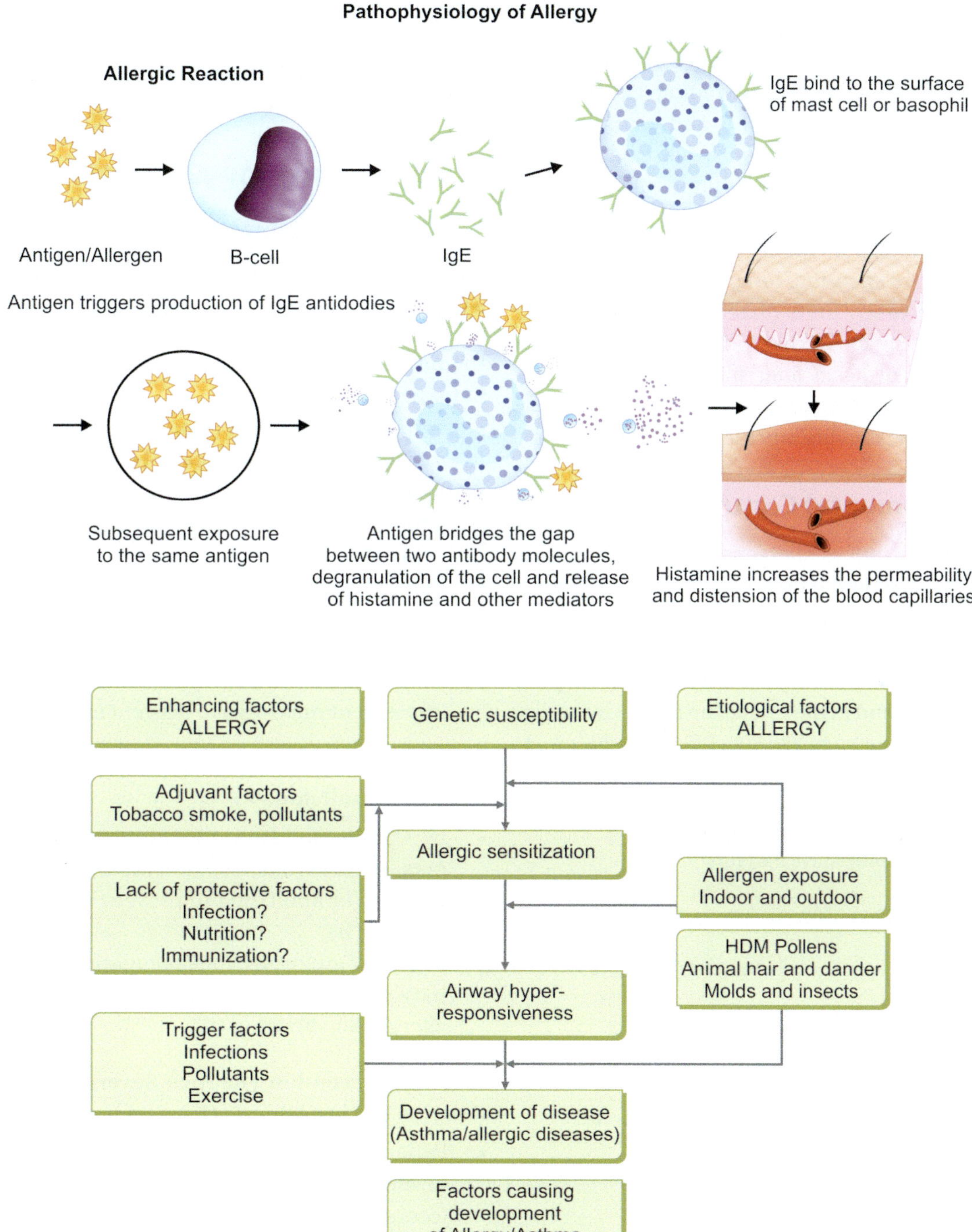

Fig. 53.1: The development of immunological sensitization, bronchial hyper-responsiveness, and further progression of various allergic diseases especially allergic rhinitis and asthma are mainly due to etiological and enhancing factors, and determined with genetic inheritance, early age, and smoking during pregnancy, etc.[5-24]

APPROACH OF ENVIRONMENTAL CONTROL

Outdoor Environmental Control

Although complete avoidance of exposure to environmental allergens and pollutants/irritants is impossible, it can be minimized by certain measures. Avoiding exposure to outdoor allergens (pollen and mold) and air pollutants (SO_2, NO_2; O_3) is an important step in all categories of prevention of allergy/asthma, but impossible due to ubiquitous nature. Pollen concentration is maximum in the morning; therefore, patients are advised to wait till the late afternoon before spending long time outside. Pollen concentration also drops immediately after a rain while mold count usually spike. Staying indoors during midday and afternoon, use of nasal filter/mask, changing work place/occupation, etc. are recommended. Keep always car windows closed while moving outside.[4,5,7,9-14,16,18-22]

Indoor Environmental Control

Avoiding exposure to indoor allergens (HDMs, pet animal dander, and mold) is required for the prevention of allergy/rhinitis/asthma. If the removal of pets from the house is not possible, frequent washing and bathing the pets will reduce the amount of dander and dried saliva on carpets, furniture, mattresses, and in the room. The indoor humidity to be maintained should be below 50% (35–50%). Frequent cleaning of beds, bathrooms, kitchen, and basement with chlorine bleach is also essential. Cleaning of mattresses, carpets, and curtains also reduces the indoor environmental pollution. HDM control is also required. Wearing masks while cleaning the house is beneficial. Removal of allergens from indoor air is done by using mechanical and electrical filters. Avoidance of indoor irritants such as tobacco smoke, wood smoke, strong odor of perfume, and fresh paints is also required. Wash your hair and clothes at night to avoid taking pollens to bed.[4,15,16,31-37]

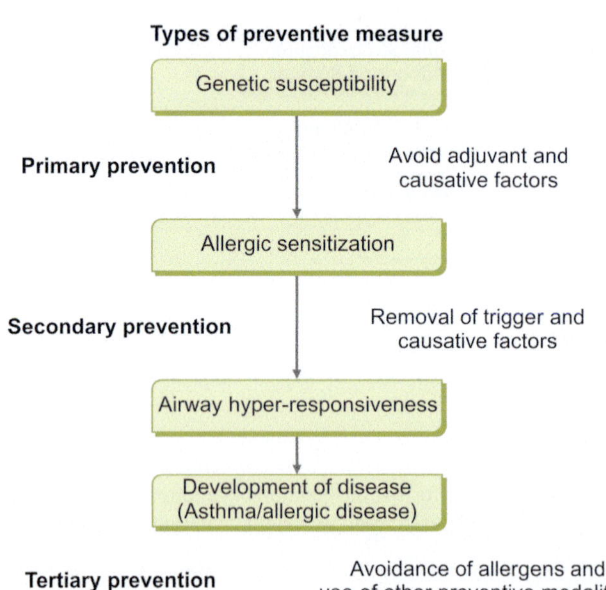

PREVENTION OF ALLERGY AND ALLERGIC ASTHMA

WHO Evidence-Based Guidelines and Strength of Recommendations[4]

Primary Prevention (To Prevent the Immunological IgE Sensitization/BHR)

- Avoid smoking and exposure to ETS, particularly during pregnancy and early childhood (B).
- Reduce exposure to inhalant allergens in young children at high risk (dust mites, cockroaches, furred pets) (B).
- Remove tobacco smoke from workplaces (B).
- Reduce indoor air pollutants (C).
- Eliminate sensitizing and highly irritating agents in occupational environments (C). If this is not possible, implement measures to prevent employee exposure.

Secondary Prevention (To Prevent Allergic Diseases in Sensitized Individuals)

- In young children already sensitized to HDMs, pets, or cockroaches, specific exposures should be reduced or abolished to prevent the onset of allergic disease (B).
- Remove employees from occupational exposure if they have developed symptoms caused by occupational allergic sensitization (C).

Tertiary Prevention (Reduce Severity of Symptoms in Patients Having Allergic Diseases)

- Patients with allergic asthma, rhinitis, conjunctivitis, or atopic eczema/atopic dermatitis who are allergic to outdoor/indoor allergens such as pollens, molds, dust mites, cockroaches, and animal danders should eliminate or markedly reduce the exposure to improve symptom control and prevent exacerbations. Bed covers are particularly useful for allergic patients sensitized to mites (A, B).

SPECIFIC ALLERGEN AVOIDANCE MEASURES

Pollen Avoidance[4,31]

Provides mechanical barriers to pollen contact

- Keep windows closed at peak pollen times, e.g., in the evening when airborne pollen descends to lower altitudes
- Wear glasses or sunglasses to prevent pollen entering the eyes
- Consider wearing a mask over nose and mouth to prevent inhalation of pollen at peak times
- Wash hair and clothes at night to avoid taking pollen to bed
- Pollen-allergic individuals should not cut grass
- Keep windows closed when the grass has been mown
- Use air-conditioning, if possible
- Install car pollen filters, if possible.

Local Sealed Allergen-Free Environment in Nose by Barrier Enforcing Measures[14]

- White vaseline
- Pollen blocker cream
- Microemulsions
- Lipid-based ointments
- Sea-water gel
- Liposomal formulations.

HOUSE DUST MITE CONTROL

House dust mite (HDM) allergen exposure is much greater in bedding than elsewhere in the home. Various studies regarding the exposure to HDM and the development of allergic sensitization, wheezing, atopic dermatitis, and asthma have been reported, and the avoidance of exposure to HDM during childhood has shown beneficial effects in the development of allergic disorders. Control of HDM in the house can be done by placing the barriers, killing or removing the mites, or making the environment less suitable for mites and/or to move the patient to dust-free environment. Placing the barriers between the patient and the reservoirs of dust mite by encasing mattresses and pillows by airtight plastic covers, expensive microporous covers are also used. Electric blankets on beds (which dry the mite environment) have also been used. Killing of mites can be achieved by weekly washing of beddings and pillows in hot water (>60°C) by using ascaricides (benzyl benzoate and tannic acid), dry heating, and lastly by using liquid nitrogen. Vacuum cleaners are used for the removal of dead mites and dust, whereas HEPA (high-efficiency particulate air) filters are used for the removal of airborne mites, and less suitable environment for mites can be achieved by avoid sleeping or lying on upholstered furniture, by reduced indoor humidity to <50%, by air-conditioning or mechanical ventilation, or by removal of carpets and dust collectors laid on concrete. Removal of the patients to the HDM-free environment is very effective but practically inconvenient and expensive. It can be adopted whenever feasible while dust busting is completed at home.[4,27,31-38]

HDM Allergen Reduction

AIMS: To Reduce the Amount of Mite Allergens in the Home

Major Strategies (WHO Strength of Recommendation A)[4]

- Wash bedding regularly (every 1–2 weeks) at 55–60°C, if possible, to kill mites (washing with cold water removes 90% of mite allergens; washing at 55–60°C kills mites)
- Wash pillows and duvets in hot water at 55–60°C and encase pillows and mattresses with documented protective coverings
- Sufficient ventilation of dwellings to decrease humidity; aim to reduce indoor relative humidity to below 50%
- avoid damp housing conditions.

Additional Strategies

- Use a good-quality vacuum cleaner (if possible, one fitted with HEPA filter)
- Use a damp duster when dusting and cleaning surfaces
- Replace wall to wall carpets with linoleum or wooden floors which can be wiped clean
- Remove/reduce curtains and soft furnishings in the bedroom
- Replace fabric-covered seating with leather or vinyl
- Remove soft toys from the bedroom; wash them at 55–60°C or freeze them (in a kitchen deep freezer) to kill HDMs
- Do not allow pets in the bedroom
- HDMs are transparent and have no natural protection against sunlight. Exposure of mattresses, rugs, and

carpets to direct strong sunlight (for more than 3 h) kills mites and can be used in appropriate regions
- A hammock, easily washable and susceptible to air and sundrying, is used in many areas of the world.

COCKROACH ALLERGEN AVOIDANCE

Removes the cockroaches, eliminates the places and conditions in which they can live, and removes allergens
- Eradicate cockroaches with appropriate insecticides
- Seal cracks in floors and ceilings
- Remove sources of food
- Control dampness
- Scrub floors with water and detergent to remove allergens
- Bedding, curtains, and clothing can be contaminated and must be washed.

PET ALLERGEN AVOIDANCE

Reduces the Amount of Pet Allergen Indoors

- If possible, find another home for the pet, and do not bring new animals into the home
- Exclude pets from bedrooms and, if possible, keep pets outdoors
- Vacuum carpets, mattresses, and upholstery regularly, if a power source and equipment are available
- Change clothes before going to school/work if you have attended your horse/cat/dog.

MOLD ALLERGEN AVOIDANCE

Prevents mold from growing, and mold spores from becoming airborne during mold removal

Indoors

- Maintain indoor humidity between 35% and 50%; use dehumidifiers in the home if relative humidity is constantly high (above 50%)
- Ensure heating, ventilation, or air-conditioning systems are properly maintained
- Use bathroom exhaust fans or open window after bathing
- Use 5% ammonia solution to remove mold from bathrooms and other contaminated surfaces
- Replace carpets with hard flooring; replace wallpaper with paint
- Wear mask during house cleaning
- Remove or wash stuff toys
- Repair indoor water damage immediately.

Outdoors

- Avoid cutting grass in late summer when mold spores are present in decaying vegetation.

High Altitude Allergen Avoidance

Various studies suggest the presence of low level of the allergens at high altitude with the development of low rate of sensitization and less allergic diseases. High altitude studies also provide a proof that substantial reduction of allergen exposure over a long period may result in better clinical improvement in allergic asthmatic patients. Therefore, one can recommend to shift patient at high altitude residential areas.[1,39]

ADHERENCE TO ALLERGEN AVOIDANCE ADVICE

Although environmental allergen avoidance is included in both the United States[40] and international treatment guidelines,[41] adherence by physicians and patients to these recommendations needs improvement. Patients often report that they are adherent, but home inspection shows much less adherence than a patient's self-reports. Without formal educational programs, no patient had installed mattress covers.[42,43] With the usual clinic-based educational efforts, Korsgaard[43] found that only 17% had installed a mattress cover. Huss et al.[42] found similar figures but also found that the adherence could be increased to 27% with repetitive clinic-based education and to 39% with a computer-based educational program. Adherence to allergen avoidance advice is generally not as good as with medication. For example, in a clinical trial that achieved better than 95% adherence to medication regimens, no more than 48% of families had installed mattress covers.[44] Thus with specific clinic-based education, between 17% and 27% of patients will adhere to recommendations for environmental avoidance, whereas more intensive clinic-based education in highly motivated patients may increase adherence to 48%. With such low rates of adherence, the therapeutic potential demonstrated in clinical trials of allergen avoidance is not likely to be realized in clinical practice without more concerted action on the part of both clinicians and patients. As with other therapies, adherence to allergen avoidance should be improved by providing more concentrated education, simplifying recommendations, and developing a partnership between the physician and the patient.

CONCLUSION

Allergen avoidance is the holistic approach to prevent the immunological sensitization, BHR, and development of disease and also reduction of the severity of symptoms in patients with allergic disorders. Environmental allergen avoidance both indoors and outdoors is an important step in the management of allergic disorders but a challenging task as practically not feasible absolutely. Presently, a wide spectrum of measures have been suggested to reduce the exposure to trigger symptomatic allergy in sensitized patients suffering from respiratory allergy. Avoidance interventions for the main allergens are not supported by robust evidence of efficacy and are still a subject of controversy. Specific control interventions could be effective as part of a holistic approach at all the three levels of preventing approach. The allergen avoidance is still widely recommended in the most recent guidelines to reduce the severity of allergic symptoms in sensitized individuals.

REFERENCES

1. Woodcock A. Allergen Avoidance: does it work? Br Med Bull. 2000;56:1071-86.
2. Leopold SS, Leopold CS. Bronchial asthma and allied allergic disorders. Preliminary report of a study under controlled conditions of environment, temperature and humidity. JAMA. 1925;84:731-5.
3. Storm van Leeuwen W, Einthoven W, Kremer W. The allergen proof chamber in the treatment of bronchial asthma and other respiratory diseases. Lancet 1927;i:1287-9.
4. Johansson SGO, Haahtela T. WAO Guidelines for prevention of allergy and allergic asthma. Allergy Clin Immunol Int- J World Allergy Org. 2004;16:176-85.
5. Becker et al. Prevention strategies for asthma—primary prevention. JAMC. 2005;173:20-4.
6. Fleischer DM, Spergel JM, Assa'ad AH, et al. Primary prevention of allergic disease through nutritional interventions. J Allergy Clin Immunol Pract. 2013:1: 29-36.
7. Primary Prevention of Asthma and Allergy. J Allergy Clin Immunol. 2005;116:3.
8. Wonderen KEV, Mark LB, Mohrs J, et al. Prediction and treatment of asthma in preschool children at risk: study design and baseline data of a prospective cohort study in general practice (ARCADE). BMC Pulm Med. 2009;9:13.
9. Illi s, Von Mutius E, Lau S, Niggemann B, et al. Perennial allergen sensitization early in life and chronic asthma in children: a birth cohort study. Lancet. 2006:368:763-70.
10. Porsbjerg C, Von Linstow ML, Ulrik CS, et al. Risk factors for onset of asthma: a 12 year prospective follow up study. Chest. 2006;129:309-16.
11. Govaere E, Van Gysel D, Massa G, et al. The influence of age and gender on sensitization to aeroallergens. Petiatr Allergy Immunol. 2007;18:671-8.
12. Silvestri M, Rossi Ga, Cozzani S, et al. Age dependent tendency to become sensitized to other classes of aeroallergens in atopic asthmatic children. Ann Allergy Asthma Immunol. 1999;83:335-40.
13. Kulig M, Bergmann R, Klettke U, et al. Natural course of sensitization to food and inhalant during the first 6 years of life. J Allergy Clin Immunol. 1999;103:1173-9.
14. Anderson M, Greiff L, Ojeda P, Wollmer P. Barrier-enforcing measures as treatment principle in allergic rhinitis: a systematic review. J Curr Med Res Opin. 2014;30:1131-7.
15. Douwes J, Van Strien R, Doekes G, et al. Does early indoor microbial exposure reduce the risk of asthma? The prevention and incidence of asthma and mite allergy birth cohort study J Allergy Asthma Immunol. 2006;117:1067-73.
16. Arshad SH, Tariq SM, Matthews S, Hakim E. Sensitization to common allergens and its association with allergic disorders at age 4 years: a whole population birth cohort study. Pediatrics. 2001;108:E33.
17. Host A, Andrae S, Charkin S, et al. Allergy testing in children: why, who, when and how? Allergy. 2003;58: 559-69.
18. Eder w, Ege MJ, Von Mutius E. The asthma epidemic. N Engl J Med. 2006;355:2226-35.
19. Lee YL, Hwang BF, Lin YC, Guo YL. Time trend of asthma prevalence among school children in Taiwan: ISAAC phase I and III surveys. Pediatr Allergy Immunol. 2007;18:188-95.
20. Hsieh KH, Shen JJ. Prevalence of childhood asthma in Taipei, Taiwan and other Asian Pacific countries. J Asthma. 1988;25:73-82.
21. Hess J, De Jongste JC. Epidemiological aspects of paediatric asthma. Clin Exp Allergy. 2004;34:680-5.
22. Halken S. Prevention of allergic disease in childhood: clinical and epidemiological aspects of primary and secondary allergy prevention. Pediatr Allergy Immunol. 2004;15:4-5, 9-32.
23. Stick SM, Burton PR, Gurrin L, et al. Effects of maternal smoking during pregnancy and a family history of asthma on respiratory function in newborn infants. Lancet. 1996;348:1060-4.
24. Tager IB, Ngo L, Hanrahan JP. Maternal smoking during pregnancy. Effects on lung function during the first 18

months of life. Am J Respir Crit Care Med. 1995;152: 977-83.

25. Stewart GA. The molecular biology of allergens. In Busse WW, Holgate ST, ed. Asthma and Rhinitis. Boston: Blackwell; 1995: 898-932.
26. Solomon WR, Platts-Mills TAE. Aerobiology of inhalant allergens. In: Middleton E Jr, Reed CE, Ellis EF, Adkinson NF Jr, Yunginger JW, Busse WW, eds. Allergy: Principles and Practice, 4th ed. St. Louis: Mosby; 1993: 469-528.
27. Tovey ER, Chapman MD, Wells CW, Platts-Mills TAE. The distribution of dust mite allergen in houses of patients with asthma. Am Rev Respir Dis. 1981;124:630-5.
28. Luczynska CM, Li Y, Chapman MD, Plats-Mills TAE. Airborne concentration and particle size distribution of allergen derived from domestic cats (Felis domesticus): measurements using cascade impactor, liquid impinger and a two-site monoclonal antibody assay for Fel d I. Am Rev Respir Dis. 1990;141:361-7.
29. Custovic A, Green R, Fletcher A, et al. Aerodynamic properties of the major dog allergen, Can f 1: distribution in homes, concentration and particle size of the allergen in the air. Am J Respir Crit Care Med. 1997;155:94-8.
30. Burge HA. Airborne allergenic fungi. Immunol Allergy Clin North Am. 1989;9:307-19.
31. Cipriani F, Calamelli E, Ricci G. Allergen avoidance in allergic asthma. Front Pediatr. 2017;5:103. doi:10.3389/fped.2017.00103
32. Ehnert B, Lau-Schadendorf S, Weber A, et al. Reducing domestic exposure to dust mite allergen reduces bronchial hyperreactivity in sensitive children with asthma. J Allergy Clin Immunol. 1992;90:135-8.
33. Murray AB, Ferguson AC. Dust-free bedrooms in the treatment of asthmatic children with housedust or house dust mite allergy: a controlled trial. Pediatrics. 1983;71: 418-22.
34. Walshaw MJ, Evans CC. Allergen avoidance in house dust mite sensitive adult asthma. QJM. 1986;226:199-215.
35. Burr ML, Dean BV, Merett TG, et al. Effects of anti-mite measures on children with mite sensitive asthma: a controlled clinical trial. Thorax. 1980;35:506.
36. Dietemann A, Bessot JC, Hoyet C, et al. A double blind, placebo controlled trial of solidified benzyl benzoate applied in dwellings of asthmatic patients sensitive to mites: clinical efficacy and effect on mite allergens. J Allergy Clin Immunol. 1993;91:738-46.
37. Kneist FM, Young E, VanPmag McG. Clinical evaluation of a double blind dust-mite avoidance trial with mite allergic patients. Clin Exp Allergy. 1991;21:39-47.
38. Platts-Mills TAE, Tovey ER, Mitchell EB, et al. Reduction of bronchial hyperreactivity during prolonged allergen avoidance. Lancet. 1982;3:675-8.
39. Peroni DG, Boner AL, Vallone G, et al. Effective allergen avoidance at high altitude reduced allergen-induced bronchial hyperresponsiveness. Am J Respir Crit Care Med. 1994;149:1442-6.
40. National Asthma Education Program. Guidelines for the diagnosis and management of asthma. National Institutes of Health; July 1997; DHHS NIH Pub no. 97-4051.
41. Sheffer AL (chairman) for the International Asthma management Project. International consensus report on diagnosis and treatment of asthma. Eur Respir J. 1992;5: 601-41.
42. Huss K, Squire EN Jr, Carpenter GB, et al. Effective education of adults with asthma who are allergic to dust mites. J Allergy Clin Immunol. 1992;89:836-43.
43. Korsgaard J. Preventive measures in house-dust allergy. Am Rev Respir Dis. 1982;125:80-4.
44. Eggleston PA, Wheeler B, Bollers N, et al. The effect of home environmental allergen control measures in asthmatic children enrolled in a prospective clinical trial [abstract]. Am Rev Respir Dis. 1992;45:213.

CHAPTER 54

Guidelines for Practice of Allergen Immunotherapy in India: 2017-An Update

SN Gaur, Raj Kumar, AB Singh, MK Agarwal, Naveen Arora

INTRODUCTION

Allergen immunotherapy (AIT) is an immunomodulatory method for the treatment of immunoglobulin E (IgE)-mediated allergic diseases to control the symptoms and decrease the sensitivity toward allergen(s) by giving sequentially increasing dose of antigen(s) to induce a shift of the immunological response from TH2 to TH1. Numerous terms have been used to describe AIT for treating allergy, including allergen-specific immunotherapy (IT), specific IT, and other terms such as hyposensitization and desensitization.[1] The term AIT is used most recently to refer to the class of therapies that aim to induce immune tolerance to allergens. AIT is a therapy with disease-modifying effects and is currently used for the treatment of allergic rhinitis, rhinoconjunctivitis, allergic asthma, and venom hypersensitivity. It is the only method to prevent the onset/progression of asthma in patients suffering from allergic rhinitis/rhinoconjunctivitis. AIT can be administered through different routes (subcutaneous, sublingual, oral, nasal, bronchial, and lymphatic), but currently, only subcutaneous IT (SCIT) and sublingual IT (SLIT) have sufficient evidence and therefore are routinely used.[1-3]

Following the international regulations, which are also relevant for India, the practice of AIT should be allowed only to those physicians who have obtained specialized training in allergy and AIT and to be practiced at a place where facilities of managing anaphylaxis are available.

Guidelines for AIT are available in Western/developed countries,[1-5] but a separate guideline focusing on India is also necessitated due to a multitude of factors. This 2017 update by the Indian College of Allergy, Asthma, and Applied Immunology (ICAAI) has been prepared to review the recent data and update the guidelines published in 2009.[6] The aim of the current guidelines is to provide clinicians comprehensive recommendations on the use of AIT in their daily practice.

How to cite this article: Gaur SN, Kumar R, Singh AB, Agarwal MK, Arora N. Guidelines for practice of allergen immunotherapy in India: 2017-An update. Indian J Allergy Asthma Immunol. 2017;31:3-33.

MECHANISM OF ACTION

Initially, it was presumed that by giving low doses of same antigen, the immune system produces IgG antibodies (blocking antibodies) instead of IgE antibodies and thus consumes the antigens, resulting in less number of IgE molecules available to produce allergic reaction. However, the changes in clinical parameters post-IT did not always correlate with the changes in IgG or IgE levels. It is now well established with a number of evidence that AIT produces a shift of TH2 response toward TH1. This brings the reduction in release of inflammatory mediators, specific IgE (sIgE) levels, and allergen-specific airway hyperresponsiveness apart from producing clinical improvement. There is an increase in specific IgG levels after AIT. However, initial increase in IgG4 level indicates poor prognosis but that of IgG1 means a better prognosis. AIT induces a decrease in interleukin-4 (IL-4) and IL-5 production by CD4$^+$ TH2 cells and a shift toward increased interferon gamma (IFN-Φ067) production by TH1 cells. Activation of TH1 subset is associated with the development of cell-mediated immunity, essential for protective immune response against the development of allergy/asthma. AIT acts by modifying TH4$^+$ T-cell responses either by immune deviation, T-cell anergy, or both. Further, a subtype of T-cells with immunosuppressive function and cytokines profiles distinct from their TH1 and TH2 cells, termed regulation/suppressor T-cell, have been described. T-regulatory (Treg) cells producing IL-10 and possibly transforming-growth-factor beta (TGF-β), CD4$^+$ CD25$^+$ T-cells, and TH3 cells play a major role in the inhibition of allergic disorders. The expression of FOXP3 on CD4$^+$ CD25$^+$ T-cells has also been demonstrated to correlate with the suppressive capacity of Treg cells and clinical efficacy following AIT. Figure 54.1 depicts the mechanism of action of AIT.[7]

SELECTION OF PATIENTS

The success of AIT depends on proper selection of patients, allergens, doses, quality of allergens, and compliance to the treatment. AIT results may reflect failure if done by an untrained person. Unnecessary testing, wrong prescription of IT, and taking advantage of psychology of patient can lead to adverse reputation in AIT practice.

AIT has proved useful in patients with IgE-mediated diseases such as allergic rhinitis, asthma, and insect sting hypersensitivity. It should be considered in a patient who had history of systemic anaphylaxis reaction after an insect sting and has documented IgE sensitivity to specific venom, and there is a likelihood of future exposure to the insect. AIT can be lifesaving in such cases with appropriate antigen. Patients with atopic dermatitis (AD) due to the aeroallergen house dust mites (HDMs) may also be an appropriate candidates for AIT (Table 54.1).[1-3,5]

Patients of allergic rhinitis, of asthma, and with history of symptoms after natural exposure to the allergen demonstrated sIgE antibodies against the offending allergens. The allergy is assessed by clinical history, skin tests, and radioallergosorbent test (RAST) or enzyme-linked immunosorbent assay (ELISA). AIT is prescribed for patients ≥5 years with no limit on the upper age, with symptoms interfering with their routine work or school performance, causing sleep disturbances, and quality of life (QoL). Patients who failed to avoid allergen exposure in spite of all efforts or had no response to allergen avoidance had poor response to drugs or tired of taking drugs or developed adverse reactions to medicines are most suitable candidates for AIT. The patients selected must assure long-term compliance for the therapy and should not have contraindications for AIT (Table 54.2).[8]

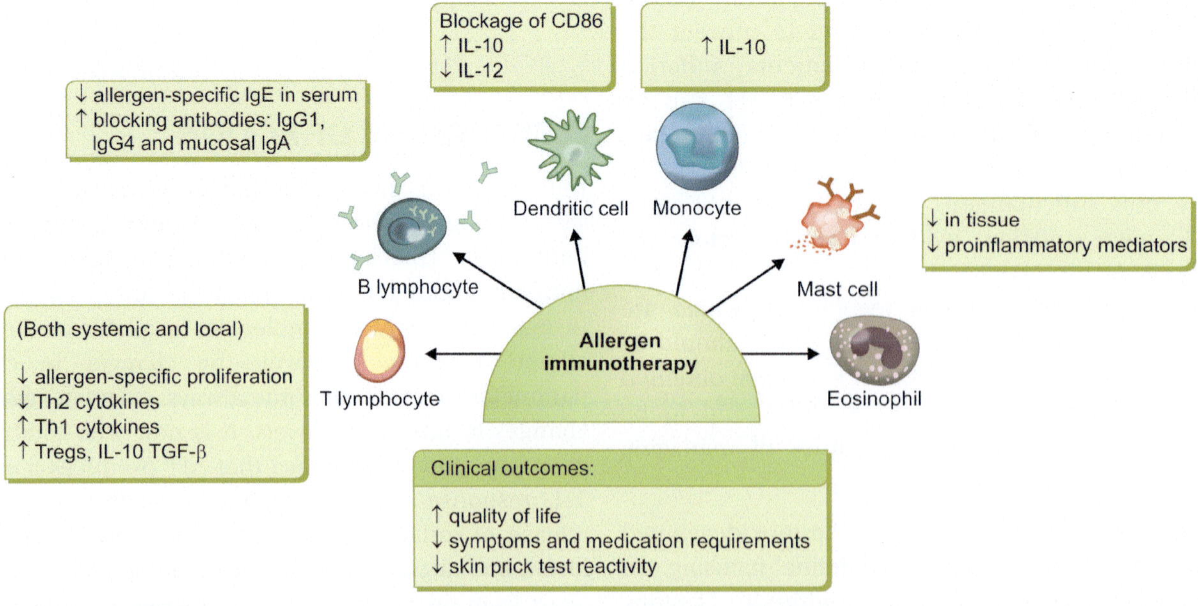

Fig. 54.1: Mechanism of AIT.

Table 54.1: Indications for allergen immunotherapy.
IgE-mediated disease in patients ≥5 years with no limit on the upper age (i.e., presence of sensitization on a skin prick test* with clinical correlation to the symptoms)
Allergic rhinoconjunctivitis
Moderate–severe intermittent rhinitis
Mild to moderate–severe persistent rhinitis Allergic asthma (controlled)
Large local reactions to insect venom
Atopic dermatitis in patients with aeroallergen sensitivity (low level of evidence)
Symptoms are of sufficient duration and severity
Allergen avoidance not possible or if symptom relief is inadequate
Availability of standardized or best as technically possible allergen extracts
Proof of efficacy of the planned AIT for the respective indication and age group

*In vitro tests may be used only in situations in which skin testing is not possible and for diagnostic work-up in children below 5 years. AIT, Allergen immunotherapy.

Table 54.2: Contraindications for allergen immunotherapy.

Absolute contraindications	*Relative contraindications*
Uncontrolled persistent	β-blockers
asthma (FEV_1<70% in spite of treatment)	Cardiovascular diseases HIV (A, B; CD4>200/μL)
Malignant neoplasias	Children (2–5 years of age)
Pregnancy (only for the initiation of AIT)	Psychiatric or mental disorders
Children (<2 years of age)	Chronic infections
AIDS	Autoimmune disorders Immunodeficiencies or use of immunosuppressives

FEV_1, forced expiratory volume 1s; AIT, allergen immunotherapy; AIDS, acquired immunodeficiency syndrome

Table 54.3: Factors that increase the clinical efficacy of allergen immunotherapy*.
Short duration of disease (early age/initiation of AIT in the course of the disease)
Minor involvement of the lower airways
Good compliance and adherence with 3–5 years of AIT
A high cumulative AIT dose (efficacy of immunotherapy is associated with a dose response curve)

*The more of these factors that apply, the higher the probability that administration of AIT will reduce symptoms and medication use, as well as decrease the likelihood of progression of allergic rhinitis to allergic bronchial asthma and increase in the number of sensitizations. AIT, Allergen immunotherapy.

A shorter disease duration and compliance to AIT improves clinical outcomes. Table 54.3 discusses additional factors associated with favorable outcomes.[5]

SELECTION OF ALLERGENS

The local flora/airborne pollens change approximately every 200 km distance in India. The soil conditions along with environment of the place may affect the protein content as well as the antigenicity of the allergens. The urban and rural setup as well as the coastal or hilly climate affects the type or antigenicity of the atmospheric pollens in our country. Currently, more data need to be generated to understand the interplay between the above-mentioned factors and allergenic properties. It is essential to select the antigens for testing in a patient based on the above points and confirming the history of exposure. Besides, it is important to have the knowledge about the geographical habitat, occupation/residence of the patient, and also the precipitating factors for his/her allergic symptoms.

A document on aeroallergens (pollens) in different parts of the country has been published[9] and can be consulted to frame the testing kit for patients residing in respective area. Physicians/allergologists are also required to consult local aerobiological studies and studies evaluating the sensitization patterns[9-33] published in relevant journals for the prevalence of airborne pollens, fungi, insects, and mite allergens. They can consult the researchers at their nearest botany, plant pathology, and entomology departments or attend training courses in identification of allergens. Relevant allergens are included in Indian allergen manufacturer's list, which are mostly common throughout the country.

Some of the allergenically important pollens are *Prosopis juliflora, Ricinus communis, Chenopodium album, Cynodon dactylon, Artemisia* species, *Alnus nitida, Amaranthus spinosus, Parthenium hysterophorus,*

Cassia siamea, and members of Poaceae.[22] While numerous references are available from the different geographical zones of India, limited evidence is available from the Himalayan area.[13,34] Among the Himalaya pollen, a high incidence of skin sensitivity was observed to pollen antigens of *Cedrus deodara, Mallotus philippensis,* and *Quercus incana* in patients of Chandigarh residing in the hills and foothills of the Himalayas while *A. nitida, Betula utilis,* and *C. deodara* were important sensitizers in New Delhi patients. Furthermore, the skin sensitization pattern against these pollens was in accordance with the level of exposure to these pollen of the subjects residing in that part of the country.[13] Two HDM species, namely *Dermatophagoides pteronyssinus* and *Dermatophagoides farinae,* are predominant in regions with high humidity, especially in coastal areas. *Blomia tropicalis* is another important mite species found to be prevalent in tropical countries, and it is found to be prevalent in about 15% of Indian patients.[35] Another mite species *Acarus siro* and *Tyrophagus* species have also been found to be present in studies published from India.[36-38] In some patients, new antigens for testing may be required, decided on individual basis after surveying patient's environment.

Studies focusing on food sensitizations in India have demonstrated the relevance of the following food allergens in patients with respiratory allergies: Rice, black gram, lentils, citrus fruits, peanut, banana, fish, soybean, chicken, wheat, etc., In a study conducted in New Delhi, patients aged 12–62 years were screened for food allergies using standard questionnaire and skin prick test (SPT). sIgE level was determined by ELISA, and allergy was established by blinded food challenges. In this study, food allergy is estimated to be 4.5% in adolescents and adults with asthma, rhinitis, or both. Rice, citrus fruits, black gram, and banana were identified as major allergens for inducing allergic symptoms.[39] Furthermore, Indian-specific data suggest that severe SPT reactions (4 mm or above) and sIgE (6.9 ng/mL) to rice are associated with positive blinded food challenge with clinical symptoms.[40] Results from the recently published EuroPrevall-INCO study which was conducted in Karnataka, South India, demonstrated a high level of sensitization (26.5%) for most of the foods in the general population, higher than that observed among adults in Europe. The highest prevalence of sensitization to individual foods was observed for shrimp and sesame and was above 13%. However, the prevalence of probable food allergy (self-reports of adverse symptoms after the consumption of food and sIgE to the same food) was 1.2%, which was mainly accounted for cow's milk (0.5%) and apple (0.5%) with very few cases, with probable food allergy to egg and banana (0.05% each) and to sesame, wheat, and tomato (0.02% each).[41]

Table 54.4: Allergens of proven efficacy in allergen immunotherapy trials globally.

Allergen	*Level of evidence*	*Availability of data*
House dust mite	A	++++
Pollen	A	++++
Mold	A	++
Animal epithelia	A	++
Hymenoptera venom	A	++
Cockroach	B	+

A, Evidence from meta-analysis of RCTs or at least 1 RCT; B, Evidence from at least 1 controlled study without randomization or at least 1 other type of quasi experimental study; ++++, Multiple long-term RCTs available; ++, Few RCTs available; +, Limited data; RCTs, Randomized controlled trials

Relevant allergens are major contributors to the safety and efficacy of the allergenic extracts used for AIT. Most of the available data address HDMs and selected pollens, whereas less is known about the efficacy and safety of mold, animal epithelia, venom, and cockroach (Table 54.4).[3,42]

Allergen extracts which have been evaluated in Indian studies include HDMs, pollen, horse dander, insects (cockroach, mosquito, and housefly), and mixes of allergen extracts.

DIAGNOSTIC TESTS FOR DETECTING SENSITIZING ALLERGEN(S)

For AIT of patients with IgE-mediated respiratory allergic disorders, identification of specific causative allergens is of paramount importance. Patient's history and clinical examination are the primary modalities for identifying an allergic etiology and identifying the likely allergens responsible for the allergic symptoms. The following in vivo and in vitro diagnostic tests are recommended[43-45] and commonly used:

In vivo tests

i. Skin tests (prick and intradermal)[46-48]
ii. Mucosal challenge tests (bronchial[49] and nasal[50] challenge, double-blind placebo-controlled food challenge[51]).

In vitro tests

It is used for the quantification of total serum IgE/ allergen-sIgE levels.

i. RAST[52,53]
ii. ELISA
iii. Multi-allergen screening assays.

In Vivo Tests

Skin Tests

Skin tests with inhalant allergens are simple and effective method for the identification of causative allergens. They are the most accurate diagnostic procedures for demonstrating that a specific allergen has induced an IgE antibody response and are regarded as the gold standard for the detection of IgE antibodies.[54] Skin tests are convenient, simple, biologically relevant, reproducible, easy and rapid to perform, with low cost and high sensitivity. Studies indicate that skin testing might be more sensitive than in vitro tests in detecting allergen-sIgE.[55-60] SPTs and intradermal tests vary in sensitivity and specificity, which depends on multiple factors such as concentration and quality of allergen solution.

Preparation of high-quality allergen extracts is essential for the diagnosis and AIT of allergic disorders. Standardized allergen extracts should be utilized as unstandardized extracts have large batch-to-batch variability (10–>100 times) and thus may have variability in the test results.[61] Recently, biological unit (BU) - used mostly in Europe, and bioequivalent allergen unit (BAU) - used mostly in the US, have come to be widely used on standardized products. While the BU is an in vivo standardization unit based on the SPT response compared with histamine, the BAU is based on intradermal skin tests. Furthermore, the global guidelines also recommend maintenance of an in-house reference standard, with which all the production batches should be compared using in vitro techniques of standardization.

A positive control (histamine diphosphate/ dihydrochloride) is always used to ensure (i) that the patient is suitable for the performance of skin tests and (ii) is not taking any medication(s) which may suppress the cutaneous response to injected allergen extracts. Similarly, test with the diluent used to prepare/ preserve the allergen extracts is also performed as negative control to rule out the possibility of getting false positive skin response due to dermographism or traumatic reactivity induced by skin test device.[62]

Skin Prick Test

The position papers on skin tests by the European Academy of Allergy and Clinical Immunology (EAACI) and the US Joint Council of Allergy, Asthma and Immunology (American Academy of Allergy, Asthma and Immunology [AAAAI], ACAAI) state that properly performed prick test is most convenient for better clinical correlation and is economical.[62,63] In addition, the World Allergy Organization (WAO) has mentioned that SPT is the best screening method for detecting sIgE antibodies.[54] They are highly reproducible when carried out by trained individuals. SPTs are minimally invasive, have high specificity, and have a lower rate of systemic effects as compared to the intradermal tests. SPT is the gold standard diagnostic method to detect allergen sensitization.

Medicines to Avoid before the Skin Prick Tests

Certain medicines are known to decrease skin reactivity, leading to false negative skin tests. Clinicians should be aware of the medicines that could interfere with allergy testing and should counsel their patients to avoid these to achieve an appropriate diagnosis (Table 54.5).[62,64]

Medicines which do not have a suppressant effect on the SPT include intranasal antihistamines, nasal and inhaled corticosteroids, leukotriene receptor antagonists (montelukast), angiotensin-converting enzyme inhibitors, β-agonists, cyclosporine, H_2-blocker, theophylline, selective serotonin reuptake inhibitors, and selective norepinephrine reuptake inhibitors.

Intradermal Test

In Western countries, allergen extract solutions for intradermal tests have been recommended to be 100-fold or 1,000-fold dilution of the concentration used for prick test. However, in India, 25–50-fold dilution of the concentration used for prick tests (1:10/1:20 weight/ volume [w/v]), i.e., 1:500 w/v, has been found suitable for intradermal tests.[46,48] Intradermal tests are more sensitive than SPT testing and thus may provide more false positive results than SPT. Furthermore, they possess a greater risk of systemic reactions (SRs) than SPT testing. Therefore, the intradermal tests are generally used when percutaneous tests are negative despite an adequate history of exposure and symptoms.[65]

Table 54.5: Medicines having a suppressant effect on the skin prick test.

Medicine	*Suppressant effect*
Antihistamines Oral first-generation H_1-blocker (hydroxyzine, etc.)	>2 days
Oral second-generation H_1-blocker (cetirizine, loratadine, etc.)	7 days
Glucocorticoids Topical (at the test sites) Systemic short-term (up to 10 days)	>7 days
<50 mg/day prednisolone-equivalent	>3 days
>50 mg/day prednisolone-equivalent	>7 days
Systemic long-term (>10 days) <10 mg/day prednisolone-equivalent	None
>10 mg/day prednisolone-equivalent	>3 weeks
Other categories Omalizumab[64]	4–6 months
Antidepressants Doxepin	7 days
Desipramine	3 days
Phenothiazine antipsychotics	10 days
UV light treatment (PUVA)	4 weeks

Mucosal Challenge Tests

Mucosal challenge tests with allergen extracts, both bronchial challenge and nasal provocation tests (NPTs), are of limited clinical value.[49,50] These tests are mostly used for research purposes as they do not give any significant clinical information, in addition to that provided by properly taken clinical history and carefully performed and graded skin tests.

The in vivo methods are summarized below for reference:

- Skin tests are followed commonly for allergy diagnosis with allergen extracts. The SPT is most convenient for better clinical correlation and is a least expensive in vivo diagnostic test
- Patient having skin diseases such as eczema, leukoderma, dermographism, severe dermatitis, and any other chronic skin disease is not fit for skin testing, and in case of fever, the test is postponed till the patient becomes normal
- For SPT, the allergens are tested in 1:10 or 1:20 w/v dilution, and in intradermal test, antigens are injected intradermally in 1:500 w/v dilution
- Antigens are administered in the volar aspect of the arm or on the back of the patient with a distance of 5 cm (intradermal) or 3 cm (prick) in between the two tests
- Globally, the wheal diameter is measured after 15–20 min and reported in "mm." A skin reaction of ≥3 mm than that produced by the negative control on the SPT is considered as a positive reaction. This is done to maintain objective assessments of the SPT responses[62,63]
- Qualitative scoring (0–4+; 0 or +) is no longer used by many clinicians because of marked interphysician variability in scoring and interpretation of this method
- The global guidelines do not support the use of grading the skin response. However, in India, some clinicians still use the grading system for documenting skin reactions. Grading of skin reaction is done after 15–20 min in comparison with negative control (phosphate buffered saline [PBS]) and positive control (histamine diphosphate/dihydrochloride). For grading of allergic reaction (skin tests), the criteria given in Tables 54.6 and 54.7 can be followed (Tables 54.6 and 54.7).[46,53,66]

Table 54.6: Grading for the skin prick test.

Wheal diameter	*Interpretation*
0–<3 mm	Negative = Negative control
3–5 mm	1+
6–8 mm	2+ = Positive control
9–11 mm	3+
>11 mm	4+

Modified.[6,53] The wheal size measured during the SPT should be the mean wheal diameter calculated by taking the sum of the horizontal and transverse diameters which is then divided by 2.
SPT, skin prick test.

Table 54.7: Grading for the intradermal test.

Wheal diameter	*Interpretation*
<6 mm	Negative = Negative control (C)
2×C	1+
3×C	2+ = Positive control
4×C	3+, with 1–2 pseudopodia
>4×C	4+, with >2 pseudopodia

The significance of allergen for considering AIT is considered only if the reaction is equal to or more than the positive control.

- Physician should be available at the time of skin testing to take care of any adverse reaction
- In case of high sensitivity (history), skin tests are performed with diluted antigen extracts
- In case of doubtful reaction, a repeat skin test is performed to confirm the reaction
- Provocation tests with allergen are recommended only at the institution level and are mainly done for research purposes.

In Vitro Tests

Most commonly used in vitro diagnostic tests[53] for the estimation of total IgE and allergen-sIgE levels in the sera of allergic patients are radio/enzyme immunoassays. The basic principle remains the same, in which a solid phase allergen/antibody binds with primary antibody which is further detected using a radio/enzyme-labeled secondary antibody. The binding signal is converted to a quantitative measurement of concentration using a standard curve, in which one reactant is added in known amounts.

To establish atopic status of the patient, total serum IgE levels are measured.[45] However, the raised IgE levels are also found in some nonatopic individuals and in patients suffering with various nonallergic diseases. An Indian study has also concluded that "the IgE levels in Indian allergic patients is significantly related to atopy; however, due to wide overlap of IgE levels in patients and healthy subjects, its diagnostic significance in Indian population seems to be limited."[67]

Measurement of allergen-sIgE levels gives reliable information about patients' clinical sensitivity to various aeroallergens. For this purpose, kits based on immunoenzymetric techniques commercially available can be used. Multiallergen screens are useful to support a more extensive clinical and immunologic investigation for allergic diseases.

In vitro tests are considered as a backup tool to SPT and should be utilized in cases when the SPT cannot be performed.

Quality assurance is very important for all these in vitro diagnostic tests. In USA, external proficiency surveys are conducted in selected laboratories for checking uniformity of results using reference samples. In India, there is an urgent need to conduct such surveys to establish indigenous quality control standards for the measurement of allergen-sIgE levels.

The AIT should not be given only on the basis of the serological tests. In vitro tests may be used only as a supportive test or in situations, in which skin testing is not possible.

A positive result (either on in vivo or in vitro testing) does not necessarily mean that the symptoms are due to an IgE-mediated allergy, and therefore, it is important to correlate results with history and examination findings.

TYPES OF ALLERGEN IMMUNOTHERAPY

Subcutaneous Immunotherapy

The subcutaneous route has been the commonly used method of administration of AIT.

Types of Allergen Extracts

In India, native extracts available as aqueous preparations are used for SCIT. These allergen extracts are prepared by aqueous extraction of allergenic materials obtained from natural sources. The composition and biologic properties may be influenced by the quality and purity of the source material, as well as their processing, extraction, and storage conditions. In addition to aqueous extracts, which are commonly used, depot extracts are primarily used in Europe for SCIT. In Europe, allergens or newer hypoallergenic preparations are physically adsorbed to a carrier, such as aluminum hydroxide (most common), tyrosine, or calcium phosphate. The concept of hypoallergenic preparations is that they possess less reactive B-cell epitopes and thus reduce IgE binding, while their T-cell epitopes and their immunogenic effect remain unaltered.[68,69] In Europe, these hypoallergenic preparations comprise up to 50% of the SCIT prescriptions.[70] Numerous studies have provided clinical efficacy and safety of the allergen extracts. Advantages of hypoallergenic preparations are lesser SRs, shorter dose build-up phase, and less frequent dosing.

Administration Regimens

Conventional regimen

Currently, in India, only aqueous extracts are available. In most of the cases, AIT is started with 1:5,000 w/v diluted antigen and the injections are given two times a week starting from and increased by 0.1 mL in every injections. The injections are given subcutaneously with graduated syringe or insulin syringe. The idea is to achieve the highest maintenance dose, i.e., 1:50 - one time a month, 1.0 mL. Usually, the maintenance dose is between 0.5 and 1.0 mL of 1:50 dilution. In cases showing high skin sensitivity with local reaction (LR)/SR after initiation (1:5,000 w/v) of AIT, it is rescheduled/started with higher dilution, i.e., 1:50,000 w/v or even higher dilution, and the first injection is administered in the hospital/clinic having facilities to manage anaphylaxis.

Fewer buildup injections are possible with the depot and hypoallergenic formulations. Furthermore, the maintenance doses may be given in a period of 4–8 weeks, thus reducing the burden of repeated injections. Randomized trials with accelerated up-dosing of hypoallergenic preparation for pollen have also been recently conducted, in which the maintenance dose is achieved in 4 weeks with safety and tolerability profiles comparable to the conventional dose escalation.

Rush immunotherapy

The advantage of rush schedule is that patients can attain the maintenance dose more quickly. Schedule for rush IT entails administering multiple injection in a row preferably in a hospital setup. Schedules using eight injections over 3 days or eight injections in a single day have been published.[71] However, these protocols need further investigation in terms of risk and benefit ratio to patient.

Cluster immunotherapy

The starting dose is similar to those of perennial AIT regimen. Here, weekly visits are necessary because, at each visit, more than one injection is given at a small interval between injections, varying from 30 min to 2 h. After the maintenance dose is reached in approximately 2 months, interval between visits is increased. The cluster regimen is advantageous to the patients who reside at a significant distance from a physician. There are similar efficacy and immunological changes in cluster regimen as observed with the perennial IT in various studies.[72] However, the initial doses are required to be given in a hospital set up able to manage emergencies associated with this form of therapy. Cluster schedule with hypoallergenic mite-SCIT has also been developed and is found to be safe and well-tolerated in routine clinical practice.

Sublingual Immunotherapy

The sublingual route has attracted the greatest interest in recent years as shown by the number of double-blind, placebo-controlled trials and the fact that SLIT has spread widely in some countries in Europe. However, further studies are needed to define the most appropriate dosage, the efficacy in pediatric patients, and to evaluate the magnitude of efficacy compared to other available treatments.[73-76]

In contrast to the subcutaneous route, SLIT requires a much higher amount of antigen to achieve clinical efficacy. On an average, SLIT requires at least 50–100 times more allergen content than SCIT to be efficacious, and consequently, low-dose SLIT is generally ineffective.[77] Furthermore, in comparison with SCIT (which is standardized in regimens and protocols), SLIT is affected by numerous variables (Table 54.8). It can be administered as drops, mono-dose vials, or tablets and with variable timings and doses. In particular, the maintenance dose is strictly dependent on the method of standardization, which varies from one manufacturer to another.[78]

In addition to above-mentioned points of variability in the doses, SLIT has also been clinically effective only for a limited number of allergens.

The SLIT is currently not approved in India but is under consideration of the drug regulatory authority.

Table 54.8: Evidence of head-to-head comparison of subcutaneous versus sublingual immunotherapy.

Study	*Number of participants*	*Treatment favoured*	
		Asthma symptoms	*Rhinitis/ rhinoconjunctivitis symptoms*
Mungan, 1999	36	SCIT	None
Yukselen, 2011	31	SCIT	SCIT
Eifan, 2010	48	SLIT	SCIT
Keles, 2011	56	SCIT	SCIT
Khinchi, 2004	48	-	SCIT
Tahamile, 2006	193	-	SCIT

SCIT, Subcutaneous immunotherapy; SLIT, Sublingual immunotherapy

Other Routes

Bronchial immunotherapy

A limited number of clinical trials have been carried out using this route of administration.[79,80] The results obtained were unimpressive in terms of efficacy, and the bronchospasm was induced in many of the patients treated. Therefore, this route of administration has been abandoned in view of an unfavorable risk-benefit ratio.

Oral immunotherapy

Although a greater number of clinical trials with a suitable design[81] have been carried out using this route of administration, a few of them achieved an acceptable level of clinical efficacy.[82,83] In some trials,[84,85] the effect was no better than that of placebo. Furthermore, adverse events including abdominal pain, vomiting, and diarrhea were recorded in some studies.[85,86] The present results do not support the oral route as an effective alternative.[87]

Nasal immunotherapy

Twenty-two studies of intranasal-administered AIT have been evaluated.[88] Sixteen used a double-blind, placebo-controlled design. Most of these trials demonstrated significant clinical efficacy in allergic rhinitis. The results are encouraging, but nasal AIT seems to be a treatment for allergic rhinitis only. Some studies also reported local adverse effects.[89,90] The only study addressing long-term efficacy demonstrated no sustained effect, following discontinuation of the treatment.[91] There are no data on the possible preventive capacity.

Additional **approaches** to AIT under active investigation include epicutaneous and intralymphatic administration. A few clinical trials with intralymphatic route have indicated that this route is efficacious and safe with a limited number of injections.[78]

DURATION OF ALLERGEN IMMUNOTHERAPY

Allergen immunotherapy is generally administered for 3–5 years; the duration and decision to discontinue it must be individualized. Some patients may require longer periods of **treatment**. It is difficult to predict that how long patients will experience symptomatic relief following discontinuation of AIT. However, prolonged remission of symptoms after discontinuation has been documented in prospective studies with grass pollen SCIT for allergic rhinitis and HDM SCIT for asthmatic patients.[92,93]

Clinical benefits which are ongoing have been documented 12 years after discontinuation of AIT as compared to pharmacotherapy only (please see the section on "Preventive and Disease Modifying Capacity" for further details). The clinical benefits may depend on the nature of the allergen extracts.

ASSESSING THE RESPONSE TO ALLERGEN IMMUNOTHERAPY

The assessment of the response to AIT is made clinically by the improvement of symptoms and reduction for the need of medications (symptom score, medication score, or combined symptom medication scores [CSMSs]) and assessment of QoL. Tests such as quantitative SPT, bronchial hyperresponsiveness test, and immunological parameters may also be used. However, these parameters may not always correlate with improvement in allergic disease status of patients. Measurement of total IgE has no value for such assessment.[2,3]

Nonquantitative skin testing (demonstrating skin test reactivity to a single dilution) or serum-sIgE antibody testing of patients during AIT is not recommended because it has not been demonstrated that they correlate with a patient's clinical response. Efficacy and clinical contraindications should be assessed regularly.[2,3] Studies have shown that AIT inhibits allergen-driven TH2 response, so the cytokines typical for TH1 versus TH2 responses could be used as markers to judge the response of AIT. The immunological markers such as Treg cells with increase in IL-10 and IgG4-blocking antibody) correlate well with reduction in immediate skin test response and decrease in late phase response, which may be used to assess the response and to decide when to stop AIT.[94]

In summary, clinical parameters (such as symptom score, medication score, or CSMSs) and assessment of QoL shall be considered to assess the response to IT.

EFFICACY: IMMUNOTHERAPY TRIALS INCLUDING COCHRANE DATABASE ANALYSIS

Subcutaneous Immunotherapy

The SCIT is effective in the treatment of allergic rhinitis, allergic conjunctivitis, and allergic asthma, in both children and adults. It is also used in the treatment of venom hypersensitivity, which is discussed separately.

The parameters that indicate clinical efficacy of a treatment are reduction in symptoms and/or drug intake of a magnitude that significantly reduces morbidity.[95] The clinical efficacy of SCIT has been validated in numerous clinical trials in children and adults. Clinical efficacy has been confirmed for allergen products from birch, grasses, mountain cedar, cypress, olive, *Parietaria*, ragweed, cat, *D. pteronyssinus*, *Alternaria*, and *Cladosporium*.

Fundamental questions on AIT are (1) whether it has potential to provide long-term benefit following its discontinuation and (2) whether it can prevent either disease progression or the onset of new allergic sensitivities.[96] Without long-term reduction in disease severity and disease-modifying capability, AIT may not be cost-effective and consequently not be a real alternative to pharmacologic treatment.[97] Previous studies on IT indicate that the treatment may have a long-lasting effect. A controlled study by Durham et al.[92] has documented the long-term efficacy of AIT after withdrawal of the treatment, following a double-blind, placebo-controlled trial.[98]

As per the WHO[99] and AAAAI recommendations,[3] at present, allergen avoidance and IT are the only treatments that modify the course of an allergic disease either by preventing the development of new sensitivity or by altering the natural history of disease or disease progression. The optimal dose for SCIT has been recommended as the maintenance target dose for all patients. Doses of 5–20 μg of the major allergen are optimal doses for domestic mites, cat dander, ragweed pollen, and hymenoptera venoms. These doses are tolerated by the majority of patients with allergic diseases without difficulty.

Allergic Rhinitis

The AIT alters allergic disease through a series of injections of clinically relevant allergens and has been recognized as the only therapeutic option known to alter the natural history of allergic rhinitis.[100,101] According to the AAAAI,[102] AIT is successful in patients with seasonal allergic rhinitis and in patients suffering with perennial allergic rhinitis. Hence, subcutaneous AIT was approved for the management of allergic rhinitis and/or allergic asthma. However, AIT is currently indicated as a supplement to allergen avoidance and to pharmacotherapy.[103] Its efficacy in the prevention of allergic march and the development of asthma among patients with allergic rhinitis has been demonstrated.[104,105] Data were extracted from 16 studies showing clinical effectiveness of SCIT in the treatment of allergic rhinitis, involving 759 patients (546 adults, 53 children, 160 all ages). In 15 (94%) of the studies, SCIT led to significant improvement in both symptoms and medication scores.[94] Its efficacy has been validated in many trials, using grass, ragweed, and birch pollen extracts.[96] Importantly, SCIT has been shown to be effective even in patients with severe seasonal rhinitis that is resistant to conventional drug therapy. There was a highly significant decrease versus median placebo (95% confidence interval [CI] for difference between medians) in total symptom scores ($p = 0.001$), total drug use ($p = 0.002$), and visual analog symptom scores ($p = 0.02$), 2.2 versus 5.5 (–4.8 to –0.5). Provocation tests after allergen IT showed a greater than 10-fold reduction in immediate conjunctival allergen sensitivity ($p = 0.001$), a 40% decrease in early phase response ($p = 0.02$), and a 57% decrease in the late phase ($p = 0.001$) cutaneous response after intradermal allergen challenge.[98]

A Cochrane review, on the meta-analysis of 51 randomized double-blind placebo-controlled trials involving 2,871 subjects with seasonal allergic rhinitis or controls, has shown that AIT results in significant improvement in overall symptoms, medication use, and QoL. Symptom score data from 15 trials were suitable for meta-analysis and showed an overall reduction in the AIT group (standardized mean difference [SMD] –0.73 [95% CI – 0.97 to –0.50, $p < 0.00001$]). Medication score data from 13 trials showed an overall reduction in the AIT group (SMD of – 0.57 [95% CI – 0.82 to –0.33, $p < 0.00001$]). Adrenaline was given in 0.13% (19 of 14,085 injections) of those on active treatment and in 0.01% (1 of 8,278 injections) of the placebo group for treatment of adverse events. There were no fatalities.[106,107]

A current meta-analysis (2013) evaluated 17 clinical trials (up to April 2011) for the efficacy of SCIT in patients with seasonal allergic rhinitis.[108] This analysis found a reduction in the symptom scores (SMD – 0.65; 95% CI – 0.85 to –0.45; $p < 0.00001$; all 17 studies), the medication scores (SMD – 0.55; 95% CI – 0.75 to –0.34; $p < 0.00001$; 16 studies), the CSMSs (SMD – 0.48; 95% CI – 0.67 to –0.29; $p < 0.00001$; 8 studies) as well as an improvement in the QoL scores (SMD – 0.53; 95% CI – 0.66 to –0.39; $p < 0.00001$; 8 studies).

The benefits of AIT for perennial rhinitis are less than for seasonal rhinitis. In part, this reflects the difficulty in determining the extent to which allergy is responsible for perennial symptoms. Nevertheless, clinical trials have shown a definite benefit in appropriately selected subjects.[109] Clearer evidence has been obtained in perennial rhinitis due to pet allergy. Several studies have shown a marked improvement in tolerance of cat exposure after SIT, validated both on challenge tests and simulated natural exposure.[110]

Bronchial Asthma

A meta-analysis of 75 SCIT trials concluded that there is a significant reduction in asthma symptoms and drug requirement as well as in bronchial hyperreactivity with SCIT.[111] SCIT has been found to maintain a persistent improvement after discontinuation of IT[92,105,112,113] and also reduces the risk of future development of asthma in rhinitis cases.[92,94,105,113-116] Successful IT prevents development of new allergen sensitivities in monosensitized individuals.[117-119]

A 2003 Cochrane review included 75 trials with a total of 3,506 participants (3,188 with asthma) for data analysis in a meta-analysis.[111] There were 36 trials of HDM allergy, 20 pollen allergy, 10 animal dander allergy, 2 *Cladosporium* mold allergy, 1 latex, and 6 for multiple allergens. Concealment of allocation was assessed as clearly adequate in only 15 of these trials. Significant heterogeneity was present in a number of comparisons. Overall, there was a significant reduction in asthma symptoms and medication and improvement in bronchial hyperreactivity following AIT. Furthermore, a significant improvement was therein asthma symptom scores (SMD – 0.72, 95% CI – 0.99 to –0.33), and it would have been necessary to treat four (95% CI 3–5) patients with SCIT to avoid one deterioration in increased medication. AIT significantly reduced allergen-specific bronchial hyperreactivity, with some reduction in nonspecific bronchial hyperreactivity as well. However, there was no consistent effect on lung function.

The 2010 updated Cochrane meta-analysis "Injection allergen IT for asthma" included 88 trials (13 new trials).[120] There were 42 trials of IT for house mite allergy; 27 pollen allergy trials; 10 animal dander allergy trials; two *Cladosporium* mold allergy, 2 latex, and 6 trials looking at multiple allergens. Overall, there was a significant reduction in asthma symptoms and medication and improvement in bronchial hyperreactivity following AIT. There was a significant improvement in asthma symptom scores (SMD – 0.59, 95% CI – 0.83 to –0.35 [$p < 0.00001$]), and it would have been necessary to treat three patients (95% CI 3–5) with IT to avoid one deterioration in asthma symptoms. Overall, it would have been necessary to treat four patients (95% CI 3–6) with IT to avoid one requiring increased medication. AIT significantly reduced allergen-specific bronchial hyperreactivity, with some reduction in nonspecific bronchial hyperreactivity as well. There was no consistent effect on lung function. If 16 patients were treated with IT, one would be expected to develop a local adverse reaction. If nine patients were treated with IT, one would be expected to develop a SR (of any severity).

A recently published meta-analysis evaluated the efficacy and safety of SCIT in mite-sensitized subjects with asthma.[121] A total of 796 subjects from 19 different randomized controlled trials (RCTs) were included in this analysis. SCIT significantly reduced the asthma symptom scores (SMD – 0.94, 95% CI – 1.58 to –0.29, $p = 0.004$) and the asthma medication scores (SMD – 1.06, 95% CI – 1.70 to –0.42, $p = 0.001$) compared with the control group. One study conducted solely in children with allergic asthma, in which SCIT was employed using an hypoallergenic extract of HDM, showed improved asthma control as well as significant reduction in the required doses of inhaled corticosteroids compared with the control group not treated with SCIT.[122]

A meta-analysis prepared by the Johns Hopkins University Evidence-based Practice Center for the Agency for Healthcare Research and Quality (AHRQ, USA) included 74 references that investigated the efficacy and safety of SCIT.[123] In this meta-analysis, the strength of evidence was high that SCIT reduces asthma symptoms, rhinitis symptoms, conjunctivitis symptoms, asthma medication use, asthma plus rhinoconjunctivitis medication use, and rhinoconjunctivitis-specific QoL. The strength of evidence is moderate that SCIT reduces rhinoconjunctivitis medication use, relative to usual care, which includes pharmacotherapy.

Atopic Dermatitis

Atopic dermatitis (AD) may respond to SCIT if the patient is sensitized to inhalant allergens although this conclusion is based on a small number of studies[3] of HDM allergic patients, including one randomized trial of 51 patients.[124,125] Negative studies also exist.[126] The impact of IT on AD in patients sensitized to pollens or other aeroallergens has not been studied. Thus, the use of SCIT to treat AD requires careful observation of the patient's clinical status, especially during the buildup phase of treatment. One randomized double-blind dose-range finding SCIT trial on 89 adult patients with a chronic form of AD and sensitization to HDMs revealed a significant improvement of the scoring atopic dermatitis (SCORAD) over a 1-year therapy course.[125] In a more recently published DBPC-Phase-III study (SCIT) on 168 adult patients, a significant improvement in the SCORAD was only demonstrated in a subgroup with severe forms of AD.[127]

Preventive and Disease-Modifying Capacity

The capacity of SCIT to prevent the development of new sensitizations has been investigated in three nonrandomized studies in monosensitized patients.[117-119] In an open retrospective study, Purello-D' Ambrosio made a follow-up of 7,182 monosensitized (to different allergens) patients treated with SCIT for 4 years and off IT for 3 years.[118] The control group consisted of 1,214 matched patients followed for 7 years. The development of sensitization to new allergens showed a clinically relevant and statistically significant difference at the 4-year follow-up, with figures of 68% in the control group versus 24% in the IT group and at the 7-year follow-up 78% and 27%, respectively. Pajno et al. followed 75 SCIT-treated children monosensitized to HDMs and 63 comparable controls treated pharmacologically for 6 years.[119] In the IT group, 74% continued to be monosensitized versus 33% in the control group. A prospective controlled prolonged follow-up study demonstrated the ongoing clinical benefit 12 years after discontinuation of hypoallergenic AIT as compared to pharmacotherapy only. Furthermore, the reduction in onset of new sensitization (58% in the AIT group and 100% in the control group) is sustained at the 12-year follow-up. In addition, there was a tendency for lower prevalence of seasonal asthma in the post-AIT group.[105] Although these studies are of interest, prospective randomized, controlled studies are needed.

In India, a double-blind placebo-controlled study showed significant improvement in clinicoimmunologic parameters in asthma and rhinitis patients after 1 year of IT with whole-body mosquito extract.[128] A placebo-controlled study demonstrated early relapse of symptoms after discontinuation of treatment in patients receiving pharmacotherapy, whereas it was 3–5 years in IT group patients.[129]

The SCIT might prevent the progression of rhinitis into asthma. A multicenter pediatric study investigated the capacity of IT in children with allergic rhinitis to downregulate the development of asthma.[130] Children allergic to birch and grass pollen and no symptoms of lower airway hyperreactivity were randomized to pharmacologic treatment. After 3 years of treatment, the number of children developing clinical asthma was statistically reduced in the IT group. The development of asthma was in 24% children in IT group versus 44% in the drug-treated group, indicating high risk of developing asthmatic symptoms in allergic rhinitis children is diminished by IT. Bronchial hyperresponsiveness to methacholine decreased significantly in IT-treated children, but only 2 out of 40 children with asthma at inclusion were free of asthma after 3 years, indicating that IT has a greater capacity for preventing than for curing asthma. Further studies are needed to clearly define the preventive capacity of SCIT.

STUDIES ON SUBLINGUAL IMMUNOTHERAPY

Due to new controlled trials in adults[131-137] and children,[138-140] some with high patient numbers, data on the efficacy of SLIT are also available. SLIT has been suggested to be a particularly attractive treatment for children where safety is paramount and outpatient, and home-based therapy is clearly preferable. However, more studies in children are urgently required because several issues remain unsolved: for example, optimal doses and duration of treatment in children, the evaluation of quality-of-life and compliance with administration, of vaccine at home. Besides, storage of the allergen product during the time family is out of home, for example, during holidays and dosing during acute, but prolonged gastroenteritis also required to be investigated. The excellent safety profile of SLIT and the fact that injections are not required with this approach raise the possibility that SLIT could be given to children below the age of 5 years, in an attempt to modify the natural course of the allergic disease. However, definitive trials are required to achieve this objective.[141,142]

Allergic Rhinitis

A meta-analysis published by the Cochrane Library on the clinical efficacy of SLIT in patients with rhinitis included 22 double-blind, placebo-controlled clinical trials, and a total of 979 patients.[143] There was significant heterogeneity for most comparisons, likely due to the use of several alternative scoring systems in different studies. However, results showed a significant reduction in rhinitis symptoms and medication requirements. Out of 22 studies, 12 included children <15 years whereas 4 studies were conducted exclusively in children. The doses of allergen used in different studies were analyzed by Canonica and Passalacqua[88] that ranged from 3-5 to 375 times the cumulative dose of SCIT. There was no clear relationship between the dose administered and clinical efficacy; hence, more dose-response studies are needed to clearly indicate the optimal therapeutic dose. A dose-response relationship has been analyzed for ragweed extract.[144]

The 2010 Cochrane update[145] included for the symptom scores 23 studies in grass pollen allergic patients (SMD – 0.35; 95% CI – 0.45 to –0.24; $p < 0.00001$), 9 studies (including 2 using birch pollen extract) in tree pollen allergic patients (SMD – 0.42; 95% CI – 0.77 to –0,06; $p = 0.02$), and 9 studies in HDM allergic patients (SMD – 0.97; 95% CI – 1.80 to –0.13; $p = 0.02$). For the use of SLIT in AR, the Cochrane meta-analysis found an advantage for AIT for all allergens ($p < 0.00001$).

A meta-analysis published earlier this year (2015) assessed the efficacy and safety of the grass pollen sublingual tablets licensed as drugs in the treatment of patients with seasonal allergic rhinoconjunctivitis to grass pollen.[146] Data were available in 13 RCTs for the symptom score (4,659 patients) and in 12 RCTs for the medication score (4,558 patients). The authors found a small treatment benefit in the symptom score (SMD, –0.28; 95% CI, –0.37 to –0.19; $p < 0.001$) and in the medication score (SMD, –0.24; 95% CI, –0.31 to –0.17; $p < 0.001$) and concluded that considering the low magnitude of the benefit, the convenience and easy administration do not seem to be sufficient reasons for the choice of SLIT.

Allergic Asthma

Compared with allergic rhinoconjunctivitis, there are only a limited number of studies on the efficacy of SLIT in patients with allergic bronchial asthma. The 2006 Cochrane Collaboration method meta-analysis data found no significance ($p = 0.07$) for the use of SLIT in allergic asthma.[147] A grass tablet study showed efficacy for SLIT in bronchial asthma in a subgroup of children with seasonal allergic asthma.[138] With regard to IT using dust mite extracts, heterogeneous results were found in clinical trials with methodological limitations.[148-151]

A recent study included 604 HDM allergic patients at least 14 years of age with mild to moderate asthma treated for a 1-year period with SLIT with HDM tablets. Compared with placebo, actively treated patients exhibited a significant reduction in the dose of inhaled corticosteroids required to maintain asthma control over the course of the study period.[152]

A meta-analysis published in September 2015 evaluated a total of 454 children with asthma/rhinitis who were sensitized to HDMs and were treated with SLIT or control for between 4 months and 3 years.[153] The analysis indicated that dust mite SLIT therapy was effective in reducing asthma symptoms and in increasing sIgG4 but did not significantly reduce medication scores or specific *D. pteronyssinus* IgE levels. The authors noted that the data are not enough to support the use of dust mite SLIT in children with asthma.

Preventive and Disease-Modifying Capacity

A randomized controlled open SLIT study in children has shown preventive effect on asthma onset.[154] In control group, 18 of 44 developed asthma versus 8 of 45 in the sublingual group after 3 years of treatment. Another randomized controlled open study demonstrated the prevention of new sensitizations in a 3-year long trial[155] whereas this effect was not observed in another open study.[156,157]

The long-term effect of SLIT was investigated in an open controlled study including 60 mite-sensitive asthmatic children aged 3–17 years.[156] Allocation to IT or pharmacotherapy group was based on parental preference. SLIT was given for 4–5 years and the children followed up for 10 years. At 10 years, there was a significant reduction in the onset of asthma, use of asthma medication, and an increase in peak expiratory flow rate as compared to control group.

Allergens to be used for SLIT are limited and no Indian clinical trial data on SLIT (i.e., randomized double-blind placebo-controlled studies) are available. The dosage of SLIT also ranges from 50-fold to 100-fold compared to the doses which are commonly given for SCIT. In addition, different manufacturers have different doses for the SLIT allergens which are not comparable.

The summary of efficacy data for AIT from Cochrane Reviews/meta-analysis is shown in Figure 54.2.[120,145,147,158]

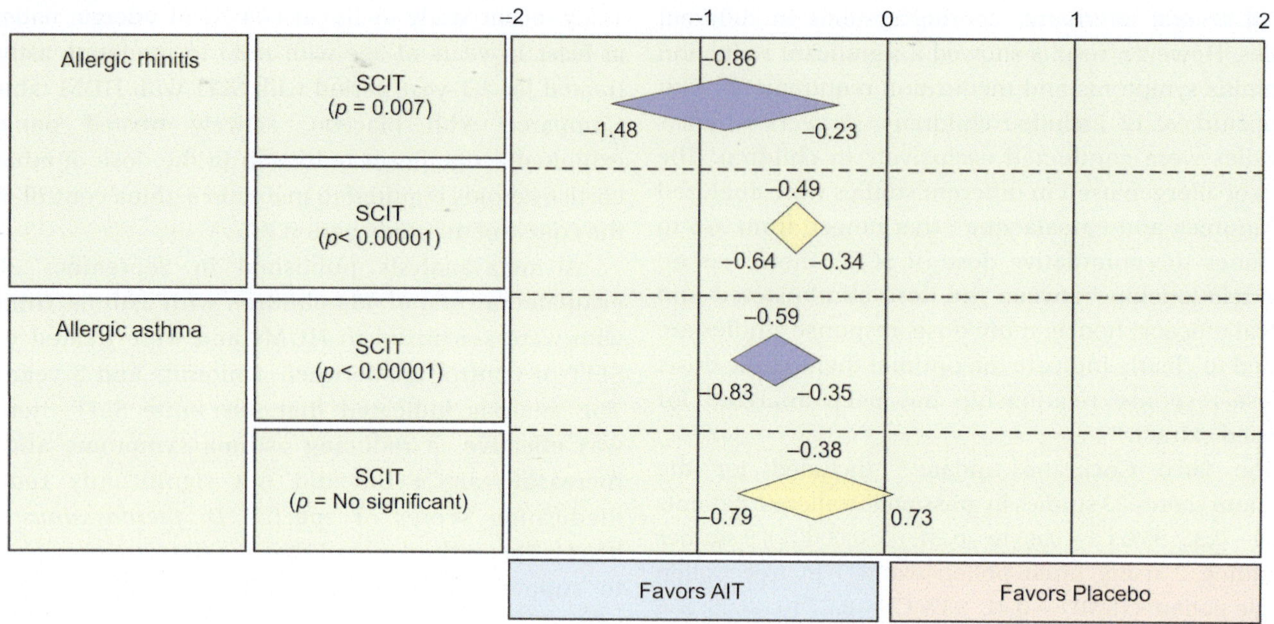

Fig. 54.2: Summary of efficacy data for allergen immunotherapy from Cochrane reviews.[120,145,147,158]

Table 54.9: Systematic reviews comparing subcutaneous and sublingual immunotherapy.

Key findings	*Chelladurai, 2013*	*Kim, 2013*
Number of RCTs	8 SCIT versus SLIT	3 SCIT vs. SLIT (only pediatric)
Symptom score	Favors SCIT (moderate-grade evidence)	Favors SCIT (low-grade evidence)
Medication score	No difference (low-grade evidence)	Favors SCIT (low-grade evidence)
Safety (reactions)	Local (frequency): SCIT: 20%; SLIT: 7%-56% Anaphylactic: SCIT: 1; SLIT: 0	Local (patients): SCIT: 3; SLIT: 3 Systemic (patients): SCIT: 4; SLIT: 0 Anaphylactic: SCIT: 1; SLIT: 0

SCIT, subcutaneous immunotherapy; SLIT, sublingual immunotherapy; RCTs, randomized controlled trials

STUDIES COMPARING SUBLINGUAL AND SUBCUTANEOUS IMMUNOTHERAPY

Both the routes of administration, SCIT and SLIT, have shown efficacy and safety in clinical trials and meta-analyses. There are few trials and meta-analyses which have compared that there are two routes of administration.

The meta-analysis prepared by the Johns Hopkins University Evidence-based Practice Center for the AHRQ, USA, investigated the efficacy and safety of subcutaneous and SLIT.[123] The researchers reviewed the head-to-head comparative trials of the two routes of administration (Table 54.8).[123] The analyses revealed:

- For allergic asthma symptom control: The studies support SCIT over SLIT (strength of evidence, low [4 studies, $n = 171$])
- For allergic nasal and/or eye symptoms: The strength of evidence was moderate that SCIT is more effective than SLIT for reducing allergic nasal and/or eye symptoms (6 RCTs, $n = 412$)
- The data were inadequate to comment on reduction of medication use, symptom and medication reduction, and QoL. The strength of evidence lowly favors SCIT for reducing asthma symptoms and for controling nasal and eye symptoms.

Other systematic reviews which have compared the two routes of administration (i.e., SCIT and SLIT) are detailed in Table 54.9.[159] These include the studies in adult as well as the pediatric population.

Systematic reviews and meta-analyses of RCTs of SCIT, SLIT, or both versus placebo (indirect and direct comparison) suggest that SCIT might provide greater clinical and immunologic efficacy. However, more studies with a greater number of patients are needed to evaluate the magnitude of the clinical efficacy and the optimal dosage. Regarding the final choice between SCIT and SLIT, the decision needs to be made individually with each patient after careful considerations of factors.

VENOM IMMUNOTHERAPY

The efficacy of venom IT (VIT) has been analyzed in three controlled and several prospective uncontrolled studies which employed a usual maintenance dose of 100 μg of venom.[160-162] In these studies, patients were monitored with sting provocation tests during IT.[163] In all controlled trials with vespid, honey bee, or ant venom allergy, comparing venom with either whole-body extract or placebo, a highly significant difference was observed in favor of VIT. Here, 75–100% of venom-treated patients tolerated resting without any allergic symptoms, while 64–75% of whole-body product and 58–72% of placebo-treated patients developed systemic allergic reactions on resting challenge. In the prospective uncontrolled studies, only 0–9% of vespid allergic and around 20% of bee venom allergic patients reacted to challenge with the respective insect. These studies suggest the superior efficacy for IT with vespid or ant venom compared to honey bee venom. The patients who reacted following a course of VIT had mild symptoms than those observed before the treatment. VIT is effective in 95% of patients allergic to wasp venom and about 80% of those allergic to bee venom.[164]

The safety of VIT is related to the nature of the venom used and the protocol. More side effects were observed during IT with honey bee venom than vespid venom.[165] In an EAACI multicenter study of 840 patients totaling 26,601 injections, 20% of patients developed mild systemic allergic reactions, corresponding to 1.9% of injections during the dose increase phase and 0.5% during the maintenance phase.[166] Rapid dose increase, especially with high cumulative daily doses of 200–500 μg in rush protocols, may increase the risk of side effects. In patients who cannot safely discontinue β-blockers but who have a history of moderate to severe sting-induced anaphylaxis, VIT is indicated because the risk of anaphylaxis related to a venom sting is greater than the risk of an IT-related SR.[3]

ALLERGEN IMMUNOTHERAPY STUDIES IN INDIA

A limited number of studies are available on AIT from our country.[128,129,167-169] IT for 1 year in cases of asthma and/or rhinitis has demonstrated >50% improvement in clinical parameters (symptoms).[167] A placebo-controlled study on AIT for 6–12 months with *Cocos nucifera* pollen extract showed significant clinical improvement (symptom-medication score), reduction in IgE, and elevation of specific IgG in posttherapeutic patients' sera than placebo.[168] Another study evaluated the immunological changes that follow SCIT in patients suffering from bronchial allergy and/or allergic rhinitis. The inflammatory makers (IL-5 and IL-6 levels) at 0, 3, and 6 months were compared, and it was noted that with an increase in duration of treatment, the levels of these markers decrease significantly ($p = 0.003$).[170]

An open comparative study of IT versus budesonide inhalation has reported almost equal improvement in asthma patients in both the groups.[129] However, the decline in benefit was rapid in drug treatment group than AIT after cessation of treatment. Another study determined the efficacy of HDM IT over a 15-year period.[171] The use of IT resulted in a statistically significant improvement in both global symptom scores and forced expiratory volume 1s in patients receiving IT when compared with those in the control group who did not receive IT. This improvement was sustained for at least 10 years after cessation of IT.[171] Another observation presented the ongoing clinical benefit for 6–9 years in 35 patients even after discontinuation of HDM (*D. farinae*/*D. pteronyssinus*) SCIT for 3 years.[172]

A recent double-blind placebo-controlled study on AIT with mosquito extract in asthma and allergic rhinitis patients has demonstrated significant clinical improvement, supported with changes in airway reactivity and immunologic parameters (IgE, IgG1, IgG4, and IFN-α) from the baseline and placebo.[128] Further, AIT with two to three mix extracts from the same allergen group is effective for insect hypersensitivity.[169] A double-blind, placebo-controlled trial of cockroach AIT was performed for 1 year in 50 patients of asthma, rhinitis, or both. AIT with cockroach extract improved clinical and immunological status of asthma and rhinitis patients.[128] A case study has also documented the successful SCIT with horse dander allergy in a patient with recurrent episodes of anaphylaxis on coming in contact with horse.[173] An open-label study evaluated the efficacy of swallow SLIT and rush SCIT (25 patients in each group, with allergic rhinitis, asthma, or both) using randomization technique and followed up for 1 year.[174] There was significant improvement in QoL in both SLIT and rush SCIT groups from baseline to end of 1 year. Another study evaluated the response to AIT in 80 patients with allergic conjunctivitis. Sixty-two percent of these showed beneficial response as documented by the symptoms and medications scores.[175]

In India, a preliminary observation has documented the steroid-sparing effect of cluster IT combined with anti-IgE, the combination being also associated with good tolerability.[176]

A retrospective analysis of a prospective symptom review in patients receiving AIT has been conducted in India to determine the type of allergens, number of allergens, and concentration of the allergens or the combination on the efficacy of AIT. Patients received AIT with a mixture of 5–8 allergens and HDM was administered separately. The authors found that only 42% of their patients improved while 58% had no improvement or had worsening of their symptoms. It was observed that 58% of the patients, who did not benefit from AIT, received the incorrect combination of allergens. The compatibility of allergens was based on the protease activity of the individual allergens. High protease-containing enzymes included dust mites, fungal, and insect allergens. These results clearly lay emphasis on the nature of allergens and their combination used for IT. Furthermore, the inclusion of all allergens to which IgE antibodies are present, without establishing the possible clinical relevance of these allergens, dilutes the content of other allergens in the vaccine and can make AIT less effective.[177] A double-blind placebo-controlled study evaluated the efficacy of single insect extract (cockroach, housefly, or mosquito) and mix allergen IT (two or three insect extracts) with placebo. In this study of insect AIT, mixed and/or single insect AIT for 1 year demonstrated significant improvement in clinical (skin reactivity, airway reactivity, and symptom score) and immunological (IgE/IgG4 and IgG1/IgG4 ratio) parameters.[169]

Another study - a double-blind, placebo-controlled trial of cockroach AIT performed for 1 year in 50 patients of asthma, rhinitis, or both - evaluated the efficacy of AIT by change in skin reactivity and clinical parameters such as symptom/drug score, airway reactivity, and immunological parameters. AIT with cockroach extract demonstrated significant improvement in clinical parameters of active group patients compared with baseline values and placebo group. sIgE levels showed a modest reduction, while IgG4 levels increased significantly in active AIT group after 1 year. IgE immunoblotting demonstrated reduction in intensity and number of specific bands, whereas IgG4 binding showed more number and distinct bands following AIT. Active group patients showed correlation between increase in IgG4/IgG1 ratio and reduction in symptom score post-AIT.[178]

A prospective nonrandomized with 6-year follow-up study evaluated the safety of SLIT in pregnancy in Indian patients.

One hundred and fifty-five patients received SLIT with either HDM (*D. farinae*) or a mixture of up to five allergens during 185 pregnancies.[179] Two control groups did not receive IT; Group A (85 patients) received budesonide 400 μg twice daily, and Group B (40 patients) received rescue salbutamol inhalation. In this study, there were no episodes of SRs, but there were 11 episodes of LRs (oral) to SLIT, consisting of mild itching in the oral cavity and/or swelling of lips. Patients, in whom LRs were noted, delivered normally. The incidence of abortion in the salbutamol group was higher than in the general population ($p < 0.05$) and was higher in both control groups when compared with the SLIT group ($p < 0.05$). The incidence of perinatal deaths, prematurity, and toxemia of pregnancy was also higher in both control groups as compared to the SLIT group, but within the expected incidence for the general population. Another study, which retrospectively analyzed the safety of SCIT in pregnancy, also concluded that IT for allergic diseases is safe in pregnancy.[180]

All these studies show substantial evidence in favor of allergen IT; however, more studies are required involving long-term clinical trials from the country.

SAFETY OF ALLERGEN IMMUNOTHERAPY: A GLOBAL PERSPECTIVE

The administration of allergens into an IgE-sensitized individual always implies a risk, however small, of inducing local and systemic side effects.[3,99,169] LRs are fairly common with both SCIT (erythema, pruritus, and swelling at the injection site) and SLIT (oropharyngeal pruritus, swelling, or both), affecting up to 82% of patients receiving SCIT[3] and 75% of patients receiving SLIT.[181] Gastrointestinal symptoms associated with SLIT can be classified as LRs (if only associated with oral mucosal symptoms) or SRs (if occurring with other systemic symptoms). LRs were "deemed not bothersome at all or only slightly bothersome" by 82% of SCIT survey respondents, with only 4% indicating that they would stop SCIT because of the LR.[182] LRs are not predictive of subsequent SRs with either AIT route.[183,184] No study found that increased frequency of large SCIT LRs increases the risk for future SRs.[185]

Table 54.10: Risk factors for systemic reactions during allergen immunotherapy.

Current allergy symptoms and potential allergen exposure
Current infections
Mast cell disease
Hyperthyroidism
Unstable or insufficiently treated asthma
A high degree of sensitization
Inadequate dose escalation during initiation
Pharmaceutical use (β-blockers)
Inadequate circulatory stress, excessive alcohol consumption, high-intensity physical exercise, sauna (shortly before and for the rest of the day of injection, augmenting factors should be avoided)
Poor technique of injection
Allergen extract overdose
Manufacturer's recommendation for dose reduction upon changing to a new production

Evidence suggests that the patients most likely to develop anaphylaxis are those who are highly sensitive as determined by skin tests or sIgE tests, patients with more severe disease (in particular with chronic and uncontrolled asthma)[186] and prior SCIT-related SRs among others (Table 54.10).[187] It must be noticed that the occurrence of adverse events with SCIT largely depends on the allergen type and preparation. Higher frequency is seen with native allergens compared to the hypoallergenic preparations and in animal dander compared to pollen and mite.[2] Systemic side effects occur more frequently in patients during the induction (up-dosing) phase of treatment compared to maintenance therapy.[188,189] SCIT-related SRs can range in severity from mild to life-threatening or fatal anaphylaxis. The incidence of SCIT SRs varies depending on the induction schedule, augmenting factors, premedication, and the degree of sensitization. In most surveys, the rate of SRs with nonaccelerated SCIT induction is approximately 0.1–0.2% of injections and 2–5% of patients.[190,191]

Compared with SCIT, the SLIT-related SR rate is significantly lower, and severe SRs are relatively uncommon. When introducing a new route of administration, safety is a priority, especially when treatment is self-administered at home.[95] Clinical trials and pharmacosurveillance studies have demonstrated a very low rate of systemic adverse effects and no life-threatening systemic side effects with SLIT.[192,193] In a comprehensive review of 104 SLIT studies published through October 2005, the SLIT-related SR rate was 0.056% of doses administered (i.e., 14 probable SLIT-related serious adverse events, which translated to 1.4 serious adverse events per 100,000 SLIT administered doses).[181] The Food and Drug Administration (FDA)-approved product information of the three SLIT tablets includes a warning about the possibility of severe allergic reactions from SLIT and a recommendation that an epinephrine autoinjector be prescribed to patients receiving allergy tablets in the event a severe allergic reaction should occur. To date, there have been no confirmed reports of SLIT-related fatalities, but SRs of a severity to be categorized as anaphylaxis have been reported.[194] Unlike SCIT, the incidence of SRs does not appear to be related to induction schedule, allergen dose, symptomatic asthma, or degree of sensitization. Because SLIT is administered in a setting without direct medical supervision, specific patient instructions should be provided regarding management of adverse reactions and the clinical scenarios when the administration of SLIT should be postponed (e.g., asthma exacerbation, acute gastroenteritis, and stomatitis or esophagitis).

- SRs (anaphylaxis) are generally rare, but facilities for its management should be available at the place of skin testing and IT. SRs are categorized into immediate SRs (occurring within 30 min) and late SRs (debut >30 min after injection)
- Important symptoms of anaphylaxis include change in voice, frequent change in posture, itching in eye and skin, redness in eye, appearance of symptoms - such as rhinitis, asthma, and urticaria, fall in blood pressure and feeble pulse, mental confusion, sinking sensation, and losing consciousness
- Early signs of a severe reaction include a burning sensation and pruritus of the palms and soles; perianal or perigenital pruritus; an urge to defecate and urinate; sneezing attacks; and generalized pruritus. In addition, further respiratory and/or cardiovascular symptoms may occur rapidly
- Sequential increase in the size of swelling at the site of injection is suggestive of impending anaphylaxis
- Other complications may include vasovagal attack.

WAO SCIT SR grading system should be utilized to identify SRs and grade them accordingly.[190]

Anaphylaxis and its Management

SRs (anaphylaxis) may occur in patients while skin testing with some antigens or initiation phase. Anaphylaxis refers to severe allergic reaction, in which prominent dermal and systemic signs including symptoms manifest. The full-blown syndrome includes urticaria (hives) and/ or angioedema with hypotension and bronchospasm. The classic form, described in 1902, involved prior sensitization to an allergen with later re-exposure, producing symptoms through an immunologic mechanism. An anaphylactoid reaction produces a very similar clinical syndrome but is not immune-mediated.

Pathophysiology of anaphylaxis is characterized by rapid onset of increased secretion from mucous membrane, increased bronchial smooth muscle tone, decreased vascular smooth muscle tone, and increased capillary permeability after exposure to an inciting substance. These effects are produced by the release of mediators, such as histamine, leukotriene C4, prostaglandin D2, and tryptase. The release of these mediators are immune mediated involving type I allergic reaction that occurs when the antigen (allergen) binds to antigen-sIgE attached to previously sensitized basophils and mast cells. The mediators are released almost immediately when the antigen binds.

The most common inciting agents in anaphylaxis are parenteral antibiotics (especially penicillins), intravenous contrast materials, hymenoptera stings, and certain foods (most notably, peanuts). Oral medications and many other types of exposures also have been implicated in anaphylaxis. Anaphylaxis may sometimes be idiopathic.

Anaphylactic reaction is clinically manifested by respiratory distress, laryngeal edema, and/or intense bronchospasm, often followed by vascular collapse or by shock without antecedent respiratory difficulty. Cutaneous manifestations exemplified by pruritus and urticaria with or without angioedema are characteristic of such systemic anaphylactic reactions. Gastrointestinal manifestations include nausea, vomiting, crampy abdominal pain, and diarrhea.

Adrenaline/epinephrine is the drug of choice for the management of anaphylaxis.

Prehospital interventions include high-flow oxygen, cardiac monitoring, and facility for intravenous line. Active airway intervention is needed in rare cases but may be difficult due to laryngeal or oropharyngeal edema. Inhaled beta-agonists are used to counteract bronchospasm and should be administered to patients having wheezing. For large-volume intravenous fluid resuscitation, isotonic crystalloid solutions (i.e., normal saline, ringer lactate) are preferred. With mild cutaneous reactions, an antihistamine alone may be sufficient. In patients with systemic manifestations of anaphylaxis, epinephrine is to be administered. Patients taking β-blockers may be resistant to the effects of epinephrine. Glucagon may be effective in this situation. Administration of corticosteroids is used in anaphylaxis primarily to decrease the incidence and severity of delayed or biphasic reactions. Corticosteroids may not influence the acute course of the disease; therefore, they have a lower priority than epinephrine and antihistamines.

Essential equipment/drugs (emergency kit) for the treatment and monitoring of systemic anaphylactic reactions[81] should be available, while skin testing and injection(s) for AIT, as follows:

- Stethoscope, blood pressure monitor
- Adrenaline (1 mg/mL) for injection
- Antihistamine, corticosteroids, and vasopressor for injection or oral treatment
- Bronchodilator (rapidly acting β-2 agonist for inhalation or intravenous injection)
- Syringes, needles, tourniquet, and equipment for infusion
- Saline for infusion
- Oxygen (with face mask/nasal cannula) and suction equipment
- Silicone mask and equipment for manual ventilation
- Forms for recording the course and treatment of anaphylaxis.

Precautions for Systemic Side Effects

Before deciding the dose of allergen, a careful evaluation of the patient suitability to receive the scheduled dose is required to avoid systemic side effects. The precautions recommended are as follows:[81,195] (1) IT should not be started during peak allergen season and (2) injections should not be administered when the patient has clinical symptoms or the symptoms should be controlled by adequate medication.[92] As a safety precaution, a reduction in allergen dose during allergen season is commonly recommended.

- AIT injections (SCIT) in patients with airway infection or other significant diseases within the last 3 days can be postponed.

- Injections (SCIT) in patients with deterioration of allergy symptoms or increased need for anti-allergic drugs due to recent allergen exposure within the last 3 days should be postponed.
- Injections (SCIT) should be postponed in patients with decreased lung function <80% of personal best value. In asthmatic patients, measuring lung function before each injection is mandatory (peak flow measurement is sufficient).
- The scheduled dose of antigen can be reduced if the interval between injections has been exceeded. The magnitude of reduction depends on the degree exceeded and should be defined in the clinical guidelines.
- The scheduled allergen dose should be reduced in case of an SR at the preceding visit. The magnitude of reduction depends on the severity of the reaction and should be defined in the clinical guidelines. In case of anaphylactic and other life-threatening reactions, the continuation of SCIT should be carefully evaluated (except in case of hymenoptera venom allergy, in which it actually reinforces the indication for IT).
- Allergen injections (vaccine) should be administered separately from other vaccination for infectious diseases by at least a gap of 1 week.

Conventionally, the late LR at the injection site is used to adjust the allergen dosage for the next allergen administration. However, studies have indicated that the late LR at the preceding injection is not related to a risk of developing an SR at the next injection.[195]

- Preinjection monitoring of patients also includes a check of any drug intake that may either increase the risk of systemic side effects or render the treatment of anaphylactic reactions more difficult. Here, the Φ062-blockers are the most important example.[196] Heavy drinking of beer may similarly increase risk due to inhibition of the histamine-converting enzyme diamine oxidase.[197]
- Antihistamine pretreatment during the initial phase of AIT has shown to reduce the frequency and severity of systemic side effects.[198] In a controlled trial of hymenoptera VIT involving a small number of patients, antihistamine pretreatment was associated with a better clinical efficacy.[199] However, further studies are required on this aspect. A potential problem is that the use of antihistamine pretreatment may mask a mild reaction, which would otherwise help in dose modification.

SPECIAL CONSIDERATIONS

Monoallergen Immunotherapy and Mix Allergen Immunotherapy

One important variable in the administration of SCIT is the use of a single or multiple allergens. For example, allergy/immunology specialists in USA generally administer mixtures of all of the major allergens (or a representative of each group of allergens) to which the patient has been shown to be sensitive. In contrast, it is common in Europe to administer only the one or two allergens that appear to cause the most symptoms for that individual patient. Most of the studies in India have also been on multiple allergen AIT. However, globally, most of the studies of SCIT efficacy used a single allergen, and thus, the efficacy of multiple allergen SCIT has not been extensively evaluated in clinical studies.[187]

The prevalence of polysensitization has been documented to increase with age, and a majority of the patients consulting an allergist are polysensitized. A polysensitized patient does not necessarily have polyallergy (Box 54.1 for their definitions).[200]

The management of patients with polysensitizations and/or polyallergy has been dealt with in a recently published review article. Understanding the sensitization and allergy profile of a patient can help the allergist provide specific AIT with greater confidence. In a patient with polysensitization, if the clinician identifies only a single allergen responsible for the most clinically relevant symptoms, then monoallergen IT with that allergen can be prescribed.[200]

If two or more allergens are recognized as clinically significant, then AIT may be initiated with parallel 2-AIT (i.e., both allergens as individual AIT) or mixed 2-AIT. The European Medicines Agency has recommended that allergists should mix nonrelated allergens as little as possible and should not mix seasonal and perennial

BOX 54.1: Definitions of polysensitization and polyallergy.

Polysensitization: Sensitization (according to standardized skin prick tests or ssIgE assays) to two or more allergens

Polyallergy: Clinically confirmed allergy to two or more sensitizing allergens (i.e., causal relationships between exposure to two or more sensitizing allergens and clinical allergy symptoms)

allergens or allergens with proteolytic activity (such as extracts of HDMs, molds, and insects) without justification. Mixing allergens clearly has an impact on pharmaceutical parameters (stability and dosing) and clinical effects (optimal dose and safety). The authors of the review article also recommend that AIT with three or more allergen sources should only be considered in the very rare cases, in which all the allergens clearly cause severe symptoms.[200]

Understanding the principles of homologous groups as suggested by Lorenz et al. can guide the clinician on the physicochemical and biological characteristics of allergen extracts that can help in defining the strategy of monoallergen IT or mixing of allergens.[201] Homologous groups have been suggested only for the mites (*Dermatophagoides* species) and the pollen allergens.

D. pteronyssinus and *D. farinae* belong to the homologous groups of HDMs. Among tree pollens, three groups have been described - the birch group or *Fagales* group, group of *Oleaceae*, and group of *Cupressaceae*. In grasses/cereals, sweet grasses of the *Poaceae* (*Gramineae*) family, subfamily of *Pooideae* have been identified as a homologous group. A group of weed pollen has also been described. Homologous groups have not been defined for insect venoms, animal dander, and molds/fungi.

Within a homologous group (such as *Dermatophagoides* species), the use of a single course of AIT with a mixture of allergens that mimic natural exposure is recommended. Use of separate AIT formulations is preferable when treating with two nonhomologous allergens.

When mixing two allergens from the homologous group, the ratios between the individual allergen sources should be the same.

Skin Test and Allergen Immunotherapy during Pregnancy

1. Do not perform skin testing in a pregnant woman
2. Do not start IT in a pregnant woman
3. Skin testing and IT are to be avoided up to 6 months after delivery or earlier if lactation is discontinued before
4. Do not discontinue IT if person is already on IT started much before pregnancy and receiving benefit from the therapy.

Allergen Immunotherapy in Children

Compliance with the injection regimen may be affected by age and may be problematic, particularly during the adolescent years. Children should accompany a parent, guardian, or other responsible person with them at each visit. It is recommended to start IT at an early age in allergic children to modify the natural course of allergic disease.

Airway remodeling may start early in life, especially in children with severe asthma,[202] and ongoing airway inflammation and remodeling in adolescents and young adults may increase the risk of asthma later in life.[203] As documented earlier, there is evidence that early-specific injection IT reduces the risk of asthma in children with allergic rhinoconjunctivitis[130] and diminishes the risk of new sensitizations in monosensitized children.[118,119]

Age limit for AIT in children:[8]

- Age <2 years is an absolute contraindication for AIT
- Age 2–5 years is a relative contraindication for AIT
- Age ≥5 years can be prescribed AIT.

QUALITY CONTROL OF ALLERGEN EXTRACTS

Several allergen vaccines (extracts) are available commercially in the country. It is recommended that allergen manufacturers should supply vaccines tested for consistency relative to an in-house reference standard. There has been significant progress in allergen standardization in recent years, and a large number of standardized allergen extracts are marketed in the US and European countries. Indian researchers have also published their work on biological standardization of pollen such as *R. communis* and *Hydrangea integrifolia*.[204]

In recent years, a lot of knowledge has been generated in India on characterization of major/minor allergen of pollen, fungi, food, and insect sources.[34,51,205-210] However, the purified proteins (major allergens) and monoclonal/polyclonal antibodies are not available for characterization based on major allergen content. Under these circumstances, allergen extracts are standardized based on weight/volume and protein estimation by modified Lowry's, bicinchoninic acid assay, or micro Kjeldahl method.[211] Researches have shown that allergen source material processed by freeze-drying gives better quality extracts.[207-209] The pollen contents in the samples/raw materials should be >90% for grasses/weeds and >95% in case of trees.

Most of the allergenic proteins (>80%) come in the solution within first few minutes of extraction. Recent studies have shown that 4–8 h extraction in PBS (pH 7.4) or ammonium bicarbonate (pH 8.0) yields extracts with optimum allergenic potency.[51,208,209] The extraction buffer should contain phenyl methyl sulfonyl fluoride and EDTA as protease inhibitors.

Fifty percent glycerol is a good stabilizer of proteins in SPT solutions. However, same concentration cannot be used for therapeutic extracts and the lower concentrations are not effective.[212] Recently, sucrose or epsilon-amino caproic acid (EACA) has been used successfully for stabilizing grass pollen and cockroach extracts.[209,212] Cool gel packs or cold chain should be used/developed for transporting the extracts throughout the country.

Allergen extract(s) vary from one manufacturer to another; hence, it is suggested that diagnostic and therapeutic allergen extracts should be procured from the same allergen manufacturer.

Drug controller of India/state unit(s) regulates the allergen manufacture in the country. Currently, the emphasis is on good manufacture practice to be implemented in these drug antigen units. However, the coordinated efforts of experts from ICAAI, Antigen Units and Drug Regulatory Authorities, are required to upgrade the quality control of allergen extracts following standard WHO/IUIS/EMA protocols. In fact, there is need to develop allergen certification centers in the country such as FDA and Centre for Biologics Evaluation and Research in USA and Paul Ehrlich Institute in Europe.

The methods for antigen preparation and quality control of extracts/vaccine are summarized below for reference:

- Allergy units (AUs) recommended for defining potency of extracts vary across different countries. Hence, at present, weight/volume, protein estimation (PNU in µg/mL), and SDS-PAGE protein profile should be followed for maintaining the quality of antigen in different batches
- Source material for antigen extraction should be freeze-dried, fungal culture (extracts) of 10–20 days should be taken, and PBS of 0.1 M, pH 7.2 has been found most suitable for antigen extraction
- For stability of aqueous extracts, addition of sucrose or EACA is recommended
- Allergen extracts should be free of contaminants including of aflatoxins and endotoxins
- Sterility test is required for each batch of antigen extracts.
- Storage of antigen:
  - The allergen extracts/vaccines should be stored at 2°C–8°C in a refrigerator
  - In case of withdrawal of more antigen from the vaccine vial, it should not be injected back in vial to avoid contamination
  - In case of electricity failure for more than 2 h, keep vaccine in an ice box or any other cooling device/pack
  - Transportation of antigen should be done using a cooling container.

STANDARD PRESCRIPTION (PROTOCOL) FOR PERENNIAL SUBCUTANEOUS IMMUNOTHERAPY

- The allergens for AIT are decided after correlating with history, evidence of exposure to the allergen in the patient environment, precipitation of symptoms after exposure, and skin test positivity preferably with an SPT
- In cases of rhinitis and sinusitis, it is important to exclude mechanical causes such as gross DNS
- Before initiating AIT, patients must be informed about the following: The practical procedure, type, and duration of treatment; expected effects; as well as possible risks of and alternatives to treatment
- Most of the published randomized controlled studies of both SCIT and SLIT are conducted with single allergen extracts. These studies dominate the meta-analyses that indicate both SCIT and SLIT are effective treatments for AR and allergic asthma. There is conflicting evidence for the effectiveness of allergen mixes.[213] The preparation of AIT with an increasing number of extracts creates a potential for interactive effects (cross-reactivity, protease activity) that can change their allergenic and immunogenic properties. Of particular importance is the contribution of proteolytic enzymes in some fungal and whole-body insect allergenic extracts. For these reasons, the number of allergens in an AIT prescription should be limited to as low as possible, never more than four.

Recent evidence demonstrates that within a homologous group (such as *Dermatophagoides* species), the use of a single course of AIT with a mixture of allergens that mimic natural exposure is recommended. When mixing two allergens from the homologous group, the ratios between the individual allergen sources should be the same (e.g., one should always use 1/2 of allergen source 1 and 1/2 of allergen source 2 in a two-allergen mixture, etc.).[200]

- However, in India, the pollen from different categories may be mixed to reduce the number of injections and to improve compliance. In such cases, the amount of individual antigen should be decided depending on their skin test positivity. The greater the positivity, the more is the amount of that antigen to be included in vaccine. These allergens shall be mixed in proportion of skin sensitivity.[214] Such mixture of extracts may be diluted 10 times or more to reduce the chances of an adverse event.

Several factors need to be considered when mixing allergens, including (1) cross-reactivity, (2) optimal dose for each allergen, and (3) potential interaction between different types of allergens (e.g., proteolytic enzymes).

- Allergens of the same group show cross-reactivity; hence, the most potent and relevant allergen should be selected from the group. If the relevance of the allergens are equivalent, then mixing of allergens may be utilized
- Allergens to be mixed in AIT should be done with precaution as certain allergens have proteolytic enzymes and thus reduce the potency of other allergens. Hence, it is recommended not to mix HDM or fungal or insect allergens with any other allergens and prescribe these preferably in separate vials. In India, practice of mixing all the allergens in single vials is done from last more than 50 years to improve compliance and acceptability. The chances of misuse or overdose due to separate vials is a more likely particularly for less illiterate patients
- AIT should be prescribed only by the physician trained in allergy and AIT and administered in his/her presence in a place having facility of managing anaphylaxis
- AIT is started usually with 1:5,000 w/v diluted antigen, and the injections are given two times a week starting from 0.1 mL and increased in every injection by 0.1 mL.
  - Use a tuberculin syringe with 26 number needle
  - The injections are given subcutaneously
  - If the dose is more than 0.5 mL, divide the injection in two sites
  - The allergen vial should be kept in a refrigerator between 2°C and 8°C
  - The schedule is as follows (Table 54.11) (detailed dosing schedule is given in Appendix 1).

The dosing regimen may be modified and patient can be initiated with a higher dilution in patients with higher positivity on the SPT.

Table 54.11: Standard dosing regimen for subcutaneous immunotherapy.

Concentration	*Frequency*	*Dose*
1:5,000	Two injections in a week	0.1–0.9 mL (increments of 0.1 mL)
1:500	Two injections in a week	0.1–0.9 mL increments of 0.1 mL)
1:50	One injection in a week	0.1–0.5 mL (increments of 0.1 mL)
1:50	One injection in 2 weeks	0.6 mL
1:50	One injection in 3 weeks	0.7 mL
1:50	One injection in 4 weeks	0.8 mL
1:50	One injection in 4 weeks	0.9 mL
1:50	One injection in 4 weeks	1.0 mL

- In cases showing high skin sensitivity or AIT with single antigen showing LR/SR at initiation of AIT, higher dilution, i.e., 1:50,000 w/v, can be selected and the first injection should be given in the hospital/clinic
- Usually, the maintenance dose is between 0.5 and 1.0 mL of 1:50 dilution in different patients
- The duration is usually 3–5 years, but in India, where it is not possible to avoid the presence of antigens (mostly pollens, dust mites, and insects), the decision has to be individualized
- AIT may be postponed if the patient is symptomatic and presents with decreased lung function (i.e., <80% of the personal best value)
- Response to AIT starts slowly; however, clinical and physiological improvement has been demonstrated very shortly after the patient reaches a maintenance dose.[3] However, the time duration and efficacy are variable among individuals
- If there is no clinical improvement observed after 1 year of therapy, the possible reasons for lack of efficacy with IT should be evaluated. The following reasons may be evaluated when there is no clinical improvement: (1) Failure to remove the causative allergen exposure (e.g. animal dander), (2) exposure to high levels of allergen, (3) continued exposure to nonallergen triggers (e.g., tobacco smoke), (4) incomplete identification and treatment of clinically relevant allergens, or (5) failure to treat with adequate doses of each allergen.

If none of the above reasons are found, discontinuation of IT should be considered and other treatment options should be pursued.[3]

In case of default, up to 1 month - no change in schedule; 1-2 months - continue with last lower dose; 2-4 months - continue with last dilution, and >4 months - restart AIT. This schedule has been advised as per the current Indian practice followed for over 50 years.

- Antigen for skin testing and for AIT should be procured from the same manufacturer, to avoid difference in potency of the allergen. The difference in potency of extracts among different manufacturers has been reported world over. Standardized extracts should be used whenever available. Studies evaluating major allergens have documented their presence in standardized allergens extracts
- The allergen extracts produced for AIT can differ in composition and allergen activity in two AIT products.[5] Thus, data from one AIT product cannot be extrapolated to other products even if they contain the same allergen sources.

FUTURE OF ALLERGY DIAGNOSIS AND ALLERGEN IMMUNOTHERAPY

Over the last 20 years, a large number of new diagnostic and therapeutic concepts have emerged in the field of allergy management.

Future of Allergy Diagnosis

In in vivo tests, one of the important future implications of allergy diagnosis includes availability and use of standardized allergen extracts which can improve the utility of allergy diagnosis. Preliminary studies have also evaluated the in vivo component-resolved diagnosis and have shown a promising approach.[215] Recombinant allergens have also been used for SPT,[216] and skin tests with recombinant and natural allergens have a similar value if the recombinant allergens have been well selected and represent all or most epitopes of the natural allergen.[216,217]

Provocation tests including nasal and conjunctival have been evaluated and recommended by international organizations for the definitive diagnosis of IgE sensitization and allergies. Specific NPT consists of controlled exposure to allergens and thereby eliciting a response from the nasal mucosa in an allergic individual. It is indicated for the diagnostic confirmation of allergic rhinitis and when discrepancies arise between medical history and the results of skin tests and/or serological tests. It is also used to evaluate sensitivity to the allergen, the efficacy and safety profile of treatment, and in research on the pathophysiological mechanisms of nasal response to allergens.[218] Similarly, the conjunctival allergen provocation test reproduces the events occurring by instilling an allergen on the ocular surface. It is indicated especially when the relevance of the allergen is not obvious or in polysensitized patients suffering from IgE-mediated ocular allergy.[219]

Another area of interest is the development of molecular allergology for the diagnosis of allergic sensitizations. Development and progress made in the field of recombinant allergens have allowed for the development of a new concept in allergy diagnosis, molecular diagnosis, or component-resolved diagnosis, which makes it possible to identify potential disease-eliciting molecules. This also presents as a new challenge for health-care professionals for appropriate interpretation of test results; clinicians must know about the basics of allergen components, their clinical implications and must always keep in mind that sensitization does not necessarily imply a clinical allergy.[220,221]

The basophil-activation test (BAT) measures basophil response to allergen cross-linking IgE. The clinical impact of BAT is due to the unique ability of these cells to degranulate on cross-linking of the sIgE bound on membrane-bound high-affinity IgE receptor (FcΦ065RI) by allergen exposure. Compared with the determination of sIgE in serum, BAT reflects a functional response as basophil activation can be induced by cross-linking of FcΦ065RI, which requires more than binding of sIgE to allergen. The clinical applications of BAT range from diagnosis to monitoring the progress of AIT. It is a multifaceted and promising tool which needs to be further well established and evaluated in clinical practice.[222]

Future of Allergen Immunotherapy

Although AIT is specific, it is associated with some side effects thereby newer treatments are under research to improve IT. The future developments in AIT would include newer routes of administration including intralymphatic IT (ILIT), epicutaneous (EPIT), and intradermal AIT. In ILIT, allergen is given directly in the lymph node with the aim for higher allergen amounts in secondary organs. ILIT requires much lower doses of allergen and fewer injections than the conventional SCIT modality, while maintaining the same efficacy. EPIT has been tested with good results for both aeroallergens and food allergens. This route currently seems particularly suitable in children[78] and has a potential for self-administration, safe, and needle free. The epicutaneous tissue has a number of antigen-presenting cells and is nonvascularized.

In addition to the newer routes, newer formulations (nanoparticles) are at early experimental stage, with positive results in animal models. Addition of adjuvants to allergen extracts is an additional possibility; crude allergen extracts can be improved by adding adjuvants, which provide an additional enhancement of the TH1 response. An organic adjuvant usually stimulates the Toll-like receptors of the innate immunity, which in turn favor the TH1-oriented response.[223] Bacterial adjuvants are commercially available for SCIT globally and have lower number of injections. DNA adjuvants are under experimental investigation, with a single human trial.[78]

Peptide-based IT is another future prospect. It is possible to give only allergenic fragments, instead of the whole allergenic proteins, because antigen-presenting cells recognize linear sequences. Encouraging results from clinical trial have been observed.[78,224] The recombinant allergens have been used to improve the IT by identifying disease-causing molecules. They have also been evaluated recently in clinical studies. However, their overall efficacy has been similar to those provided by the crude extracts.[78] Further, pretreatment with anti-IgE before AIT may reduce the systemic allergic reactions in patients unable to reach the targeted maintenance dose for IT.

The future of AIT would also incorporate newer and upcoming indications–food allergy, being the predominant one. A Cochrane review of egg allergy reviewed four RCTs with a total of 167 recruited individuals (oral IT [OIT] 100; control 67 participants), all of whom were children (aged 4–15 years).[225] The evidence suggested that OIT can desensitize a large number of egg allergic patients although it remains unknown whether long-term tolerance develops. In addition, there are no standardized protocols for OIT and the "data" remains experimental. Other important food allergens for which research is still ongoing include peanut and cow's milk.[226]

Position statements

- AIT should be practiced only by allergy-trained doctors (physicians [MD], pediatricians, ENT surgeon, pulmonologists, dermatologists) and in a clinical setting where instruments and medications for the management of anaphylaxis are available
- The treatment of allergic diseases is based on patient education, allergen avoidance, pharmacotherapy, and AIT
- SPT is the gold standard for the detection of allergen sensitization
- The treating physicians should be aware of local and regional allergens prevailing in patient's environment
- AIT is indicated for the treatment of patients (≥5 years with no limit on the upper age) with allergic rhinitis/conjunctivitis, allergic asthma, and allergic reaction against insect sting/venom. AIT might have positive effects in selected sensitized patients with AD; the best evidence is available for HDM AIT
- Age <2 years is an absolute contraindication for AIT while the age of 2–5 years is a relative contraindication for AIT[8]
- AIT should be used in properly selected cases with a history of precipitation of attack after allergen exposure and positive SPT to clinically relevant allergens. The response of AIT is antigen-specific administered to the patient. Unrelated/irrelevant antigens based on skin text (sensitization) alone should not be included in allergen vaccine
- Most of the randomized controlled studies of both SCIT and SLIT are with single allergen extracts
- Mixing of allergens (after looking at homologous groups, dose, and compatibility) may be required if the patient suffers from allergic disease due to ≥2 clinically relevant allergens
- When mixing two allergens from the homologous group, the amount of the individual allergen extract should be equal or select only most important allergen based on highest skin positivity
- When mixing allergens from the nonhomologous groups, the amount of individual antigen should be decided depending on their skin test positivity. Compatibility of the allergens (cross-reactivity and enzymatic degradation) should be remembered before mixing allergens
- Do not mix allergens with high proteolytic enzyme activities (such as dust mites, fungal, and insects) with any other allergen and prescribe these preferably in separate vials
- SCIT and SLIT both have clinical efficacy proven in trials. However, SLIT is currently not approved in India
- AIT is used in combination with pharmacotherapy to control the symptoms which would decrease with the increasing efficacy of AIT
- AIT should be started at an early age as it has the potential to modify the natural course of allergic disease

- AIT can be continued in pregnancy but is usually not initiated in a pregnant woman
- Response to AIT starts slowly; however, clinical and physiological improvement has been demonstrated very shortly after the patient reaches a maintenance dose. This should be explained to the patient
- If there is no clinical improvement observed after 1 year of therapy, the possible reasons for lack of efficacy with IT should be evaluated. If no reasons are found, discontinuation of IT should be considered, and other treatment options should be pursued
- The optimal duration of AIT is still debated. According to reports, AIT can be administered for 3–5 years in patients with a good therapeutic response. However, the decision to discontinue AIT after 5 years should be based on individual patient basis
- AIT for food is in the experimental stages and should not be practiced until it has shown to have clinical efficacy and safety
- Studies suggest that VIT can be discontinued after 3–5 years in most of the patients. However, decision to discontinue VIT should be taken on the response of patient to treatment
- AIT is cost-effective based on clinical response with reduction in medicine requirements and also persistence of benefit for 5–6 years after discontinuation of IT
- Skin testing as well as AIT can give severe SR (anaphylaxis) at times. Therefore, skin testing and/or IT should be administered under the supervision of a trained physician who can recognize early symptoms and signs of anaphylaxis and administer requisite treatment in emergency unit
- Adrenaline is the drug of choice for IT-induced SRs
- Allergens for diagnosis and AIT should be preferably from the same manufacturer
- Standardized allergen extracts should be used both for allergy diagnosis and IT to obtain better response. Efforts are required to upgrade the standardization of allergen extracts so that they can be defined in BUs, for example, BAU, AUs, therapeutic unit, standardized BUs. However, in India, following parameters are mandatory for manufacturers - protein content, protein profile, and biopotency
- Allergen extracts/vaccine (diagnostic/therapeutic antigen) should be stored at 2°C–8°C and transported using cool device to maintain the allergenic potency.

Acknowledgments

We are thankful to all the core committee members, contributors for providing their valuable inputs in framing the revised guidelines, 2017.

Financial Support and Sponsorship

Nil.

Conflicts of Interest

There are no conflicts of interest.

REFERENCES

1. Burks AW, Calderon MA, Casale T, et al. Update on allergy immunotherapy: American Academy of Allergy, Asthma & Immunology/European Academy of Allergy and Clinical Immunology/PRACTALL consensus report. J Allergy Clin Immunol. 2013;131:1288-96.e3.
2. Zuberbier T, Bachert C, Bousquet PJ, et al. GA^2 LEN/EAACI pocket guide for allergen-specific immunotherapy for allergic rhinitis and asthma. Allergy. 2010;65:1525-30.
3. Cox L, Nelson H, Lockey R, et al. Allergen immunotherapy: a practice parameter third update. J Allergy Clin Immunol. 2011;127: S1-55.
4. Scadding GK, Durham SR, Mirakian R, et al. BSACI guidelines for the management of allergic and non-allergic rhinitis. Clin Exp Allergy. 2008;38:19-42.
5. Pfaar O, Bachert C, Bufe A, et al. Guideline on allergen-specific immunotherapy in IgE-mediated allergic diseases: S2k Guideline of the German Society for Allergology and Clinical Immunology (DGAKI), the Society for Pediatric Allergy and Environmental Medicine (GPA), the Medical Association of German Allergologists (AeDA), the Austrian Society for Allergy and Immunology (ÖGAI), the Swiss Society for Allergy and Immunology (SGAI), the German Society of Dermatology (DDG), the German Society of Oto- Rhino-Laryngology, Head and Neck Surgery (DGHNO-KHC), the German Society of Pediatrics and Adolescent Medicine (DGKJ), the Society for Pediatric Pneumology (GPP), the German Respiratory Society (DGP), the German Association of ENT Surgeons (BV-HNO), the Professional Federation of Paediatricians and Youth Doctors (BVKJ), the Federal Association of Pulmonologists (BDP) and the German Dermatologists Association (BVDD). Allergo J Int. 2014;23:282-319.
6. Gaur SN, Singh BP, Singh AB, et al. Guidelines for practice of allergen immunotherapy in India. Indian J Allergy Asthma Immunol. 2009;23:1-21.
7. Moingeon P, Mascarell L. Novel routes for allergen immunotherapy: safety, efficacy and mode of action. Immunotherapy. 2012;4:201-12.

8. Pitsios C, Demoly P, Bilò MB, et al. Clinical contraindications to allergen immunotherapy: an EAACI position paper. Allergy. 2015;70:897-909.
9. Singh BP, Singh AB, Gangal SV. Pollen Calendars of Different States, India. CSIR Centre for Biochemicals, Delhi, and National Botanical Research Institute, Lucknow; 1992.
10. Singh AB, Kumar P. Common environmental allergens causing respiratory allergy in India. Indian J Pediatr. 2002;69:245-50.
11. Singh AB, Kumar P. Aeroallergens in clinical practice of allergy in India: an overview. Ann Agric Environ Med. 2003;10:131-6.
12. Singh AB, Kumar P. Aerial pollen diversity in India and their clinical significance in allergic diseases. Indian J Clin Biochem. 2004;19:190-201.
13. Bist A, Kumar L, Roy I, et al. Clinico-immunologic evaluation of allergy to Himalayan tree pollen in atopic subjects in India – a new record. Asian Pac J Allergy Immunol. 2005;23:69-78.
14. Singh AB, Deval R. Aerobiology of fungi associated with allergy. In: Mould Allergy, Biology and Pathogenesis. USA: Research Signpost; 2005: 105-36.
15. Singh AB, Dahiya P. Pollen aerobiology and allergy: an integrated approach. Indian J Aerobiology. 1992;5:1-19.
16. Singh AB, Dahiya P. Allergens in India – we are different from the West. In: Sheikh W, ed. Principles and Practice of Tropical Allergy and Asthma. Mumbai: Vikash Medical Publishers; 2006: 61-92.
17. Bisht V, Kukreja N, Singh BP, et al. Current status of fungal allergens. Indian J Allergy Asthma Immunol. 2003;17:9-19.
18. Rajeshwari IR, Reddy PS, Jaju M, et al. Allergens in nasobronchial allergy as determined by skin testing. Lung India. 1985;4:167-70.
19. Goyal M, Parikh R, Goyal N. Identification of common allergens by skin prick test associated with common respiratory allergic disorders in the city of Jaipur, Rajasthan. Indian J Allergy Asthma Immunol. 2010;24:1-6.
20. Raju BV, Kotilingam K, Raghavendra Rao M, et al. Allergenic skin tests in extrinsic asthmatics in Visakhapatnam – a pilot study. Lung India. 1990;8:79-83.
21. Jerath V, Nishchal R, Sood M. Prevalance of skin reactivity to fungal antigens in patients of nasobronchial allergy of Jalandhar and neighbouring area in Punjab. Indian J Allergy Asthma Immunol. 2012;26:73-6.
22. Singh AB. Pollen and fungal aeroallergens associated with allergy and asthma in India. Glob J Immunol Allerg Dis. 2014;2:19-28.
23. Agrawal RL, Chandra A, Jain S, Agrawal G. Identification of common allergens by skin prick test associated with United airway disease in Allahabad, Uttar Pradesh, India. Indian J Allergy Asthma Immunol. 2008;22:7-13.
24. Jerath VP, Sood M, Jerath P, Jerath A. Sensitization to pollen antigens in 1420 patients of Jalandhar and neighbouring area in Punjab. Indian J Allergy Asthma Immunol. 2010;24:69-73.
25. Dave L, Srivastava N. A study of sensitisation pattern to various aero-allergens by skin prick test in patients of United airway disease (UAD) in Bhopal, Madhya Pradesh, India. Res J Pharm Biol Chem Sci. 2014;5:1397-403.
26. Kumar R, Kumar M, Sharan N, et al. Pattern of skin sensitivity to various aeroallergens in patients of bronchial asthma and/or allergic rhinitis in India. Indian J Allergy Asthma Immunol. 2012;26:66-72.
27. Wani NA, Shah ZA, Hameed M. Different types of aero-allergens causing nasobronchial allergy in District Kupwara of Jammu and Kashmir State, India. J Public Health Epidemiol. 2012;4:101-4.
28. Patel A, Choudhary S. Prevalence of allergen sensitivity in nasobronchial allergy in Gujarat, India. Natl J Med Res. 2012;2:431-4.
29. Awasthi A, Singh R. Determination of aerobiological flora associated with allergic rhinitis by skin prick test in a tertiary care hospital in the West Coast of Southern India. Clin Epidemiol Glob Health. 2014;2:143-8.
30. Moitra S, Sen S, Datta A, et al. Study of Allergenicity spectrum to aero allergens by skin prick testing. Austin J Allergy. 2014;1:1-4.
31. Donthi S, Sivasai KS, Lakshmi VV. Prevalence of inhalant allergens in nasobronchial allergy in Hyderabad region: India. E Int Sci Res J. 2011;3:192-9.
32. Singhal P, Kumar R. A study of skin sensitivity to various allergens by intradermal test in patients with respiratory allergy (bronchial asthma and allergic rhinitis) in India. Intern Med J Thai. 2003;19:202-6.
33. Mishra M, Chakarwati A, Kumar R. Skin sensitivity to aeroallergens in allergic rhinitis. Clin Rhinol. 2013; 6:64-6.
34. Rawat A, Singh A, Singh AB, et al. Clinical and immunologic evaluation of *Cedrus deodara* pollen: a new allergen from India. Allergy. 2000;55:620-6.
35. Thomas WR. Geography of house dust mite allergens. Asian Pac J Allergy Immunol. 2010;28:211-24.
36. Sharma D, Dutta BK, Singh AB. Dust mites population in indoor houses of suspected allergic patients of South Assam, India. ISRN Allergy. 2011;2011:576849.
37. Kaur N, Kaur H. A study on the occurrence, prevalence and species composition of mite fauna in human dwellings of Patiala city, Punjab (India). Indian J Sci Res. 2014; 8:91-7.
38. Tripathi DM, Parikh KM. Mite fauna and other allergens present in the house dust in Bombay. Lung India. 1983;4:147-51.
39. Kumar R, Kumari D, Srivastava P, et al. Identification of IgE-mediated food allergy and allergens in older children and adults with asthma and allergic rhinitis. Indian J Chest Dis Allied Sci. 2010;52:217-24.
40. Kumar R, Srivastava P, Kumari D, et al. Rice (*Oryza sativa*) allergy in rhinitis and asthma patients: a clinico-immunological study. Immunobiology. 2007;212:141-7.
41. Mahesh PA, Wong GW, Ogorodova L, et al. Prevalence of food sensitization and probable food allergy among adults in India: the EuroPrevall INCO study. Allergy. 2016;71:1010-9.

42. Kleine-Tebbe J, Bufe A, Ebner C, et al. Specific immunotherapy (hyposensitization) for IgE-mediated allergic diseases. Allergo J. 2009;18:509-37.
43. Dreborg S. Methods for skin testing. Allergy. 1989;44: 22-30.
44. Shankar J, Singh BP, Gaur SN, Arora N. Recombinant glutathione-S-transferase a major allergen from *Alternaria alternata* for clinical use in allergy patients. Mol Immunol. 2006;43:1927-32.
45. Kumar R, Singh BP, Srivastava P, et al. Relevance of serum IgE estimation in allergic bronchial asthma with special reference to food allergy. Asian Pac J Allergy Immunol. 2006;24:191-9.
46. Agarwal MK, Jhamb S. Immunodiagnosis of type I respiratory allergic disorders. Cardiothorac J. 1995;1:36.
47. Demoly P, Piette V, Bousquet J. In vivo methods for study of allergy. In: Adkinson NF Jr, Yunginger JW, Busse WW, Bochner BS, Holgate ST, Simons FER, eds. Middleton's Allergy Principles and Practice. Philadelphia, USA: Mosby Inc.; 2006:631-43.
48. Agarwal MK. Skin testing and respiratory allergic disorders. Indian J Chest Dis Allied Sci. 1986;28:179-82.
49. Fish JE, Peters SP. Bronchial challenge testing. In: Adkinson NF Jr, Yunginger JW, Busse WW, Bochner BS, Holgate ST, Simons FER, eds. Middleton's Allergy Principles and Practice. Philadelphia, USA: Mosby Inc.; 2006:657-70.
50. Rajakulasingam K. Nasal provocation testing. In: Adkinson NF Jr, Yunginger JW, Busse WW, Bochner BS, Holgate ST, Simons FER, eds. Middleton's Allergy Principles and Practice. Philadelphia, USA: Mosby Inc.; 2006:644-55.
51. Kumari D, Kumar R, Sridhara S, et al. Sensitization to blackgram in patients with bronchial asthma and rhinitis: Clinical evaluation and characterization of allergens. Allergy. 2006;61:104-10.
52. Hamilton RG. Laboratory tests for allergic and immunodeficiency diseases. In: Adkinson NF Jr, Yunginger JW, Busse WW, Bochner BS, Holgate ST, Simons FER, eds. Middleton's Allergy Principles and Practice. Philadelphia, USA: Mosby Inc.; 2006:611-30.
53. Kausar MA, Vijayan VK, Bansal SK, et al. Mosquitoes as sources of inhalant allergens: Clinicoimmunologic and biochemical studies. J Allergy Clin Immunol. 2007;120: 1219-21.
54. Pawankar R, Canonica G, Holgate S, Lockey R. WAO White Book on Allergy 2011-2012. United States of America: World Allergy Organization; 2012.
55. Berg TL, Johansson SG. Allergy diagnosis with the radioallergosorbent test: A comparison with the results of skin and provocation tests in an unselected group of children with asthma and hay fever. J Allergy Clin Immunol. 1974;54:209-21.
56. van der Zee JS, de Groot H, van Swieten P, et al. Discrepancies between the skin test and IgE antibody assays: Study of histamine release, complement activation in vitro, and occurrence of allergen-specific IgG. J Allergy Clin Immunol. 1988;82:270-81.
57. Wood RA, Phipatanakul W, Hamilton RG, Eggleston PA. A comparison of skin prick tests, intradermal skin tests, and RASTs in the diagnosis of cat allergy. J Allergy Clin Immunol. 1999;103:773-9.
58. Bernstein DI, Biagini RE, Karnani R, et al. In vivo sensitization to purified Hevea brasiliensis proteins in health care workers sensitized to natural rubber latex. J Allergy Clin Immunol. 2003;111:610-6.
59. Koskela H, Taivainen A, Tukiainen H, Chan HK. Inhalation challenge with bovine dander allergens: Who needs it? Chest. 2003;124:383-91.
60. Sharma HP, Wood RA, Bravo AR, Matsui EC. A comparison of skin prick tests, intradermal skin tests, and specific IgE in the diagnosis of mouse allergy. J Allergy Clin Immunol. 2008;121:933-9.
61. American Academy of Allergy, Asthma and Immunology (AAAAI). J Allergy Clin Immunol. 1997;99:583-6.
62. Heinzerling L, Mari A, Bergmann KC, et al. The skin prick test - European standards. Clin Transl Allergy. 2013;3:3.
63. Bernstein IL, Li JT, Bernstein DI, et al. Allergy diagnostic testing: an updated practice parameter. Ann Allergy Asthma Immunol. 2008;100 3 Suppl 3:S1-148.
64. American Academy of Otolaryngic Allergy (AAOA). Clinical Care Statement: Medicines to Avoid Before Allergy Skin Testing; January, 2015. http://www.aaoaf.org/PDF/Clinical%20Statements/2015%20Clinical%20Care%20Statements%20Medicines%20to%20Avoid%20Before%20Allergy%20Skin%20Testing.pdf. Last accessed on July 5, 2016.
65. Fatteh S, Rekkerth DJ, Hadley JA. Skin prick/puncture testing in North America: a call for standards and consistency. Allergy Asthma Clin Immunol. 2014;10:44.
66. Shivpuri DN, Agarwal MK. Studies on the allergenic fungal spores of the Delhi, India, Metropolitan area. Clinical aspects. J Allergy. 1969;44:204-13.
67. Sharma S, Kathuria PC, Gupta CK, et al. Total serum immunoglobulin E levels in a case-control study in asthmatic/allergic patients, their family members, and healthy subjects from India. Clin Exp Allergy. 2006;36:1019-27.
68. Grammer LC, Shaughnessy MA, Patterson R. Modified forms of allergen immunotherapy. J Allergy Clin Immunol. 1985;76:397-401.
69. Brehler R, Kahlert H, Thum-Oltmer S. Hypoallergenic preparations in SCIT. Allergo J. 2010;19:477-84.
70. Calderon M. Presentation on: European Survey on Adverse Systemic Reactions in Allergen Immunotherapy (EASSI). At: Annual Congress of the European Academy of Allergy and Clinical Immunology, June 6-10, 2015, Barcelona, Spain.
71. Cox L. Accelerated immunotherapy schedules: review of efficacy and safety. Ann Allergy Asthma Immunol. 2006;97:126-37.
72. Durham SR. Immunotherapy Mechanism, Planary Immunotherapy: is it a Shot in the Dark, or Just a Drop, Do We Know When to Start and When to Stop? American College of Allergy, Asthma and Immunology 2006, Annual Meeting November 6-15, 2006, Philadelphia, USA.
73. Brown JL, Frew AJ. The efficacy of oromucosal immunotherapy in respiratory allergy. Clin Exp Allergy. 2001;31:8-10.

74. Malling HJ. Is sublingual immunotherapy clinically effective? Curr Opin Allergy Clin Immunol. 2002;2:523-31.
75. Nelson HS. Advances in upper airway diseases and allergen immunotherapy. J Allergy Clin Immunol. 2003;111:S793-8.
76. Khinchi MS, Poulsen LK, Carat F, et al. Clinical efficacy of sublingual and subcutaneous birch pollen allergen-specific immunotherapy: a randomized, placebo-controlled, double-blind, double-dummy study. Allergy. 2004;59:45-53.
77. Demoly P, Passalacqua G, Calderon MA, Yalaoui T. Choosing the optimal dose in sublingual immunotherapy: rationale for the 300 index of reactivity dose. Clin Transl Allergy. 2015;5:44.
78. Passalacqua G, Canonica GW. Allergen Immunotherapy: history and Future Developments. Immunol Allergy Clin North Am. 2016;36:1-12.
79. Crimi E, Voltolini S, Troise C, et al. Local immunotherapy with *Dermatophagoides* extract in asthma. J Allergy Clin Immunol. 1991;87:721-8.
80. Tari MG, Mancino M, Monti G. Immunotherapy by inhalation of allergen in powder in house dust allergic asthma - a double-blind study. J Investig Allergol Clin Immunol. 1992;2:59-67.
81. Bousquet J, Lockey R, Malling HJ. Allergen immunotherapy: therapeutic vaccines for allergic diseases. A WHO position paper. J Allergy Clin Immunol. 1998;102:558-62.
82. Möller C, Dreborg S, Lanner A, Björkstén B. Oral immunotherapy of children with rhinoconjunctivitis due to birch pollen allergy: a double blind study. Allergy. 1986;41:271-9.
83. Giovane AL, Bardare M, Passalacqua G, et al. A three-year double-blind placebo-controlled study with specific oral immunotherapy to *Dermatophagoides*: evidence of safety and efficacy in paediatric patients. Clin Exp Allergy. 1994;24:53-9.
84. Cooper PJ, Darbyshire J, Nunn AJ, Warner JO. A controlled trial of oral hyposensitization in pollen asthma and rhinitis in children. Clin Allergy. 1984;14:541-50.
85. Oppenheimer J, Areson JG, Nelson HS. Safety and efficacy of oral immunotherapy with standardized cat extract. J Allergy Clin Immunol. 1994;93:61-7.
86. Mosbech H, Dreborg S, Madsen F, et al. High dose grass pollen tablets used for hyposensitization in hay fever patients. A one-year double blind placebo-controlled study. Allergy. 1987;42:451-5.
87. Nowak-Wegrzyn A, Albin S. Oral immunotherapy for food allergy: mechanisms and role in management. Clin Exp Allergy. 2015;45:368-83.
88. Canonica GW, Passalacqua G. Noninjection routes for immunotherapy. J Allergy Clin Immunol. 2003;111:437-48.
89. Nickelsen JA, Goldstein S, Mueller U, et al. Local intranasal immunotherapy for ragweed allergic rhinitis. I. Clinical response. J Allergy Clin Immunol. 1981;68:33-40.
90. Welsh PW, Butterfield JH, Yunginger JW, et al. Allergen-controlled study of intranasal immunotherapy for ragweed hay fever. J Allergy Clin Immunol. 1983;71:454-60.
91. Passalacqua G, Albano M, Pronzato C, et al. Long-term follow-up of nasal immunotherapy to *Parietaria*: Clinical and local immunological effects. Clin Exp Allergy. 1997;27:904-8.
92. Durham SR, Walker SM, Varga EM, et al. Long-term clinical efficacy of grass-pollen immunotherapy. N Engl J Med. 1999;341:468-75.
93. Des Roches A, Paradis L, Knani J, et al. Immunotherapy with a standardized *Dermatophagoides pteronyssinus* extract. V. Duration of the efficacy of immunotherapy after its cessation. Allergy. 1996;51:430-3.
94. Van Bever HP, Stevens WJ. Evolution of the late asthmatic reaction during immunotherapy and after stopping immunotherapy. J Allergy Clin Immunol. 1990;86:141-6.
95. Malling HJ. Immunotherapy as an effective tool in allergy treatment. Allergy. 1998;53:461-72.
96. Bousquet J, Van Cauwenberge P, Khaltaev N; Aria Workshop Group; World Health Organization. Allergic rhinitis and its impact on asthma. J Allergy Clin Immunol. 2001;108: S147-334.
97. Malling HJ, Weeke B. EAACI Immunotherapy position paper. Allergy. 1993;48:9-35.
98. Varney VA, Gaga M, Frew AJ, et al. Usefulness of immunotherapy in patients with severe summer hay fever uncontrolled by antiallergic drugs. BMJ. 1991;302:265-9.
99. Bousquet J, Lockey R, Malling HJ. Allergen immunotherapy: therapeutic vaccines for allergic diseases. A WHO position paper. J Allergy Clin Immunol. 1998;102(4 Pt 1):558-62.
100. Till SJ, Francis JN, Nouri-Aria K, Durham SR. Mechanisms of immunotherapy. J Allergy Clin Immunol. 2004;113: 1025-34.
101. Seidman MD, Gurgel RK, Lin SY, et al. Clinical practice guideline: allergic rhinitis. Otolaryngol Head Neck Surg. 2015;152: S1-43.
102. Joint Task Force on Practice Parameters. Allergen immunotherapy: a practice parameter. American Academy of Allergy, Asthma and Immunology. American College of Allergy, Asthma and Immunology. Ann Allergy Asthma Immunol. 2003;90:1-40.
103. Alvarez-Cuesta E, Bousquet J, Canonica GW, et al. Standards for practical allergen-specific immunotherapy. Allergy. 2006;61 Suppl 82:1-20.
104. Ross RN, Nelson HS, Finegold I. Effectiveness of specific immunotherapy in the treatment of allergic rhinitis: an analysis of randomized, prospective, single- or double-blind, placebo-controlled studies. Clin Ther. 2000; 22:342-50.
105. Eng PA, Borer-Reinhold M, Heijnen IA, Gnehm HP. Twelve-year follow-up after discontinuation of preseasonal grass pollen immunotherapy in childhood. Allergy. 2006;61: 198-201.
106. Calderon MA, Alves B, Jacobson M, et al. Allergen injection immunotherapy for seasonal allergic rhinitis. Cochrane Database Syst Rev. 2007; (1):CD001936.
107. Calderon MA, Alves B, Jacobson M, et al. Cochrane review: allergen injection immunotherapy for seasonal allergic rhinitis. Evid Based Child Health. 2010;5:1279-379.
108. Dretzke J, Meadows A, Novielli N, et al.. Subcutaneous and sublingual immunotherapy for seasonal allergic rhinitis: a

systematic review and indirect comparison. J Allergy Clin Immunol. 2013;131:1361-6.

109. Stokes JR, Casale TB. Allergy immunotherapy for primary care physicians. Am J Med. 2006;119:820-3.
110. Varney VA, Edwards J, Tabbah K, et al. Clinical efficacy of specific immunotherapy to cat dander: a double-blind placebo-controlled trial. Clin Exp Allergy. 1997;27:860-7.
111. Abramson MJ, Puy RM, Weiner JM. Allergen immunotherapy for asthma. Cochrane Database Syst Rev. 2003;(4):CD001186.
112. Jacobsen L, Nuchel Petersen B, Wihl JA, et al. Immunotherapy with partially purified and standardized tree pollen extracts. IV. Results from long-term (6-year) follow-up. Allergy. 1997;52:914-20.
113. Marogna M, Bruno M, Massolo A, Falagiani P. Long-lasting effects of sublingual immunotherapy for house dust mites in allergic rhinitis with bronchial hyperreactivity: a long-term (13-year) retrospective study in real life. Int Arch Allergy Immunol. 2007;142:70-8.
114. Johnstone DE, Dutton A. The value of hyposensitization therapy for bronchial asthma in children - a 14-year study. Pediatrics. 1968;42:793-802.
115. Jacobsen L. Preventive aspects of immunotherapy: prevention for children at risk of developing asthma. Ann Allergy Asthma Immunol. 2001;87 1 Suppl 1:43-6.
116. Niggemann B, Jacobsen L, Dreborg S, et al. Five-year follow-up on the PAT study: specific immunotherapy and long-term prevention of asthma in children. Allergy. 2006;61:855-9.
117. Des Roches A, Paradis L, Ménardo JL, et al. Immunotherapy with a standardized *Dermatophagoides pteronyssinus* product. VI. Specific immunotherapy prevents the onset of new sensitizations in children. J Allergy Clin Immunol. 1997;99:450-3.
118. Purello-D'Ambrosio F, Gangemi S, Merendino RA, et al. Prevention of new sensitizations in monosensitized subjects submitted to specific immunotherapy or not. A retrospective study. Clin Exp Allergy. 2001;31:1295-302.
119. Pajno GB, Barberio G, De Luca F, et al. Prevention of new sensitizations in asthmatic children monosensitized to house dust mite by specific immunotherapy. A six-year follow-up study. Clin Exp Allergy. 2001;31:1392-7.
120. Abramson MJ, Puy RM, Weiner JM. Injection allergen immunotherapy for asthma. Cochrane Database Syst Rev. 2010;(8):CD001186.
121. Lu Y, Xu L, Xia M, et al. The efficacy and safety of subcutaneous immunotherapy in mite-sensitized subjects with asthma: a meta-analysis. Respir Care. 2015;60:269-78.
122. Zielen S, Kardos P, Madonini E. Steroid-sparing effects with allergen-specific immunotherapy in children with asthma: a randomized controlled trial. J Allergy Clin Immunol. 2010;126:942-9.
123. Lin SY, Erekosima N, Suarez-Cuervo C, et al. Allergen-Specific Immunotherapy for the Treatment of Allergic Rhinoconjunctivitis and/or Asthma: Comparative Effectiveness Review. Comparative Effectiveness Review No. 111. (Prepared by the Johns Hopkins University Evidence-based Practice Center under Contract No. 290-2007-10061-I.) AHRQ Publication No. 13-EHC061-EF. Rockville, MD: Agency for Healthcare Research and Quality; March, 2013. http://www.effectivehealthcare.ahrq.gov/reports/final.cfm. Last accessed on December 10, 2016.
124. Bussmann C, Maintz L, Hart J, et al. Clinical improvement and immunological changes in atopic dermatitis patients undergoing subcutaneous immunotherapy with a house dust mite allergoid: a pilot study. Clin Exp Allergy. 2007;37:1277-85.
125. Werfel T, Breuer K, Ruéff F, et al. Usefulness of specific immunotherapy in patients with atopic dermatitis and allergic sensitization to house dust mites: a multi-centre, randomized, dose-response study. Allergy. 2006;61:202-5.
126. Glover MT, Atherton DJ. A double-blind controlled trial of hyposensitization to *Dermatophagoides pteronyssinus* in children with atopic eczema. Clin Exp Allergy. 1992; 22:440-6.
127. Novak N, Bieber T, Hoffmann M, et al. Efficacy and safety of subcutaneous allergen-specific immunotherapy with depigmented polymerized mite extract in atopic dermatitis. J Allergy Clin Immunol. 2012;130:925-31.e4.
128. Srivastava D, Singh BP, Sudha VT, et al. Immunotherapy with mosquito (*Culex quinquefasciatus*) extract: a double-blind, placebo-controlled study. Ann Allergy Asthma Immunol. 2007;99:273-80.
129. Shaikh WA. Immunotherapy vs inhaled budesonide in bronchial asthma: an open, parallel, comparative trial. Clin Exp Allergy. 1997;27:1279-84.
130. Möller C, Dreborg S, Ferdousi HA, et al. Pollen immunotherapy reduces the development of asthma in children with seasonal rhinoconjunctivitis (the PAT-study). J Allergy Clin Immunol. 2002;109:251-6.
131. Dahl R, Stender A, Rak S. Specific immunotherapy with SQ standardized grass allergen tablets in asthmatics with rhinoconjunctivitis. Allergy. 2006;61:185-90.
132. Dahl R, Kapp A, Colombo G, et al. Efficacy and safety of sublingual immunotherapy with grass allergen tablets for seasonal allergic rhinoconjunctivitis. J Allergy Clin Immunol. 2006;118:434-40.
133. Didier A, Malling HJ, Worm M, et al. Optimal dose, efficacy, and safety of once-daily sublingual immunotherapy with a 5-grass pollen tablet for seasonal allergic rhinitis. J Allergy Clin Immunol. 2007;120:1338-45.
134. Worm M. Efficacy and tolerability of high dose sublingual immunotherapy in patients with rhinoconjunctivitis. Eur Ann Allergy Clin Immunol. 2006;38:355-60.
135. Durham SR, Yang WH, Pedersen MR, et al. Sublingual immunotherapy with once-daily grass allergen tablets: a randomized controlled trial in seasonal allergic rhinoconjunctivitis. J Allergy Clin Immunol. 2006;117: 802-9.
136. Worm M, Rak S, de Blay F, et al. Sustained efficacy and safety of a 300IR daily dose of a sublingual solution of birch pollen allergen extract in adults with allergic rhinoconjunctivitis: results of a double-blind, placebo-controlled study. Clin Transl Allergy. 2014;4:7.

137. Bergmann KC, Demoly P, Worm M, et al. Efficacy and safety of sublingual tablets of house dust mite allergen extracts in adults with allergic rhinitis. J Allergy Clin Immunol. 2014;133:1608-14.e6.
138. Bufe A, Eberle P, Franke-Beckmann E, et al. Safety and efficacy in children of an SQ-standardized grass allergen tablet for sublingual immunotherapy. J Allergy Clin Immunol. 2009;123:167-73.e7.
139. Wahn U, Tabar A, Kuna P, et al. Efficacy and safety of 5-grass-pollen sublingual immunotherapy tablets in pediatric allergic rhinoconjunctivitis. J Allergy Clin Immunol. 2009;123:160-6.e3.
140. Wahn U, Klimek L, Ploszczuk A, et al. High-dose sublingual immunotherapy with single-dose aqueous grass pollen extract in children is effective and safe: a double-blind, placebo-controlled study. J Allergy Clin Immunol. 2012;130:886-93.e5.
141. Marogna M, Spadolini I, Massolo A, et al. Randomized controlled open study of sublingual immunotherapy for respiratory allergy in real-life: clinical efficacy and more. Allergy. 2004;59:1205-10.
142. Scheinmann P, Ponvert C, Rufin P, de Blic J. Immunotherapy in young children. In: Lockey RF, Bukantz SC, Bousquet J, editors. Allergens and Allergen Immunotherapy. New York: Marcel Dekker; 2004:567-83.
143. Wilson DR, Lima MT, Durham SR. Sublingual immunotherapy for allergic rhinitis: systematic review and meta-analysis. Allergy. 2005;60:4-12.
144. André C, Perrin-Fayolle M, Grosclaude M, et al. A double-blind placebo-controlled evaluation of sublingual immunotherapy with a standardized ragweed product in patients with seasonal rhinitis. Evidence for a dose-response relationship. Int Arch Allergy Immunol. 2003;131:111-8.
145. Radulovic S, Calderon MA, Wilson D, Durham S. Sublingual immunotherapy for allergic rhinitis. Cochrane Database Syst Rev. 2010;(12):CD002893.
146. Di Bona D, Plaia A, Leto-Barone MS, et al. Efficacy of grass pollen allergen sublingual immunotherapy tablets for seasonal allergic rhinoconjunctivitis: a systematic review and meta-analysis. JAMA Intern Med. 2015;175:1301-9.
147. Calamita Z, Saconato H, Pelá AB, Atallah AN. Efficacy of sublingual immunotherapy in asthma: systematic review of randomized-clinical trials using the Cochrane Collaboration method. Allergy. 2006;61:1162-72.
148. Bousquet J, Scheinmann P, Guinnepain MT, et al. Sublingual-swallow immunotherapy (SLIT) in patients with asthma due to house-dust mites: A double-blind, placebo-controlled study. Allergy. 1999;54:249-60.
149. Pajno GB, Morabito L, Barberio G, Parmiani S. Clinical and immunologic effects of long-term sublingual immunotherapy in asthmatic children sensitized to mites: a double-blind, placebo-controlled study. Allergy. 2000;55:842-9.
150. Hirsch T, Sähn M, Leupold W. Double-blind placebo-controlled study of sublingual immunotherapy with house dust mite extract (D.pt.) in children. Pediatr Allergy Immunol. 1997;8:21-7.
151. Bahçeciler NN, Isik U, Barlan IB, Basaran MM. Efficacy of sublingual immunotherapy in children with asthma and rhinitis: a double-blind, placebo-controlled study. Pediatr Pulmonol. 2001;32:49-55.
152. Mosbech H, Deckelmann R, de Blay F, et al. Standardized quality (SQ) house dust mite sublingual immunotherapy tablet (ALK) reduces inhaled corticosteroid use while maintaining asthma control: a randomized, double-blind, placebo-controlled trial. J Allergy Clin Immunol. 2014;134:568-75.e7.
153. Liao W, Hu Q, Shen LL, et al. Sublingual Immunotherapy for asthmatic children sensitized to house dust mite: a meta-analysis. Medicine (Baltimore) 2015;94:e701.
154. Marogna M, Tomassetti D, Bernasconi A, et al. Preventive effects of sublingual immunotherapy in childhood: an open randomized controlled study. Ann Allergy Asthma Immunol. 2008;101:206-11.
155. Novembre E, Galli E, Landi F, et al. Coseasonal sublingual immunotherapy reduces the development of asthma in children with allergic rhinoconjunctivitis. J Allergy Clin Immunol. 2004;114:851-7.
156. Di Rienzo V, Marcucci F, Puccinelli P, et al. Long-lasting effect of sublingual immunotherapy in children with asthma due to house dust mite: a 10-year prospective study. Clin Exp Allergy. 2003;33:206-10.
157. Marogna M, Spadolini I, Massolo A, et al. Long-lasting effects of sublingual immunotherapy according to its duration: a 15-year prospective study. J Allergy Clin Immunol. 2010;126:969-75.
158. Calderón MA, Carr VA, Jacobson M, et al. Allergen injection immunotherapy for perennial allergic rhinitis. Cochrane Database Syst Rev. 2008;2:CD007163.
159. Li JT, Bernstein DI, Calderon MA, et al. Sublingual grass and ragweed immunotherapy: Clinical considerations-a PRACTALL consensus report. J Allergy Clin Immunol. 2016;137:369-76.
160. Hunt KJ, Valentine MD, Sobotka AK, et al. A controlled trial of immunotherapy in insect hypersensitivity. N Engl J Med 1978 27;299:157-61.
161. Müller U, Thurnheer U, Patrizzi R, et al. Immunotherapy in bee sting hypersensitivity: bee venom versus whole body product. Allergy. 1979;34:369-78.
162. Brown SG, Wiese MD, Blackman KE, Heddle RJ. Ant venom immunotherapy: a double-blind, placebo-controlled, crossover trial. Lancet. 2003;361:1001-6.
163. Ruëff F, Przybilla B, Müller U, Mosbech H. The sting challenge test in Hymenoptera venom allergy. Position paper of the Subcommittee on Insect Venom Allergy of the European Academy of Allergology and Clinical Immunology. Allergy. 1996;51:216-25.
164. Krishna MT, Ewan PW, Diwakar L, et al. Diagnosis and management of hymenoptera venom allergy: British Society for Allergy and Clinical Immunology (BSACI) guidelines. Clin Exp Allergy. 2011;41:1201-20.
165. Müller U, Helbling A, Berchtold E. Immunotherapy with honeybee venom and yellow jacket venom is different regarding efficacy and safety. J Allergy Clin Immunol. 1992;89:529-35.

166. Mosbech H, Müller U. Side-effects of insect venom immunotherapy: results from an EAACI multicenter study. European Academy of Allergology and Clinical Immunology. Allergy. 2000;55:1005-10.
167. Gaur SN, Gupta S. Clinical response of immunotherapy in cases of nasobronchial allergy. Indian J Allergy Asthma Immunol. 1996;10:65-8.
168. Karmakar PR, Das A, Chatterjee BP. Placebo-controlled immunotherapy with *Cocos nucifera* pollen extract. Int Arch Allergy Immunol. 1994;103:194-201.
169. Srivastava D, Singh BP, Arora N, Gaur SN. Clinico-immunologic study on immunotherapy with mixed and single insect allergens. J Clin Immunol. 2009;29:665-73.
170. Kumar R, Gupta N, Bisht I. Inflammatory response to subcutaneous allergen-specific immunotherapy in patients with bronchial asthma and allergic rhinitis. Indian J Allergy Asthma Immunol. 2015;29:7-13.
171. Shaikh WA. Long-term efficacy of house dust mite immunotherapy in bronchial asthma: a 15-year follow-up study. Allergol Int. 2005;54:443-9.
172. Kathuria PC, Kathuria N. Nine Yrs Follow-up in 35 Patients of Persistent Allergic Rhinitis & intermittent Br. Asthma after discontinuation of H.D. Mites (*D. farinae/D. pteronyssinus*) Immunotherapy (SCIT). Abstr Presentation ICAAICON; 2013.
173. Gaur SN, Bhati G. Successful allergen immunotherapy with horse dander allergy. Indian J Allergy Asthma Immunol. 2014;28:47-8.
174. Parasuramalu BG, Gangaboraiah, Balaji R, Someswara GM. Assessment of quality of life among patients with respiratory allergy, receiving sublingual and subcutaneous immunotherapy. Indian J Allergy Asthma Immunol. 2011;25:21-7.
175. Prakash OM, Murthy KR. Immunotherapy in allergic conjunctivitis. Indian J Ophthalmol. 1992;40:9-10.
176. Kathuria PC. Safety of Accelerated Schedules of Cluster Allergen Immunotherapy with House Dust Mites in Sixty Five Patients with Perennial BR. Asthma. Poster (2083) Presented at 2012 WAO International Scientific Conference; 2012.
177. Susmita J, Vijayalakshmi V, Suman Latha G, Murthy KJ. Combination of allergens in specific immunotherapy for IgE mediated allergies. Lung India. 2007;24:3-5.
178. Srivastava D, Gaur SN, Arora N, Singh BP. Clinico-immunological changes post-immunotherapy with *Periplaneta americana*. Eur J Clin Invest. 2011;41:879-88.
179. Shaikh WA, Shaikh SW. A prospective study on the safety of sublingual immunotherapy in pregnancy. Allergy. 2012;67:741-3.
180. Shaikh WA. A retrospective study on the safety of immunotherapy in pregnancy. Clin Exp Allergy. 1993; 23:857-60.
181. Cox LS, Larenas Linnemann D, Nolte H, et al. Sublingual immunotherapy: a comprehensive review. J Allergy Clin Immunol. 2006;117:1021-35.
182. Coop CA, Tankersley MS. Patient perceptions regarding local reactions from allergen immunotherapy injections. Ann Allergy Asthma Immunol. 2008;101:96-100.
183. Kelso JM. The rate of systemic reactions to immunotherapy injections is the same whether or not the dose is reduced after a local reaction. Ann Allergy Asthma Immunol. 2004;92:225-7.
184. Tankersley MS, Butler KK, Butler WK, Goetz DW. Local reactions during allergen immunotherapy do not require dose adjustment. J Allergy Clin Immunol. 2000;106:840-3.
185. Roy SR, Sigmon JR, Olivier J, et al. Increased frequency of large local reactions among systemic reactors during subcutaneous allergen immunotherapy. Ann Allergy Asthma Immunol. 2007;99:82-6.
186. Bousquet J, Hejjaoui A, Dhivert H, et al. Immunotherapy with a standardized *Dermatophagoides pteronyssinus* product. III. Systemic reactions during the rush protocol in patients suffering from asthma. J Allergy Clin Immunol. 1989;83:797-802.
187. Jutel M, Agache I, Bonini S, et al. International consensus on allergy immunotherapy. J Allergy Clin Immunol. 2015;136:556-68.
188. Tabar AI, Garcia BE, Rodriguez A, et al. A prospective safety-monitoring study of immunotherapy with biologically standardized products. Allergy. 1993;48: 450-3.
189. Wells JH. Systemic reactions to immunotherapy: comparisons between two large allergy practices. J Allergy Clin Immunol. 1996;97:1030-2.
190. Cox L, Larenas-Linnemann D, Lockey RF, Passalacqua G. Speaking the same language: The World Allergy Organization Subcutaneous Immunotherapy Systemic Reaction Grading System. J Allergy Clin Immunol. 2010;125:569-74.
191. Epstein TG, Liss GM, Murphy-Berendts K, Bernstein DI. AAAAI/ACAAI surveillance study of subcutaneous immunotherapy, years 2008-2012: An update on fatal and nonfatal systemic allergic reactions. J Allergy Clin Immunol Pract. 2014;2:161-7.
192. Grosclaude M, Bouillot P, Alt R, et al. Safety of various dosage regimens during induction of sublingual immunotherapy. A preliminary study. Int Arch Allergy Immunol. 2002;129:248-53.
193. Lombardi C, Gargioni S, Melchiorre A, et al. Safety of sublingual immunotherapy with monomeric allergoid in adults: multicenter post-marketing surveillance study. Allergy. 2001;56:989-92.
194. Calderón MA, Simons FE, Malling HJ, et al. Sublingual allergen immunotherapy: mode of action anditsrelationship with the safety profile. Allergy. 2012;67:302-11.
195. Adkinson NF Jr., Eggleston PA, Eney D, et al. A controlled trial of immunotherapy for asthma in allergic children. N Engl J Med. 1997;336:324-31.
196. Malling HJ. Minimising the risks of allergen-specific injection immunotherapy. Drug Saf. 2000;23:323-32.

197. Javeed N, Javeed H, Javeed S, et al. Refractory anaphylactoid shock potentiated by beta-blockers. Cathet Cardiovasc Diagn. 1996;39:383-4.
198. Ciprandi G, Buscaglia S, Pesce G, et al. Minimal persistent inflammation is present at mucosal level in patients with asymptomatic rhinitis and mite allergy. J Allergy Clin Immunol. 1995;96:971-9.
199. Nielsen L, Johnsen ER, Mosbech H, et al. Antihistamine premedication in specific cluster immunotherapy: a double-blind, placebo-controlled study. J Allergy Clin Immunol. 1996;97:1207-13.
200. Demoly P, Passalacqua G, Pfaar O, et al. Management of the polyallergic patient with allergy immunotherapy: a practice-based approach. Allergy Asthma Clin Immunol. 2016;12:2.
201. Lorenz AR, Lüttkopf D, May S, et al. The principle of homologous groups in regulatory affairs of allergen products - a proposal. Int Arch Allergy Immunol. 2009;148:1-17.
202. Müller U, Hari Y, Berchtold E. Premedication with antihistamines may enhance efficacy of specific-allergen immunotherapy. J Allergy Clin Immunol. 2001;107:81-6.
203. Delacourt C, Benoist MR, Waernessyckle S, et al. Relationship between bronchial responsiveness and clinical evolution in infants who wheeze: a four-year prospective study. Am J Respir Crit Care Med. 2001;164(8 Pt 1): 1382-6.
204. Singh AB, Malik P, Parkash D, Gupta CK. Biological standardization of pollen allergens from India. Asian Pac J Allergy Immunol. 1992;10:103-9.
205. Singh BP, Verma J, Arora N, Sridhara S. Status of Allergen Standardization in India. Arbeiten aus dem Paul Ehrlich Institute Band 93, 9th International Paul-Ehrlich-Seminar (1999), GIT Verlag, Dermstadt, FRG; 2000: 41-5.
206. Singh BP, Gangal SV. Defined allergen extracts; need for efficient diagnosis of allergy and immunotherapy. Indian J Allergy Appl Immunol. 2001;15:67-72.
207. Gupta R, Singh BP, Sridhara S, et al. Allergen of *Curvularia lunata* during cultivation in different media. J Allergy Clin Immunol. 1999;104:857-62.
208. Thangam Sudha V, Arora N, Sridhara S, et al. Biopotency and identification of allergenic proteins in *Periplaneta americana* extract for clinical applications. Biologicals. 2007;35:131-7.
209. Bijli KM, Singh BP, Sridhara S, et al. Effect of various stabilizing agents on *Imperata cylindrica* grass pollen allergen extract. Clin Exp Allergy. 2003;33:65-71.
210. Singh BP, Kukreja N, Arora N. Clinically relevant allergens from fungi imperfecti and yeast. In: Kurup VP, editor. Mold Allergy, Biology and Pathogenesis. Trivandrum, India: Research Signpost; 2005:77-92.
211. Singh BP, Sridhara S, Arora N, Gangal SV. Evaluation of protein assay methods for pollen and fungal spore extracts. Biochem Int. 1992;27:477-84.
212. Sudha VT, Srivastava D, Arora N, et al. Stability of protease-rich *Periplaneta americana* allergen extract during storage: Formulating preservatives to enhance shelf life. J Clin Immunol. 2007;27:294-301.
213. Nelson HS. Multiallergen immunotherapy for allergic rhinitis and asthma. J Allergy Clin Immunol. 2009;123: 763-9.
214. Shivpuri DN. Treatment of naso-bronchial allergy. Indian Pract. 1976;29:407-32.
215. Asero R, Jimeno L, Barber D. Preliminary results of a skin prick test-based study of the prevalence and clinical impact of hypersensitivity to pollen panallergens (polcalcin and profilin). J Investig Allergol Clin Immunol. 2010;20:35-8.
216. Bousquet J, Heinzerling L, Bachert C, et al. Practical guide to skin prick tests in allergy to aeroallergens. Allergy. 2012;67:18-24.
217. Barbosa MC, Santos AB, Ferriani VP, et al. Efficacy of recombinant allergens for diagnosis of cockroach allergy in patients with asthma and/or rhinitis. Int Arch Allergy Immunol. 2013;161:213-9.
218. Dordal MT, Lluch-Bernal M, Sánchez MC, et al. Allergen-specific nasal provocation testing: Review by the rhinoconjunctivitis committee of the Spanish Society of Allergy and Clinical Immunology. J Investig Allergol Clin Immunol. 2011;21:1-12.
219. Fauquert JL, Jedrzejczak-Czechowicz M, Rondon C, et al. Conjunctival allergen provocation test: guidelines for daily practice. Allergy. 2017;72:43-54.
220. Riccio AM, De Ferrari L, Chiappori A, et al. Molecular diagnosis and precision medicine in allergy management. Clin Chem Lab Med. 2016;54:1705-14.
221. Sastre J. Molecular diagnosis in allergy. Clin Exp Allergy. 2010;40:1442-60.
222. Hoffmann HJ, Santos AF, Mayorga C, et al. The clinical utility of basophil activation testing in diagnosis and monitoring of allergic disease. Allergy. 2015;70:1393-405.
223. Pfaar O, Cazan D, Klimek L, et al. Adjuvants for immunotherapy. Curr Opin Allergy Clin Immunol. 2012;12:648-57.
224. Creticos PS. Advances in synthetic peptide immuno-regulatory epitopes. World Allergy Organ J. 2014;7:30.
225. Romantsik O, Bruschettini M, Tosca MA, et al. Oral and sublingual immunotherapy for egg allergy. Cochrane Database Syst Rev. 2014;(11):CD010638.
226. Le UH, Burks AW. Oral and sublingual immunotherapy for food allergy. World Allergy Organ J. 2014;7:35.

APPENDIX: IMMUNOTHERAPY DOSING CHART (VALLABHAI PATEL CHEST INSTITUTE, NEW DELHI)

Instructions

1. Use tuberculin syringe, needle number 26
2. Give subcutaneous injections
3. After 0.5 mL, divide the injection in two sites
4. Keep the vial under refrigeration
5. Place next order before the last vials exhausts

Date	*Dose (mL)*	*Severity and frequency of asthma or rhinitis*	*Doses and frequency of using steroids and/or bronchodilators*
I	1:5,000 (twice a week) 0.1 0.2 0.3 0.4 0.5 0.6 0.7 0.8 0.9		
II	1:500 (twice a week – after I) 0.1 0.2 0.3 0.4 0.5 0.6 0.7 0.8 0.9		
III	1:50 (once a week – after II) 0.1 0.2 0.3 0.4 0.5 0.5 0.5 0.5 0.5 0.5 0.5 0.5		

(Contd...)

(Contd...)

Date	*Dose (mL)*	*Severity and frequency of asthma or rhinitis*	*Doses and frequency of using steroids and/or bronchodilators*
IV	1:50 (once in 2 weeks – after III) 0.6 0.6 0.6 0.6 0.6 0.6 0.6 0.6		
V	1:50 (once in 3 weeks – after IV) 0.7 0.7 0.7 0.7 0.7 0.7 0.7		
VI	1:50 (once in 4 weeks – after V) 0.8 0.8 0.8 0.8 0.8 0.8		
VII	1:50 (once in 4 weeks – after VI) 0.9 0.9 0.9 0.9 0.9 0.9		
VIII	1:50 (once in 4 weeks – after VII) 1.0 1.0 1.0 1.0 1.0		
Maintenance dose with 1.0 mL of 1:50 should be continued once in 4 weeks till discontinuation of allergen immunotherapy is considered.			

Flowchart 1a: Algorithm for allergy management.

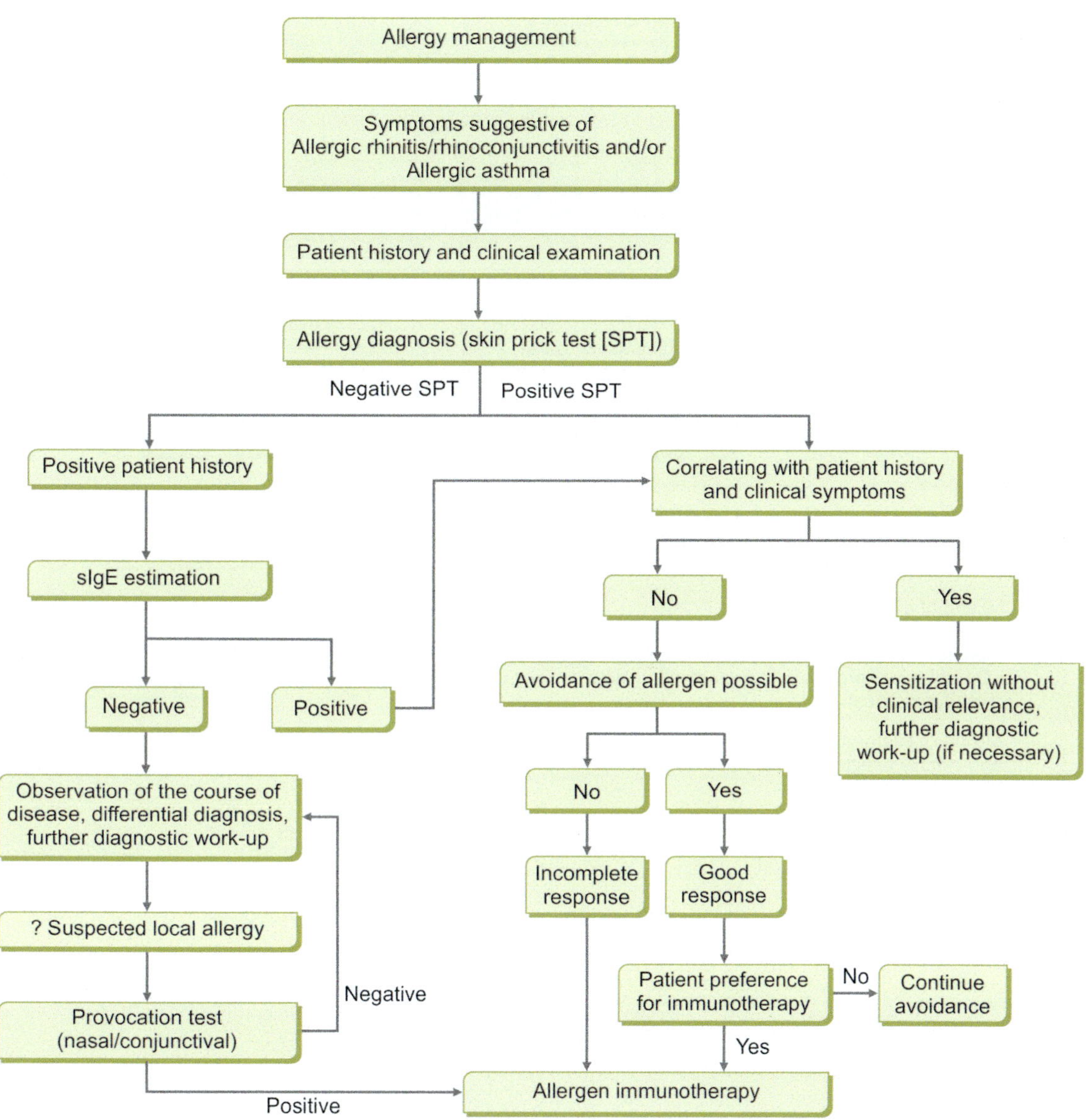

Pharmacotherapy may be initiated following the initial visits and SPT (skin prick test)
AIT (allergen immunotherapy) should not be given only on the basis of serum specific IgE

Flowchart 1b: Algorithm for Allergy Management *(Contd...)*.

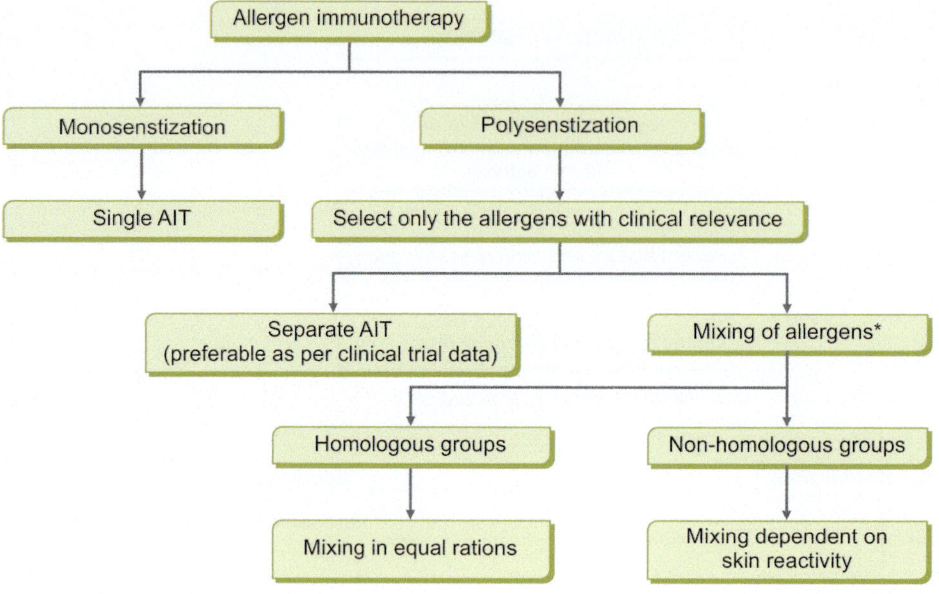

Mixing of allergens*

- Allergists should mix non-related allergens as little as possible
- Do not mix seasonal and perennial allergens
- Do not mix allergens with proteolytic activity (such as extracts of HDMs, molds, and insects) without justification

Mixing of allergens has an impact on their pharmaceutical parameters (stability and dosing) and clinical effects (optimal dose and safety)

Index

Page numbers followed by *b* refer to box, *f* refer to figure, *fc* refer to flowchart, and *t* refer to table

B

C

D

E

N

O

P

Q

R

T

U